SILENT SCARS BOLD REMEDIES

Cutting-Edge Care and Healing From Post-Traumatic Stress Injuries

Dino Garner & Liz Fetter

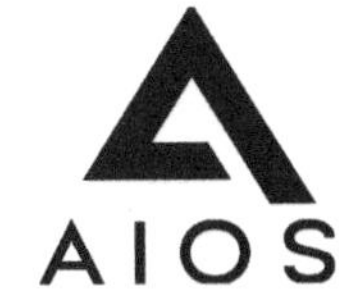

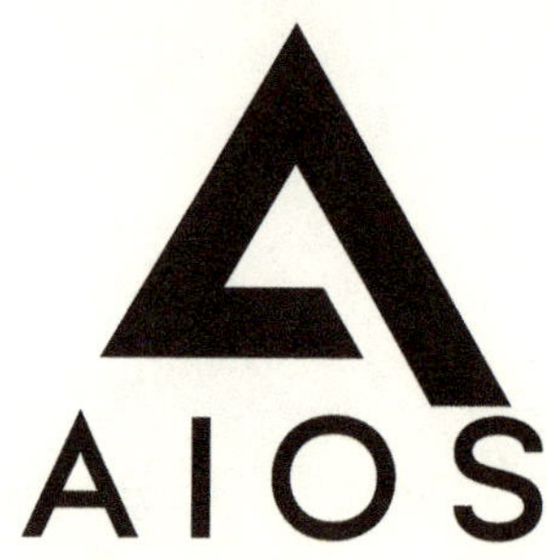

AIOS is an imprint of Frontier Insights LLC
http://FrontierInsightsLLC.com

Published in America by AIOS
AIOS and its colophon are trademarks of
AIOS and Frontier Insights LLC

Library of Congress Catalog Number: 2024947647

Hardback ISBN: 978-1-7373880-9-8
Paperback ISBN: 978-1-7373880-8-1
eBook ISBN: 978-1-7373880-2-9

Contact: AIOSeditorial@gmail.com

AIOS-20251111HPE

First release: VETERANS DAY 2025
Bozeman, Montana 59715

Contents

PART TWO: Challenges and Impacts

PART THREE: Therapies and Treatments

PART FOUR: Foundational Healing Approaches

PART FIVE: Emerging Science and Innovation

PART SEVEN: The Molecular Basis of PTSX

PART EIGHT: A Curated Library

The Beginning

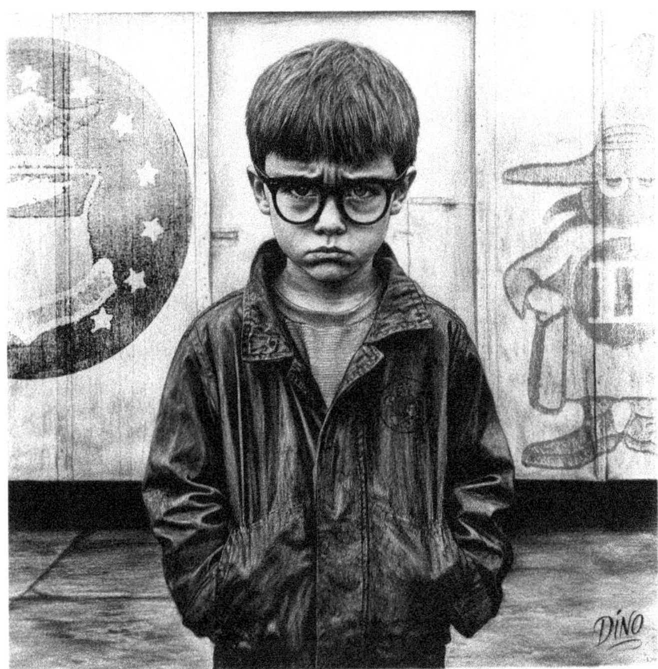

This is a glimpse into the motivation behind the conception and writing of *Silent Scars, Bold Remedies*. In author Dino Garner's own words: I sketched the image above from memories I have of growing up in Europe. This one was outside a hangar at Bitburg Air Force Base, Germany, where I used to play and hang out with fighter pilots, maintenance personnel and in the cockpits and guts of each fighter aircraft. My dream was to become a fighter pilot and fly the F-4 Phantom II like my dad. Seventeen years later, half of my dream would materialize and change my life forever.

My dad was an Air Force fighter pilot who flew the F-4D Phantom II in the Vietnam War. Like most fighter-pilot fathers, he was largely absent during my childhood, except for brief appearances at baseball games and to escort me onto the flightlines and his squadrons at various fighter bases in Europe. My mother was there full time, making her my primary caregiver. And also my tormentor. And mentor in combat.

WARNING: “The Beginning” contains stories of childhood abuse and trauma, and stories of violence, though not overly graphic. They may trigger deep emotions in certain readers. Despite the seemingly negative energy of some content, my story is meant to be an inspiration to all, especially to those who experienced trauma at a young age. It is about resilience and perseverance in the face of fear, trauma and violence. And it encourages you to keep going, though the future may look bleak at the moment.

I knew one day I would write a book about my experiences, but I had no idea it would be a long and deep journey into post-traumatic stress injuries and their underlying mechanical, molecular and physiological foundations. I don't blame my parents for anything, though I sometimes lament over what could have been had I retained my once-perfect eyesight, destroyed by my mother's severe beatings to the back of my head as a child. My deep-seated dream of becoming a fighter pilot was stolen from me by my mom, the woman who should've been cheering me on as I pursued my wishes and dreams.

After decades of deep thinking and personal hypnosis, I was able to figure out, too, how I got those deep scars on my head and the back of my neck: mom's beatings with a blunt instrument. She also punched and slapped me in the mouth many times and shifted my once-perfect teeth. When I was 10, it took three oral surgeries to get those crooked teeth to line up well enough so I could brush my teeth well. Still, I don't blame her for a thing.

As I wrote this "Journey of a Thousand Pages" to heal myself, I used chapters to open up and be vulnerable, enabling me to relax and accept certain things about myself. I hope it works for you, too. Remember: The negative energy from pain and suffering can, with work and dedication, be converted to something entirely positive and useful. The "absolute value" principle I live by.

The Art of Cussing and Psychological Warfare

My mother taught me how to cuss like a motherf***. Not the kind you hear when someone stubs their toe or gets cut off in traffic. No, my mother's cussing was a passionate art form. She could tear you down with words so vicious and surgically precise, you didn't even realize you'd been gutted until your blood was already pooling on the floor. She wielded sarcasm and profanity like King Arthur's sword, leaving wounds that healed slowly, leaving permanent scars.

By the time I was seven, I was her apprentice in verbal warfare. She didn't need fists to knock someone out—she could do it with a smile and a well-placed word. It wasn't just about cussing for the sake of it. Hers was about control, establishing dominance, and tearing someone down to the bone before they knew what hit them. That woman unleashed her torrents at my dad from atop bridges in Holland and Italy, made famous during spectacular battles in WWII.

They became her stage so the whole town could feel her vitriol. Sadly, I was often her target, for whatever reason, and while it might sound cruel, I've come to realize she was preparing me for something bigger. She was teaching me survival in a way only someone who had endured the worst kind of trauma could. I didn't know it then, but she was preparing me for combat long before I'd ever set foot on a battlefield.

Preparing for Combat

At seven years old, I already knew how to navigate her moods, reading her like a soldier reads terrain for hidden landmines and snipers. The look in her eyes, the clench of her jaw, the subtle tightening of her fingers around a book—all signals that it was time to get out of the line of fire. Our house was a war zone, and she was the unpredictable, merciless commander. Surviving that kind of environment sharpens you in ways you don't understand until later in life, even as you're going through the often-dangerous kinetics.

It forces you to develop an instinct for survival, an ability to read people and situations with a clarity most people never have to learn. My mother was the drill sergeant of my childhood, and our home was the battlefield. I had to be ready for anything at any time.

Years later, when I found myself in actual combat, I realized that nothing the military or the [REDACTED] could throw at me was more intense than what I had already been through. My mother had trained me well—how to survive, stay sharp, and strike back when the moment was right. The Army Rangers taught me how to use weapons, but my mother taught me how to wage war unlike anything Sun Tzu or Clausewitz wrote about.

A History of Abuse

But here's the part that most people, and even I, didn't know—the part that explains why she was the way she was. Before my mother met my father, she had already lived through a hell most people can't even imagine. She grew up in a small house in San Antonio, Texas, where abuse was an everyday reality. Her father—my grandfather—was her first abuser. He violated her, beat her and attempted to break her spirit before she even had a chance to know what it meant to be safe or loved.

My mom escaped that nightmare only to fall into the hands of another monster, a former US Army helicopter pilot. Her first husband—my older brother's father—was no better than her father. In fact, he was worse. He didn't protect her like he'd vowed. He had other men use my dear mother for money that went into his pocket. She was his pawn, his whore. And that piece of crap was her pimp. Disappointingly, he died before I could *visit* him.

The humiliation and degradation broke something in my mom that could never be fixed, though she concealed it behind a unique façade. By the time she met my father, she was already too damaged to ever fully recover, a hard fact my father discovered all too late. My dad tried to give her stability, but it wasn't enough because he wasn't present enough to monitor her progress and modulate her terrible moods. The wounds were too deep, the trauma too ingrained. She couldn't heal, and so she gifted that pain down to me, her baby boy. In later years, she figured out how to end her pain.

I recall finding an old letter in an old box in our basement in Maryland, It was dated 1957 and was from the Staff Judge Advocate at Laredo Air Force Base, Texas, where I would be born two years later in 1959. The lieutenant stated that his investigation didn't suggest my mother was unfaithful, but he advised my dad to get as far away from her as he could because she was nothing but trouble. He also mentioned that my dad's mom called my mom a "bitchy woman." That's rich, coming from a backwoods North Carolina woman who was beyond that term, bitch.

Turning Trauma into Power

When I joined the military, everything my mother had drilled into me—the instincts, the survival tactics, the knack for reading people and staying ten steps ahead—clicked into place like a finely tuned machine. Combat was just the physical manifestation of the emotional and

When I joined the military at age 35, I realized that everything I had learned growing up—how to survive, how to anticipate danger, how to think ten steps ahead—was developed well before combat and general Ranger training. The Rangers taught me how to shoot, how to move as

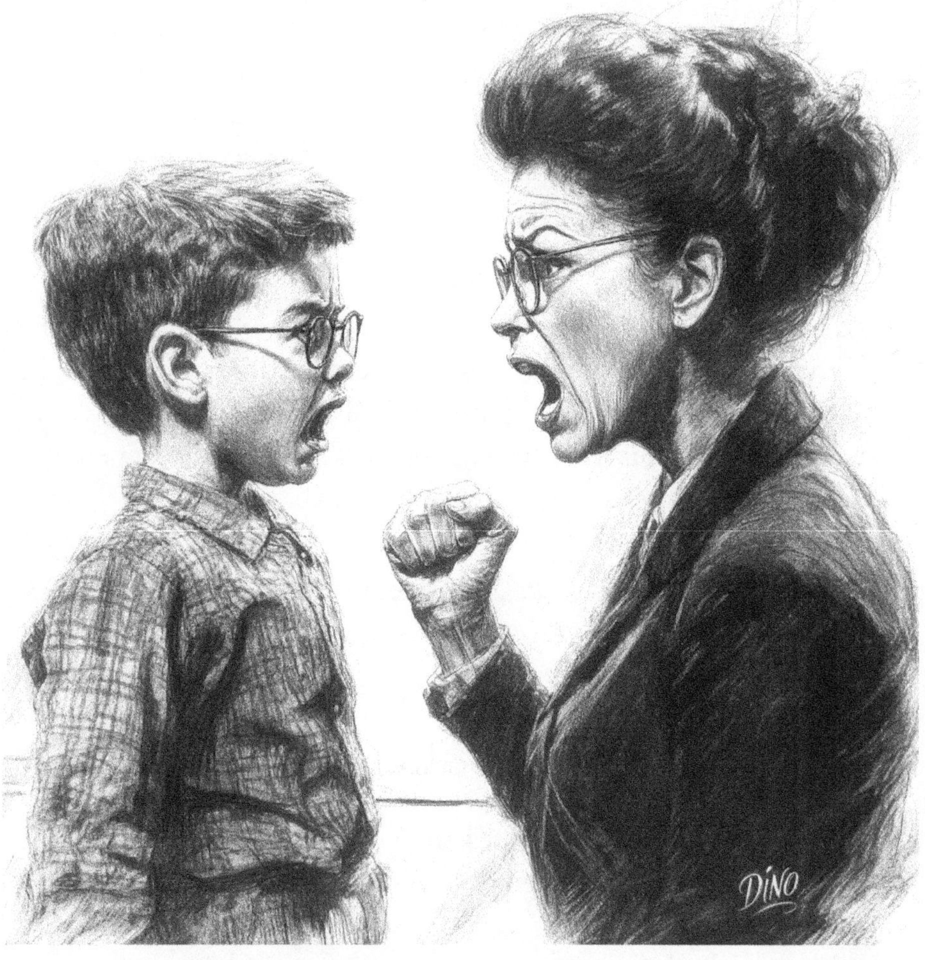

a unit, how to follow orders. But my mother taught me how to stay calm in the face of chaos, how to read people, how to strike when the time was right. She was a better tactician and strategist than any US Army Airborne Ranger, or ST6 / Delta Force operator I knew.

psychological battles I had already been fighting for years. The military taught me how to pull a trigger, but my mother taught me how to wait—how to bide my time, how to know when to strike with deadly precision. She gave me the instincts.

There's something twisted about knowing your mother's survival tactics translate directly into combat zones, but it's the shocking truth. My childhood was the training ground, and the military was just the next level of the deadly game I signed on for. There were moments in the field where I felt more at home than I ever had under my mother's roof. The chaos made sense to me. The fear, the blood, the raw intensity of life and death—none of that felt foreign. It was actually peaceful, in a malignant way.

I wasn't the baddest or strongest, I wasn't the toughest, and I wasn't the fastest—most people could probably whoop me in a fistfight—but I was always thinking five, ten steps ahead, strategizing before anyone else had even considered the first move. And I always had one rule of engagement (ROE): *Anything goes*. I learned that I was not a fighter. I was something else entirely.

It wasn't about youth or brute-force strength, either. It was about mental agility and elasticity, especially in combat training. It was about knowing when to wait, when to attack, and when to simply walk/run away. It was about harnessing the chaos inside and turning it into a lethal weapon against people who were truly scary-badass dudes, tough men who gave me the shivers, which I transduced into lethal electrical energy.

Proving Myself, One Stride at a Time

The real proof that I had earned combat skills from my mom was born out when I joined the US Army and became an Airborne Ranger. Every day I was in Battalion, I proved to those kids that I was just as good at being a Ranger as they were. I proved myself early on by graduating #2 in my class of 75 at the Ranger Indoctrination Program (RIP).

We originally had 150 of the Army's toughest recruits, and most of them left in disgrace, going "worldwide," i.e. to units well beyond the hallowed halls of the 75th Ranger Regiment. We soon got down to 75, and I was out front with this skinny Vietnamese-American recruit who could run a 10-minute 2-mile. That's the only reason he beat me for Distinguished Graduate of RIP.

As an outstanding graduate, number two, though, I got my choice of duty station and I chose the 1st Ranger Battalion at Hunter Army Airfield in Savannah, Georgia. There the Rangers of 1/75 had already been training for weeks for the Expert Infantryman Badge competition, the most coveted award an Army infantryman could earn. Besides the Medal of Honor, Distinguished Service Cross and Silver Star.

I was told I would have details (scut work) in support of those Rangers who were participating in the competition. I called bullshit and requested to see Charlie Company's First Sergeant immediately. First Sergeant Van Houten listened to my impassioned speech about how I was fully prepared to go through this competition, and how I was an old man who had been around the block a few times.

I told him I would not take NO for an answer and that I promised I would make him look good. He took it all in, lowered his head for a minute, then looked over at my Team Leader, SGT M, said, "Let him." SGT M was seething. He hated me and made my life a living hell, which later became a blessing. And I loved him for it, though he never knew it. He was a young kid from Indiana so I held nothing against him. In fact, I felt sad for him, he was so angry all the time.

And that was the beginning of a beautiful and illustrious career as an Army Ranger. Not only had I not been able to train for this grueling competition that consisted of 50 very difficult stations, I had only been a Ranger for 24 hours. I had no experience being a soldier, let alone a US Army Airborne Ranger. I had no idea how to conduct myself around Rangers. Kids half my age would soon remedy that, smoking my bags every few minutes. Transduction of demonic mechanical energy into useful electrical energy for me to use at will.

The Art of Hazing and Hatred, Ranger Style

In short, I didn't know much of anything useful. I was the lowest of humanity to these guys and they let me know it 24/7, smoking and hazing me every chance they got. It turned out to be another blessing two years later when I prepared for Ranger School. I could do more pushups and situps than anyone in Battalion because of all those punishing smokings they heaped on me. What doesn't kill you only makes you stronger.

My Team Leaders hated me the whole time, judging from how they treated me and talked down to me to all their buddies. When someone hates you and everything you stand for, you can't get any lower in their eyes. And I took advantage of that fact and pushed the boundaries each week, mostly to test their resolve and to learn what I could get away with. After all, I was there to learn new skills that I would take with me into the next phase of life: overseas civilian specops work.

In the end, I earned the 1st Ranger Battalion's highest score in the Expert Infantryman Badge competition, earning a perfect score of 50 out of 50 stations. No one else got that high a score without a "Christmas-GO," i.e. a free pass on a station.

Those Rangers were beginning to wonder who the hell I was and how I could be this proficient at the jobs they'd been doing a lot longer than I had. And I hadn't even trained for this. Though I didn't know it, there was a planned celebration for all EIB awardees. It was a huge event and more than 500 people attended.

Twice My Hero: Colonel Ralph Puckett

I was told at the last minute that I would represent the entire enlisted corps of Army Rangers for the 1st Ranger Battalion, and I was ordered to go screaming down the line of Rangers in formation until I got to the presenter, Colonel Ralph Puckett, whose Distinguished Service Cross in Korea would later be upgraded to the Medal of Honor.

He had previously presented my certificate of graduation at #2 from RIP and asked how old I was. When I told him I was 35, he was incredulous. He remembered me at the EIB ceremony and said something like, "Ranger Garner, we meet again. Congratulations. Good luck with your career."

Unfortunately, I ran into very few good men, especially officers, like Colonel Puckett in the US Army, and yet I learned a lot from the others, as well.

Never a Badass, And Always Proficient

It goes without saying that I wasn't the baddest or strongest or fastest Ranger, and I wasn't the most popular or well liked, but I proved to be very skilled at many things, especially innovating new tactics and building improvised explosives and demolitions over the years I served honorably at 1st Bat. It gave me new confidence to carry on bravely and learn even more in my subsequent work in mercenary duties overseas and later hunting [REDACTED], regardless of how difficult the situations became.

Distraction as a Tool

One of the greatest weapons my mother taught me wasn't violence, but kindness. She knew how to kill with a smile, how to use charm to disarm people, making them think they were in control when, really, she was the one pulling the strings. I watched her do it over and over again—lure people into a false sense of security with a laugh, a compliment, a soft touch. And just when they were completely off guard, she'd strike.

Her strikes sometimes were simple "asks," like having the ambassador of a foreign country permit her to redecorate his country's embassy. My mom was an otherworldly witch who cast spells over others. She did decorate six foreign embassies in Washington, DC. They all loved the spell-caster in her, though they weren't aware of mom's secret weapon.

She also designed and implemented The Emerald Ball at the Kennedy Center in DC, and The International Fair in Rock Creek Park in the early 1980s. The fair brought in dozens of foreign embassies and their cultural events. My favorite was all that otherworldly food they shipped in especially for mom's event. She'd insisted on it. I learned that skill, spell-casting, from her too, but I learned to keep it under wraps until needed. In my line of work—whether it was in the military or in civilian special ops—usually it wasn't about brute force. Mostly, it was about finesse.

People expect violence from a stereotypical predator or prospective threat, but they never expect kindness, wit and humor. That's what makes that tool so dangerous, and turned me into an effective hunter. I could be laughing with some bad guy one moment, making him feel like my best friend, and in the next second, I'm "doing my job." That ability to switch so fluidly from charm to lethal force was one of the most valuable tools I had, and it came in handy in certain countries and in [REDACTED] against poachers who did not value life on any level. Psychological jiu jitsu became my favorite workout routine.

The Hunt

There was one mission where I was deep in poacher territory, surrounded by animals who wanted to consume me. I wasn't the biggest guy in the bush, and I wasn't the most intimidating. But I didn't need to be. I just needed them to underestimate me. Why? The biggest killer in the world is not cancer or heart disease. It's *arrogance*. And when some arrogant bad guy underestimated me, that gave me leverage to strike.

From 300 meters away, I spotted the poachers' small camp and slowly and carefully made my way toward them. At 100 meters, I waved my arms and yelled something unintelligible but very friendly sounding, ensuring I was not a threat to them. They permitted me to get closer until, at 20 meters, I . . . did what I had to do. The incredulous look on each face is still emblazoned deep in my mind, and offers a painful reminder about how arrogance kills.

So, I did what my mother taught me. I charmed those poachers. In other instances, I got even closer— right into their camp—and laughed, told jokes, acted like I was just some ignorant or inexperienced American hunter who didn't know anything, was taking a Sunday stroll in [REDACTED]. And for a moment, they let their guard down, curious to meet this idiot white boy. I hiked out of there alive and escaped not because I was faster or stronger, but because I knew how to use kindness as a weapon. I knew how to make them feel safe just long enough for me to do my job. It's a brutal way to live, but in my world it was absolutely necessary. The saddest yet most compelling part of this story is that I had developed the foundation of being this way from my mom.

My Mother's Contradictions

My mother was a walking contradiction. She could be brutally violent one minute and heartbreakingly tender and loving the next. One moment, she was tearing into me for leaving one item in my room out of place or not finishing my math homework. The next, she was stroking my hair and dressing me in the latest European fashion, telling me I was her whole world.

That kind of emotional whiplash messes with the head of anyone, let alone a young boy who, with his father absent, needed a mother, a child desperate for validation. It makes you question everything—what's real, what's not and whether love is supposed to hurt as much as it does. To me, pain and love were synonyms that coexisted symbiotically in the same boiling cauldron. There was a part of her that was so deeply damaged, so tortured by her past, that she couldn't fully love anyone, especially herself. Yet despite all that, she had moments of pure kindness, of genuine warmth that made you believe, for just a second, that she could be the mother you needed. But it was ephemeral. The tenderness would always give way to the rage.

I remember one time—I was eight or nine—we were sitting at a restaurant in San Antonio, Texas, my mom and dad and me. Dad was home on leave from the Vietnam War. I'd ordered hot chocolate with my spicy Mexican food. I was a kid, so I didn't know better. I just loved hot chocolate. And I loved spicy Mexican food. I thought they paired well. I was proud of my choice. She looked at me like I'd just committed the greatest crime against humanity. Then, out of nowhere, she exploded: screaming, cussing, telling me I was an idiot for not knowing what drinks paired with food. The thing was, she wasn't just mad about the hot chocolate.

That was just the surface. Beneath it, there was so much more. There was the pain of her past, the unresolved trauma, the scars she carried from her father and her first husband. That's what was really driving the rage. The hot chocolate was just the trigger.

And yet, I loved her, even admired her tenacity and resilience. I couldn't help it. Despite everything she put me through, despite the violence and the emotional abuse, she was still my mother. And in her own way, she loved me too. She just didn't know how to show it without hurting me.

Inheriting Trauma DNA (tDNA)

The thing about trauma is that it doesn't just stay with the person who experienced it. It gets passed down, generation after generation, a twisted inheritance. I coined the term "trauma DNA" (tDNA) to describe it in molecular terms.

My mother's pain became mine. I didn't ask for it, didn't want it, but it was there—in the way she raised me, in the way she loved me with one hand and hurt me with the other. I grew up under the weight of her trauma, and it shaped me in ways I'm still figuring out. Her love was violent, unpredictable and often terrifying. One minute, she was praising me, telling me I was the smartest, most talented boy in the world. The next, she was berating me for something as small as leaving a dirty dish in the sink.

But I didn't let any of it destroy me. I refused to let her trauma define me. Instead, I took it and turned it into something else. I used it as fuel to push myself further, to be better, to prove to myself that I could rise above the chaos and live the life I dreamed of from all those books of action and adventure I'd read during my formative years. Ironically, it was mom who gave me a photo album with the inscription by Goethe: "Become the one you dream you can be." What do you call her gifting me this—cognitive dissonance?—because that is an understatement.

It was then that I learned about "absolute value" in math class and how to apply the concept to my life: Anything negative was placed between those two little brackets that stripped away all negativity and created infinite positivity. Still burdened with all that toxic tDNA, I didn't begin to practice this until my later years. Since then, I've lived a life of "absolute value."

Turning Trauma into Strength

When I joined the military at age 35, I realized that everything I had learned growing up—how to survive, how to anticipate danger, how to think ten steps ahead—was developed well before combat and general Ranger training. Again, the Rangers taught me how to shoot, how to move, how to follow orders. But my mother taught me how to stay calm in the face of chaos, how to read people, how to strike when the time was right. She was a better tactician and strategist than any US Army Airborne Ranger, ST6 or Delta Force operator I knew.

The battlefield was just another version of home. The bullets, the blood, the extreme violence, the fear—it was all familiar. I had been living in a war zone my entire life. The only difference was that in the military, I had imposed-upon discipline and control. I wasn't the one being beaten down. I was the one with the power to destroy. And that's where I found further strength. I became a soldier, a leader and later, a civilian special operations guru because I knew how to harness and manipulate the chaos, what I later termed "fluidics," i.e. navigating among the unpredictable obstacles. I knew how to take the pain without complaining, the rage without losing control, and the trauma without losing my cool, and turn it into something productive. Something powerful against the bullies of the world.

The Poet and the Artist

For all the violence and brutality I've witnessed and participated in, there's a part of me that craves beauty, that demands peace.

That's a part of me my mother gave me, too. She taught me how to study and appreciate the color and texture of a fabric, a Old Master paintings in the Louvre, a drape or tapestry in a foreign embassy. She taught me how to respect the brush strokes of Titian and Rembrandt in their paintings. How they used artificial light to create the illusion of dancing light in their artwork. Layers upon layers were here favorite, as they brought a two-dimensional painting to 3-D life. She was like those Old Masters, too: creating a multilayer façade to enhance what lay beneath.

She taught me to love reading books, to seek refuge in the pages where words offered escape. For all her contradictions, she knew the power of knowledge and the magic of stories. She devoured books like they were her lifeline, a way out of the cursed reality she couldn't escape.

At ages seven through ten, I read the poetry of Lord Byron and James Dickey, *Portnoy's Complaint*, *Catch-22*, all the Agatha Christie novels—my favorite was *The Murder of Roger Ackroyd*. No one ever saw Dr. Sheppard coming and they severely underestimated him, tactics I used on overseas missions against bad actors—and the *Stars and Stripes* newspaper each week. I read the entire *Encyclopedia Britannica.* Twice. I devoured *The National Enquirer*, which my mom said had tidbits of information you couldn't find in mainstream news.

Finding refuge in the stories of brave and courageous people, both men and women, became second nature to me. When the world was too chaotic, too painful, I turned to books, to poetry, to writing. It was where I could make sense of the madness, where I could find some peace and learn things no teacher could ever expose me to.

Over the years, all the spirits of men and women in those books I read inspired me to capture moments of beauty amid the chaos. It's how I've balanced the violence in my life. It's how I remind myself that there's more to this world than pain and bloodshed. I discovered that creating what I called "Tranquil Impressionism" brought me a deep sense of calm. Painting became my refuge, and after completing 100 pieces—some of which ended up in high-end galleries, yacht clubs and restaurants—I just stopped.

It wasn't planned. It felt like I had within me just enough energy to do exactly 100 paintings, as if each one was part of a larger process, and once I reached the end, there was nothing more to express in that form. It was as though the creative journey had naturally completed itself, and I had said everything I needed to say through those works. Didn't Forrest Gump stop running in the middle of the great American Southwest over a similar situation? He turned around and went home.

Later, I turned to poetry and crafted 100 poems, some of which were praised by distinguished professors and lecturers at renowned universities. But just like with painting, it felt as though I had exactly 100 in me. Once I reached that number, the words no longer came.

It was as if each poem was part of a natural cycle, and when I had expressed everything I needed, the creative well ran dry. The work had served its purpose, and once fulfilled, there was no need to continue—almost as if I instinctively knew when the journey was complete. Something about being a work in progress, particularly in family and personal relationships. Incidentally, for our book, *AEROMASTERS: Celebrating a Century of the American Fighter Pilot*, Vol. I, which was nominated for a Pulitzer Prize, I got to resurrect my painting and poetry skills. Quite an honor to contribute them to such a beautiful volume and honor our heroes of the past and present.

While researching for and writing *Silent Scars, Bold Remedies*, I also discovered the healing art of a worldclass Licensed Clinical Social Worker (LCSW) and several scientists and physicians, and treatments: Eugene Lipov, Stellate Ganglion Block, Mark Gordon, hyperbaric oxygen therapy, vagal nerve stimulation, and whole-body vibration.

The Legacy of My Mother

My mother wasn't perfect or even average by any standard. She was deeply flawed, broken in ways that can never be fully understood, even by modern abnormal psychology work. But she gave me something invaluable: resilience, the unique ability to bounce back after a tragic loss or event, and move on without dragging the previous baggage with me.

What I did carry with me were all the lessons learned and how to implement them in just the right moment. Moving every 2-3 years and starting over again added to the gift of becoming resilient. She taught me how to survive, how to fight, how to harness my pain and turn it into true positive power and energy. And in her own way, she taught me how to love with unconditional kindness.

Mom was a wanderer and she passed that trait to me, in addition to loving and appreciating arts and crafts, ballet and the symphony, and attending grand balls and galas, parties and other events.

It would be unfair if I didn't share this, too: my mom taught me to travel and explore and absorb all I could. Growing up in Europe in the 1960s and '70s, I lived in several cities and towns in Germany and Italy, and traveled to many others in all countries. Thanks to her, I traveled to more than 100 countries and learned multiple languages over the decades.

The countless people who touched, influenced and inspired me? Thanks, mom. The great cultures and cuisines and drink? Thanks, mom. She may have been a walking contradiction—kind and cruel, loving and violent—but she was mine. And part of who I am today, I owe to dear Olga Marie Ramirez-Garner, bless her restless and troubled soul. That's her legacy. And now it is mine. I hope this chapter serves as inspiration and encouragement to you and those you share our book with. If you find something useful that changes your life in some way, please pay it forward.

I'll leave you with a poem I wrote to honor the woman who inspired me on all levels and taught me the art of living a full and rich life, and to share it with others. . . .

Diamonds by the Yard, Shadows of a Soul

Olga always wanted a decorative von or van before Ramirez,
some advance PR to trumpet her grand entrance,
something she thought would upmarket her ghetto roots.
Always ashamed of being Mexican, she re-invented herself Spanish.
Patrician flamenco dancer from Spain.
Descended from some tree aristocratic,
according to her counterfeit provenance.
Never acknowledged her starving littermates in Meh-hee-co,
let alone the land that designed her DNA,
where my epic hero, the archvillain Pancho Villa, was considered royalty by convention.
No, Olga made up everything in her short, miserable life,
from the heels of her Ferragamo kicks
waaay up to her Elsa Peretti Diamonds by the Yard licks.
Lies always sounded sexier to her own ear, even if only a casual smear.
And when she was done writing her sad narrative,
passed her shit onto me to complete it, her little dear.
When she passed in Ninety-Two, tears didn't roll down, much

less even birth.
I dismissed it for decades, thinking . . .
I don't really know what the hell I was thinking.
Until she came to me in a dream last eve,
asked me kindly "Por favor, Mejo,"
to grant her that special nobiliary preposition,
something befitting a Spanish Princess of the High Court.
So I rose this little a.m., the rock bottom of the thirteenth of
May in the 2,024th year after whatshisname kicked,
and eight days after the death of Count Cinco de Mayo, and
granted her final wish, betricked:
"Prinzessin Olga Marie von Ramirez."
Only now do the rains come,
deepest sorrow for this lonely Mexican girl,
who only wanted to feel important
to those who didn't matter:
the Crowd von This, the Clan van That.
What she never knew, though:
Olga was deeply loved, admired and respected by us little,
unimportant people
from the darkest
caves and farthest huts
in the land of Meh-hee-co and A-meh-ree-ca!

—Dino Garner ibn Prinzessin Olga Marie von Ramirez

Dedication

This book is for anyone who has faced trauma and continues to struggle with its various forms.

US Air Force Chief Ramon "CZ" Colon-Lopez, SEAC (ret.).

US Air Force Chief Wayne "Lao Tzu" Fisk (ret.).

CIA Paramilitary Officer/Senior Operations Officer Ric "Archilochus" Prado (ret.).

US Air Force Chief Ivan Ruiz (ret.).

US Navy Lieutenant Kegan "Smurf" Gill, who redefined *resilence.*

Active-duty US military personnel and veterans of all wars, foreign and domestic, who have served our country.

Leil Yvette, who keeps storming along because she's having entirely too much fun and because she needs to see how it all ends.

A very special human being in Dino's life, someone who never gives up and who is always loving, upbeat, positive and super-productive.

Dino's brother John who taught him the art of making The List and how to shoot the feathers off a bird mid-flight.

For Liz's siblings and the childhood trauma they shared.

Foreword

As a former Senior Enlisted Advisor to the Chairman of the Joint Chiefs of Staff (SEAC), I've been privileged to serve alongside some of the most dedicated and resilient warriors in our armed forces. Like many of them, I too have faced the physical and emotional scars that come from a lifetime of service.

For years, I dealt with the effects of traumatic brain injury and post-traumatic stress injuries (new term is PTSX), and like many of my brothers and sisters in arms, I tried to push through it, thinking I could handle it on my own. For too long, I acted like nothing was wrong—like many of us are trained to do.

We are taught to be tough, to never show weakness, and to always put the mission first. But the truth is, by refusing to acknowledge the problem I was making things worse. The symptoms of PTSX— sleepless nights, irritability, flashbacks—were starting to take over my life. I had to admit that I was struggling and needed help.

That's when I found Stellate Ganglion Block (SGB) therapy, which provided me with much-needed relief and allowed me to regain control over my life. You will read about SGB in Dino and Liz's book, so take note. The most important thing I've learned from my journey is this: the earlier you recognize the signs of PTSX, the sooner you can start healing. Don't wait until it feels like your world is falling apart. Don't suffer in silence. PTSX is a real, treatable condition, and there are resources available to help. Admitting you need help is not a sign of weakness—it's a sign of strength.

Reach out to the VA, your fellow veterans, or any trusted support system. As long as you make an effort to talk with someone who is in a position to assist you and get you the help you need. You are not alone in this fight. The sooner you seek assistance, the sooner you can reclaim your life, and avoid the tragic path so many of us have seen—losing friends to suicide.

You may need to read this manual of wisdom many times to extract the nuggets from within. My suggestion: look through the whole book, cover to cover, the first time to familiarize yourself with its contents.

Then, going slowly, read and study each chapter, one at a time, for comprehension. Jot down notes as you go along, explore concepts that pertain to your own struggles and things that interest you personally.

Dino and Liz have written the most comprehensive, important and accessible book on PTSX in veterans, active-duty personnel and anyone who's experienced any form of lasting trauma, especially of the brain. This will be the go-to book for all-things Post-Traumatic Stress Injuries for years to come.

—SEAC Ramón "CZ" Colón-López (ret.)
4th Senior Enlisted Advisor to the Chairman of the Joint Chiefs of Staff (2019-2023) and bestselling author of *CARNIVORE LEADERSHIP: Taking Charge Instead of Taking Shit*
Washington, DC

Introduction

Welcome. Whether you are a scientist exploring the molecular basis of trauma, a clinician seeking to expand your therapeutic toolkit, or a policymaker hoping to build a better system of care, there are sections in this book written specifically for you.

If you are a veteran, a first responder, or anyone who carries the silent scars of a life altered by trauma, this book is, first and foremost, a testament to your resilience and a guide for your journey forward. If you are a spouse, a family member, or a friend walking alongside a survivor, these pages offer a map to help you navigate the path with compassion and understanding.

Silent Scars, Bold Remedies was written to be a multi-layered resource. While some chapters delve into deep and complex science, they are balanced by personal stories, practical step-by-step guides, and messages of hope.

The separate companion volume to *Silent Scars, Bold Remedies* features only chapter summaries, illustrations, personal stories, plus If-Then Guidance, Take the Next Step and Through Their Eyes sections. We have removed all the dense technical, scientific and medical information, making it an easier and more gentle read for those not familiar with the science and technology underlying post-traumatic stress injuries.

We invite you to engage with the sections that speak most directly to you. This is not a book to be read in a single sitting, but a long-term companion for a journey we believe no one should have to walk alone.

Below is a list of the readers who will benefit most from this book, ordered from the broadest audience to the most technically specialized.

Veterans, Active-Duty Military Personnel, and First Responders: This is the heart and soul of the book's audience. The raw personal stories, practical guidance, and overarching message of hope will resonate deeply and provide a tangible roadmap for healing.

Clinical Practitioners, Therapists, and Counselors: Psychologists, Licensed Clinical Social Workers (LCSWs), nurse practitioners, and counselors will benefit greatly from the detailed chapters on specific therapeutic modalities, trauma-informed care, and healing secondary trauma in caregivers.

Family Members, Spouses, and Caregivers of Veterans: The chapters on the toll of PTSX on relationships and "Healing the Healers" are written directly for them, offering understanding, validation, and crucial coping strategies.

Veteran Advocates and VSO Representatives: This group will find the practical guides—especially the detailed chapter on navigating the VA system—to be an indispensable resource for their work.

General Readers and Trauma Survivors: Anyone who has been touched by trauma or is interested in resilience, the science of healing, and the future of mental healthcare will find the book accessible, inspiring, and profoundly educational.

Specialist MD Practitioners: Psychiatrists, neurologists, endocrinologists and anesthesiologists who will find immense value in the advanced chapters on TBI, the vagus nerve, and emerging therapies like SGB and ketamine.

PhD Researchers and Medical Scientists: Particularly those in biophysics, neurobiology, immunology, endocrinology, and molecular biology. They are the primary audience for the deep scientific dives in Part Seven and will appreciate the book's rigorous, evidence-based foundation.

Policymakers, Legislators, and Healthcare Administrators: The chapters on systemic challenges, navigating the VA, the open letters to Congress, and the final "Gentle Revolution" chapter are written to inform and persuade this influential group.

This book does not contain medical advice, nor is it meant to offer it on any level. We do not present personal opinions. Rather, we show facts based on sound scientific research, including a thorough review of the literature, interviews with experts and those who suffer from post-traumatic stress injuries, and our own personal experiences.

The landscape of PTSX diagnosis, care, therapy and treatment changes every week, so please consult with trusted healthcare specialists and practitioners about the latest developments that may affect you. Our book is up to date as of November 2025, and will be further updated every six months.

For those who love great movies, think of this book in "Hollywood shorthand" terms:

American Sniper meets Brené Brown: *The Call to Courage.*

That shorthand captures the essence of this book's balance between the raw realities of trauma and the courageous journey toward healing.

American Sniper represents the intense and honest portrayal of a veteran's experience and the lasting impact of trauma.

Brené Brown: *The Call to Courage* adds the layer of emotional vulnerability required for resilience and growth.

Silent Scars, Bold Remedies is both an unflinching look at the real struggles survivors face and an inspiring guide toward emotional resilience, recovery and the courage to heal.

Trauma may not wear a uniform or arrive on a battlefield, but it can alter a life with equal ferocity. It is an invisible wound that can lie dormant for years, only to surface when triggered by memory, sensory input, or biological stress. It is a full-spectrum disruption—a systems-level injury that does not respect the artificial boundaries between mental and physical health.

This book grew out of a deep concern for the military service members, veterans, first responders, and civilians whose sacrifices often leave these lasting, silent scars. Throughout this volume, you will encounter leading research, innovative treatments, and powerful personal stories. The common thread is a commitment to compassionate, evidence-based care, however new and emerging.

A New Language for Invisible Wounds

Words build worlds. They also build clinics, policies and self-concepts. For this reason, we have moved beyond the term PTSD and replaced it with PTSX: Post-Traumatic Stress Injury.

This shift is intentional. The "X" signifies inclusivity, encompassing a broad range of post-traumatic effects beyond a single diagnosis, such as anxiety, depression, neuroinflammation, and traumatic brain injury.

Framing the condition as an "injury" highlights the real, physical harm caused by trauma, suggesting something that can be healed rather than a permanent "disorder" that must be managed. By moving away from the word "disorder," PTSX avoids negative connotations, making it less stigmatizing and more approachable. This new language helps survivors declare, "Something happened to me—and it can be mended."

Guiding the Reader Through an Interdisciplinary Journey

This book is structured in eight parts, each serving as a waypoint on the journey from understanding the roots of trauma to envisioning a future where PTSX is not only treatable but preventable.

- Part One: Understanding PTSX and Trauma lays the foundation, mapping out the spectrum of trauma-related conditions and examining how PTSX develops, from childhood adversity to the unique complexities faced by women in the military .
- Part Two: Challenges and Impacts casts light on the tangible hurdles survivors face, exploring suicide risk, the societal cost to families, the reality of an inadequate system of care, and the interpersonal toll trauma exacts.
- Part Three: Therapies and Treatments delves into cutting-edge methods, including psychedelic-assisted therapies, MDMA clinical trials, ketamine infusions, and the use of stellate ganglion block for trauma-related dysregulation.
- Part Four: Foundational Healing Approaches focuses on holistic care. Nutrition, rest, spirituality, animal-assisted interventions, and community support are explored as essential components of healing, alongside the transformative potential of post-traumatic growth.
- Part Five: Emerging Science and Innovation provides a forward-looking view of where the field is heading. Brain imaging, the gut microbiome, and the potential of artificial intelligence in mental healthcare are examined.
- Part Six: Stories, Guidance and Support turns to the voices of real people and practical resources. Personal narratives are paired with step-by-step guides for navigating the complexities of the

VA system and finding support.

- Part Seven: The Molecular Basis of PTSX details the latest research into the physical, molecular basis of trauma-related injuries, offering new hope for those struggling with the "a pill for every ill" practice of medicine.
- Part Eight: The Compass at the End: Essential References serves as a toolkit—an organized library of the peer-reviewed sources, articles, and studies that inform this volume, empowering you to continue your own research.

Take This Compass, Traveler

We invite you to approach this book as a long-term guide. We have filled it with charcoal sketches, personal narratives, and actionable tools—"If-Then Guidance," "Take the Next Step," and "Through Their Eyes"—to help you engage at your own pace. A reader once described our approach as a Campfire Compass, and we believe that captures our intent perfectly.

The map is written as we walk. Trauma may be ubiquitous, but so is human ingenuity. What begins as pages can blossom into practice, and practice into policy—so the circle widens until every survivor sees their reflection in a system built to heal, not to judge.

Your participation in that widening circle starts now—on the next page, in the next breath, in the quiet decision to heal.

—Dino Garner and Liz Fetter

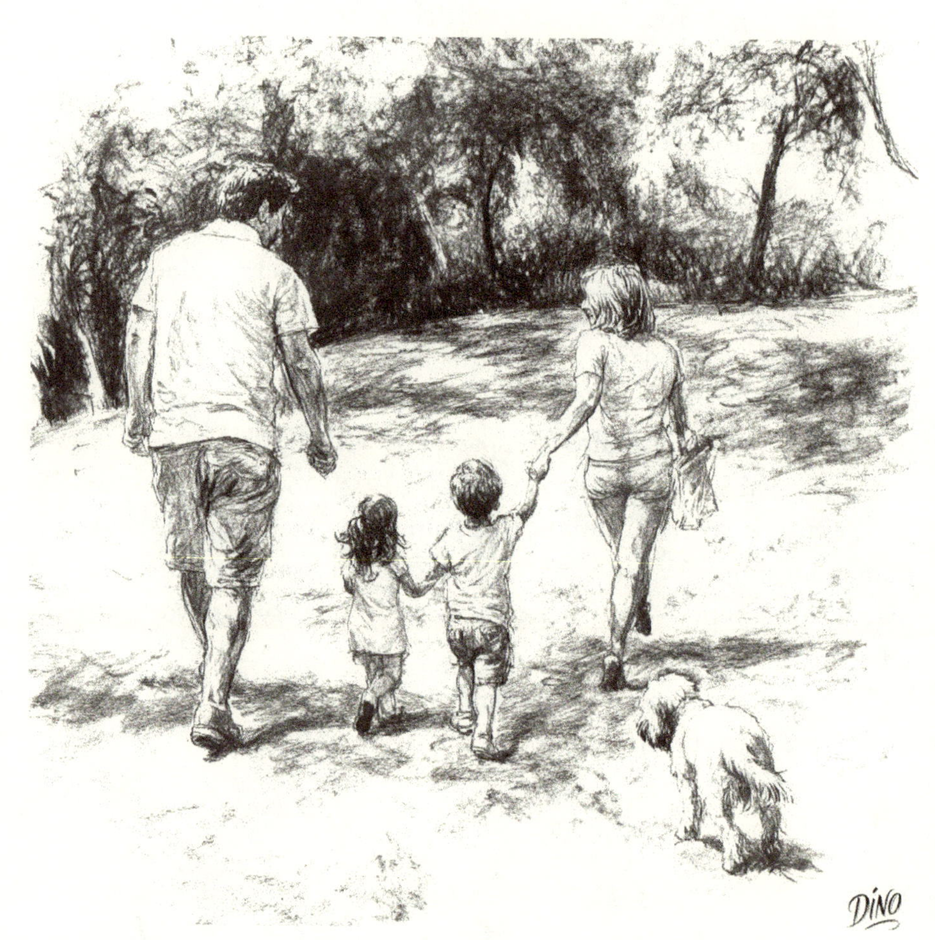
DINO

PART ONE

Understanding PTSX and Trauma

1

Understanding PTSX in the Context of War and Combat-Related Events

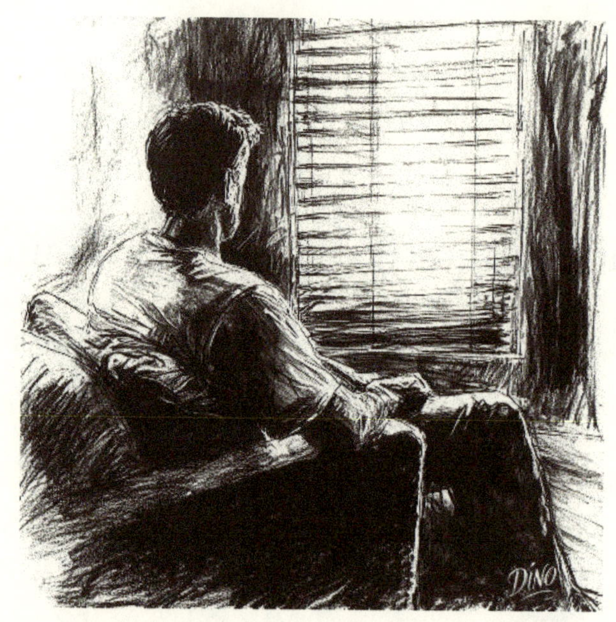

Jake sat alone in his living room, the afternoon sun slipping through the blinds. He had come back from his third deployment six months ago, but it felt like yesterday. Little noises still made him jump. A car door slamming might set his heart racing. At times, he wondered if he was the only one feeling this way.

He remembered older veterans talking about something called "shell shock." His grandfather, who had fought in World War II, never liked fireworks on the Fourth of July. Later, folks said it was "battle fatigue" or "combat stress."

But whatever name it took, the story was always the same: good men and women came home changed, weighed down by experiences they could not forget.

In more recent years, we have learned that these wounds are not just "in the mind." They affect the brain and body. They can surface in the middle of a quiet conversation or when you're trying to fall asleep at night. It is not a sign of weakness or failure. It is a common response to extreme stress.

Jake found solace when he learned that he was not alone. He heard that firefighters, police officers, and others who face daily danger sometimes felt the same. PTSX, as we are calling it, crosses every boundary. It does not care about rank, gender or background.

But with understanding comes hope. There are new treatments and better ways to help those carrying these silent scars. Jake began to see a path forward when he started talking with other veterans. He realized this was not an end but a turning point. He heard stories of people who had learned to sleep through the night again, to smile, to feel alive.

This chapter explores that legacy—from the early label of "shell shock" to the modern view of PTSX. Dive into these pages, for there is light ahead, just as Jake found.

Historical Context of PTSX in Military Personnel

The understanding of Post-Traumatic Stress Injuries (PTSX) has evolved significantly over time, especially within the military context. While the original acronym, PTSD, as a clinical term was officially recognized by the American Psychiatric Association in 1980, the psychological effects of war have been observed for centuries. From the ancient accounts of soldiers' struggles in battle to the clinical discussions following World Wars I and II, the history of PTSX in military personnel has been commonly overlooked.

During World War I, the term "shell shock" was used to describe soldiers who were severely affected by the trauma of combat. Many of these soldiers displayed symptoms such as uncontrollable tremors, anxiety, nightmares and a general inability to function. While early hypotheses attributed these symptoms to the physical effects of exploding shells and artillery, it soon became evident that the prolonged stress of warfare was the primary cause. Nevertheless, shell shock was poorly understood and many soldiers who displayed these symptoms were often labeled as cowards or malingerers or "Embusqué" (slackers), a stigma that has continued in some form even today.

The psychological toll of war continued to be a concern through World War II, where the term "combat fatigue" or "battle fatigue" replaced "shell shock." However, the understanding of the disorder remained limited and the resources available to address the mental health needs of soldiers were minimal.

Approach these pages slowly and thoughtfully. Let knowledge land the way a medic's hand settles on a wound. Patient reading plus deliberate rest will help you heal over time.

Following the Vietnam War, there was a marked increase in awareness about the long-term psychological effects of combat, particularly as veterans began to report recurring nightmares, flashbacks and difficulties adjusting to civilian life. This led to the eventual formal recognition of PTSX as a psychiatric disorder.

Today, PTSX is widely recognized as a consequence of traumatic exposure, particularly in military personnel. However, the understanding of its causes, symptoms and treatments continues to evolve. What remains consistent is that PTSX represents a profound challenge to those who experience it and understanding its roots within the military context is crucial for effective treatment.

Causes of PTSX in Military Settings

PTSX in military personnel is typically associated with direct combat experiences, but the causes are far more complex. Some of these also apply to civilians, especially first-responders. The trauma experienced by just about anyone can stem from various sources:

Combat-Related Trauma: The most widely recognized cause of PTSX in military personnel is exposure to combat. This includes being directly involved in firefights, bombings or ambushes, witnessing death and injury among fellow soldiers, and experiencing near-death situations. Combat-related trauma is often characterized by extreme violence and unpredictability, which creates an environment where servicemembers are constantly at risk. The intensity of combat, combined with the physical and emotional toll of survival, leaves many soldiers psychologically wounded. We now know that these psychological wounds are actually physical. And they can manifest themselves as undesirable behaviors.

Moral Injury: Moral injury refers to the psychological distress that results from actions or inactions that go against an individual's moral beliefs. In combat, soldiers may be forced to make split-second decisions that result in harm to others, including civilians. The sense of guilt, shame or betrayal that arises from these experiences can lead to a deep moral injury, which complicates PTSX. Veterans often struggle to reconcile their actions with their personal values, leading to feelings of anger, self-loathing and depression.

Witnessing Atrocities: Even when military personnel are not directly involved in combat, witnessing acts of violence, death, or suffering can lead to PTSX. This is particularly true for medics and healthcare workers in war zones who treat severe injuries and deal with death on a regular basis. The continual exposure to human suffering can take a heavy toll on their mental health.

Non-Combat Stressors: Not all military-related trauma is combat-related. Military personnel often face extended deployments, long periods of separation from their families and the stresses of living in hostile or unstable environments, or even being stuffed into a submarine for long periods.

These non-combat stressors, including the fear of injury or death, extreme weather conditions and limited resources, can contribute to the overall psychological burden that may develop into PTSX.

Sexual Assault and Harassment: Military sexual trauma (MST) is another significant cause of PTSX in servicemembers. Both men and women in the military can experience sexual assault or harassment during their service, leading to severe emotional trauma. MST is a unique risk factor for PTSX and requires targeted interventions to address the specific psychological and subsequent physical wounds it inflicts.

Symptoms of PTSX

The symptoms of PTSX can vary greatly from person to person and they often manifest in ways that are difficult to identify, especially in veterans who are accustomed to suppressing their emotions and maintaining control. The four main categories of PTSX symptoms are:

Unwelcome, Intrusive Thoughts: Veterans with PTSX often experience intrusive thoughts, memories or flashbacks related to their traumatic experiences. These may occur without warning and can be triggered by sights, sounds or smells that remind the individual of their trauma. Nightmares and disturbing dreams are also common and can severely disrupt sleep patterns.

Avoidance: Veterans with PTSX may go to great lengths to avoid reminders of their trauma. This can include avoiding certain places, people or activities that might trigger memories of their experiences. Emotional numbing is another form of avoidance, where individuals distance themselves from feelings of joy and love, or connections in an attempt to shield themselves from pain.

Negative Changes in Thinking and Mood: PTSX often leads to persistent negative beliefs about oneself or the world. Veterans may feel guilty, ashamed or unworthy and struggle with distorted thoughts about their own actions during combat. They may also experience depression, detachment from loved ones, or a diminished interest in activities they once enjoyed.

Hyperarousal and Reactivity: Hypervigilance, irritability and an exaggerated startle response are common symptoms of PTSX. Veterans may feel constantly on edge, as though danger is always imminent, even in safe environments. Sleep disturbances, trouble concentrating and angry outbursts are also common and can make daily life difficult to manage.

Comorbidity of PTSX with Other Conditions

PTSX rarely occurs in isolation. Veterans with PTSX often experience other mental-health conditions, such as depression, anxiety and substance-abuse disorders. The comorbidity of PTSX with these conditions complicates treatment and can lead to more severe health outcomes if left unaddressed. Substance abuse is particularly common among veterans with PTSX, as many turn to drugs or alcohol to cope with their symptoms.

Self-medication can provide temporary relief but often exacerbates the problem in the long run. Similarly, depression and anxiety disorders can develop alongside PTSX, further impacting a veteran's ability to function in daily life and maintain healthy relationships.

Recognizing and treating these comorbid conditions is essential for a comprehensive approach to PTSX care. Treating PTSX without addressing other mental health issues may leave veterans vulnerable to ongoing struggles with their mental health.

If-Then Guidance

- If you are a veteran or service member experiencing symptoms of PTSX, such as nightmares, flashbacks or heightened anxiety, then recognize that these are common responses to the trauma of war. Seeking help is crucial, as early intervention can provide relief and prevent long-term psychological challenges.
- If you feel stigma or shame around PTSX due to military culture or historical perceptions of mental health (e.g., "shell shock" or "combat fatigue"), then remind yourself that PTSX is now widely recognized as a legitimate and treatable physical and mental-health condition. You are not alone, and seeking help is a courageous step toward recovery.
- If you are unsure whether your experiences align with PTSX, then review the symptoms and causes of PTSX within the context of war, such as exposure to traumatic combat events. PTSX symptoms can include intrusive memories, avoidance behaviors, hypervigilance and emotional numbness. Consult with a mental-health professional to explore a proper diagnosis.

- If you are struggling with the long-term psychological effects of combat, particularly with difficulties adjusting to civilian life, then seek support from veteran organizations, mental-health services, or counseling. PTSX often manifests after the transition from military to civilian life, and addressing it early can aid in reintegration.
- If you believe that PTSX only affects modern soldiers, then understand that the psychological effects of war have been documented throughout history, from ancient warriors to soldiers in World Wars I and II.
- The evolution of terms like "shell shock" and "combat fatigue" illustrates that PTSX has long been an issue in military settings, even if it was misunderstood in the past. While the names have been changed, the science and medicine behind them have improved dramatically.
- If you are currently receiving treatment for PTSX but feel that your symptoms are not improving, then explore newer therapeutic approaches. The understanding of PTSX continues to evolve, and treatments such as cognitive behavioral therapy (CBT), exposure therapy, and emerging treatments like EMDR or MDMA-assisted therapy may offer more effective solutions. We discuss all these later in this book.
- If you are supporting a veteran who is showing signs of PTSX, then encourage them to seek professional help. PTSX is a recognized mental-health disorder that responds well to treatment, and early intervention can make a significant difference in your loved one's quality of life.

Take the Next Step

- Reflect on Your Symptoms: Take a moment to assess how you feel. Are you experiencing flashbacks, nightmares, or anxiety after combat or traumatic events? Acknowledge any symptoms you may have.
- Talk to a Fellow Veteran: Reach out to a trusted fellow veteran or a peer-support group. Sharing your experiences a step to healing.

- Seek a Mental-Health Evaluation: Contact your local VA or military healthcare provider to schedule an evaluation if you suspect you may have suffered from some form of trauma and may have PTSX.
- Explore PTSX Resources: Visit the VA's PTSX website or a reputable resource for more information on symptoms and treatments.

Through Their Eyes

"When you step off the battlefield, no one tells you that the war keeps fighting inside your head. They trained us for every threat out there—but not for the one inside. 'Shell shock,' 'combat fatigue,' or whatever they called it back then . . . it's PTSX now, and it's as real as the bullets and bombs we faced. You don't have to be ashamed of it.

I didn't ask for these nightmares or the endless overactive vigilance, and neither did you. It took me years to realize it, but getting help isn't a sign of weakness—it's a different kind of fight, one that takes guts. If you're in that fight right now, know that you're not alone. We've all been there, and together, we'll keep pushing forward. Hooah!"

—Staff Sergeant Matthew L., US Army (ret.)

2

Childhood Trauma and PTSX: Understanding the Deep Impact of Early Adversity

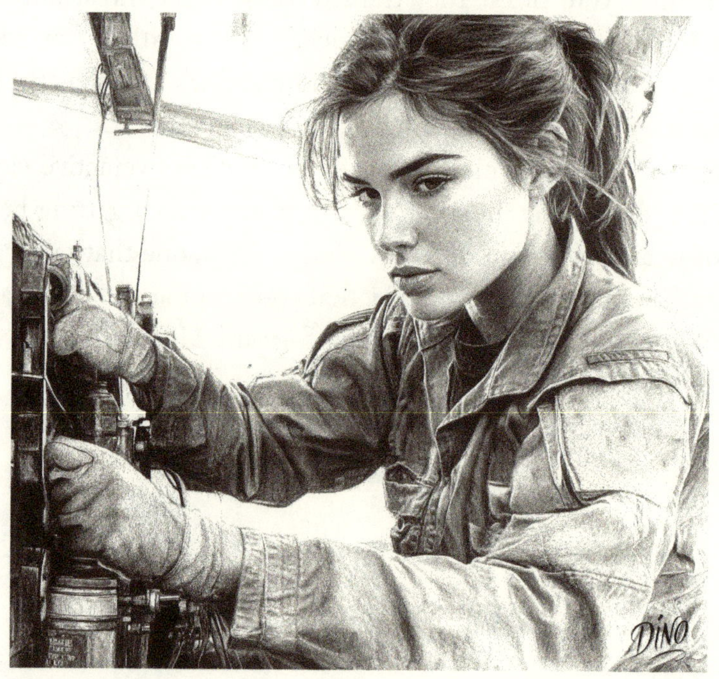

Elena turned the wrench until her hands ached. She liked it that way. A job finished, hands sore, and the metal bird ready to scream into the sky. She didn't mind the noise on the flight line. It drowned out everything else.

She was thirty now, but the noise had always been there. As a girl, she heard her father's voice cut through the house like the jets she would one day fix. He taught her about engines—how to keep them humming. And how to keep quiet. She was quick with the tools, better than him by fourteen. It made him angrier. When she joined the Air Force, she thought she'd left all that behind. But her father's lessons followed her.

She carried his hands in her hands, his anger in her chest, his silence in her mouth. Every plane she fixed flew, but she stayed grounded, carrying the weight of years that wouldn't take off.

After the Air Force, she went through the motions: a job at a civilian hangar, an apartment that stayed neat, and nights that felt too long. One night, staring at the glow of a computer screen, she clicked a link to a veterans' center. It offered therapy, something she'd always ignored. She made the call anyway.

The therapist's office was quiet, too quiet, but Elena kept showing up. She talked about her father, about engines, about what it meant to live with ghosts you couldn't fix.

Weeks turned into months, and the heaviness began to lift. She learned to recognize the old anger and let it pass, like a jet roaring overhead. It didn't vanish, but it didn't own her anymore.

One morning, Elena walked onto the flight line, the sun just starting to rise. Same wrench, same noise, same sky. But she was lighter now. She couldn't change the past, but she could build something new. She smiled, gripping the wrench, ready to begin.

This chapter is about how childhood trauma (0-18 years of age) leaves deep imprints, shaping who we are and how we navigate the world—but also about how resilience and healing can transform even the most fractured lives. Some of the material on neurobiology is dense, so please read carefully and vow to learn something new with each reading.

Before an adult enters the US military, they have already lived a life of at least 18 years. And some of those years may have been traumatic, even though most see childhood as a time of innocence and growth, a period of life where the foundation for future wellbeing is built. Yet for countless individuals, these formative years are marked by adversity that leaves an indelible imprint. Childhood trauma, in all its forms, has a profound ability to reshape lives—not only in the immediate aftermath of events but often well into adulthood.

The impacts of childhood trauma can also extend far beyond the individual, influencing families, communities, and society as a whole. This ripple effect underscores why addressing childhood trauma must be a public health priority. Early adversity can lead to patterns of dysfunction in relationships, employment struggles, and cycles of intergenerational trauma. However, recognizing these patterns provides an opportunity to intervene and creates healing not only for survivors but for entire communities.

The Scope of Early Life Trauma

Childhood trauma is a vast and multifaceted issue, one that is far more common than many realize. Studies reveal that nearly 60% of adults report experiencing at least one adverse childhood experience (ACE), with a significant number facing multiple sources of trauma. Adverse experiences can include physical, emotional, or sexual abuse, neglect, domestic violence, parental substance abuse, or the incarceration of a parent. Each of these experiences carries its own unique challenges, yet all share the potential to disrupt a child's development.

Acute trauma: Singular, overwhelming events such as accidents, natural disasters, or sudden losses. These incidents create clear before-and-after moments that can forever alter a child's sense of safety.

Chronic trauma: Prolonged exposure to neglect or repeated abuse, weaving itself into the fabric of daily life. This form of trauma is often insidious, making it harder to identify and address.

Complex trauma: Harm that arises within caregiving systems—where those meant to protect become sources of fear or harm. This form of trauma is particularly damaging, as it undermines foundational trust and security.

What makes childhood trauma particularly impactful is that it strikes during critical developmental periods, shaping not only how children see the world but how their minds and bodies function. Trauma creates a lens through which children perceive themselves, others, and their environment, often leading to distorted beliefs such as "I am unworthy" or "The world is dangerous." These beliefs, if unaddressed, can become deeply ingrained, influencing every aspect of life.

The prevalence of childhood trauma also makes it a significant public health issue. The ACE study—a landmark investigation into the long-term effects of early adversity—revealed a strong correlation between childhood trauma and poor health outcomes in adulthood. Individuals with high ACE scores are more likely to suffer from chronic illnesses, mental health disorders, and even premature death.

Understanding these connections highlights the urgent need for trauma-informed care and prevention strategies. By examining the scope of early life trauma, we begin to see not just the depth of the issue but the opportunities for intervention. Through education, policy changes, and compassionate care, we can mitigate the effects of trauma and support children in building healthier, more resilient futures.

Elena learned to feel her father's anger rise, watch it roar overhead like a jet, then fade. The engine still exists, but it no longer owns the sky inside her. Find the source of your trauma.

Understanding Childhood Trauma: Origins and Impact

Childhood trauma leaves its initial mark in ways that are deeply personal yet remarkably universal. A single traumatic event can sear itself into memory, leaving vivid flashbacks and triggers. By contrast, chronic neglect or abuse often embeds itself more subtly, creating what some clinicians call a "survival brain"—a heightened state of vigilance that prioritizes safety above all else.

Acute trauma, such as a natural disaster or a severe accident, often creates what experts describe as "frozen moments." These events are so overwhelming that the mind struggles to process them fully, leading to fragmented memories and heightened responses to reminders of the event.

For example, a child who survives a car accident may later experience fear and anxiety every time they hear screeching tires or see a similar vehicle. This response is the brain's way of protecting itself from future harm, and it also interferes with daily life and creates ongoing distress.

Chronic trauma—the kind that arises from persistent neglect or repeated abuse—affects children in more pervasive ways. Unlike acute trauma, which often has a clear beginning and end, chronic trauma becomes an ongoing reality. Children exposed to chronic trauma often develop a state of hypervigilance, where their nervous systems remain on high alert. This state, while adaptive in the moment, can lead to long-term challenges, including difficulty concentrating, disrupted sleep patterns, and struggles with emotional regulation.

Perhaps the most complex form of trauma is that which arises within caregiving relationships. When the very people meant to provide safety and nurture instead become sources of harm, the impact is profound. This type of trauma undermines a child's ability to form secure attachments, leaving them with deep-seated trust issues and an inability to seek comfort or support from others. Over time, this can lead to a sense of isolation and difficulty forming healthy relationships in adulthood.

Compounding the issue are environmental factors that increase vulnerability. Socioeconomic hardship, for example, not only increases the likelihood of trauma but magnifies its impact. Children living in poverty are four times more likely to experience adversity. When coupled with systemic challenges such as racial discrimination, the risk intensifies further, creating what researchers describe as "perfect storms of vulnerability."

The timing of trauma matters immensely. Early childhood—a period of rapid brain development—is particularly sensitive. Trauma during this time disrupts the formation of secure attachments, undermines emotional regulation, and sets the stage for future behavioral patterns. By understanding these early impacts, we can better anticipate the needs of trauma survivors and craft interventions that meet them where they are.

The Neurobiology of PTSX in Childhood Trauma Survivors

The following sections should inspire you to become familiar with basic neuroscience. Some are technical, others dense with new material and unfamiliar acronyms. We encourage you to dig deep into the neurosciences, because PTSX has its basis at the molecular level. In the least, please have on hand a diagram of basis brain anatomy so you can follow along as you read these sections. Also knowing very basic functions of each brain region allows you to better appreciate the following information.

When trauma occurs in childhood, its effects are not just emotional or psychological; they are profoundly biological. Trauma rewires the developing brain in ways that reflect adaptation to chronic stress but often come at a cost. Recent advances in neuroimaging provide a window into this process:

The hippocampus, essential for memory and learning, often shows reduced volume in trauma survivors, affecting their ability to contextualize experiences. The hippocampus is critical for processing and storing memories, particularly those tied to time and place. In trauma survivors, chronic exposure to stress hormones such as cortisol can impair neurogenesis, leading to reduced hippocampal volume.

This shrinkage affects the ability to distinguish between past and present, often manifesting as flashbacks or intrusive memories. Survivors may struggle to consolidate new information, impacting academic performance and decision-making skills. Results from long-term studies suggest that early intervention with therapies promoting neuroplasticity, such as mindfulness or cognitive training, can partially reverse these deficits, underscoring the importance of timely support.

With trauma, the amygdala, the brain's threat detection center, becomes hyperactive, leading to heightened fear responses and an overactive stress response system. The amygdala serves as the brain's alarm system, scanning the environment for potential threats. In trauma-exposed children, repeated activation of this system leads to structural and functional changes, including increased size and heightened sensitivity.

Hyperactivity primes survivors to perceive danger even in safe contexts, contributing to hypervigilance and anxiety. Elevated amygdala activity also perpetuates the dysregulation of the hypothalamic-pituitary-adrenal (HPA) axis, resulting in chronic stress responses. The term "axis" means there's a direct connection between or among different body parts and regions. Emerging interventions, such as trauma-focused cognitive behavioral therapy and neurofeedback, recalibrate the amygdala's overactivity and build a more adaptive response to perceived threats.

The prefrontal cortex, which governs executive function and emotional regulation, may show decreased connectivity, leaving survivors less equipped to manage emotions and impulses. The prefrontal cortex (PFC) plays a pivotal role in regulating behavior, planning, and decision-making. In children exposed to trauma, the connectivity between the PFC and other brain regions, such as the amygdala, is often weakened.

Reduced connectivity compromises the brain's ability to dampen emotional outbursts and control impulsive behaviors. Additionally, trauma can hinder the maturation of the PFC, delaying the development of skills like self-regulation and problem-solving.

Recent studies highlight the potential of interventions like mindfulness-based stress reduction (MBSR) and aerobic exercise to enhance PFC connectivity and functionality, offering hope for improved emotional and cognitive outcomes in trauma survivors.

These changes are not merely transient. They represent a "toxic stress adaptation." The brain's development during childhood is uniquely susceptible to environmental input, and persistent stress reshapes neural pathways to prioritize survival over higher-order functions like reasoning and problem-solving. This adaptive mechanism ensures immediate survival but can hinder long-term emotional and cognitive growth.

Stress-related changes also extend beyond individual brain regions to the interconnectedness of neural networks. For instance, the limbic system, which governs emotional responses, becomes hyperactive and poorly regulated, creating a cascade of challenges in managing fear, anxiety and mood. These imbalances often manifest in symptoms like heightened reactivity, difficulty calming down, and persistent feelings of threat.

The body's primary stress response system, the HPA axis, also undergoes significant changes in trauma survivors. Chronic activation of this axis leads to dysregulated cortisol levels, either too high or too low, contributing to a state of constant physiological arousal or emotional numbness. Over time, this dysregulation impacts immune function, inflammation, and even metabolic processes, further embedding trauma's chemical and molecular effects in the body.

Beyond the brain and HPA axis, any type of trauma leaves a distinct molecular imprint. Epigenetic modifications, changes to how genes are expressed without altering DNA itself, have been observed in survivors of childhood trauma. These changes influence stress-related genes, effectively "programming" the body's response to future stressors and even passing these adaptations to the next generation. Understanding this transgenerational impact highlights the urgency of early intervention, as untreated trauma does not merely affect one individual but can reverberate through families and communities.

Despite these profound effects, the brain's remarkable plasticity offers a foundation for healing. Neuroscience research has revealed that targeted interventions, from trauma-focused therapy to mindfulness practices, can create new neural pathways and repair disrupted connections.

The challenge lies not in the brain's ability to recover but in ensuring survivors have access to the resources and support they need to begin that process. Remember: actions and behaviors (like trauma) affect brain chemistry and underlie PTSX. In turn, changing the brain's chemistry with various types of treatments and therapies also affects and changes behaviors.

Psychological Manifestations of Childhood Trauma

Trauma's psychological impact is complex and far-reaching, often manifesting as a tapestry of emotional, cognitive, and behavioral challenges. Trauma survivors frequently struggle with emotional regulation, finding it difficult to process and manage their feelings in ways that create stability.

For many, the experience of "emotional tsunamis"—sudden and overwhelming waves of intense emotion— becomes a hallmark of their trauma response. These emotional surges can arise without warning, leaving survivors feeling out of control and consumed by feelings of fear, anger or sadness.

Emotional flashbacks are another pervasive symptom, distinct from the visual flashbacks often associated with trauma. These flashbacks push survivors into the emotional states they experienced during the trauma, often without conscious awareness of the connection to past events. This can make the emotional intensity feel inexplicable and isolating, further compounding the difficulty of managing daily life.

Cognitive impacts of trauma are equally significant. Survivors often develop deeply ingrained beliefs about themselves and the world, shaped by the need to make sense of their experiences. These beliefs— such as "I am unworthy," "The world is unsafe," or "I cannot trust anyone"—form the foundation of trauma-related cognitive schemas. These negative schemas influence thought patterns, decision-making and interactions with others, perpetuating a cycle of fear, shame and withdrawal.

Memory systems also bear the impact of trauma. Traumatic memories are often fragmented and stored differently from ordinary memories, making them difficult to integrate into a cohesive narrative. This disjointed processing leads to intrusive thoughts, difficulty recalling events accurately, or "blackouts" where portions of traumatic experiences seem to vanish from memory entirely. Advances in neuroscience suggest this fragmentation arises from disruptions in the hippocampus and its role in contextualizing and organizing memories.

Behaviorally, trauma survivors may exhibit patterns driven by survival instincts rather than conscious choice. Hypervigilance, avoidance and impulsive reactions are common adaptations to perceived threats. These behaviors, while protective during trauma, often become maladaptive in safe environments, leading to strained relationships and difficulty achieving personal or professional goals.

Interpersonal relationships are particularly fraught for trauma survivors. Attachment research indicates that individuals with childhood trauma often exhibit disorganized attachment patterns, simultaneously craving closeness and fearing vulnerability. This creates a paradox where survivors struggle to maintain meaningful connections, oscillating between dependency and withdrawal.

Dissociation—a protective mechanism that allows individuals to "escape" unbearable emotional or physical pain—is another hallmark of severe trauma. While dissociation can provide relief in the short term, it complicates long-term healing by creating fragmented experiences of self and reality.

Survivors may feel detached from their emotions, bodies or identities, making it challenging to integrate their experiences and develop a cohesive sense of self. Healing from these behavioral manifestations requires an integrated approach that addresses emotional regulation, cognitive restructuring and relational repair. Evidence-based therapies such as eye movement desensitization and reprocessing (EMDR) and trauma-focused cognitive behavioral therapy (TF-CBT) have demonstrated significant efficacy in helping survivors process and integrate their experiences.

Somatic therapies that focus on reconnecting with the body, such as yoga or somatic experiencing, also play a crucial role in addressing the physical and emotional disconnection that trauma often creates.

Ultimately, understanding the psychological manifestations of childhood trauma underscores the need for compassionate and comprehensive care. By addressing the multifaceted impact of trauma, survivors can move from merely surviving to thriving, reclaiming their sense of agency and possibility.

Physiological Consequences of Childhood Trauma

The body bears the burden of trauma as much as the mind. Chronic stress leaves physiological traces that can affect health across a lifetime. Childhood trauma sets off a cascade of biological changes, many of which endure far beyond the traumatic experiences themselves. This somatic legacy reflects the body's attempt to adapt to extreme stress, but these adaptations often come at a significant cost.

<u>The Immune System and Inflammation</u>: One of the most well-documented consequences of childhood trauma is a state of chronic inflammation. The body's stress response, designed for short-term activation, becomes persistently engaged when stress is unrelenting. This chronic activation results in elevated levels of inflammatory markers like C-reactive protein (CRP) and interleukin-6 (IL-6). Over time, these pro-inflammatory states increase the risk of autoimmune diseases like rheumatoid arthritis, lupus and multiple sclerosis. They also contribute to the development of chronic illnesses, including cardiovascular disease, diabetes, and even certain types of cancer.

Research has shown that adults with high Adverse Childhood Experiences (ACE) scores are significantly more likely to experience these conditions, pointing to the long-term health impact of early adversity. The ACE is a measure used to quantify the amount of childhood trauma or adversity an individual experienced during their first 18 years of life.

This scoring system originated from the Adverse Childhood Experiences Study (ACE Study), a landmark research project conducted by Kaiser Permanente and the CDC in the late 1990s.

An ACE score is derived from a questionnaire covering 10 types of traumatic events experienced in childhood:

- Abuse:
  - -Physical abuse
  - -Emotional abuse
  - -Sexual abuse
- Neglect:
  - -Physical neglect
  - -Emotional neglect
- Household Dysfunction:
  - -Parental mental illness
  - -Substance abuse in household
  - -Domestic violence
  - -Parental separation or divorce
  - -Incarceration of a family member

Each event experienced counts as one point, with scores ranging from 0 (no adversity) to 10 (highest adversity).

Research shows a strong correlation between high ACE scores and increased risks of:

Mental Health:

- Depression and anxiety
- PTSD/PTSX
- Suicide attempts

Physical Health:

- Heart disease
- Diabetes
- Stroke
- Obesity
- Chronic obstructive pulmonary disease (COPD)

Behavioral and Social Outcomes:

- Substance abuse

- Smoking
- Risky sexual behaviors
- Poor educational and employment outcomes

The ACE Study demonstrated that individuals with an ACE score of 4 or higher are significantly more likely to suffer from chronic diseases, mental health disorders, and engage in risky and dangerous behaviors. Those with an ACE score of 6 or higher have reduced life expectancy by up to 20 years compared to individuals with a score of zero.

This means that, even though their lifespan is the same of their peers, say, 82 years for males, the number of years they are expected to live is significantly decreased. What's worse, these individuals may also experience a life of pain and suffering, adding to the insult of a shorter life.

Early trauma and adversity can have lifelong consequences because they disrupt normal neurological, hormonal and emotional development, contributing to long-term issues with health, stress management and interpersonal relationships.

Addressing and preventing ACEs through early intervention, trauma-informed care, counseling, and supportive relationships significantly mitigates the long-term adverse effects.

Early screening and intervention are critical strategies to improve long-term outcomes for individuals with high ACE scores.

The Endocrine System and HPA Axis Dysregulation: The HPA axis is the body's primary stress response system. In individuals exposed to childhood trauma, this system often becomes dysregulated.

Some survivors exhibit hyperactivation of the HPA axis, resulting in persistently high cortisol levels, while others show blunted cortisol responses, reflecting an exhausted stress response system. Both patterns are associated with a range of physical and mental health issues, including anxiety, depression, obesity and metabolic syndrome. Dysregulation of the HPA axis also affects sleep, energy levels, and overall resilience to stress.

Neurological Consequences Beyond the Brain: The nervous system—

particularly the autonomic nervous system (ANS)—plays a crucial role in the body's response to trauma. Survivors of childhood trauma often exhibit an overactive sympathetic nervous system (the "fight or flight" response) and an underactive parasympathetic nervous system (responsible for rest and recovery).

An imbalance can lead to symptoms such as increased heart rate, digestive issues, chronic or persistent pain, and heightened sensitivity to environmental stimuli. These somatic expressions of trauma are particularly common in individuals with complex trauma histories, as the body continuously perceives danger even in safe environments.

Epigenetic Changes and Transgenerational Impact: At the molecular level, childhood trauma leaves its mark through epigenetic modifications. These changes alter how genes related to stress, inflammation and emotional regulation are expressed, without altering the DNA sequence itself. Epigenetic changes are not confined to the individual. They can be passed down to subsequent generations, creating a biological legacy of trauma.

For example, studies of WWII trauma survivors and their descendants have revealed altered stress hormone regulation in children and grandchildren, even when these individuals did not directly experience the original trauma. Understanding these transgenerational effects emphasizes the need for systemic and family-oriented approaches to healing.

Telomere Shortening and Accelerated Aging: Telomeres, the protective caps at the ends of chromosomes, naturally shorten with age. However, chronic stress accelerates this process, leading to premature cellular aging. Shortened telomeres are associated with an increased risk of chronic diseases, reduced immune function and shorter lifespans.

Studies have shown that individuals with high ACE scores often exhibit telomere shortening equivalent to several years of additional biological aging. This highlights the urgent need for interventions that can mitigate the physiological toll of early adversity.

Somatic Symptoms and Cultural Expression: Trauma often manifests as physical symptoms that vary across cultures. In some Western contexts, survivors may report chronic pain, gastrointestinal distress or unexplained fatigue, while in other cultural settings, distress may be expressed through specific physical complaints that reflect local understandings of illness. Recognizing these variations is crucial for accurate diagnosis and treatment, as culturally sensitive approaches can significantly improve outcomes for trauma survivors.

The Path to Physical Healing: Addressing the physiological consequences of childhood trauma requires a holistic approach that integrates physical and mental health and healthcare. Evidence-based interventions like mindfulness-based stress reduction (MBSR), yoga, and biofeedback have demonstrated efficacy in calming the nervous system and reducing inflammation. Trauma-informed primary care, which incorporates an understanding of how trauma affects the body, is essential for providing comprehensive treatment.

Pharmacological interventions may also play a role, particularly in addressing HPA axis dysregulation or co-occurring conditions like chronic pain. However, medication is most effective when combined with therapies that address the root causes of trauma, rather than solely managing symptoms.

Emerging research on the use of psychedelics and other novel treatments for trauma-related conditions offers promising new avenues for addressing both the physical and emotional legacies of childhood adversity. Also, now that we know PTSX in all its forms has a molecular basis, new treatments and therapies that target molecular-level symptoms will be beneficial, if not provide total healing.

Ultimately, healing the body from the effects of trauma is an integral part of the broader journey to recovery. By addressing the physiological imprints of trauma, survivors can begin to reclaim a sense of safety and well-being, paving the way for holistic healing and resilience.

Healing Pathways and Treatment Modalities

Childhood trauma—with its profound ability to disrupt emotional, physical, and psychological development—does not have to consign individuals to a lifetime of suffering. The study of neuroplasticity, or the brain's capacity to reorganize and heal, underscores an empowering truth: recovery is not only possible but achievable. With the right therapeutic interventions and support, survivors can transform their pain into a pathway of growth and resilience.

Trauma-Focused Therapies: Reprocessing and Integration

One of the most effective means of addressing childhood trauma is through trauma-focused psychotherapies. These evidence-based methods help survivors reframe and integrate their traumatic experiences, reducing the emotional charge associated with distressing memories.

Trauma-Focused Cognitive Behavioral Therapy (TF-CBT): TF-CBT combines traditional cognitive-behavioral strategies with trauma-sensitive interventions. This approach equips individuals with tools to challenge distorted beliefs, manage distressing emotions, and confront their trauma narrative in a safe, gradual manner. Over time, survivors learn to reinterpret their experiences, reducing feelings of shame, guilt, and fear. These behavioral changes, in turn, directly affect the underlying chemistry, though we don't yet know to what extent.

Eye Movement Desensitization and Reprocessing (EMDR): EMDR offers a nontraditional yet highly effective way to process trauma. By engaging in bilateral stimulation—such as guided eye movements—while recalling traumatic memories, individuals can reprocess these experiences, diminishing their intensity and reframing their meaning. Research shows that EMDR not only alleviates symptoms of PTSX but also facilitates lasting cognitive and emotional shifts, promoting healing at a deeper level.

Somatic Interventions: Reconnecting with the Body

Trauma lives in the body as much as it does in the mind. For many survivors, dissociation—a coping mechanism developed in response to overwhelming stress—creates a disconnect between their physical and emotional selves.

Trauma-Sensitive Yoga: Unlike traditional yoga practices, trauma-sensitive yoga emphasizes safety, choice and body awareness. Survivors are encouraged to move at their own pace, reconnecting with their bodies in a way that feels empowering rather than triggering. Studies have shown that trauma-sensitive yoga can reduce symptoms of hyperarousal, anxiety and dissociation, helping individuals regain a sense of agency over their physical selves.

Mindfulness and Meditation: Mindfulness-based practices cultivate present-moment awareness, enabling individuals to observe their thoughts and emotions without judgment. For trauma survivors, mindfulness provides a grounding tool to counteract flashbacks, intrusive thoughts and emotional overwhelm. Over time, these practices strengthen emotional regulation and resilience, laying the groundwork for lasting recovery. Future work likely will reveal how this and other behavioral therapies affect the brain and body at the molecular level.

The Phase-Based Approach to Healing

Recovery from childhood trauma often unfolds in distinct phases, each addressing a specific aspect of the healing journey. This structured approach ensures that survivors progress at a pace that respects their individual needs and readiness.

Phase One: Safety and Stabilization

The foundation of trauma recovery lies in establishing a sense of safety—both internal and external. Many survivors enter therapy in a state of dysregulation, marked by heightened arousal, emotional numbing or chaotic relationships. The initial phase focuses on:

Building a secure environment: Collaborating with a trusted therapist to establish boundaries, routines, and coping strategies.

Regulating the nervous system: Employing grounding techniques, breathing exercises, and somatic practices to manage symptoms of hyperarousal and dissociation.

Establishing trust: Creating a therapeutic alliance that builds a sense of safety, validation and nonjudgment.

This phase may also involve addressing immediate concerns like housing instability, financial insecurity or medical needs, ensuring that survivors have the stability necessary to engage in deeper work.

Phase Two: Trauma Processing

Once safety and stabilization have been achieved, survivors can begin the delicate process of confronting and processing their traumatic memories. This phase often involves:

Gradual exposure: Revisiting traumatic experiences in a controlled, supportive setting to desensitize triggers and reduce avoidance.

Narrative reconstruction: Developing a coherent, empowering narrative that reframes trauma as a part of the survivor's story rather than its defining element.

Emotional expression: Safely expressing feelings of grief, anger or loss that may have been suppressed or avoided.

Therapeutic modalities such as TF-CBT, EMDR and art therapy play a pivotal role in this phase, allowing survivors to process trauma in ways that align with their personal needs and preferences.

Phase Three: Integration and Growth

The final phase of trauma recovery focuses on integration—bringing together the fragmented pieces of the survivor's identity—and encouraging growth. In this stage:

Reclaiming a sense of self: Exploring and embracing their values, strengths, and aspirations outside the context of trauma.

Building resilience: Developing adaptive coping strategies and support networks to navigate future challenges.

Pursuing meaningful goals: Engaging in activities that promote personal fulfillment, such as education, creative expression or advocacy.

This phase often marks a shift from surviving to thriving, because survivors harness their newfound sense of agency to lead empowered, purpose-driven lives.

The Role of Community and Support

Healing from childhood trauma is rarely a solitary journey. Social support—whether from family, friends, or therapeutic groups—is a cornerstone of recovery. For many survivors, connecting with others who share similar experiences provides validation, reduces isolation, and creates hope. Community-based resources, such as peer-support groups or trauma-informed organizations, can also play a vital role in sustaining progress and building resilience.

Embracing Hope and Possibility

While the journey of healing from childhood trauma is neither linear nor easy, it is profoundly transformative. Each step—from establishing safety to processing trauma to reclaiming identity— represents a victory over adversity. As survivors harness the brain's remarkable ability to heal and adapt, they discover that their trauma, while a part of their story, does not define them.

Recovery is a testament to the resilience of the human spirit, a process through which survivors not only mend the wounds of the past but also forge a future of strength, connection, and possibility. By embracing evidence-based interventions, supportive relationships, and their own inherent capacity for growth, survivors of childhood trauma can move from merely surviving to truly thriving.

Addressing Stigma and Barriers to Healing

Childhood trauma, despite its prevalence and profound impact, is often shrouded in stigma. This stigma arises from deeply entrenched societal misconceptions that frame trauma responses as personal failings rather than natural adaptations to extraordinary stress. These harmful narratives perpetuate silence, delay treatment, and exacerbate the suffering of survivors. Overcoming these barriers requires a multifaceted approach that addresses cultural misconceptions, systemic inequities, and the broader need for trauma-informed care across all sectors.

Breaking the Cycle of Silence and Shame

Stigma surrounding trauma often stems from a lack of understanding about its origins and manifestations. In many cultures, behaviors associated with trauma—such as emotional dysregulation, hypervigilance or withdrawal—are misinterpreted as weakness, moral failure or willful defiance. These judgments serve no practical purpose other than to cause further trauma. They may:

<u>Perpetuate isolation</u>: Survivors may feel compelled to hide their struggles for fear of judgment, further entrenching feelings of shame and unworthiness.

<u>Delay intervention</u>: Mislabeling trauma responses as character flaws

can prevent individuals from seeking or receiving appropriate support.

Reinforce harmful stereotypes: Cultural stigmas disproportionately affect marginalized groups, where trauma responses may intersect with prejudices related to race, gender or socioeconomic status.

Efforts to dismantle stigma must begin with education. Public awareness campaigns, trauma-informed media portrayals, and open dialogue can help normalize discussions about trauma and its effects.

Schools, workplaces and community organizations should provide training that encourages empathy, reduces judgment, and equips individuals with the tools to support survivors effectively.

Equity in Access to Trauma-Informed Care

While trauma impacts individuals across all demographics, access to treatment remains deeply unequal. Marginalized communities—including people of color, low-income families, and LGBTQ+ individuals—often face disproportionate barriers to care. These barriers include:

Economic constraints: The cost of therapy, lack of insurance coverage, and limited access to affordable care prevent many survivors from seeking treatment.

Geographic disparities: Rural and underserved areas frequently lack trauma-informed providers, forcing individuals to travel long distances or forgo care altogether.

Cultural and linguistic mismatches: Survivors may struggle to connect with providers who lack an understanding of their cultural context or who do not speak their language. Addressing these inequities requires systemic change.

Policymakers, healthcare providers and community leaders must collaborate:

- Training programs should actively recruit individuals from underrepresented backgrounds, ensuring that survivors can access care from professionals who share or understand their cultural experiences.
- Investing in public-health initiatives and community-based programs can make trauma-informed care more accessible and

affordable.

- Telehealth services and mobile applications can bridge gaps in care, particularly in remote or underserved regions.

Integrating Trauma-Informed Practices

Trauma-informed care extends beyond individual therapy sessions. To create environments where survivors can thrive, trauma-informed principles must be woven into the fabric of schools, healthcare systems, workplaces and community services. Key components of this integration include:

Trauma-Informed Education: Schools are often the first point of contact for children experiencing trauma. Educators and administrators can play a pivotal role in creating resilience by:

- Recognizing the signs of trauma and responding with compassion rather than punishment.
- Implementing restorative practices that prioritize healing and relationship-building over punitive discipline.
- Providing mental-health resources like school counselors trained in trauma-informed approaches.

Healthcare System Reform: Medical professionals frequently encounter trauma survivors, often without realizing it. Integrating trauma-informed care into healthcare systems involves:

- Training providers to approach patients with sensitivity, avoiding re-traumatization during medical procedures or consultations.
- Screening for trauma as part of routine assessments, ensuring that survivors receive timely referrals to mental health services.
- Collaborating with community organizations to address social determinants of health, such as housing instability or food insecurity, that exacerbate trauma.

Workplace Support: Trauma does not disappear in professional settings. Employers can support their staff by:

- Offering employee assistance programs (EAPs) that include access to trauma-informed counseling.
- Building a culture of flexibility and understanding, allowing employees to prioritize their mental health without fear of stigma

or reprisal.

- Providing training for managers and HR professionals on recognizing and responding to trauma in the workplace.

The Power of Community Advocacy

Community-based efforts are essential in overcoming stigma and barriers to healing. Grassroots organizations, peer-support groups, and advocacy campaigns amplify survivor voices, challenge harmful narratives, and create spaces where individuals feel seen and valued. Examples include:

- Empowering survivors to share their stories can inspire others to seek help and combat feelings of isolation.
- Connecting with others who have experienced similar challenges builds validation and mutual understanding.
- Lobbying for legislative reforms, such as increased funding for mental health services or the implementation of trauma-informed policies, can create lasting systemic impact.

Addressing stigma and barriers to healing requires collective effort. It demands that we challenge ingrained misconceptions, advocate for equitable access to care, and integrate trauma-informed principles into every aspect of society. By doing so, we create a world where survivors of childhood trauma are met with compassion, understanding and the resources they need to heal.

Building a World Where Every Child Can Thrive

The ultimate goal of a trauma-informed world is to prevent childhood trauma wherever possible and to mitigate its effects when it does occur. Achieving this vision requires:

<u>Investing in prevention</u>: Supporting families and communities to address the root causes of trauma, such as poverty, violence and systemic inequities.

<u>Promoting early intervention</u>: Ensuring that children and families have access to resources and support before challenges escalate.

<u>Creating a culture of empathy</u>: Shifting societal attitudes to prioritize understanding, compassion, and inclusion.

In this new world, no child—and no survivor—would walk their journey alone. Instead, they would be surrounded by a network of care and support, empowered to heal and thrive.

Creating a trauma-informed world is not the work of a single individual or organization. It is a collective responsibility that requires courage, dedication, and an unwavering commitment to change. Each of us has a role to play, whether by supporting a survivor, advocating for policy reform, or creating trauma awareness within our own spheres of influence.

Together, we can transform silent scars into stories of hope and renewal. By recognizing the profound impact of early adversity and embracing the principles of trauma-informed care, we take meaningful steps toward a world where every child has the opportunity to thrive. This vision, though ambitious, is within reach—and its realization is a testament to the power of empathy, resilience, and shared humanity.

If-Then Guidance

- If you suspect a child is struggling with trauma-related memory issues, then encourage structured routines and cognitive exercises to support hippocampal development.
- If a child exhibits hypervigilance or heightened fear responses, then provide reassurance and create predictable, safe environments to reduce amygdala overactivation.
- If you notice a child struggling with emotional regulation, then introduce mindfulness techniques or breathing exercises to strengthen prefrontal cortex functionality.
- If the child's symptoms appear to interfere with daily functioning, then seek professional help from a trauma-informed therapist who can provide targeted interventions.
- If caregivers or teachers are uncertain about a child's behavior, then provide education about how trauma affects brain development and behavior.
- If you observe signs of chronic stress in a child, then explore calming activities such as yoga, art therapy or guided relaxation to reduce their overall stress response.

- If a child seems withdrawn or disconnected, then prioritize building trust through consistent, compassionate interactions.
- If trauma-related symptoms worsen over time, then advocate for a comprehensive evaluation by a multidisciplinary team.
- If a child shows difficulty focusing or learning, then consider introducing memory games and structured tasks to support cognitive recovery.
- If caregivers feel overwhelmed by a child's trauma responses, then connect them with support groups or trauma-informed resources for guidance.

Take the Next Step

- Educate yourself about the biological impacts of trauma and how they manifest in behavior and cognition.
- Seek out a trauma-informed therapist to address specific symptoms and provide tailored interventions.
- Encourage children to participate in mindfulness or relaxation exercises to build emotional regulation skills.
- Create a consistent and safe environment for children, reducing unpredictability that may trigger stress responses.
- Integrate grounding techniques, such as deep breathing or sensory exercises, into daily routines to help manage hypervigilance.
- Advocate for trauma-informed practices in schools and community programs to ensure supportive environments for children.
- Introduce activities that promote neuroplasticity, such as problem-solving tasks, memory exercises, or creative outlets.
- Use nonjudgmental language when discussing trauma to reduce stigma and encourage open dialogue.
- Connect with community organizations offering resources or support for families dealing with childhood trauma.
- Encourage children to express themselves through art, storytelling, or other creative means to process their experiences.

Through Their Eyes

"I wear two hats—as a nurse practitioner and a Licensed Clinical Social Worker (LCSW). For over a decade, I've worked with adults whose childhoods were clouded by trauma, and I've learned to see the world through their eyes. Each day, I am reminded that while scars may fade from the skin, they often remain etched on the soul.

"When I sit across from my patients, I see the remnants of battles they fought long before they could understand what war was. There's a fragility in their posture, a hesitance in their voice. Yet, there's also a strength—a quiet defiance against the wounds that tried to define them. One of my patients, Sarah, once described it as feeling like a house that had been burned to its foundation but somehow still managed to stand.

"Many of my patients struggle to articulate what happened to them, and I've come to learn that the silence often says more than words ever could. Childhood trauma, especially in its severe forms, has a way of stealing language. Memories become fragmented, buried under layers of shame and self-preservation. For some, those memories are like ghosts: fleeting, haunting and ever-present. For others, they're like locked doors—barriers built to keep the pain out but which also trap them inside.

"I once worked with a man named James, who had grown up in a household riddled with domestic violence. He told me that as a boy, he would sit in the corner of his room, pressing his hands to his ears, trying to drown out the sound of his parents' fighting. Decades later, James still struggled to sleep, his body jolting awake at the faintest noise. 'I feel like I'm always bracing for impact,' he confessed one day. His amygdala, I explained, had become a hyperactive sentinel, always scanning for threats that weren't there. Science had a name for it. James only called it 'the monster in my mind.'

"For many of my patients, the trauma of childhood was not just a moment but an entire landscape they grew up in. It was the air they breathed, the water they drank. It shaped the way they saw themselves and the world around them. They grew up believing they were unworthy, broken or invisible. And while those beliefs may have helped them survive back then, they became chains that held them back as adults.

"One woman, Maria, carried an immense burden of guilt. Her mother had been emotionally abusive, constantly belittling her, calling her "useless" and "unlovable." As a child, Maria internalized those words. As an adult, she found herself in toxic relationships, always trying to prove her worth to people who mirrored her mother's cruelty. 'Why do I keep choosing people who hurt me?' she asked tearfully during one session.

"I told Maria what I tell many of my patients: that the brain often seeks familiarity, even when it's harmful. It's not a weakness. It's a pattern—one that can be understood and, with time, unlearned. Helping her recognize the roots of her pain was the first step toward her reclaiming her life. Slowly, Maria began to see herself not as the sum of her mother's words but as someone deserving of love and kindness.

"As a practitioner, my work is as much about creating a safe space as it is about clinical expertise. Trauma survivors often walk into my office guarded, their walls built high. My job isn't to dismantle those walls but to give them the tools to lower them at their own pace. Sometimes that means validating their pain. Other times, it means sitting in silence, holding the space for emotions too heavy to name.

"There are days when the weight of my patients' stories stays with me long after I leave the clinic. I've cried in my car after sessions, not because I felt hopeless, but because I felt the enormity of what they had endured. It's humbling to witness their courage—to see them face their pain, day after day, even when the progress feels agonizingly slow.

"But there are also moments of light. I've seen patients reconnect with parts of themselves they thought were lost forever. I've watched them find their voices, set boundaries, and redefine what safety means. I remember the day James told me he'd slept through the night for the first time in years. Or the time Maria stood up to her boss and realized she didn't have to shrink herself to be worthy of respect. Those victories, no matter how small they may seem, are monumental.

"Working with survivors of childhood trauma has taught me that healing is not about erasing the past but about learning to live with it in a way that doesn't consume you. It's about finding strength in vulnerability and courage in connection. It's about transforming pain into purpose, one step at a time.

"When I look into the eyes of my patients, I see resilience. I see people who have been to the depths of despair and still found a way to reach for the light. They remind me every day why this work matters. Because no one—not a child, not an adult—should have to face their journey alone. And together, we can build a path toward healing, one story at a time."

—Major Lana S., US Air Force (ret.), LCSW

3

Understanding Post-Traumatic Stress Injuries in Veterans

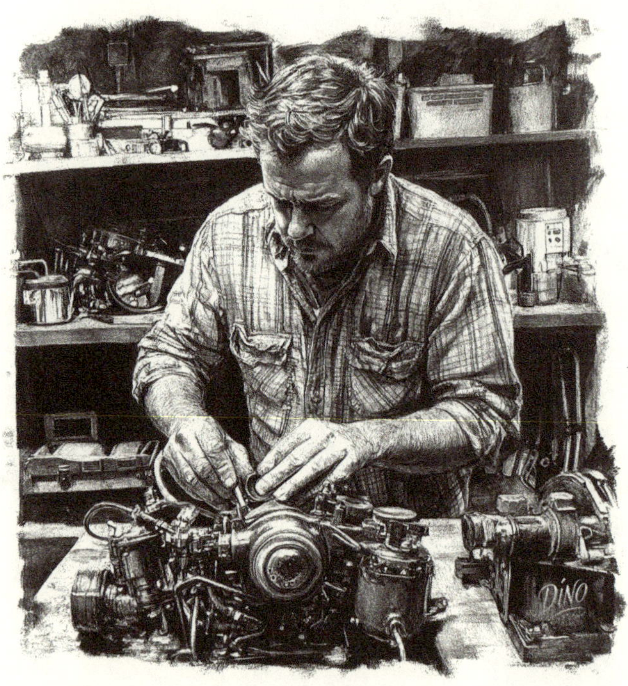

On a rainy afternoon, Jon was in his garage tinkering with an old motorcycle engine— something to keep his hands busy. A few weeks earlier, a slammed door at the supermarket had sent his heart racing and his mind rushing back to a desert road overseas. He'd laughed it off at first, but deep down, he knew his military experiences were still following him home. His wife Megan noticed he'd been distant— waking up in the middle of the night, eyes wide, struggling to remember where he was. Their young daughter started drawing pictures of "Dad looking scared," and that hurt him more than he cared to admit. Yet each time he thought about seeking help, the old voices in his head told him to tough it out. Then he ran into an old battle buddy at a local Veterans' Center. They grabbed coffee and talked about things neither had shared with anyone else.

His friend mentioned he'd started an alternative therapy program: a blend of talk sessions, family workshops, and even some new treatments like ketamine infusions and neurofeedback. "It's different," his buddy said, "but it makes sense when you think about how the brain wires itself after trauma."

Jon felt relief just hearing about it. Maybe there was more to healing than another bottle of pills. He knew families carried a big part of the burden, and it mattered that Megan and his daughter were part of the conversation. Learning about new options—like research on psychedelics or specialized nerve-block treatments—sparked his curiosity.

This chapter dives into that same journey: the impacts of PTSX, its effect on veterans and families, and how understanding the brain leads to better solutions. Most of all, it highlights that true recovery means breaking old barriers, finding fresh therapies, and involving the people who matter most along the way.

The Impacts of PTSX

Military leadership must recognize the importance of creating a culture that prioritizes mental health, allowing servicemembers to seek help without fear of judgment. By creating an environment of openness and support, the military can play a pivotal role in the recovery journey of its personnel.

The US military has a long history of producing and maintaining brave, stoic warriors. The very notion of asking for assistance for a mental-health issue counters the military's storied history. It is becoming clear that the US military is slow to address the issues of imbalanced mental health in its warriors.

On a societal level, the impact of PTSX is felt in various ways, including increased healthcare costs, lost productivity and familial and social disconnection. As veterans struggle to reintegrate into civilian life, the need for effective treatment becomes paramount. Innovative therapies like psychedelic-assisted treatments, cannabinoid integration and stimulation techniques like stellate ganglion block and ketamine offer hope for many.

These alternative approaches are not just scientific advancements. They represent a shift toward more compassionate and comprehensive healthcare models that prioritize the unique needs of veterans. By embracing these innovative therapies, mental healthcare professionals can empower individuals on their path to recovery.

> "Shell shock" became "combat fatigue," now PTSX, yet the frontline truth stays brutal: split-second choices collide with lifelong values, and the body and soul pay the price.

Finally, the integration of community-based support systems is essential for veterans undergoing alternative therapies. Building networks that connect veterans with peers, mental healthcare resources and holistic treatment options creates a sense of belonging and shared experience.

This collaborative approach not only enhances individual recovery but also strengthens the fabric of our society by ensuring that those who have served are honored, understood and supported, especially when they return home and become active in our society once again.

It is our responsibility to advocate for these systems, ensuring that veterans receive the comprehensive care they deserve and paving the way for a more resilient future. In doing so, we honor their sacrifices and reaffirm our commitment to their healing journey.

The Neurobiological Basis of PTSX

The neurobiological basis of post-traumatic stress injuries, anxiety, depression and other challenges is a complex fabric woven from genetic predispositions, environmental triggers and the brain's structural and functional changes from trauma.

For military personnel and veterans, these conditions often arise from the unique stresses of combat and military life, leading to profound impacts on mental health.

Understanding the neurobiology behind these issues is crucial for developing effective treatment strategies that resonate with the lived experiences of those who have served. By exploring these mechanisms, mental healthcare professionals can better tailor interventions that not only address symptoms but also create resilience and promote recovery.

At the core of PTSX and related disorders lies the dysregulation of the HPA axis (including the amygdala), which governs the body's response to stress. When exposed to trauma, the brain's fear circuitry, particularly within the amygdala, becomes hyperactive, leading to heightened anxiety and fear responses.

Traumatic brain injury (TBI) also changes the concentration of certain brain hormones and other molecules, manifesting as changes in a person's behaviors and personality. When a TBI occurs, there's a cascade of events that result in what we finally see and define as PTSX. The upcoming chapter on "The Mechanics of the Mind: Cellular Mechanotransduction" details what goes on following TBI.

Concurrently, the prefrontal cortex, responsible for decision-making and emotional regulation, often shows decreased activity. This imbalance can manifest as intrusive memories, hypervigilance and emotional numbness.

Of course, there are many different parts of brain anatomy, and neural pathways and cascades of events that affect the brain during and after trauma. Our aim is not to discuss them in detail here, but to introduce you to some of them.

Author Dino Garner spent many years doing research in neuroscience and found it fascinating. Perhaps you will explore more on your own, as well. Recognizing these neurobiological responses allows clinicians to better understand their patients' struggles and empowers them to implement targeted therapies that can recalibrate these disrupted pathways.

Emerging therapies, including psychedelic-assisted treatments, cannabinoid integration, stellate ganglion block and ketamine therapy offer exciting avenues for addressing these neurobiological issues. Research has shown that substances like MDMA and psilocybin can promote neurogenesis and synaptic plasticity, facilitating new and improved emotional processing and trauma resolution.

For veterans, these innovative approaches can unlock new pathways to healing that conventional therapies do not address. As the understanding of these neurobiological mechanisms deepens, it encourages the adoption of holistic treatment models that consider the interplay of mind and body in the healing journey. For true success, we must seek new holistic paths.

In addition to pharmacological interventions, stimulation techniques such as stellate ganglion block have shown promise in alleviating symptoms of PTSX. By targeting specific neural pathways, these techniques can help restore balance to the nervous system, providing relief from the debilitating effects of trauma.

It is essential for mental healthcare professionals to stay informed about these advances and integrate them into treatment protocols, ensuring that veterans have access to a comprehensive array of options that cater to their unique needs and experiences. Ultimately, the goal of understanding the neurobiological basis of PTSX, anxiety and depression is to create a more compassionate and effective mental healthcare system for military personnel and veterans. By creating a collaborative environment among these professionals, civilian providers and the military community, we can cultivate a culture of support that prioritizes evidence-based practices and innovative therapies.

If-Then Guidance

- If you are unfamiliar with how PTSX manifests in veterans and the connection between PTSX and physical diseases, then consider speaking with a healthcare provider or researching reliable sources to understand the symptoms and impacts of PTSX. Learning about the emotional, cognitive and physical effects of PTSX can help you identify signs in yourself or others and seek timely support.

- If you are experiencing symptoms of PTSX (such as flashbacks, nightmares, hypervigilance or emotional numbness), then seek help from a healthcare professional as soon as possible. Early intervention can prevent the condition from worsening and help you manage symptoms before they lead to more severe mental health issues or physical health problems.
- If you are aware of your PTSX diagnosis but have noticed physical health problems (e.g., heart disease, gastrointestinal issues, chronic pain, etc.), then discuss these symptoms with your healthcare provider. PTSX is associated with higher rates of physical diseases, and your provider can help you explore treatments that address both mental and physical health.
- If you believe that PTSX is only a psychological condition (hint: it is not), then understand that PTSX can affect both mental (i.e. thinking and cognition) and physical health. And the underlying mechanisms are all physical, right down to the molecular level within cells. Research shows that veterans with PTSX are at a higher risk for conditions such as cardiovascular disease, hypertension and autoimmune disorders.
- If you are not sure how PTSX may be impacting your overall health, then ask your healthcare provider for a full physical and mental-health evaluation. Understanding the broader effects of PTSX on your body and mind can lead to more comprehensive treatment options that address both psychological and physical symptoms.
- If you are managing PTSX but have not explored how it may be linked to physical health conditions, then consider integrating treatments that address both aspects. This could include lifestyle changes (such as diet and exercise), stress-reduction techniques, and collaboration between your mental-health providers and primary-care physicians to ensure holistic care.

Take the Next Step

- Understand Your Condition: Learn the basics of PTSX and how it affects the brain and body. Knowledge empowers you to take control of your healing process.
- Connect with a Counselor: If you haven't already, make an appointment with a counselor or therapist experienced in treating veterans. They can guide you through a personalized treatment plan.
- Journal Your Symptoms: Start tracking your PTSX symptoms, noting any triggers, emotional reactions or improvements. This can help both you and your healthcare provider better understand your condition.
- Watch the Amazon Prime film *Quiet Explosions*. Then contact The Millennium Health Centers. The film is empowering. Dr. Gordon's practice is healing. Just do it.

Through Their Eyes

"After coming home from deployment, everything felt different. I knew about PTSX—I'd heard the stories, seen the stats—but I didn't expect it to take over my life the way it did. The flashbacks, the constant anxiety, it was like I was still in combat, even when I was sitting at home.

"It wasn't just in my head, though. My body felt it too. My heart was always racing, and I'd get these sharp pains in my chest. At first, I thought it was all part of the PTSX, but then I learned that PTSX isn't just mental—it's physical too.

"That's when I realized I needed a different kind of help. I started seeing a therapist who specialized in working with veterans, and she explained how trauma affects the whole body. I started taking care of myself in ways I hadn't thought about before—sleeping better, exercising more, even changing my diet.

"There are ways to heal, ways you might not even know about yet. You just have to take that first step and reach out for help."

—Sergeant David W., US Army Veteran

4

PTSX and Its Complex Comorbidities: Diagnostic Challenges

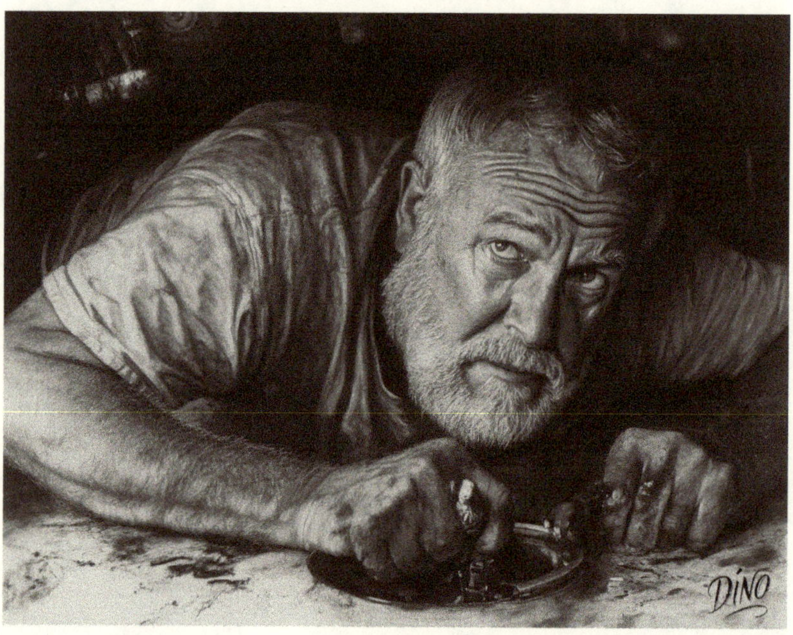

Jason woke up every morning feeling like his body and mind were at war. Thirty-two, former Marine, and now a mechanic at a bustling shop, he didn't have a name for the chaos inside him. He just knew it was there.

Some days, it was the constant edge of panic, like his heart couldn't slow down. Other days, it was the fog—the kind that made everything feel far away, like he was watching his life from the outside. His back hurt, his head hurt, his temper flared over nothing. He drank too much at night, then stared at the ceiling when he should have been sleeping.

The VA doctor had diagnosed PTSD, but the pills didn't help much, and the therapy felt like wading through mud. Then came the migraines, the stomach problems, and the days when his hands trembled so badly he couldn't hold a wrench steady. His boss started looking at him sideways. Jason couldn't blame him.

It wasn't until a new therapist asked about everything—the pain, the drinking, the sleepless nights, the way his mind felt scrambled—that Jason started to understand. She talked about trauma like it wasn't just one thing but a whole storm that could rip through your body, your brain, your life. She called it PTSX.

Intersectionality reminds us that every veteran arrives carrying race, gender, orientation and faith. When care sees those layers, stigma shrinks and recovery starts speaking every dialect of bravery and courage.

For the first time, Jason felt like someone saw all of him. The pieces started fitting together. Therapy became less about fixing one thing and more about untangling the knots. It wasn't fast, and it wasn't easy. But Jason stuck with it. He stopped looking for a cure and started looking for balance. One night, after a long shift, he sat on his porch, the cool air filling his lungs. The storm inside wasn't gone, but it was quieter now. He could live with that.

This dense chapter delves into the intricate web of psychiatric, neurological, physical, behavioral, cognitive and social comorbidities that interact with PTSX, making accurate diagnosis and treatment a challenging task. PTSX represents a comprehensive understanding of the myriad ways individuals process and respond to traumatic experiences. Unlike traditional diagnoses such as PTSD, PTSX accounts for a broader spectrum of symptoms and complications. A significant challenge in diagnosing and treating PTSX arises from the high prevalence of comorbid conditions. These comorbidities complicate symptomatology, often obscuring the primary diagnosis and leading to misdiagnosis or delayed treatment.

Psychiatric Comorbidities

Major Depressive Disorder (MDD) is one of the most frequently observed comorbidities in individuals with PTSX. Symptoms such as persistent sadness, lack of interest in activities, and hopelessness often overlap with the emotional numbness and withdrawal seen in PTSX. This overlap can mask the presence of trauma-induced stress, leading clinicians to focus solely on treating depression while overlooking the underlying molecular trauma.

Depression in PTSX can also manifest uniquely, with symptoms such as heightened irritability or guilt stemming directly from traumatic experiences. For example, a survivor of combat trauma may not only experience sadness but also an acute sense of failure in protecting others, which fuels depressive symptoms.

Effective treatment requires distinguishing these trauma-related features from those of standalone MDD. Furthermore, depression exacerbates the sense of isolation often felt in PTSX, creating a feedback loop where avoidance behaviors deepen depressive states. Understanding these nuances is crucial for targeted interventions.

Anxiety Disorders

<u>Generalized Anxiety Disorder (GAD)</u>: Excessive worry about daily life may mirror hypervigilance, a hallmark of PTSX. Individuals with PTSX often anticipate danger in benign situations, a behavior that can be misinterpreted as generalized anxiety. For example, a trauma survivor may constantly worry about safety, finances, or relationships due to unresolved trauma triggers.

<u>Panic Disorder</u>: Recurrent panic attacks with physical symptoms like chest pain and dizziness may be misattributed solely to panic disorders. In PTSX, these attacks are often triggered by trauma reminders, such as a loud noise resembling gunfire.

Social Anxiety Disorder: Intense fear of social situations, common in PTSX survivors, often stems from trauma-related shame or hyperawareness. This is particularly pronounced in individuals who have experienced interpersonal violence, leading to avoidance of social interactions. Each subtype of anxiety requires careful evaluation to differentiate whether the symptoms are rooted in trauma or represent standalone anxiety disorders. Treatment plans should integrate trauma-focused therapies to address underlying causes.

Substance Use Disorders (SUDs)

Many individuals with PTSX turn to substances like alcohol, opioids, or stimulants to cope with intrusive memories or emotional pain. This maladaptive coping mechanism frequently leads to addiction, further complicating the diagnostic picture. For instance, veterans with PTSX may use alcohol to suppress memories of combat, only to develop dependency that worsens sleep disturbances and irritability.

Similarly, individuals exposed to prolonged trauma may rely on opioids to dull physical and emotional pain, creating a cycle of avoidance and addiction. The interplay between PTSX and SUDs is particularly challenging because substance use can exacerbate trauma symptoms, such as impulsivity or mood instability. Effective treatment must address both conditions simultaneously, using trauma-informed care and evidence-based addiction treatments.

Bipolar Disorder

Trauma can exacerbate or even trigger the onset of Bipolar Disorder. Individuals may oscillate between manic episodes, characterized by impulsivity and hyperactivity and depressive lows. These mood swings can mirror the emotional instability of PTSX, making differentiation challenging yet critical.

For example, a person with trauma-induced hyperarousal may be misdiagnosed as experiencing mania, while trauma-related numbing may be mistaken for bipolar depression. The overlap of symptoms often leads to misdiagnosis, resulting in inappropriate treatments that fail to address the underlying trauma. Effective care requires a good understanding of the individual's trauma history and its influence on mood regulation.

Obsessive-Compulsive Disorder (OCD)

Intrusive thoughts in OCD can resemble the flashbacks and intrusive memories associated with PTSX. Similarly, compulsive behaviors may emerge as a method of controlling trauma-induced anxiety. For instance, a trauma survivor might engage in repetitive checking behaviors to ensure safety, stemming from a deeply ingrained sense of vulnerability. This can lead to misdiagnosis if the compulsions are interpreted as standalone OCD symptoms rather than trauma responses. Addressing the trauma origin of these behaviors is essential for effective treatment.

Personality Disorders

Borderline Personality Disorder (BPD): Emotional dysregulation, a hallmark of BPD, often overlaps with the mood instability seen in PTSX. Trauma is frequently a precursor to both conditions. For example, individuals with PTSX may display intense fear of abandonment or self-harming behaviors, which can be mistaken for BPD.

Antisocial Personality Disorder: Severe trauma histories can manifest as distrust, aggression, and rule-breaking behaviors, complicating treatment. These behaviors are often rooted in survival mechanisms developed during trauma, such as a need to assert control or avoid vulnerability. Differentiating between trauma-induced personality traits and personality disorders requires careful assessment and a trauma-informed approach to care.

Dissociative Identity Disorder (DID): Depersonalization and derealization disorders often arise from severe trauma. These conditions involve disruptions in identity and perception, which can be mistaken for psychosis or other psychiatric illnesses. For example, individuals with DID may exhibit different personality states as a coping mechanism for trauma, while those with depersonalization may feel detached from their surroundings. Understanding the trauma context of these symptoms is critical for accurate diagnosis and effective treatment.

Neurological Comorbidities

Common among combat veterans and survivors of physical trauma, Traumatic Brain Injury (TBI) shares cognitive and emotional symptoms with PTSX, such as memory impairment and mood instability. Differentiating between the two is critical for effective treatment. For example, a veteran with both TBI and PTSX may experience difficulty concentrating and irritability, which can be attributed to either condition. Advanced neuroimaging and cognitive assessments can help clarify the overlap and guide appropriate interventions.

Chronic Pain Syndromes

Conditions like fibromyalgia are linked to prolonged stress and hypervigilance. Chronic pain exacerbates the emotional burden of PTSX, creating a vicious cycle of distress and physical discomfort. For instance, a trauma survivor with chronic back pain may experience heightened anxiety, worsening both the pain and PTSX symptoms. Integrated treatment approaches that address both pain management and trauma processing are essential for improving outcomes.

Migraines

PTSX patients often report increased frequency and intensity of migraines, likely due to heightened stress responses and hyperarousal. Migraines can significantly impair daily functioning, adding to the challenges faced by individuals with PTSX. Stress management techniques and trauma-focused therapies can help reduce migraine severity and improve overall quality of life. Interestingly, several patients experiencing migraines throughout life found total relief from migraines after undergoing Dual Sympathetic Reset, a recent type of stellate ganglion block, developed by Dr. Eugene Lipov in Chicago. We discuss his therapies in detail, in later chapters.

Physical Health Comorbidities

Chronic stress and hyperarousal in PTSX increase the risk of cardiovascular disease: hypertension, heart disease and stroke. Elevated cortisol levels and heightened sympathetic nervous system activity play pivotal roles. For example, a trauma survivor experiencing frequent flashbacks may have consistently elevated heart rates, contributing to long-term cardiovascular strain. Lifestyle modifications and stress-reduction interventions are critical components of care.

Gastrointestinal Disorders

Functional GI disorders like Irritable Bowel Syndrome (IBS) are common in individuals with PTSX. Stress-related dysregulation of the gut-brain axis is a significant contributor. For instance, a trauma survivor may experience abdominal pain and digestive disturbances triggered by anxiety or hypervigilance. Addressing both the physical and emotional aspects of GI disorders is essential for effective treatment.

Autoimmune Disorders

Conditions such as rheumatoid arthritis and lupus are associated with chronic inflammation, which may be exacerbated by trauma-induced stress. For example, individuals with PTSX may have heightened immune responses that contribute to autoimmune flare-ups. Holistic care that addresses both immune health and trauma recovery is vital in managing these conditions.

Metabolic Disorders

Hormonal imbalances caused by chronic stress can lead to Type 2 Diabetes and metabolic syndrome, compounding the physical health challenges faced by PTSX patients. Prolonged exposure to cortisol can contribute to insulin resistance and weight gain. Comprehensive care plans should also include dietary and lifestyle interventions.

Respiratory Disorders

Asthma and other breathing-related conditions are frequently worsened by the anxiety and panic symptoms prevalent in PTSX. For example, a trauma survivor may experience panic-induced hyperventilation, exacerbating asthma symptoms. Integrating breathing exercises and anxiety management techniques into treatment can improve respiratory health and overall wellbeing.

Behavioral Comorbidities

Trauma often triggers disordered eating behaviors like anorexia, bulimia or binge eating, as a way to regain a sense of control or cope with emotional pain. For instance, a survivor of sexual violence may develop restrictive eating habits to exert control over their body. Addressing the trauma underlying these behaviors is critical for sustainable recovery.

Sleep Disorders

Insomnia, nightmares and obstructive sleep apnea are almost universal among PTSX patients. Sleep disturbances exacerbate emotional dysregulation and impair daily functioning. For example, a combat veteran with PTSX may experience recurrent nightmares that prevent restful sleep, leading to daytime fatigue and heightened irritability. Trauma-focused treatments combined with sleep hygiene practices can improve outcomes.

Self-Harm and Suicidal Behavior

Individuals with PTSX are at an elevated risk for suicide attempts and self-injurious behaviors, driven by overwhelming emotional pain and hopelessness. For instance, a trauma survivor who feels trapped by flashbacks may resort to self-harm as a temporary release. Providing a supportive and trauma-informed environment is essential for reducing this risk and promoting recovery.

Developmental and Cognitive Comorbidities

Childhood trauma significantly increases the risk of Attention-Deficit/ Hyperactivity Disorder (ADHD), with symptoms like inattention and impulsivity often masking trauma-related hypervigilance. For example, a child exposed to domestic violence may struggle to focus in school due to constant worry about their safety. Trauma-informed approaches in educational and clinical settings can help differentiate ADHD from trauma responses and guide appropriate support.

Learning Disabilities

Trauma can disrupt cognitive development, leading to difficulties in memory, attention and processing speed, which are often mislabeled as learning disabilities. For instance, a child who has experienced neglect may struggle with reading comprehension due to impaired working memory. Addressing the trauma underlying these challenges is critical for improving educational outcomes.

Neurocognitive Disorders

Older adults with a history of trauma may experience memory impairments and executive dysfunction, complicating the distinction between PTSX and neurodegenerative conditions. For example, a trauma survivor with PTSX may appear to have early dementia due to difficulty concentrating and recalling information. Comprehensive assessments that consider trauma history are essential for accurate diagnosis and care planning.

Social and Relational Comorbidities

Attachment Disorders

Trauma can disrupt the ability to form and maintain healthy relationships, resulting in attachment disorders that exacerbate feelings of isolation and distrust. For instance, a survivor of childhood abuse may struggle to trust others, leading to difficulties in forming close relationships. Therapy focused on building secure attachments is crucial for recovery.

Domestic Violence and Interpersonal Conflicts

Unresolved trauma can perpetuate cycles of abuse or conflict, further compounding emotional and relational challenges. A survivor of intimate partner violence may struggle to set boundaries, leading to repeated patterns of victimization. Trauma-informed interventions can help break these cycles and promote healthier relationships.

Homelessness

High rates of PTSX are observed in homeless populations, where trauma and stress are compounded by lack of stability and resources. A veteran with PTSX who experiences job loss may become homeless, further exacerbating their symptoms. Support services that address both trauma and practical needs are essential for care and a full recovery.

Public Health Considerations

High-risk behaviors and lack of access to preventive care in trauma survivors contribute to an increased prevalence of sexually transmitted diseases like HIV/AIDS and other STDs. For instance, a trauma survivor engaging in substance use may neglect safe sex practices, increasing their risk. Providing trauma-informed sexual health education and care can help mitigate these risks.

Chronic Fatigue Syndrome (CFS)

Persistent fatigue often arises from trauma-related dysfunction in the HPA axis, exacerbating physical and emotional distress. For example, a trauma survivor with CFS may struggle to complete daily tasks due to overwhelming fatigue. Integrated care that addresses both the physical and emotional aspects of CFS is essential for improving quality of life.

Cancer

Prolonged stress and immune dysregulation may increase susceptibility to certain cancers, underscoring the need for holistic care in PTSX patients. For instance, a trauma survivor with chronic stress may experience reduced immune function, increasing their risk. Comprehensive care plans that include stress management and preventive screenings can improve outcomes.

Diagnostic Challenges

The pervasive nature of these comorbidities highlights the need for nuanced diagnostic approaches. Many symptoms of PTSX mimic or overlap with those of its comorbid conditions, making it challenging to identify the root cause of distress. This diagnostic complexity often leads to a number of issues:

Misdiagnosis

Misdiagnosis is a common consequence of the overlapping

symptomatology between PTSX and its comorbidities. Depressive symptoms like persistent sadness and hopelessness may be attributed solely to Major Depressive Disorder (MDD) without recognizing their roots in trauma.

Similarly, hypervigilance and exaggerated startle responses might be mistaken for Generalized Anxiety Disorder, while intrusive memories could be labeled as symptoms of Obsessive-Compulsive Disorder.

These diagnostic errors are often exacerbated by the siloed nature of healthcare systems, where specialists may focus exclusively on their domain without considering the broader trauma-related context. Misdiagnosis not only delays appropriate treatment but can also lead to the prescription of ineffective or even counterproductive therapies, such as the use of anxiolytics for trauma-induced dissociation.

Delayed Treatment

The intricate presentation of PTSX and its comorbidities often results in delayed treatment. Patients may spend years cycling through various specialists—from neurologists to endocrinologists to psychiatrists—without receiving an accurate diagnosis. For example, a patient with chronic migraines and gastrointestinal issues linked to PTSX may undergo extensive medical testing for physical conditions while their underlying trauma remains unaddressed.

This delay can compound the severity of symptoms, as untreated trauma often leads to further psychological and physical deterioration. Delayed treatment also erodes patient trust in the healthcare system, making them less likely to seek help in the future.

Fragmented Care

Fragmented care is another significant challenge in managing PTSX. Patients often receive piecemeal treatment for individual symptoms rather than an integrated approach that addresses the root cause. For example, a patient with co-occurring substance use disorder and PTSX might receive addiction treatment without trauma therapy, leaving the underlying cause of their substance use unaddressed. Similarly, a patient with insomnia and chronic pain may be referred to separate specialists for each issue, resulting in disconnected care plans that fail to recognize the interplay between these symptoms.

Fragmented care not only reduces treatment efficacy but also increases the burden on patients, who must navigate a complex and disjointed healthcare system. To overcome these diagnostic challenges, clinicians must adopt a holistic and trauma-informed approach that prioritizes understanding the full spectrum of a patient's experiences and symptoms.

An Integrated Approach

Accurate diagnosis of PTSX requires a multidisciplinary approach that considers the interplay of psychiatric, physical, neurological and social factors. This integrated approach involves several key strategies:

Comprehensive Patient History Study

Gathering a detailed patient history is foundational to accurate diagnosis. Clinicians should inquire not only about current symptoms but also about the patient's trauma history, including childhood experiences, interpersonal violence, combat exposure or significant losses. Understanding the timeline of symptom development can help differentiate between trauma-related conditions and other disorders.

For example, identifying that a patient's anxiety symptoms began after a traumatic event can shift the diagnostic focus from generalized anxiety to PTSX. Clinicians should also be attuned to indirect signs of trauma, such as reluctance to discuss certain topics or inconsistent accounts of past events.

Use of Validated Screening Tools

Validated screening tools are essential for identifying trauma and its comorbidities. Instruments such as the Clinician-Administered PTSX Scale (CAPS) and the Trauma Symptom Checklist (TSC) can help quantify the severity of trauma-related symptoms and differentiate them from similar conditions.

These tools can also guide further evaluation, such as neuroimaging for suspected traumatic brain injury or laboratory tests for stress-related hormonal imbalances. Incorporating routine trauma screening into primary care settings can help identify PTSX early, even in patients who may not initially present with overt psychiatric symptoms.

Collaboration Among Healthcare Providers

Effective diagnosis and treatment of PTSX require collaboration among mental-health professionals, primary care providers, neurologists, endocrinologists and other specialists. A patient with PTSX and autoimmune symptoms may benefit from a care team that includes a rheumatologist to manage inflammation, a psychiatrist to address trauma-related distress, a therapist trained in trauma-focused cognitive behavioral therapy (TF-CBT), and a molecular neurobiologist to suggest new molecular treatments.

Regular communication among providers is crucial to ensure that care plans are aligned and mutually reinforcing. Integrated care models, such as those used in veterans' healthcare systems, provide a useful framework for coordinating multidisciplinary teams.

Holistic Treatment Plans

Treatment plans for PTSX should address both the core trauma and its associated conditions. This requires a combination of evidence-based psychotherapies, such as Eye Movement Desensitization and Reprocessing and prolonged exposure therapy, alongside interventions for comorbidities. For example, a patient with co-occurring PTSX and substance use disorder might benefit from trauma-focused therapy combined with medication-assisted treatment for addiction.

Similarly, patients with chronic pain and PTSX may benefit from integrative approaches that combine physical therapy, mindfulness-based stress reduction, and trauma-focused psychotherapy. Addressing social determinants of health, like housing instability or access to healthcare, is also critical for supporting long-term recovery.

By adopting an integrated approach, clinicians can provide more effective and compassionate care for individuals with PTSX. This not only improves patient outcomes but also empowers survivors to reclaim their lives and achieve a greater sense of wellbeing.

If-Then Guidance

- If a patient presents symptoms of depression overlapping with trauma, then explore trauma history alongside depressive symptoms to identify PTSX as a potential root cause.
- If anxiety symptoms resemble generalized or social anxiety disorder, then evaluate for hypervigilance or trauma triggers to determine whether anxiety stems from PTSX.
- If a patient demonstrates substance use behaviors, then consider substance use as a coping mechanism for unresolved trauma and address both conditions simultaneously.
- If bipolar symptoms such as mood swings are observed, then differentiate between trauma-induced emotional dysregulation and manic-depressive cycles to avoid misdiagnosis.
- If dissociative behaviors are detected, then assess for underlying trauma that might indicate dissociative identity disorder or related conditions linked to PTSX.
- If a patient reports chronic physical pain or migraines, then investigate stress-related triggers and potential connections to hypervigilance or trauma-induced physiological responses.
- If a patient presents with comorbidities like IBS or cardiovascular issues, then assess for trauma's role in exacerbating these physical health conditions.
- If diagnostic challenges arise from fragmented care, then advocate for multidisciplinary collaboration to create a unified treatment plan addressing PTSX and its comorbidities.
- If a patient struggles with sleep disturbances or disordered eating, then prioritize trauma-informed interventions to address behavioral symptoms rooted in PTSX.

Take the Next Step

- Screen for Trauma: Use validated tools like the Clinician-Administered PTSX Scale (CAPS) during initial evaluations.
- Build a Comprehensive History: Collect detailed accounts of trauma exposure, symptom onset, and contextual factors impacting the patient's health.

- Distinguish Overlapping Symptoms: Use differential diagnostic strategies to separate PTSX symptoms from similar psychiatric or physical conditions.
- Refer to Specialists: Engage neurologists, endocrinologists, and other experts to address physical and neurological manifestations of PTSX.
- Coordinate Multidisciplinary Care: Encourage communication among providers to ensure treatment plans are cohesive and holistic.
- Prioritize Trauma-Focused Therapies: Recommend evidence-based approaches such as EMDR, TF-CBT, or prolonged exposure therapy to address core trauma.
- Implement Lifestyle Interventions: Incorporate mindfulness, physical activity and dietary adjustments to manage stress-related physical health conditions.
- Address Social Determinants: Assist patients in accessing housing, financial support or social services to improve stability and recovery outcomes.
- Educate the Patient: Provide resources on PTSX and its impacts to empower patients to actively participate in their care journey.

Through Their Eyes

"I served as a nurse practitioner in the United States Air Force for over three decades. During my tenure, I had the privilege—and often the challenge—of working closely with service members who carried invisible wounds from their time in uniform. As a medical officer specializing in PTSX and its numerous comorbidities, my role extended beyond diagnoses and treatments. It was about understanding the intricate stories behind the symptoms and bringing a team together to deliver comprehensive care.

"From the moment I joined, I knew mental health would play a pivotal role in my career. Early on, I worked with service members returning from conflict zones, often displaying symptoms that couldn't be neatly categorized into a single diagnosis. A young airman might come to me struggling with crippling migraines, gastrointestinal distress, and insomnia. On paper, it might seem straightforward: treat the physical complaints. But the longer I listened, the clearer it became that these symptoms often traced back to an unresolved trauma—a near miss during a mission, the loss of a comrade, or even childhood adversity brought to the surface by the stress of military life.

"PTSX rarely walked into my office alone. It brought friends: depression, anxiety, substance use disorders, and chronic pain. Each case was like a puzzle, requiring not just my clinical expertise but also a collaborative approach with neurologists, endocrinologists, mental health professionals and social workers. My responsibility was to identify how these pieces fit together so we could address the root causes instead of just treating symptoms.

"One case that stands out involved a senior non-commissioned officer—let's call him Sergeant J. He'd served multiple deployments in the Middle East and came to me complaining of debilitating back pain. Traditional treatments hadn't worked, and he was frustrated, to say the least. As we talked, he revealed he was barely sleeping due to nightmares.

"He'd started drinking heavily to dull the pain and the memories. What others might have labeled as a 'simple' chronic pain case quickly unfolded into a complex web of PTSX and substance use. By involving a multidisciplinary team, we were able to develop a comprehensive plan: physical therapy for his pain, trauma-focused cognitive behavioral therapy for his PTSX, and a support program to address his alcohol use.

"Women in the Air Force often presented a different set of challenges. I recall one young captain who came to me with severe gastrointestinal issues. She'd been diagnosed with irritable bowel syndrome, but nothing seemed to alleviate her symptoms. During a routine check-up, she broke down and shared that she'd been the victim of military sexual trauma years earlier.

"Her symptoms weren't just physical. They were her body's way of holding onto unprocessed pain. Helping her involved more than medication—it required safety, trust, and patience. Over time, through a combination of trauma therapy and medical care, she began to reclaim her health and her voice. Throughout my career, I've seen how the military's approach to mental health has evolved. When I started, admitting to psychological struggles often came with stigma, especially in a high-pressure environment like the Air Force. Servicemembers feared their careers would suffer if they sought help. Thankfully, the culture has shifted.

"Programs like embedded mental health teams and trauma-informed care training for providers have made it easier for airmen and women to seek support without fear of judgment. I'm proud to have been part of that change, advocating for policies that prioritize mental health as a cornerstone of readiness and resilience.

"Now in retirement, I carry the stories of those I served and treated. Each one reminds me that healing from PTSX is not linear. It's a journey, often messy, but always worth pursuing. If I could leave one message for providers stepping into this field, it would be this: Listen deeply. Behind every symptom is a story, and behind every story is a human being yearning to be seen, heard and healed. That's what it truly means to serve.

—Lieutenant Colonel Marlene F., US Air Force (ret.)

5

The Ripple Effect: PTSX and Its Impact on the Human Body

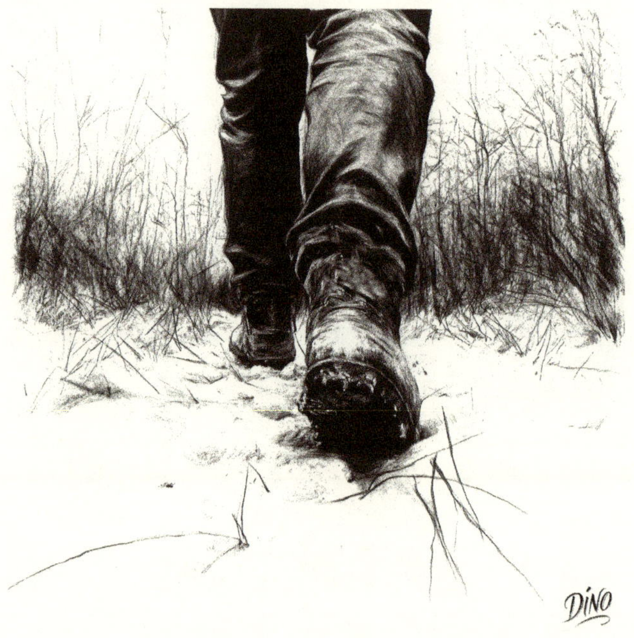

Barry had no idea that PTSX was often inaccurately viewed through the lens of psychology and psychiatry, with its hallmark symptoms like flashbacks, hypervigilance, and emotional dysregulation attributed solely to the mind. He was well familiar with the fact that trauma impacts the body just as deeply, if not more so, weaving its effects through every organ, tissue and system.

The ripple effect of PTSX within him extended far beyond his brain, altering cardiovascular health, immune function, digestion, musculoskeletal balance, and even hormonal and reproductive health. It took many years for someone to explain to him that these interconnected effects reveal that PTSX is not merely a mental-health condition. It is a very real multisystem disorder with a molecular basis and one that requires comprehensive treatment.

His new primary care physician told him: at its core, trauma activates the body's stress response—a survival mechanism designed to protect us in the face of danger. While this system is effective in short bursts, chronic activation due to unresolved trauma creates widespread physiological disruptions. Prolonged exposure to stress hormones like cortisol and adrenaline affects cellular repair, impairs organ function, and fuels inflammation, setting the stage for a cascade of health issues.

Barry now knew how his body had broken down over the decades, and everything was interconnected. His mind-body connection ensured that the body's systems did not function in isolation. For instance, the gut-brain axis illustrates how stress-related changes in the brain influence digestive health and vice versa.

Similarly, the intricate balance of Barry's immune system and endocrine system had been disrupted under the chronic strain of trauma over many years, even well after he left the military. The physical symptoms of PTSX—ranging from chest pain and gastrointestinal distress to chronic pain and fatigue—are not isolated complaints but interconnected manifestations of a body trying to cope with a traumatic past. Now that Barry knew this, he began the long, slow process of teasing apart all the various symptoms and treating each of them holistically.

This chapter dives into the ripple effect of PTSX, exploring the distinct ways in which trauma reshapes each bodily system. By illuminating the complex interplay between mental health and physical health, we aim to create a better understanding of PTSX as a holistic condition. Armed with this knowledge, clinicians, researchers, and patients alike can advocate for integrated care models that treat the whole person, not just isolated symptoms.

The Cardiovascular System: Stress on the Heart and Vessels

The cardiovascular system is highly sensitive to the effects of chronic stress, making it one of the primary bodily systems affected by PTSX. The body's fight-or-flight response, mediated by the sympathetic nervous system, triggers an immediate surge in stress hormones like adrenaline and cortisol. While these hormones are beneficial for short-term survival, their chronic release in individuals with PTSX places immense strain on the heart and blood vessels.

Studies consistently show that individuals with PTSX are at a significantly higher risk of developing cardiovascular diseases, including hypertension, arrhythmias, heart attacks and stroke. Elevated resting heart rates and persistently high blood pressure are common among those with PTSX, reflecting the body's inability to deactivate its stress response. This chronic activation damages the endothelium, the inner lining of blood vessels, which leads to atherosclerosis—a condition marked by the buildup of plaques that restrict blood flow.

Inflammation further exacerbates cardiovascular risks in PTSX. Elevated levels of pro-inflammatory cytokines, such as interleukin-6 (IL-6) and tumor necrosis factor-alpha (TNF-alpha), have been observed in individuals with trauma-related disorders. These inflammatory biomarkers contribute to vascular dysfunction and cardiac remodeling, increasing the risk of adverse cardiac events.

Behavioral factors associated with PTSX also contribute to cardiovascular strain. Many individuals with PTSX turn to coping mechanisms like smoking, excessive alcohol consumption or a sedentary lifestyle, all of which compound cardiovascular risks. Sleep disturbances, another hallmark of PTSX, further impair heart health by disrupting circadian rhythms and preventing the restorative processes essential for cardiovascular repair.

Treatment strategies for mitigating cardiovascular risks in PTSX include a combination of lifestyle modifications, medical interventions, and trauma-focused therapies. Regular aerobic exercise like walking, jogging or swimming, has been shown to improve heart health while reducing PTSX symptoms.

Mindfulness-based interventions, including yoga and tai chi, help regulate the autonomic nervous system, reducing the physiological impact of chronic stress on the heart. For individuals with severe cardiovascular conditions, pharmacological interventions like beta-blockers may be necessary to control heart rate and blood pressure.

Addressing cardiovascular health in PTSX is not just about preventing disease but also about improving quality of life. A well-regulated cardiovascular system supports better sleep, enhanced energy levels, and improved emotional resilience, creating a positive feedback loop for recovery.

The Immune System: Inflammation and Immune Dysregulation

The immune system is intricately tied to the body's stress response, and in PTSX, this relationship becomes profoundly dysregulated. The HPA axis, a key component of the stress response, normally modulates immune activity by releasing cortisol. However, in PTSX, chronic stress alters cortisol production, leading to either an overactive or suppressed immune system.

One of the most significant findings in PTSX research is the elevated levels of systemic inflammation and neuroinflammation. Pro-inflammatory cytokines like interleukin-1 beta (IL-1-beta), IL-6 and C-reactive protein (CRP) are often elevated in individuals with PTSX.

These molecules, while crucial for fighting infections and healing injuries, become harmful when persistently activated. Chronic inflammation has been linked to a wide range of health conditions, including cardiovascular disease, diabetes and neurodegenerative disorders like Alzheimer's disease.

At the same time, the immune dysregulation seen in PTSX makes individuals more susceptible to infections. This susceptibility is particularly concerning for veterans and others with high exposure to environmental toxins or pathogens, as their immune systems are already compromised. For example, impaired natural killer cells (NK) activity, a marker of immune dysfunction, has been observed in individuals with chronic trauma histories.

Emerging evidence also highlights the role of the gut microbiome in immune regulation. Dysbiosis, or an imbalance in gut bacteria, is common in PTSX and contributes to systemic inflammation through the gut-brain axis. Restoring a healthy microbiome using dietary interventions, probiotics and prebiotics can modulate immune activity and reduce inflammation. As you will see in an upcoming chapter, the gut microbiome plays a much larger role in the body's health and wellbeing than previously thought.

Therapeutic strategies targeting immune dysregulation in PTSX are increasingly multidisciplinary. Anti-inflammatory diets rich in omega-3 fatty acids, fruits, vegetables and whole grains have been shown to reduce systemic inflammation. Mind-body practices like meditation and tai chi can lower inflammatory markers by promoting HPA axis balance. For severe cases, pharmacological interventions targeting specific inflammatory pathways, such as TNF-alpha inhibitors, may be explored.

Understanding the immune dimensions of PTSX underscores the need for holistic care. Treating inflammation and immune dysfunction not only reduces physical symptoms but also alleviates the emotional and cognitive challenges that accompany PTSX.

The Gastrointestinal System: The Brain-Gut Connection

The gastrointestinal (GI) system is often referred to as the body's "second brain" due to its intricate relationship with the central nervous system (CNS). This connection, known as the gut-brain axis, plays a pivotal role in both mental and physical health.

In PTSX, disruptions to this axis manifest as gastrointestinal disorders, exacerbating the condition's complexity. Chronic stress alters gut motility, leading to conditions like irritable bowel syndrome (IBS), functional dyspepsia, and gastroesophageal reflux disease (GERD).

These issues cause symptoms like abdominal pain, bloating, diarrhea, and constipation, which are frequently reported by those with PTSX.

Stress-induced changes in gut motility can also disrupt the intestinal barrier, resulting in a "leaky gut." This condition allows harmful substances like lipopolysaccharides (LPS) to enter the bloodstream, triggering systemic inflammation and exacerbating PTSX symptoms.

The gut microbiome, comprising trillions of microorganisms, is another critical player. Studies have shown that individuals with PTSX often have reduced microbial diversity and an overgrowth of pro-inflammatory bacteria. This dysbiosis impacts not only digestion but also mental health, as gut bacteria produce neurotransmitters like serotonin, dopamine and gamma-aminobutyric acid (GABA), which regulate mood and stress responses.

Treating GI issues in PTSX requires a multifaceted approach. Dietary interventions emphasizing high-fiber foods, fermented products, and omega-3 fatty acids can restore microbial balance and reduce inflammation. Probiotic and prebiotic supplements offer additional support for gut health. Stress-reduction techniques like mindfulness meditation and yoga have been shown to improve gut motility and enhance vagal tone, promoting better communication along the gut-brain axis.

Emerging therapies targeting the gut-brain axis hold promise for PTSX treatment. For example, fecal microbiota transplantation (FMT) is being explored as a way to reset the microbiome in individuals with severe dysbiosis. Additionally, vagus nerve stimulation devices, which enhance parasympathetic nervous system activity, are showing potential for alleviating both GI and psychological symptoms.

Addressing the GI dimensions of PTSX highlights the interconnected nature of trauma's impact on the body. By prioritizing gut health, individuals can experience improvements in both their physical and emotional well-being, paving the way for comprehensive recovery.

The Musculoskeletal System: Chronic Pain and Tension

The musculoskeletal system often bears the brunt of trauma's physical manifestations, with chronic pain and tension serving as hallmark symptoms in individuals with PTSX. This connection between trauma and the body's physical framework is deeply rooted in the physiological changes induced by prolonged stress and hypervigilance.

One primary mechanism involves the constant activation of the fight-or-flight response. When the body perceives a threat, muscles tighten as part of the stress response, preparing for immediate action. For individuals with PTSX, this heightened state of arousal becomes chronic, leading to persistent muscle tension, joint discomfort, and even musculoskeletal disorders such as tension headaches, temporomandibular joint dysfunction (TMJ), and myofascial pain syndrome.

Chronic inflammation also plays a significant role in musculoskeletal issues associated with PTSX. Elevated levels of pro-inflammatory cytokines contribute to joint pain and stiffness, mirroring the inflammatory patterns seen in autoimmune conditions. Additionally, individuals with trauma histories often experience reduced physical activity due to depression or fatigue, which exacerbates musculoskeletal issues by weakening the muscles and joints over time.

Treatment strategies for musculoskeletal symptoms in PTSX are diverse and integrative. Physical therapy is a cornerstone of care, focusing on improving mobility, reducing pain, and restoring function through targeted exercises.

Complementary therapies like yoga and tai chi combine gentle movements with mindfulness, and address both physical tension and psychological stress. Massage therapy and myofascial release techniques are particularly effective in alleviating chronic muscle tightness, providing immediate relief and promoting relaxation. Endermologie is a non-aesthetic skin treatment that uses gentle massage and suction to improve the flow of lymph, improve skin texture and suppleness, and tighten saggy skin. The overall result is a general feeling of wellbeing and relief, mostly from improving lymph flow.

Emerging interventions like dry needling and acupuncture offer additional avenues for pain management, targeting specific trigger points to release tension and improve blood flow. Additionally, anti-inflammatory diets and supplements, such as turmeric and omega-3 fatty acids, support musculoskeletal health by reducing systemic inflammation. Addressing the musculoskeletal impact of PTSX underscores the need for a whole-body approach to care. By treating chronic pain and tension, individuals can regain physical functionality and improve their overall quality of life, creating a foundation for holistic recovery.

Whole-body vibration (WBV) therapy is emerging as a novel, non-invasive approach with potential relevance for individuals living with PTSX. Devices such as the LifePro Rumblex generate multi-axis mechanical stimulation that engages muscles, enhances circulation, modulates stress hormones, and supports recovery metabolism—all within short daily sessions. Early results show that WBV can reduce cortisol, elevate endorphins, and improve cognitive function, while also promoting anti-inflammatory pathways. These combined effects may lessen hyperarousal, improve mood regulation, and reduce systemic stress loads that intensify PTSX symptoms. Though still under active investigation, WBV shows promise as a safe, accessible adjunct to established therapies.

The Endocrine System: Hormonal Imbalances and Their Effects

The endocrine system, responsible for regulating hormones throughout the body, is profoundly affected by the chronic stress associated with PTSX. Hormones like cortisol, noradrenaline and adrenaline are central to the body's stress response, and their dysregulation has far-reaching consequences.

In PTSX, the HPA axis often becomes hyperactive, leading to persistently elevated cortisol levels. While cortisol is essential for managing acute stress, its prolonged elevation disrupts homeostasis, impairing metabolic functions, immune responses, and even brain health. Over time, this chronic activation can lead to HPA axis fatigue, characterized by reduced cortisol production and an inability to respond effectively to new stressors.

Hormonal imbalances also extend to the thyroid and reproductive systems. Dysregulation of the thyroid, which governs metabolism, contributes to symptoms like fatigue, weight fluctuations and difficulty concentrating, commonly reported by individuals with PTSX. Similarly, disruptions in sex hormone levels, including testosterone, estrogen and progesterone, can affect mood, libido and overall reproductive and sexual health.

Emerging research highlights the bidirectional relationship between trauma and hormonal health. For instance, imbalances in oxytocin—a hormone linked to bonding and stress regulation—may exacerbate feelings of isolation and mistrust in individuals with PTSX. Understanding these connections provides valuable insights into the systemic impact of trauma.

Treatment strategies for endocrine dysregulation in PTSX involve both medical and lifestyle interventions. Endocrinologists may prescribe hormone replacement therapies or medications to stabilize thyroid and cortisol levels. Lifestyle modifications, such as regular physical activity and stress management techniques, also play a critical role in restoring hormonal balance. Practices like yoga, meditation and tai chi have been shown to enhance HPA axis function, promoting resilience against chronic stress, not to mention greatly improving overall wellbeing.

Sexual and Reproductive Health: Trauma's Hidden Toll

PTSX often casts a shadow over sexual and reproductive health, areas that are deeply personal and frequently overlooked in trauma care. The physiological and psychological effects of PTSX create barriers to intimacy, fertility, and overall reproductive health, underscoring the need for a sensitive and holistic approach to treatment.

One significant factor is the impact of chronic stress on the hypothalamic-pituitary-gonadal (HPG) axis, which regulates reproductive hormones. In individuals with PTSX, dysregulation of this axis can lead to hormonal imbalances, affecting menstrual cycles, libido, and fertility. Women with trauma histories may experience irregular periods, while men often report reduced testosterone levels, contributing to erectile dysfunction and low libido.

Psychological impacts of PTSX can hinder the ability to form and maintain intimate relationships. Intrusive memories and flashbacks may be triggered during physical intimacy, creating a cycle of avoidance and strain in partnerships. Additionally, the stigma surrounding sexual health issues often prevents individuals from seeking help, exacerbating feelings of isolation.

Emerging evidence also links trauma to adverse pregnancy outcomes. Women with PTSX are at higher risk for complications such as preterm labor, low birth weight, and postpartum depression, highlighting the systemic impact of unresolved trauma on reproductive health.

Treatment strategies in this domain require a multidisciplinary approach. Trauma-informed counseling provides a safe space to address the emotional barriers to intimacy and relationships. Hormonal therapies and fertility treatments may be necessary for individuals facing reproductive challenges. Mind-body interventions like mindfulness and somatic therapy, help individuals reconnect with their bodies in a positive and empowering way.

Education and open communication are vital for addressing the stigma surrounding sexual and reproductive health in PTSX care. By creating a supportive environment, individuals can access the resources they need to heal both physically and emotionally, paving the way for healthier relationships and improved quality of life.

Axis by Axis: A Multisystem Approach to Understanding PTSX

The gut-brain axis is a bidirectional communication system between the gastrointestinal system and the brain, and is mediated by neural, hormonal, immune and microbial pathways. Dysbiosis (imbalance in gut microbiota) can influence stress response, neuroinflammation, and emotional regulation. Trauma-induced stress disrupts gut microbiota diversity, impairing production of short-chain fatty acids (SCFAs) that support brain health. Microbial metabolites directly impact the brain through the vagus nerve, contributing to mood dysregulation in PTSX.

Hypothalamic-Pituitary-Adrenal (HPA) Axis

The endocrine pathway regulates the body's response to stress through the release of cortisol. Dysregulation of the HPA axis leads to abnormal cortisol levels, contributing to hyperarousal, anxiety and emotional dysregulation. Prolonged trauma exposure causes chronic activation and eventual exhaustion of this axis, impairing the body's ability to respond to stress effectively. Cortisol dysregulation also disrupts sleep and emotional resilience in individuals with PTSX.

Immune-Brain Axis

Communication between the immune system and the brain is mediated by cytokines, immune cells and inflammation. Trauma-induced neuroinflammation and overactivation of pro-inflammatory cytokines (e.g., IL-6, TNF-alpha) disrupt neural circuits involved in emotion and memory. Sustained inflammation not only exacerbates PTSX symptoms but also increases vulnerability to neurodegenerative conditions. Targeting inflammation may improve emotional regulation and cognitive function in trauma survivors.

Neuroendocrine Axis

Interaction between the nervous and endocrine systems to regulate stress, mood, and behavior. Dysregulation in neurohormones like norepinephrine, dopamine,and serotonin impacts mood, attention and arousal in PTSX. Imbalances in oxytocin, a hormone critical for social bonding, can impair trauma recovery and relational trust. Addressing these hormonal pathways is crucial for restoring emotional stability.

Vagus Nerve Axis

The vagus nerve connects the brain to key organs, including the heart and gut, playing a large role in parasympathetic regulation. Impaired vagal tone can contribute to heightened stress responses, reduced emotional regulation, and increased inflammation. Trauma diminishes vagal activity, prolonging states of hyperarousal. Vagus nerve stimulation (VNS) and breath-focused therapies have shown promise in restoring balance and reducing PTSX symptoms.

Cardiovascular-Brain Axis

The connection between cardiovascular health and brain function includes the impact of blood flow and heart rate on cognitive and emotional regulation. PTSX is associated with autonomic dysregulation, increased heart rate variability, and heightened risk of cardiovascular diseases. Chronic stress and trauma impair brain perfusion, affecting executive functions and emotional control. Interventions aimed at improving heart-brain coherence, like biofeedback, can mitigate these impacts.

Microbiota-Immune Axis

The interactions between gut microbiota and the immune system help to regulate systemic and neuroinflammation. Dysbiosis can trigger immune activation, influencing brain function and exacerbating PTSX symptoms. SCFAs and bacterial metabolites play a role in regulating immune responses and neuroinflammation. Maintaining microbial balance is key to reducing systemic inflammation and improving mental health outcomes.

Gut-Liver-Brain Axis

The gut, liver and brain interact via metabolic and inflammatory pathways. Trauma-related stress can impact liver function, increasing systemic inflammation and oxidative stress that affect brain health. Bile acids produced by the liver influence gut microbiota composition and are linked to mood regulation, highlighting the importance of this axis in trauma recovery.

Amygdala-Prefrontal Cortex Axis

Neural circuits involve the amygdala (fear and emotional processing) and the prefrontal cortex (executive functions and emotion regulation). Overactivation of the amygdala and underactivation of the prefrontal cortex lead to hyperarousal, fear responses and impaired emotional control. Trauma-focused therapies, such as EMDR, target this imbalance to reduce overactivation and strengthen prefrontal regulation, improving emotional resilience.

Brain-Heart-Mind Axis

There is a strong connection between emotional states, heart functions and cognitive processes. PTSX-related emotional dysregulation impacts heart rate variability and stress resilience. Interventions like heart rate variability biofeedback and mindfulness practices help improve autonomic balance and enhance cognitive-emotional integration, building greater stability.

Psychoneuroimmunology Axis

Chronic stress in PTSX dysregulates immune responses and contributes to neuroinflammation. Psychological therapies that reduce stress—like CBT or mindfulness-based stress reduction—indirectly modulate this axis, alleviating inflammation and improving emotional health.

HPG Axis

The endocrine axis regulates reproductive hormones (e.g., estrogen, testosterone). Hormonal imbalances, especially in women, can amplify PTSX symptoms. Trauma exposure disrupts hormonal cycles, affecting stress reactivity and emotional regulation. Addressing HPG axis dysfunction can improve resilience and recovery in trauma survivors.

Bone-Brain Axis

Connections between bone metabolism and brain function are mediated by hormones like osteocalcin. Osteocalcin, produced by bone, has been linked to stress response and memory processes. PTSX-related dysregulation of this pathway can contribute to cognitive and metabolic challenges, making it a potential target for holistic interventions.

Skin-Brain Axis

Bidirectional communication between the skin and brain via immune, neural, and endocrine signaling. Trauma-related stress exacerbates inflammatory skin conditions (e.g., eczema, psoriasis), impacting quality of life and mental health. Addressing stress and inflammation simultaneously can alleviate skin symptoms and improve overall wellbeing.

A Holistic Approach to PTSX Care

The ripple effect of PTSX underscores its profound impact on the entire body and the various axes of communication with the brain, transcending the boundaries of traditional mental healthcare paradigms. From the cardiovascular and immune systems to the musculoskeletal, endocrine and gastrointestinal systems, trauma leaves no organ or tissue untouched. By understanding these interconnected effects, we can move toward a more holistic model of care that addresses the full spectrum of trauma's consequences.

Because of this complex interconnection, integrated care is essential for treating PTSX as a multisystem condition. This approach combines trauma-focused therapies, medical interventions and lifestyle modifications to address both the psychological and physical dimensions of the disorder. By prioritizing the body-mind connection, individuals can experience more comprehensive healing and resilience.

This discussion serves as a call to action for clinicians, researchers and policymakers to expand their understanding of trauma's impact. Only by addressing the full ripple effect of PTSX can we hope to provide the compassionate and effective care that survivors deserve.

If-Then Guidance

- If you are experiencing cardiovascular symptoms like rapid heartbeat, high blood pressure or chest discomfort alongside your PTSX symptoms, then consult a healthcare provider for a comprehensive cardiovascular evaluation. These symptoms may be linked to chronic stress, and addressing them early can prevent long-term health complications.
- If you notice recurring joint pain, muscle stiffness or tension headaches, then consider incorporating gentle physical activities like yoga, tai chi or stretching routines into your daily schedule. These exercises can alleviate musculoskeletal tension and provide mental relaxation, supporting both physical and emotional recovery.
- If you struggle with frequent illnesses or prolonged recovery times, then speak with your healthcare provider about evaluating your immune health. Stress from PTSX can suppress the immune system, and interventions like a balanced diet, stress management techniques and immune-boosting supplements may help restore resilience.
- If you are dealing with fatigue, difficulty concentrating or unexpected weight changes, then explore the possibility of hormonal imbalances with your doctor. These symptoms could be signs of endocrine system dysregulation, and targeted treatments or lifestyle adjustments can help rebalance your body.
- If intimacy issues or changes in reproductive or sexual health are affecting your relationships, then seek support from a trauma-informed therapist or counselor. Open conversations about sexual and reproductive health are essential for addressing emotional and physical challenges, paving the way for improved relationships.

- If gastrointestinal distress such as bloating, cramping or irregular bowel movements is interfering with your daily life, then evaluate your diet and stress levels with the help of a nutritionist or gastroenterologist. Chronic stress can disrupt gut health, and small dietary changes or relaxation techniques can make a significant difference.
- If you notice a decline in overall energy or motivation to engage in daily activities, then explore integrative therapies like acupuncture, mindfulness or physical rehabilitation programs. These approaches can help restore vitality and improve your overall quality of life.

Take the Next Step

- Schedule a comprehensive health check-up to address any physical symptoms that may be linked to PTSX. Inform your provider about your trauma history to ensure a holistic evaluation.
- Consult with specialists in areas where you experience persistent symptoms, for example, a cardiologist for heart issues or an endocrinologist for hormonal imbalances. Targeted care can provide clarity and relief.
- Explore community-based programs offering complementary therapies like yoga, massage therapy or tai chi to address musculoskeletal and emotional tension in a supportive environment.
- Keep a symptom journal to track patterns and triggers in your physical health. This record can guide discussions with healthcare providers and highlight areas requiring intervention.
- Join a support group that focuses on holistic recovery for individuals with PTSX. Shared experiences can create understanding and offer practical advice for managing interconnected physical and emotional symptoms.
- Educate yourself about the ripple effect of trauma on the body. Knowledge empowers you to advocate for comprehensive care and make informed decisions about your treatment journey.
- Prioritize self-care practices that address both your mind and body. Set aside time each day for relaxation, movement, and mindfulness to promote healing and resilience.

Through Their Eyes

"I spent 27 years in the United States Army, serving most of my career as the head of supply at Fort X [Installation name withheld.]. My journey has been one of resilience, strength and determination. As a Black woman in a role dominated by men, I had to earn respect every single day, but I wouldn't trade those years for anything. They made me who I am today—a survivor, a leader and now a mentor for others walking the path I once traveled.

"Growing up, my parents, strong and principled, taught me to stand tall and never let anyone undermine me. My father, a retired firefighter, instilled in me a sense of discipline and the importance of integrity.

"My mother, a nurse with an iron will, showed me how to face challenges with grace. My brothers, taller, faster,and stronger, never went easy on me. They taught me how to box, wrestle and, most important, how to carry myself so people would think twice before trying anything. That foundation carried me through my life, especially in the Army, where challenges came thick and fast.

"In my early years at Fort X, I quickly realized that respect wouldn't be given—it had to be earned. I was young, ambitious and determined not to be seen as anything less than capable. There were moments when men underestimated me or, worse, crossed boundaries they should have known better than to approach. But I wasn't one to let things slide.

"If someone made an inappropriate comment, I shut it down. If anyone tried to intimidate me, they were met with a forcefulness they hadn't anticipated. I remember one incident vividly—a superior officer who thought his rank gave him the right to cross the line. Let's just say, after a private conversation, he never tried it again, and word spread quickly that I wasn't someone to mess with. Shortly after, younger enlisted subordinates would come to me for assistance, and I was honored to guide them and, in some cases, protect them from bullies in our own Army.

"After a few years, the tide turned. My competence, combined with my refusal to tolerate nonsense, earned me respect across the board. People came to admire my work ethic and the results I delivered. Running supply for an entire post isn't glamorous, but it's vital. I ensured that every soldier had what they needed, when they needed it. Equipment, food, fuel, uniforms—everything passed through my hands. It was a high-pressure job, and the weight of responsibility was constant. But I thrived on the challenge, especially during the very difficult years overseas in war zones.

"Still, the stress took its toll. I kept a rigorous exercise routine—running, weightlifting and yoga— which kept me grounded and healthy. It was my sanctuary, a space where I could process the day's challenges and steel myself for the next. Even so, years of unrelenting pressure left their mark.

"Nightmares crept in, flashbacks to intense moments where everything had to be perfect, or the mission would fail. I found myself waking in the middle of the night, heart pounding, drenched in sweat.

"When I retired at 45, I was at a crossroads. On paper, I was successful. I had an MBA, was offered seats on several corporate boards, and had the admiration of my peers. But inside, I felt hollow, frayed. My husband, a kind and patient man who understood me better than anyone, encouraged me to seek help. I resisted at first—after all, I'd handled everything else on my own. But deep down, I knew I needed it.

"Counseling was my first step. Talking through the years of stress, the weight of responsibility, and the silent burdens I carried helped me make sense of my feelings. But the real breakthrough came with Dr. Eugene Lipov and his PTSX-killing tool, stellate ganglion block. I'd heard about it from a fellow veteran and decided to try it. The results were nothing short of miraculous. The anxiety, the flashbacks, the sleepless nights, the constant low-grade buzz of anxiety in my head—they melted away. For the first time in years, I felt free.

"Today, at 47, I'm thriving. I sit on the boards of several leading supply-chain companies, bringing my military expertise to the civilian world. I mentor young women, especially those in male-dominated industries, teaching them how to navigate challenges with confidence and strength.

Most important, I spend time with my family—my husband, my two daughters, and my extended family of nieces and nephews. Life is full and rich. My story isn't one of invincibility—it's one of resilience. I didn't escape challenges or pain, but I faced them head-on. If I can leave you with one piece of advice, it's this: strength isn't just about enduring it is also about knowing when to seek help and allowing yourself to heal.

I owe much of it to Dr. Lipov and his team of brilliant nurses and techs at Stella Center in Oak Park, Illinois, outside Chicago. While ketamine therapy helped me understand my stressors, it was really Dr. Lipov and his therapy that took away those stressors. My only regret, if I have any at all, is that I didn't see him sooner."

—Sergeant Major Olivia G., US Army (ret.)

6

PTSX and Intersectionality: Addressing Cultural, Gender and Racial Disparities

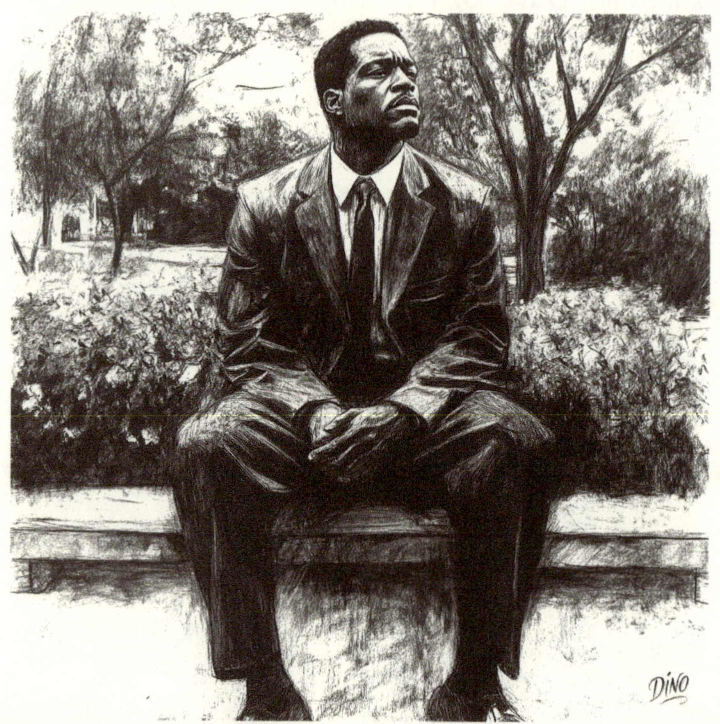

William sat alone on the worn bench in the park, his back rigid, his eyes scanning the horizon with practiced vigilance. It was instinct now, a habit formed in warzones where every shadow could conceal a threat. But here, in the quiet of his own neighborhood, it only made the silence heavier.

He had fought for his country, carried brothers off battlefields, and endured hellish nights of combat. Yet this—this invisible war inside his mind—felt insurmountable. The Army had taught him resilience, but not how to process the ghosts that haunted him.

Growing up, William had learned that vulnerability was weakness. In his community, men didn't cry. They shouldered their burdens in silence. When he left the service, the stigma of weakness followed him, wrapping around his throat like a noose. Therapy? That wasn't for men like him. He kept pushing through, anger simmering just beneath the surface, erupting when he least expected it.

It wasn't until William met another veteran, a guy who'd served in the same endless sands, that something shifted. "You're not alone," the man had said, handing William a flyer for a support group for veterans of color. William hesitated for weeks, but one night, when the walls of his apartment felt too close and the memories too loud, he went.

In that room, he found men and women who looked like him, spoke like him, understood him. They talked about PTSX, about stigma, about the quiet strength in seeking help. It wasn't easy, not at first. But as William shared his story, the weight began to lift. He found a culturally competent therapist through the group, someone who respected his experiences and his identity. Slowly, the fog began to clear.

This chapter explores how intersectionality, or the interconnected nature of social categorizations like race, gender and sexual orientation, influences the experience of PTSX. It delves into the critical need for culturally sensitive care, showing how tailored support can transform the lives of veterans like William, ensuring no one is left to fight their battles alone. By understanding these nuances, we can create a more inclusive approach to care that honors the diverse identities of those who serve.

For many veterans, the transition from military to civilian life is fraught with challenges, especially for those living with PTSX. While all who serve face unique struggles, the experience of PTSX is not universal.

This chapter acknowledges that veterans from diverse racial, ethnic, gender and sexual identity backgrounds often encounter additional hurdles, shaped by systemic inequities, cultural stigmas and underrepresentation in mental health care. Here we address these disparities as a crucial step toward effective and compassionate treatment for all.

Understanding Intersectionality in PTSX

Intersectionality is a framework that examines how overlapping identities interact with systems of power and oppression. For veterans, these identities might include race, ethnicity, gender, sexual orientation, socioeconomic status, and religious beliefs. When it comes to PTSX, these intersecting identities can shape a number of important factors:

How trauma is experienced and processed: Cultural and societal norms influence how individuals understand and cope with trauma.

Barriers to seeking help: Stigma, mistrust of institutions, and lack of culturally competent care deter many from accessing treatment.

Outcomes of care: Veterans who do seek help often face disparities in the quality and effectiveness of treatment due to systemic inequities.

By recognizing these intersections, we can better understand the unique challenges faced by diverse groups and tailor support to meet their specific needs.

"You're not alone," Marcus heard, and in a room of veterans of color he felt the weight lift. Shared stories melted silence. Culturally competent therapy turned weakness into strategic retreat.

Challenges Faced by Diverse Groups

Racial and Ethnic Minorities

Veterans from racial and ethnic minority groups often face additional layers of trauma rooted in systemic racism and discrimination. These experiences can compound the effects of military-related trauma, leading to higher rates of PTSX and other mental health conditions.

Stigma and Cultural Expectations: In some cultures, discussing mental health is taboo, leading veterans to internalize their struggles rather than seeking help.

Historic Mistrust: Marginalized communities may distrust healthcare institutions due to historical mistreatment, much like with the Tuskegee syphilis study. Lasting mistrust of medical institutions persists, rooted in abuses like Tuskegee. Such history fuels skepticism, lowers participation in clinical care and research, and continues to shape how marginalized communities view healthcare systems today.

Underrepresentation: Mental healthcare professionals often lack cultural competence, making it difficult for minority veterans to feel understood and supported.

LGBTQ+ Veterans

LGBTQ+ veterans face unique stressors, including discrimination and a history of exclusion within the military. These challenges can exacerbate PTSX symptoms and create barriers to care.

Military Policy and Trauma: Policies like "Don't Ask, Don't Tell" forced many to hide their identities, adding layers of stress and shame to their military experience.

Fear of Discrimination: Many LGBTQ+ veterans fear judgment or rejection from healthcare providers, leading to delays in seeking treatment.

Higher Rates of Mental Health Issues: Studies show that LGBTQ+ veterans experience higher rates of depression, anxiety, and suicidal ideation compared to their heterosexual and cisgender peers.

Disparities in Access to Care

Disparities in mental healthcare access and outcomes are pervasive, and they disproportionately affect marginalized veterans. Key barriers include:

Geographic Inequities: Veterans in rural areas, particularly those from Native American communities, often lack access to nearby mental health services.

Financial Barriers: Socioeconomic disparities can prevent veterans from affording out-of-pocket costs for care not covered by the VA.

Lack of Representation: The mental health workforce lacks diversity, making it difficult for veterans to find providers who understand their cultural or lived experiences. And with the elimination of protections for diversity and inclusivity, more than ever we must demand support from those in power.

Implicit Bias: Even well-intentioned providers hold unconscious biases that affect how they diagnose and treat veterans from diverse ethnic and cultural backgrounds. At a superconscious level (the current term, subconscious, is inaccurate), people have hidden demons that often obscure what we see on the surface, their veneer.

Briefly, the dated term subconscious was developed in the early 1700s and then brought into the mainstream in the late 1800s. We now know that the "subconscious" is actually a much more intricate and powerful entity within us, so we choose the term *superconscious* to better describe this often elusive entity within ourselves.

Creating Inclusive and Equitable Care Models

To address these disparities, we must develop care models that prioritize inclusion, equity, and cultural competence. Here are key strategies:

Train Providers in Cultural Competence: Ensure that mental-health professionals understand the unique experiences of diverse veterans. Training should include implicit bias recognition, culturally specific communication and an understanding of intersectionality.

Expand Representation in the Workforce: Recruit and support mental health professionals from diverse backgrounds to reflect the populations they serve.

Tailor Outreach Efforts: Design outreach campaigns that address cultural stigmas around mental health and highlight stories of resilience from veterans within marginalized communities.

Improve Accessibility: Increase telehealth options, mobile clinics, and community-based programs to reach veterans in underserved areas.

Build Peer-Support Networks: Peer-led programs can provide culturally relevant support and create safe spaces for veterans to share their experiences.

Brad's Story

Brad, a Black Army veteran, avoided seeking mental health care for years due to cultural stigma and distrust of the VA system. Growing up, Brad had internalized the belief that discussing mental health struggles was a sign of weakness. His military service compounded these feelings, as he was taught to "push through" and suppress emotions.

After his transition to civilian life, Brad found himself grappling with flashbacks, insomnia and overwhelming anger. Despite these challenges, he resisted seeking help, fearing judgment from his community and skeptical about receiving adequate care from the VA. Everything changed when Brad met a fellow veteran who encouraged him to attend a peer support group tailored for veterans of color. Initially hesitant, Brad decided to give it a try. In this group, he found a safe space where he could share his experiences without fear of judgment. Hearing others' stories of resilience helped him feel less alone, and he began to see therapy not as a weakness but as a strength.

Through the group's encouragement, Brad sought out a culturally competent therapist who understood the unique challenges faced by Black veterans. With consistent support and therapy, Brad began to heal, eventually becoming an advocate for mental health in his community. Today, Brad works to reduce stigma around mental health and mentors younger veterans, ensuring they know they're not alone.

Elena's Story

Elena served in the US Navy during the "Don't Ask, Don't Tell" era, a policy that forced her to conceal her identity as a lesbian. The constant stress of hiding who she was added a layer of trauma to her military experience. Elena feared that being outed would jeopardize her career, so she distanced herself from others, avoiding close relationships and suppressing her true self.

This isolation took a toll on her mental health, leaving her feeling disconnected and deeply lonely. After her service ended, Elena's PTSX symptoms, including nightmares and hypervigilance, worsened. The shame and fear she had carried for years made it difficult for her to trust others, let alone seek professional help.

Eventually, Elena discovered an LGBTQ+-focused veterans group through a local organization. For the first time, she met other veterans who had faced similar challenges and who understood her pain. This connection gave her the courage to seek therapy with a counselor specializing in LGBTQ+ issues.

Her therapist provided a nonjudgmental space where Elena could process her trauma and begin to rebuild her sense of self-worth. Through therapy and the support of her newfound community, Elena found healing and a renewed sense of purpose. She now speaks publicly about her experiences, advocating for inclusive policies and resources for LGBTQ+ veterans.

Asha's Story

Asha, a first-generation immigrant from India and an Air Force veteran, struggled to reconcile her cultural upbringing with the Western approach to mental health care. In her community, mental health issues were often stigmatized, and seeking therapy was seen as a last resort.

After her deployment, Asha experienced intense anxiety and intrusive memories but felt unable to share her struggles with her family, who encouraged her to "be strong" and focus on her responsibilities.

Traditional therapy sessions felt impersonal and disconnected from her values, making her hesitant to continue.

A turning point came when Asha found a therapist who was not only culturally competent but also willing to integrate elements of her heritage into the healing process. This therapist encouraged Asha to incorporate mindfulness practices rooted in her cultural traditions, such as yoga and meditation, alongside evidence-based treatments like cognitive-behavioral therapy (CBT).

They also explored storytelling as a therapeutic tool, allowing Asha to frame her experiences within the context of her cultural values. This approach created a deep sense of trust and collaboration. Over time, Asha began to feel more comfortable discussing her trauma and found strength in blending her cultural identity with her recovery journey. Today, she shares her story to inspire other immigrant veterans to seek care tailored to their unique experiences.

Moving Forward: A Call to Action

Addressing intersectionality in PTSX care requires systemic change and individual commitment.

Advocate for Policy Changes: Push for policies that increase funding for culturally competent mental health programs and expand access to care for underserved populations.

Promote Education and Awareness: Actively encourage discussions about intersectionality in mental health to reduce stigma and encourage understanding.

Listen to Diverse Voices: Create platforms for veterans from marginalized communities to share their stories and shape the future of PTSX care.

Collaborate Across Sectors: Partner with community organizations, faith-based groups, and cultural institutions to provide holistic support.

Intersectionality reminds us that every veteran's experience with PTSX is shaped by their unique identities and circumstances. By acknowledging and addressing the challenges faced by diverse groups, we can create a more inclusive, equitable, and effective approach to care. Veterans from all backgrounds deserve to feel seen, heard, and supported on their journey to healing. Together, we can build a system that honors the service of every individual and leaves no one behind.

If-Then Guidance

- If you feel misunderstood by your current therapist, then seek a provider with cultural competence. Look for someone who is trained to understand and respect your unique background and experiences, as this will build a stronger therapeutic alliance. Don't hesitate to ask potential therapists about their training and experience working with veterans who share your cultural or personal identity.
- If stigma within your community prevents you from seeking help, then connect with a peer support group. Share your experiences with others who have faced similar challenges can reduce isolation and build confidence in pursuing professional care. Peer groups also offer a space where cultural norms and experiences

are understood, helping to normalize discussions around mental health.

- If you are an LGBTQ+ veteran hesitant about therapy, then seek out LGBTQ+-affirming mental health resources. These spaces provide a safe and welcoming environment where your identity will be respected and celebrated. Affirming providers are trained to address the unique challenges LGBTQ+ veterans face, making it easier to open up and engage in healing.
- If language or cultural differences make traditional therapy feel inaccessible, then explore culturally adapted approaches. Therapists who integrate cultural traditions, such as storytelling or mindfulness, can make treatment feel more relevant and effective. These approaches honor your identity and ensure that therapy aligns with your personal values.
- If financial barriers are preventing you from accessing care, then research VA benefits, telehealth options or community-based programs. Many organizations offer free or low-cost services specifically for veterans. Financial aid programs and sliding-scale fees are also available through some mental health providers.
- If systemic inequities have caused you to mistrust healthcare institutions, then consider working with veteran-led organizations. These groups are often more attuned to the specific needs and concerns of diverse veterans. They can act as bridges, helping you find resources and care providers you can trust.
- If you live in a rural area without nearby mental health services, then explore telehealth options. Virtual therapy can connect you with specialists who understand your unique needs, regardless of location.
- Many telehealth platforms also provide access to culturally competent providers who might not be available locally.
- If you are unsure where to start, then reach out to a veteran advocacy organization. These groups can help you navigate available resources and find the support that aligns with your identity and values. They often offer tailored services and can connect you with peer mentors for guidance.

Take the Next Step

- Reflect on Your Journey: Take time to reflect on your unique experiences and the challenges you've faced. Acknowledging your story is an important first step in the healing process. Whether it's the trauma of combat, systemic barriers, or personal struggles, recognizing what you've endured can help you move forward.
- Seek Support from Trusted Resources: If you're struggling, don't hesitate to reach out to organizations that specialize in veteran care. Groups like the VA, peer support networks or community organizations can connect you with professionals who understand your needs. Support is not a sign of weakness; it's a path to strength.
- Explore Inclusive-Care Options: Look for therapists and programs that emphasize cultural competence and inclusivity. Finding care tailored to your background and identity can make a significant difference in your recovery journey. Your voice and experience matter—choose providers who honor them.
- Connect with Your Community: Surround yourself with individuals who understand and respect your journey. Whether through veteran-focused groups, cultural organizations or faith communities, finding connection will combat isolation and build healing, thus encouraging you to do more.
- Focus on Small, Positive Changes: Healing doesn't happen overnight. Start with manageable goals, like establishing a consistent routine, practicing mindfulness, or seeking therapy. Each small step builds resilience and brings you closer to recovery.
- Celebrate Your Resilience: Take pride in your strength and perseverance. Every step you take toward healing is a testament to your courage. Reflect on your accomplishments and remind yourself that your journey matters.
- Pay It Forward: Consider sharing your experiences to inspire others. Whether mentoring fellow veterans, volunteering, or simply being a source of support, your story can make a profound difference in someone else's life.
- Advocate for Change: Use your voice to advocate for more

inclusive and equitable systems of care. By raising awareness and challenging inequities, you can contribute to a better future for all veterans.

Through Their Eyes

"I don't think I ever set out to be a hero. Not even as a boy who played 'war' with brothers and friends. I was always looking after everyone else. So, to me, what I did on that day in Iraq was simply part of being a Marine. My name is Staff Sergeant Ronald J., and for ten years, I served in the United States Marine Corps as a squad leader. I am a Black and Puerto Rican man—a large man, I suppose, standing at 6'3" and weighing 225 pounds. I share this because it's part of who I am and part of the reason I was able to carry my fellow Marines when they needed me most. But my story is not about my size or my strength. It's about perseverance, pain and, ultimately, purpose.

"My time in the Corps was marked by a constant tension. On one hand, I was committed to my men, my mission and the values of the Marine Corps. On the other hand, I often felt like an outsider. Some of my fellow Marines saw my ethnicity before they saw my rank or my loyalty. I endured slurs, whispers and outright dismissals. When I needed help or support, it often wasn't there. Yet, when they needed me, I was always ready to serve. It wasn't about them. It was about the oath I took and the brotherhood I believed in, regardless of how they saw and treated me. My mother used to tell us kids: 'Be better than the bullies.'

"That day in Iraq is seared into my memory. We were ambushed while on patrol, pinned down by heavy enemy fire. The chaos was deafening—gunfire, explosions and the shouts and screams of my men. I saw fear in their eyes, but I remained calm. It's strange how clear everything becomes in moments like that. I remember yelling orders, assessing the situation, and making a plan to get my men out of there alive. No one else stepped up, so I did. That's what leadership means to me—not rank or authority, but responsibility in the face of extreme life-death danger.

"I was the first to move. I spotted a young Marine, barely 20, frozen in place. He was one of the ones who never had a kind word for me, but in that moment, none of that mattered. I grabbed him, threw him over my shoulder, and ran through enemy fire to cover. The weight didn't bother me—adrenaline has a way of numbing pain—but the bullets whizzing past did concern me. When I got him to safety, I turned back. There were six more out there, and I wasn't leaving anyone behind.

"I carried each of them, one by one. Some were unconscious, others screaming in pain. I was hit three times—once in the leg, once in the arm, and once in the back. The pain was sharp, but I didn't stop. I couldn't stop. Marines look out for each other, even when they don't act like it.

By the end of it, I was covered in blood—some mine, some theirs—and barely able to stand. But every single one of my men was alive. When we finally made it back to base, the medics patched me up.

"I remember sitting there, exhausted and in pain, when my commanding officer came in. He told me I'd been recommended for the Navy Cross, one of the highest honors a Marine can receive. But weeks later, I found out it had been downgraded to a Silver Star. No one said it outright, but I knew why. My ethnicity had always been a barrier, even in moments when it shouldn't have mattered.

"I wish I could say that recognition didn't mean anything to me, but it did. I didn't need a medal, but I wanted my men to see that what I did mattered. Instead, many of them returned to treating me the same way they always had—cold, dismissive, indifferent.

"After I left the Corps, I struggled. The memories of Iraq haunted me, not just that firefight but the years of being treated like less than I was. I turned to alcohol to numb the pain and, for a while, it worked.

But it wasn't sustainable. I was spiraling and I knew it. The turning point came when I met a VA nurse named Taneeka. She didn't just see me as another patient. She saw me as a person. She listened without judgment and helped me find the resources I needed. For the first time, I felt like someone cared.

"Taneeka connected me with a therapist who specialized in veterans of color, especially mixed race. That therapist changed my life. He helped me process my trauma, not just from Iraq but from the years of racism and mistreatment I had endured. He also encouraged me to find a purpose beyond the pain. That's when I decided to go to medical school.

"Becoming a trauma physician wasn't easy. I had to relearn how to focus, how to study, how to believe in myself. But every step of the way, I remembered the men I carried off that battlefield. I thought about their families and how much it meant to them that their sons, brothers and fathers came home. That kept me going.

"Today, I work in an ER, where I see people on the worst days of their lives. I do my best to bring them hope, to show them compassion, and to let them know they're not alone. My journey has taught me that pain and purpose can coexist. It's not about erasing the scars but finding a way to live with them and use them to help others.

"I still think about Iraq, about the men I saved and the ones who never thanked me. But I've let go of the anger. It doesn't serve me anymore. What serves me is knowing that, despite everything, I did what I set out to do—I lived up to the values of the Marine Corps. And I've found peace in that."

—Staff Sergeant Ron, MD, US Marine Corps Veteran

7

PTSX in Female Military Personnel and Veterans: Unique Challenges and Approaches

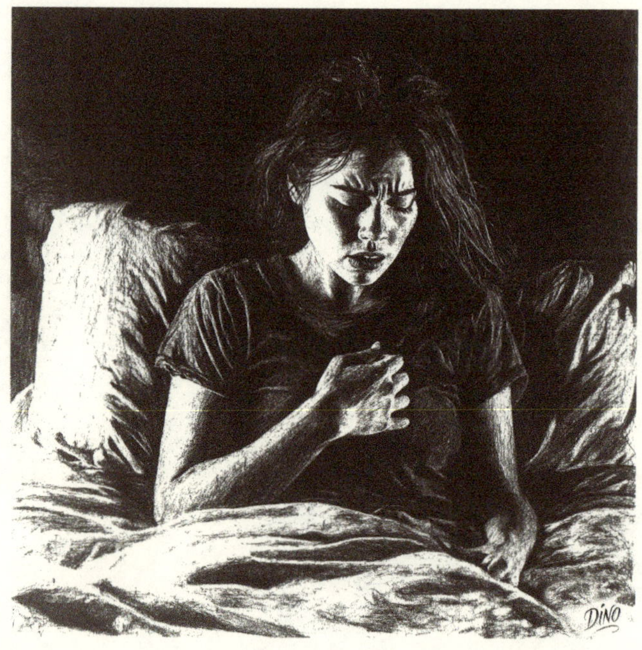

Monica stared at the rows of decorations, medals and commendations she'd earned during her time in the Army, including a Distinguished Flying Cross and a Bronze Star with V device for valor. Even with those accolades, the memories that kept her awake at night weren't tied to combat.

They circled back to an assault from someone who should have had her back. She'd tried to push past it—focusing on her duties, staying busy, never letting her guard down. Yet sleepless nights and bursts of anger became her new normal. Eventually, a family friend nudged her to seek help at a nearby veterans' clinic. She expected the same old routine: sign in, wait, maybe get medication.

Instead, a counselor sat her down and asked about things no one else had—her sense of safety, her support system, the dual struggles of balancing service obligations and family life. It felt odd at first, talking about experiences that were deeply personal, but Monica felt seen, not judged.

She discovered that other women veterans there had similar stories. Some grappled with combat stress, some with Military Sexual Trauma, and many had navigated both. Through group sessions, they shared how specialized therapy and holistic practices—like yoga and art—helped them reconnect with themselves. Monica took a hesitant step into these activities, and to her surprise, she found genuine relief.

Today, she's part of a peer-support circle. She helps women who arrive with the same haunted look she once wore, reminding them that healing is possible—even after betrayal, fear or isolation. This chapter shines a light on the unique challenges women like Monica face in uniform and after service, and how tailored strategies—from trauma-informed care to community support—can help them reclaim their lives.

This chapter shows that PTSX is a significant health concern affecting countless military personnel and veterans. And while PTSX has been extensively studied in male servicemembers, there is a growing recognition of the unique challenges faced by female military personnel and veterans.

Women in the military encounter specific stressors that can contribute to the development of PTSX, including higher rates of Military Sexual Trauma (MST), gender-specific combat experiences, and the need for tailored treatment approaches. We explore these unique issues, emphasizing the importance of understanding and addressing the distinct needs of female servicemembers and veterans with compassion and respect.

When you watch the Amazon Prime film *Quiet Explosions,* you will meet a young former Navy Midshipman who was twice raped at the Naval Academy. Her story will bring on the tears, not to mention anger and shock at how the Annapolis brass handled her cases. She was treated by Dr. Mark Gordon, whose therapy healed this courageous woman.

The Increasing Role of Women in the Military

Over the past few decades, women have become an integral part of military forces worldwide. In the United States, women now constitute approximately 17% of the active-duty military and are the fastest-growing group within the veteran population. They serve in various roles, from combat positions to leadership roles, breaking barriers and challenging traditional military norms.

> Accurate diagnosis is less detective work than deep listening: map trauma history, run molecular panels, then connect the dots before prescribing—because fragmented care never heals an integrated wound.

The inclusion of women in all aspects of military service has led to their increased exposure to combat-related stressors and traumatic events. As women take on roles traditionally held by men, they face the same risks of combat exposure, injury and psychological trauma. However, they also confront additional challenges unique to their gender, which can impact their mental health and wellbeing.

Military Sexual Trauma (MST)

One of the most significant factors contributing to PTSX among female servicemembers is MST. It's defined by the VA as sexual assault or repeated, threatening sexual harassment that a veteran experienced during military service.

Unfortunately, MST is a pervasive issue that disproportionately affects women in the military, at the service academies and also within college and university ROTC units. Survivors often describe MST as uniquely damaging because it occurs in an environment where cohesion, loyalty, and trust are supposed to be absolute. When betrayal happens inside the ranks, it undermines the very foundation of safety and belonging on which military culture is built.

Prevalence of MST Among Female Servicemembers

Studies have shown that approximately one in four female veterans report experiencing MST during their service. This rate is significantly higher than that of their male counterparts. The actual prevalence is even higher due to underreporting caused by stigma, fear of retaliation or lack of trust in the reporting process.

The US military is struggling to be a satisfactory protector and supporter of females within its ranks, so it not surprising that most women don't trust their chain of command. Retaliation—ranging from career sabotage to social isolation—is frequently cited by survivors, and the lack of consistent accountability within military justice systems reinforces silence.

This dynamic not only perpetuates trauma but also diminishes morale, weakens readiness, and contributes to long-term health disparities among women who continue to serve or have served.

Impact of MST on Mental Health

MST can have profound and long-lasting effects on a woman's mental health. Survivors of MST are at a higher risk of developing PTSX compared to those who have experienced other types of trauma. The trauma of sexual assault or harassment by fellow servicemembers can lead to feelings of betrayal, loss of trust and isolation.

Over the past several years, some encounters saw males murdering female servicemembers. Not an encouraging thought when you're a female servicemember in need of help. In addition to PTSX, MST survivors may experience depression, anxiety, substance abuse and difficulties with interpersonal relationships. The trauma can disrupt their sense of safety and belonging within the military community, exacerbating feelings of vulnerability and distress.

Barriers to Reporting and Seeking Help

Many women do not report incidents of MST due to various barriers, including:

Fear of Retaliation: Concerns about negative repercussions on their careers or personal safety.

Stigma and Shame: Internalized feelings of guilt or shame associated with the trauma.

Lack of Trust in the System: Doubts about the effectiveness of reporting mechanisms and support services.

Cultural Norms: A military culture that discourages reporting or minimizing the severity of sexual harassment and assault. In some units, it even encourages sexual assault.

These barriers often prevent women from accessing the support and treatment they need, leading to even worse outcomes.

Gender-Specific Stressors in the Military

Beyond MST, female service-members face additional gender-specific stressors that contribute to the development of PTSX.

Combat Exposure and Role Challenges

With the lifting of the ban on women in combat roles, female servicemembers are increasingly exposed to direct combat situations. While female combat participation represents a significant advancement in gender equality, it also means that women are now facing the same intense combat stressors as men, often without the same level of preparation or support. Women may also experience challenges related to:

Proving Themselves: Feeling the need to demonstrate their capabilities in a male-dominated environment.

Isolation: Being one of the few women in a unit can lead to feelings of isolation or exclusion.

Lack of Role Models: The scarcity of female leaders can impact mentorship opportunities and career development.

Balancing Military and Family Responsibilities

Many female servicemembers juggle the dual responsibilities of military service and family care. The demands of deployment, training and relocation can create significant stress for women who are mothers or primary caregivers. The strain of separation from children and managing family obligations can exacerbate stress and contribute to mental-health issues.

Gender-Based Discrimination and Harassment

Gender-based discrimination and harassment remain challenges within the military. Experiences of sexism, unequal treatment and harassment undermine a woman's confidence and sense of belonging. Such negative experiences compound the stress of military service and contribute to the development of PTSX.

Worse still is when a trusted commander abuses their authority and tries to undermine a woman's call for help. Those commanders have the unique authority to access a person's healthcare records and use any results against that servicemember, if they so choose.

Examples include removing or restricting them from duty, punishing them administratively or, worst of all, having them discharged from the military with a dishonorable discharge or less than honorable discharge, thus ruining the reputation of a good person who served their country.

The Need for Tailored Treatment Approaches

Given the unique challenges faced by female servicemembers and veterans, it is essential to develop and implement treatment approaches that address their specific needs.

Trauma-Informed Care

Trauma-informed care involves understanding, recognizing and responding to the effects of all types of trauma. For female veterans, this means:

<u>Creating a Safe Environment</u>: Ensuring that treatment settings are welcoming and free from potential triggers.

<u>Empowering Patients</u>: Involving women in their treatment planning

and respecting their choices. We also must encourage women to learn how to speak up respectfully yet firmly.

List Cultural Sensitivity: Acknowledging the impact of gender, culture and personal history on their experiences and needs.

Empowering Women: Involving women in their treatment planning and respecting their choices.

Evidence-Based Therapies

Several therapeutic approaches have proven effective in treating PTSX in female veterans. These therapies can be adapted to address issues specific to MST and gender-related stressors:

Cognitive Processing Therapy: Helps patients challenge and modify unhelpful beliefs related to the trauma.

Prolonged Exposure Therapy: Involves repeated, detailed imagining of the trauma to reduce the power of traumatic memories. It's called "habituation" and it works by having your mind and body get "bored" or accustomed to reliving the traumatic event. So much so that the trauma is lessened.

Eye Movement Desensitization and Reprocessing: Uses bilateral stimulation to process and integrate traumatic memories.

Written Exposure Therapy (WET): A brief, evidence-based intervention designed to help individuals process distressing memories associated with posttraumatic stress. Typically delivered over five sessions, WET involves writing about the traumatic event(s) in a structured, repeated manner. This therapeutic approach aims to reduce avoidance, encourage emotional processing, and create a sense of self-efficacy.

Research shows that WET can be as effective as more intensive treatments, with lower dropout rates. It is time-efficient, cost-effective and accessible, making it suitable for a variety of clinical settings.

By systematically confronting traumatic narratives, WET facilitates understanding, reframes negative cognitions, and promotes posttraumatic growth in many individuals.

Integrating Holistic and Alternative Therapies

Holistic approaches can complement traditional therapies and address the mind-body-spirit connection:

Mindfulness and Meditation: Practices that promote relaxation and present-moment awareness can reduce anxiety and improve emotional regulation.

Yoga and Physical Activity: Can help reconnect women with their bodies and promote physical wellbeing.

Art and Music Therapy: Provide creative outlets for expression and processing of emotions. These activities create a sense of connection and grounding.

Support Groups and Peer Support

Connecting with other female veterans can provide validation, reduce feelings of isolation, create a sense of community, and realign one's values. Support groups offer a safe space to share experiences and coping strategies. They also share legal aspects of their case and, in solidarity, can seek legal assistance without the fear of command retribution.

Addressing Co-occurring Conditions

Many female veterans with PTSX also experience other mental-health conditions like depression, anxiety or substance-use disorders. Integrated treatment plans that address all co-occurring conditions are essential for comprehensive care.

Systemic Changes and Advocacy

Addressing the unique challenges faced by female servicemembers requires systemic changes within the military and society at large.

Improving the processes for reporting MST is critical: Confidential Reporting Options: Providing safe and confidential avenues for reporting incidents.

Protecting Against Retaliation: Implementing strict policies to prevent retaliation against those who report MST.

Accountability: Holding perpetrators accountable to create a culture of zero tolerance for sexual harassment and assault. More people must step up and deal with these perpetrators, or they will continue harming others.

Promoting Gender Equality and Inclusion

Efforts to promote gender equality within the military can help reduce gender-specific stressors:

Leadership Opportunities: Encouraging and supporting women in leadership roles.

Education and Training: Implementing training programs that address bias and promote respectful interactions.

Policy Reforms: Updating policies to reflect the needs and contributions of female servicemembers.

Improving Access to Gender-Specific Care

Ensuring that female veterans have access to care that addresses their unique needs is essential:

Specialized Clinics: Establishing clinics focused on women's health and mental health issues.

Training Providers: Educating healthcare professionals on the specific challenges faced by female veterans.

Telehealth Services: Expanding telehealth options to reach women who have difficulty accessing care due to geographic or logistical barriers.

The Importance of Family and Community Support

Family members and communities play a vital role in supporting female veterans with PTSX. Providing education about PTSX and MST can help families understand what their loved one is experiencing and how best to support them.

Encouraging open communication and involving family members in the healing process can strengthen relationships and provide additional support. Community organizations and veterans' groups can offer resources, social connections and opportunities for engagement that promote healing and wellbeing.

In The End. . . .

Female military personnel and veterans face unique challenges that contribute to the development and persistence of PTSX. Higher rates of Military Sexual Trauma, gender-specific combat stressors, and systemic barriers highlight the need for tailored treatment approaches that are compassionate, respectful and effective. By acknowledging and addressing these unique challenges, we can improve outcomes for female servicemembers and veterans.

This requires a concerted effort to implement trauma-informed care, develop gender-specific treatment programs, promote systemic changes within the military, and provide comprehensive support networks.

As we continue to support women in the military, it's essential to recognize their contributions and ensure they receive the care and support they deserve. By creating an environment of inclusivity, compassion and empowerment, we honor the service of female veterans and contribute to a stronger, more resilient military community.

If-Then Guidance

- If you are a female servicemember or veteran experiencing PTSX, then it's important to recognize that your experiences and challenges may be unique due to factors like MST, combat exposure and gender-specific stressors.
- If you feel alone, then recognize these challenges. This is the first step toward healing. Seeking support from professionals who are trained to address the specific needs of female veterans can help you navigate these issues with compassion and respect.
- If you have experienced MST, then know that this can significantly impact your mental health and increase your risk of PTSX. MST can lead to feelings of betrayal, isolation and distrust within the military system.
- If you are hesitant to report incidents due to fear of retaliation or stigma, consider exploring confidential support options through veteran organizations or MST-specific resources. Reaching out for help is critical, and it's important to connect with trauma-informed care providers who understand the unique impact of MST on mental health. Allowing it to continue only prolongs the pain.
- If you are struggling with feelings of guilt or shame related to MST, then consider engaging with a therapist who specializes

in trauma-focused therapies like Cognitive Processing Therapy or Eye Movement Desensitization and Reprocessing. These evidence-based approaches can help you process the trauma, reframe negative beliefs about yourself, and reduce the emotional weight of the experiences. Reaching out to a mental-health professional can help you reclaim your sense of safety and self-worth.

- If you are hesitant to seek help because of barriers like stigma, isolation or lack of trust in the system, then try exploring peer-support groups specifically for female veterans. These groups provide a safe space to share experiences with others who have been through similar challenges. Hearing the stories of others can validate your feelings and reduce the sense of isolation. These support networks can also help you find practical solutions and emotional coping strategies, making it easier to seek professional care. They may also encourage you to see legal counsel, if necessary, to discuss a possible case against another servicemember.
- If you are facing gender-specific combat stressors, such as feeling the need to prove yourself or experiencing isolation in a male-dominated unit, then recognize that these pressures can exacerbate PTSX symptoms. It is essential to connect with mentors or counselors who understand these dynamics and can provide guidance in navigating them. Seeking mentorship from female leaders within or outside of the military can provide the support you need to overcome these challenges.
- If you are balancing military duties with family responsibilities, then consider reaching out for support that addresses both your military and caregiving roles. The stress of managing deployments, relocations, and family life can be overwhelming, particularly for mothers or primary caregivers. Family support programs or military family services may offer practical assistance, counseling, and stress-relief resources to help you cope with these dual demands and challenges.
- If you are experiencing gender-based discrimination or harassment in the military, then know that these experiences can undermine

your mental health and contribute to PTSX. Speaking with a trusted advocate like a military equal opportunity officer or a legal advisor can help you address these challenges. Seeking help from professionals trained in trauma-informed care can also provide the emotional support needed to process these experiences and move toward healing.

- If you feel that traditional treatment approaches do not fully address your needs, then consider exploring holistic and alternative therapies as part of your recovery plan. Practices like mindfulness meditation, yoga and art or music therapy can complement traditional PTSX treatments. They promote relaxation, reduce anxiety and create a sense of connection with your body and emotions. Incorporating these practices into your routine can provide additional tools to help you manage stress and regain a sense of control over your mental and physical wellbeing.
- If you are experiencing co-occurring mental health conditions like depression, anxiety or substance-use disorders, then seek integrated care that addresses all of your needs. Many female veterans with PTSX face additional mental-health challenges, and comprehensive treatment plans that target multiple issues simultaneously are essential for effective healing. Talk to your healthcare provider about developing a plan that addresses your mental health holistically, ensuring that all co-occurring conditions are treated in a coordinated and supportive manner.
- If you are reluctant to seek help due to the stigma surrounding MST or PTSX, then try connecting with resources that provide confidential or anonymous support. Many organizations offer MST-specific hotlines, virtual-support groups, and telehealth services that can help you receive care while maintaining privacy. Taking the first step toward help, even in a confidential setting, can make a significant difference in your healing process.
- If you feel isolated or disconnected from your family and community, then consider involving your loved ones in your healing process. Educating family members about PTSX, MST and the unique challenges faced by female veterans can help in

understanding and support. Encouraging open communication with your family can also help strengthen your relationships and provide a solid foundation of support during your recovery.

- If you have difficulty accessing care due to geographic or logistical barriers, then explore telehealth options that can bring professional mental-health support directly to you. Many healthcare providers now offer virtual therapy sessions, making it easier for all veterans to receive care regardless of their location. This can be especially beneficial for those who live in rural areas or have responsibilities that make in-person visits challenging.
- If you feel the military system has not provided adequate support, then consider advocating for systemic changes that address the needs of female servicemembers. Joining efforts to improve reporting mechanisms for MST, promote gender equality, and ensure accountability within the military can empower you and others. By advocating for change, you can contribute to a safer and more inclusive environment for future female servicemembers.
- If you are seeking support tailored to female veterans, then look for specialized clinics or programs that focus on women's health and mental-health issues. Many VA hospitals and veteran organizations now offer gender-specific care that addresses the unique experiences of female veterans, including MST and PTSX. These clinics often provide a range of services, including mental-health counseling, medical care, and support groups designed to meet your specific needs.
- If you are ready to begin your healing journey, then remember that recovery from PTSX is possible with the right support and treatment. Whether through trauma-informed care, evidence-based therapies or holistic approaches, you can find a path that works for you. Seek out compassionate healthcare providers who respect your experiences and involve you in your treatment planning.

Healing is not a one-size-fits-all process, and by exploring different treatment options, you can discover the approach that helps you reclaim your wellbeing and sense of purpose. By addressing the unique challenges faced by female servicemembers and veterans with PTSX, you can create a personalized, compassionate and effective plan for recovery.

Whether you focus on traditional therapies, alternative treatments, or a combination of both, healing is within your reach. The journey may be challenging, and with the right support, you can move toward a stronger, more empowering future.

Take the Next Step

- Acknowledge Unique Stressors: Recognize the unique challenges women in the military face, like MST. If this applies to you, consider seeking help through VA programs designed for women veterans.
- Seek Gender-Specific Support: Join a support group specifically for female veterans. These groups can provide a safe space to discuss experiences and coping strategies.
- Find a Female Veteran Mentor: Look for a peer mentor or advisor who has gone through similar experiences and can offer guidance and support.

Through Their Eyes

"When I joined the military, I knew it would be tough. I was ready for that. But I wasn't ready for the other battles—the ones I couldn't see coming. The ones where you feel you have to prove yourself just because you're a woman, the isolation of being the only female in your unit, and the way people look the other way when things go wrong. And then there was the sexual trauma—something I never thought I'd have to deal with, but I did. It shattered me in ways I still have a hard time explaining.

"At first, I didn't say anything. I was afraid of how it might affect my career, afraid no one would believe me. Even after I left the service, it haunted me. I didn't want to face it. But eventually, the nightmares and anxiety were too much, and I knew I needed help.

"Finding a support group for female veterans was the first real breakthrough for me. Hearing the stories of other women who had gone through similar things—it made me feel like I wasn't alone anymore. I started therapy that focused on my trauma, and for the first time, I began to process what had happened. It wasn't easy, but over time I learned to rebuild myself. Yoga and mindfulness helped me reconnect with my body, something I didn't even realize I had been disconnected from. Slowly, I began to feel like myself again—strong, capable and worthy.

"If there's one thing I can say to other women in the military or who've left it, it's this: don't wait to get help. It's out there. You're not alone, and you don't have to carry this on your own. There are people who understand what you've been through and who will stand by you as you heal."

—Lieutenant Sarah D., US Navy Veteran

8

Genetic Research and Epigenetics in PTSX

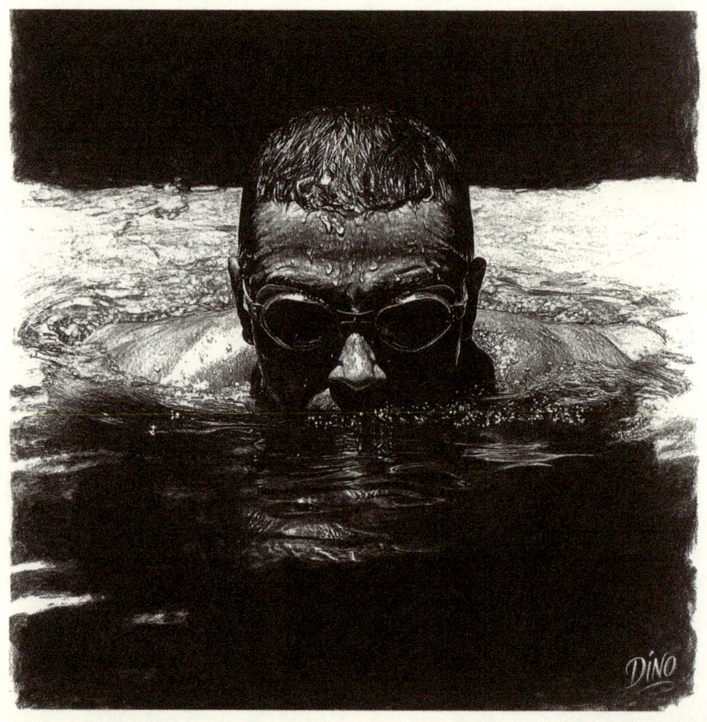

Stephen slid into the pool at 5 a.m., the water cold and invigorating against his skin. He adjusted his goggles, took a deep breath and pushed off the wall. The first few strokes always felt stiff, but by the time he reached the other end, his body had found its rhythm.

Back and forth, he swam, counting his laps. The water was his sanctuary, the one place where the noise in his head quieted. He wasn't the Navy man he once was—an underwater demolition specialist, built for endurance and precision. That life ended when the depression became too heavy to hide. Years later, a doctor had told him why. Genetic testing revealed he was predisposed to depression. No cure, they'd said. Just tools. Swim, they told him. Move. Talk. Try ketamine treatments. And stellate ganglion block—the injection into his neck that helped calm his nerves when everything felt too much.

Stephen swam harder, cutting through the water. He remembered the missions, the camaraderie, the pride he'd felt in the Navy. It was a life he missed, but the pool was where he found some of that purpose again.

The laps piled up, each one a little easier than the last. By the time he finished, his muscles burned, his chest heaved, but his mind was quiet. Stephen pulled himself out of the water and sat at the edge, letting the crisp air hit his damp skin.

He may not be able to change the way his brain was wired, but he could keep the darkness at bay. The work was never-ending, but he'd learned how to fight back—with discipline, sweat and sheer will.

Tomorrow, he'd be back at the pool, the water a welcome friend, waiting for him. Stephen smiled, just a little. He was still swimming.

This chapter delves into the interplay between inherited vulnerabilities and trauma-induced changes, highlighting the opportunities and challenges of leveraging these insights for healing and resilience. In understanding trauma, genetics and epigenetics hold immense promise for transforming PTSX care. Yes, it's technical. Consider it an invitation to up your genetics game.

The Genetic and Epigenetic Landscape of PTSX

PTSX is a deeply complex condition that profoundly affects individuals on psychological, emotional and physiological levels. While it is traditionally and incorrectly seen as a disorder of the non-physical mind, cutting-edge research in genetics and epigenetics reveals that PTSX has biological roots that interact dynamically with environmental factors.

This dual influence makes PTSX a unique condition, one that bridges inherited predispositions and the lasting biological imprints of traumatic events. Genetics provides insight into the inherent vulnerabilities that may predispose some individuals to PTSX. Certain genes influence the body's stress response systems like the HPA axis, and variations in these genes can make individuals more reactive to stress.

For example, the FKBP5 gene has been closely associated with the regulation of cortisol, a hormone critical for managing stress. When certain polymorphisms of this gene are present, the body may produce excessive cortisol in response to trauma, overwhelming the system and increasing the likelihood of developing PTSX.

> From shell fragments to micro-gliosis, modern imaging proves that the invisible is physical. Every flashback traces a pathway through inflamed cells and synapses that call for molecular study.

Epigenetics, on the other hand, explores how life experiences—particularly traumatic ones—can modify gene expression without altering the underlying DNA sequence. Trauma often leads to changes in DNA methylation, histone modification and other epigenetic markers, effectively "turning on" or "turning off" certain genes. These changes can disrupt critical systems involved in emotion regulation, memory processing and the immune response, contributing to the long-term symptoms of PTSX.

The implications of genetic and epigenetic research are far-reaching. These fields provide not only a deeper understanding of PTSX but also practical applications in early diagnosis, prevention and personalized therapies.

By identifying genetic markers and epigenetic changes, we can better predict who is most at risk, tailor treatments to individual needs, and even explore novel interventions like gene editing and epigenetic therapies.

Understanding Genetic Contributions to PTSX

Genetics plays a foundational role in shaping how individuals respond to trauma. While not everyone exposed to traumatic events develops PTSX, research with twins has demonstrated that genetic predisposition accounts for approximately 30-40% of the variance in risk. This means that certain inherited traits can significantly influence whether a person either develops PTSX or demonstrates resilience.

One of the most studied genes in PTSX research is FKBP5, which directly affects the HPA axis, the body's central stress-response system. Variants of FKBP5 are associated with dysregulation of cortisol, the hormone responsible for managing acute stress. People with high-risk FKBP5 variants may experience prolonged cortisol release, which can damage brain regions like the hippocampus over time, impairing memory and emotional regulation.

Another key genetic factor is the serotonin transporter gene (SLC6A4). Variations in this gene influence serotonin levels, which play a critical role in mood stability, fear processing and stress tolerance. The short variant of SLC6A4 has been linked to heightened sensitivity to stress and increased susceptibility to PTSX. Imaging studies show that individuals with this variant often exhibit hyperactivity in the amygdala, the brain's fear-processing center, making them more reactive to potential threats.

Dopaminergic genes, such as DRD2 and DRD4, are also under scrutiny. These genes influence dopamine signaling, which is crucial for motivation, reward processing, and emotional regulation. Variants that reduce dopamine receptor availability may contribute to the anhedonia (inability to feel pleasure) and emotional numbness often observed in PTSX.

Recent advancements in genome-wide association studies (GWAS) have identified additional genetic markers linked to PTSX, including genes involved in inflammation, neuroplasticity and synaptic function. These discoveries are expanding our understanding of how genetic vulnerabilities intersect with environmental triggers to shape PTSX risk. By identifying genetic markers, researchers aim to develop predictive tools that could identify individuals at higher risk for PTSX before any symptoms emerge. Such tools could enable targeted prevention strategies, such as stress inoculation training or early therapeutic interventions, tailored to an individual's genetic profile.

The Role of Epigenetics in Trauma and PTSX

While genetics provides a blueprint, epigenetics determines how that blueprint is executed in response to environmental influences. Epigenetic changes act as a biological memory of trauma, altering gene expression without changing the DNA sequence itself. These modifications can persist for years, contributing to the chronic nature of PTSX. One of the most well-documented epigenetic changes in PTSX involves the NR3C1 gene, which encodes the glucocorticoid receptor. This receptor regulates the HPA axis and the body's stress response.

Trauma-induced hypermethylation of NR3C1 reduces glucocorticoid receptor sensitivity, leading to dysregulated cortisol levels and prolonged stress responses. Studies in both humans and animal models have confirmed that this epigenetic change is strongly associated with PTSX symptoms, including hypervigilance, anxiety, and intrusive memories.

Histone modification is another critical epigenetic mechanism. Traumatic experiences can alter histone acetylation, affecting the accessibility of genes related to fear extinction and emotional regulation. For example, reduced acetylation in genes associated with memory consolidation may impair the ability to differentiate between past and present threats, perpetuating flashbacks and heightened arousal.

Non-coding RNAs, including microRNAs, are emerging as important regulators of gene expression in PTSX. These molecules influence post-transcriptional processes, modulating the production of proteins involved in neural plasticity and stress response. Dysregulated microRNA profiles have been observed in individuals with PTSX, disrupting pathways critical for resilience and recovery.

One fascinating aspect of epigenetics is its potential reversibility. Behavioral interventions like cognitive behavioral therapy (CBT) and mindfulness practices, have been shown to reverse trauma-induced epigenetic changes. Similarly, lifestyle factors like exercise and a healthy diet can influence epigenetic markers, providing a non-invasive means of mitigating PTSX symptoms. Epigenetics also offers a window into the intergenerational effects of trauma. Studies in survivors of historical traumas, such as those seen in WWI and WWII, show that trauma-induced epigenetic changes can be passed down to subsequent generations. Understanding these mechanisms is critical for breaking cycles of trauma and building resilience across families and communities.

Gene-Environment Interactions in PTSX

The interaction between genetics and environment is central to understanding PTSX. While genes lay the groundwork, environmental factors such as trauma exposure, social support and access to resources determine whether those genetic predispositions manifest as symptoms. This dynamic interplay—known as gene-environment interaction—helps explain why two individuals with similar genetic profiles may respond differently to the same traumatic event.

Take, for instance, the FKBP5 gene, which plays a critical role in regulating the HPA axis. Research shows that childhood trauma can amplify the effects of high-risk FKBP5 variants, increasing the likelihood of dysregulated stress responses and PTSX development. Conversely, individuals with the same genetic predisposition who experience nurturing, stable environments are less likely to exhibit these vulnerabilities.

The serotonin transporter gene (SLC6A4) provides another example. Studies reveal that individuals with the short variant of this gene are more likely to develop PTSX when exposed to severe trauma, such as combat or abuse. However, those who benefit from strong social support networks are less affected, as supportive environments can buffer against the gene's risk-enhancing effects.

Socioeconomic and cultural factors also shape these interactions. Chronic stressors like poverty, discrimination or lack of access to mental-health services can exacerbate genetic vulnerabilities. On the flip side, culturally relevant interventions and community support can mitigate risk, even in genetically predisposed individuals.

Understanding gene-environment interactions is crucial for designing preventative strategies. For example, programs that focus on building resilience, such as stress management workshops or peer support groups, may be especially effective for individuals with genetic risk factors. Similarly, early interventions in high-risk populations—such as trauma-informed care in schools—can disrupt the pathways leading to PTSX, ensuring that genetic predispositions do not become a determinant of outcomes.

Advances in Epigenetic and Genetic Research

Technological advancements have revolutionized genetic and epigenetic research, offering unprecedented insights into the biological underpinnings of PTSX. Genome-wide association studies (GWAS) have identified a multitude of genetic variants associated with trauma susceptibility, expanding our understanding of the pathways involved in stress regulation, neuroplasticity and inflammation.

Epigenome-wide association studies (EWAS) have mapped trauma-induced epigenetic changes across the genome. These studies have highlighted specific regions, such as the NR3C1 and BDNF genes, that are consistently altered in individuals with PTSX. These findings are helping to create a comprehensive picture of how trauma reshapes the epigenome, providing potential targets for therapeutic intervention.

The emergence of CRISPR-Cas9 technology has opened new frontiers in gene editing. While its application in PTSX research is still in its infancy, CRISPR offers the potential to correct genetic and epigenetic abnormalities at their source.

CRISPR-Cas9 enables precise modifications to DNA by cutting at targeted sites. This technology has shown transformative potential in treating genetic diseases and advancing neuroscience research. CRISPR is not yet used clinically for PTSX, but it is being explored in preclinical (mostly animal model) studies. Researchers are investigating how CRISPR can help:

- Modulate stress-response genes (e.g., FKBP5, NR3C1) known to influence trauma-related conditions.
- Study epigenetic modifications that may be reversible via CRISPR-based editing or interference systems (like CRISPR-dCas9 targeting histone modifiers or DNA methylation).

• Create more accurate animal models of PTSX to understand gene-environment interactions better.

CRISPR-Cas9 has opened new frontiers and holds theoretical potential for targeting PTSX-related genetic/epigenetic mechanisms. But its application is still experimental, primarily in laboratory settings.

Artificial intelligence (AI) and machine learning are transforming how researchers analyze complex genetic and epigenetic datasets. These tools can identify patterns and predict treatment outcomes, enabling a more personalized approach to PTSX care.

For instance, AI-driven algorithms can match patients to therapies based on their genetic and epigenetic profiles, optimizing treatment effectiveness. These advancements are paving the way for precision medicine in PTSX care. By integrating genetic and epigenetic insights with cutting-edge technologies, researchers and clinicians can develop targeted interventions that address the unique needs of each individual.

Potential Applications of Genetic and Epigenetic Knowledge

The practical applications of genetic and epigenetic research in PTSX are vast and transformative. One of the most promising areas is the development of biomarkers for early diagnosis.

Blood tests that detect trauma-related DNA methylation patterns could identify at-risk individuals before symptoms become debilitating. This proactive approach could enable earlier interventions, improving outcomes and reducing the societal burden of PTSX.

Gene-based therapies are another exciting avenue. Pharmacogenomics, which tailors medication to an individual's genetic profile, is already improving outcomes in mental health care and holds promise for PTSX. Individuals with specific serotonin transporter gene variants might benefit from personalized dosing of selective serotonin reuptake inhibitors (SSRIs). Similarly, epigenetic drugs targeting DNA methylation or histone modification are being explored as potential treatments.

Behavioral interventions informed by genetic and epigenetic research are gaining traction. Mindfulness-based stress reduction (MBSR), for instance, has been shown to reverse trauma-induced epigenetic changes in stress-related genes. Similarly, lifestyle modifications like exercise and dietary interventions can positively influence gene expression, providing a non-invasive complement to medical treatments.

By integrating these approaches, clinicians can offer a more personalized and effective care model, ensuring that treatments address both the biological and psychological aspects of PTSX.

Ethical and Social Implications

The promise of genetic and epigenetic research comes with ethical and social challenges that must be carefully navigated. Privacy is a significant concern, as genetic information is highly sensitive and vulnerable to misuse. Ensuring robust data protection measures and informed consent processes is essential to maintain trust and protect patient rights.

Stigmatization is another potential issue. Labeling individuals as genetically predisposed to PTSX could lead to discrimination, particularly in professions that prioritize mental resilience, e.g. the military and law enforcement. Public education campaigns will be vital to combat misconceptions and emphasize that genetic predispositions are not deterministic.

Equity is also a critical consideration. Access to genetic testing and gene-based therapies must be ensured for all populations, regardless of socioeconomic status. This requires addressing systemic barriers and ensuring that advancements benefit underserved communities as much as they do affluent ones.

Policymakers, researchers and clinicians must work collaboratively to address these challenges. By establishing ethical guidelines and promoting inclusivity, we can harness the potential of genetic and epigenetic research while safeguarding individual rights and societal wellbeing.

If-Then Guidance

- If you have a family history of mental-health disorders, then discuss genetic screening or counseling with your healthcare provider. Understanding potential genetic predispositions can help you and your medical team craft a more personalized approach to managing your mental health.

- If you are experiencing PTSX symptoms and suspect environmental factors or trauma in your past may have contributed, then consider consulting a specialist in trauma-informed care or epigenetics. They can guide you in exploring how life experiences might have influenced your genetic expression and recommend targeted interventions.
- If you are pregnant or planning to start a family and have a personal or family history of PTSX, then prioritize stress reduction techniques and a healthy lifestyle. Reducing stress during pregnancy may help prevent adverse epigenetic changes that could affect your child's health.
- If you are undergoing treatment for PTSX and not seeing significant progress, then ask your healthcare provider about emerging treatments that consider genetic and epigenetic factors. Tailored therapies, like pharmacogenetics-based medication adjustments, could be more effective for you.
- If you are concerned about passing PTSX-related vulnerabilities to your children, then explore intergenerational trauma education programs. Understanding how trauma may influence epigenetic inheritance can empower you to take preventive steps and promote resilience in your family.
- If you are interested in cutting-edge research, then stay informed about developments in gene-based therapies for PTSX. Clinical trials and emerging treatments may offer additional options for managing your condition.

Take The Next Step

- Schedule a genetic consultation. Meet with a genetic counselor or healthcare provider to explore how your genetic background and personal history may influence your mental health and response to treatment.
- Incorporate lifestyle changes to support healthy epigenetic expression. Regular physical activity, a nutritious diet and mindfulness practices like meditation can positively influence gene expression and reduce PTSX symptoms.

- Research epigenetic therapies. Stay informed about the latest studies and clinical trials in epigenetics and PTSX, which may lead to innovative treatments tailored to your genetic profile.
- Consider family-focused interventions. If intergenerational trauma is a concern, explore therapy or educational programs that address family dynamics and promote healing across generations.
- Advocate for precision medicine. Join patient-advocacy groups or participate in discussions that support the integration of genetic and epigenetic research into mainstream PTSX treatment.
- Collaborate with specialists. Work with a multidisciplinary team, including mental-health professionals, geneticists and trauma specialists, to develop a comprehensive care plan based on your unique needs.
- Educate yourself and others. Learn about genetic and epigenetic contributions to PTSX and share this knowledge with your community to raise awareness and reduce stigma around trauma and mental health.

Through Their Eyes

"I never thought I'd see the day when my own mind would betray me. I serve aboard the USS *R* [Ship name withheld.], a US Navy destroyer. Life at sea is demanding, but I've always thrived under the structure and camaraderie of Navy life. That is, until one night about a year ago when everything changed.

"I was on duty during a quiet night watch, scanning the horizon as the ship cut through the waves. Out of nowhere, my chest tightened, and my breath became shallow. A cold sweat broke out across my body, and I felt a wave of fear unlike anything I'd ever experienced. It didn't make sense. We weren't in danger. There was no reason to feel panic. But my heart pounded as though I were facing an unseen threat.

"That night marked the beginning of what felt like a spiral. The episodes started coming more frequently—uncontrolled anxiety, shivers and relentless night sweats. I couldn't sleep, couldn't eat, and started feeling like I was losing control. I confided in the ship's physician, who, at first, chalked it up to the stress of life at sea. We ran the usual tests—a full blood panel, urinalysis, hormone levels—but everything came back normal except my cortisol levels, a clear indicator of stress. Other than the cortisol result, it didn't make sense, and the lack of answers only made my anxiety worse.

"The doc decided to dig deeper. He started researching conditions that might explain my symptoms and came across studies linking genetics to mental health. He recommended I head back to port for a comprehensive genetic test. At first, I was skeptical. Genetics? I didn't think something like anxiety could be written into my DNA. But I trusted him, and I wanted answers.

"When the test results came back, they revealed something I hadn't expected: a genetic predisposition to anxiety and depression. It was like a lightbulb went off. Suddenly, everything made sense—my unexplained episodes, my heightened sensitivity to stress, even some struggles I'd seen in my family. The doctor explained how genetics could influence my brain's response to stress and how my environment might have triggered these dormant tendencies.

"Armed with this knowledge, we developed a treatment plan. I started with a stellate ganglion block, a procedure the doctor described as a "reset button" for the fight-or-flight system. To my surprise, it worked. The overwhelming anxiety diminished, and I felt like I could breathe again. I also tried a mild anti-anxiety medication, but the side effects were rough, so I stopped taking it after a few weeks.

"Instead, I focused on natural ways to manage my symptoms—exercise, lots of sunlight, and staying connected with my shipmates. I made it a point to get fresh air on deck whenever possible and worked out daily in the ship's gym. Over time, these changes made a world of difference. The fear that had once consumed me was now a distant memory.

"Today, I'm back on the USS *R*, standing watch with a clear mind. I still carry the knowledge of my genetic predisposition, but instead of feeling trapped by it, I feel empowered."

—Petty Officer Second Class Jeremy E., US Navy

9

Exercise as Medicine: Physical Activity in PTSX Recovery

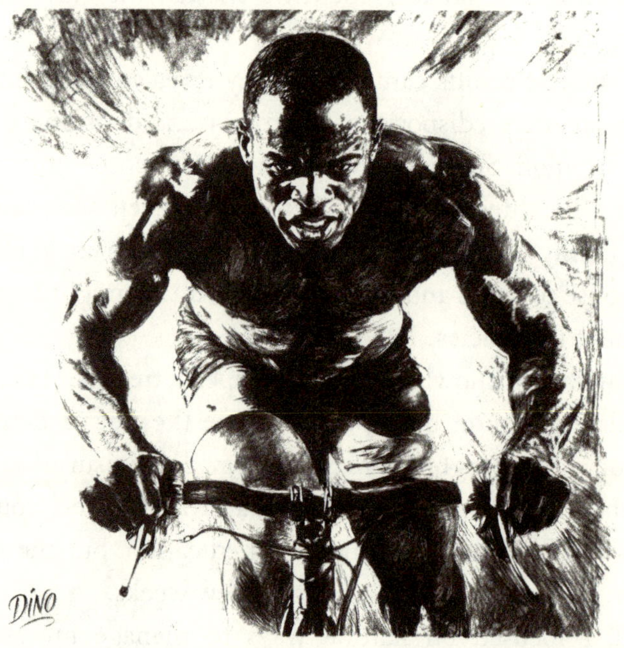

Robert gripped the handles of the bike, sweat dripping down his face, his breath ragged. The fan roared with each turn of the pedals as his legs pumped furiously. He focused on the rhythm, the steady burn in his muscles, and the feel of his heart pounding in his chest.

His therapist had told him exercise might help. At first he thought it was a joke. How could riding a bike do anything about the nightmares, the flashbacks, or the guilt that sat like a stone in his chest? But Robert was out of options, and so he showed up.

The first week had been hell. Every push of the pedals reminded him of what he'd lost—friends, sleep, and the sense of peace he hadn't felt in years. He'd nearly quit. But now, three months in, something was different. He didn't dread the bike anymore. The pain didn't scare him. It was real, tangible, and for once, something he could control.

Robert gritted his teeth, leaning forward, pouring everything into the pedals. He wasn't running from the memories anymore. He was burning through them.

The timer beeped. Ten minutes. He slowed, chest heaving, his shirt drenched in sweat. Robert leaned back, staring at the ceiling as his breath steadied. The gym was loud, but he felt calm, grounded in a way he hadn't been for years.

He wiped his face and stood, legs shaky but steady enough. The pain hadn't left his mind entirely, but it felt manageable now, like something he could keep pushing through.

Tomorrow, he'd be back. He wasn't fixed—he might never be—but he was moving forward. And for now, that was enough.

This chapter explores how exercise serves as a powerful complementary intervention alongside professional therapy and treatments for individuals recovering from PTSX. By enhancing neuroplasticity, reducing inflammation, and balancing neurotransmitters, physical activity addresses the physiological and psychological roots of trauma.

While therapies like cognitive behavioral therapy and medications are foundational in PTSX treatment, exercise has emerged as a powerful complementary intervention. Physical activity is not merely a tool for improving physical fitness. It has profound effects on brain health, emotional resilience and overall wellbeing.

Beyond the science, we delve into practical applications, including specific exercise types, their unique benefits, and real-world success stories that demonstrate the transformative power of movement. Whether through aerobic exercise, yoga, or martial arts, incorporating physical activity into PTSX recovery offers a holistic pathway to healing.

The Science Behind Exercise and PTSX Recovery

Neuroplasticity refers to the brain's ability to adapt and reorganize itself by forming new neural connections. In PTSX, neuroplasticity is often impaired, particularly in regions like the hippocampus and prefrontal cortex. Exercise, particularly aerobic activity, stimulates the production of brain-derived neurotrophic factor (BDNF), a protein essential for promoting neuroplasticity. BDNF enhances the growth of new neurons and strengthens existing neural pathways, helping repair trauma-induced damage.

Studies reveal that individuals who engage in regular aerobic exercise show significant improvements in hippocampal volume and prefrontal cortex activity—areas heavily affected by PTSX. For example, a 2018 study found that veterans who participated in a 12-week aerobic exercise program exhibited measurable increases in cognitive function and emotional regulation. These findings underscore how exercise can help the brain adapt and heal, offering hope to those living with PTSX.

Suicide rates demonstrate a bitter statistic—veterans dying at double civilian numbers—but behind every data point stands a life still within reach of hope, if we dare to intervene sooner.

Reducing Inflammation

Chronic inflammation is increasingly recognized as a contributor to PTSX symptoms. Elevated levels of pro-inflammatory cytokines have been linked to heightened anxiety, depression and cognitive impairments. Exercise acts as a natural anti-inflammatory agent by reducing the levels of these cytokines and promoting the release of anti-inflammatory chemicals like interleukin-10 (IL-10).

A landmark study in 2020 demonstrated that participants who engaged in moderate-intensity exercise three times a week showed significant reductions in inflammatory markers. This reduction was associated with improved mood and decreased hyperarousal symptoms. For individuals with PTSX, lowering inflammation through exercise can mitigate some of the physiological underpinnings of the disorder, providing a foundation for overall recovery.

Balancing Neurotransmitters

PTSX often disrupts neurotransmitter systems, particularly serotonin, dopamine, and endorphins—chemicals critical for mood regulation and emotional resilience. Exercise boosts the production and release of these neurotransmitters, helping to counteract the imbalances caused by trauma.

For instance, running and other forms of aerobic exercise increase serotonin levels, alleviating anxiety and depression. Strength training has been shown to enhance dopamine production, improving motivation and focus. Additionally, the endorphin release triggered by exercise produces a natural "runner's high," offering immediate mood elevation and stress relief. These neurochemical shifts contribute to a sense of calm, wellbeing, and control, which are often elusive for individuals with PTSX.

Types of Exercise and Their Specific Benefits

Aerobic activities like running, cycling, swimming and brisk walking are foundational in PTSX recovery. These exercises elevate heart rate and improve cardiovascular fitness while also promoting brain health. Research has consistently shown that 20-30 minutes of moderate aerobic exercise, performed three to five times a week, significantly reduces symptoms of anxiety, depression, and hyperarousal.

One study found that veterans who engaged in regular aerobic activity reported reduced flashbacks and better sleep quality. Aerobic exercise also improves oxygen flow to the brain, which enhances cognitive function and emotional regulation—critical areas affected by trauma. The accessibility and scalability of aerobic activities make them an ideal starting point for many individuals recovering from PTSX.

Yoga: Cultivating Mind-Body Awareness

Yoga uniquely combines physical movement, breathwork and mindfulness, making it a powerful tool for addressing PTSX. Trauma-sensitive yoga programs have gained popularity for their ability to reduce hyperarousal and improve emotional regulation. By focusing on gentle, controlled movements and deep breathing, yoga calms the autonomic nervous system and increases vagal tone, helping individuals shift from a fight-or-flight state to one of safety and relaxation.

A 2014 study highlighted the efficacy of yoga in reducing PTSX symptoms. Participants who attended weekly trauma-sensitive yoga sessions reported decreased intrusive thoughts, improved mood and greater self-awareness. Yoga's emphasis on reconnecting with the body is particularly beneficial for individuals who feel disassociated due to trauma.

Martial Arts: Building Confidence and Emotional Regulation

Martial arts such as Brazilian jiu-jitsu, tai chi and karate offer structured environments where individuals can develop self-discipline, focus, and physical confidence. These practices emphasize controlled movements, respect and mindfulness, which can help individuals regain a sense of control and agency.

For example, tai chi's slow, deliberate movements promote relaxation and enhance balance—both physical and emotional. Brazilian jiu-jitsu enhances problem-solving and perseverance, as practitioners learn to navigate challenging situations on the mat. These disciplines also create supportive communities, reducing feelings of isolation and building connections that are essential for recovery.

Strength Training: Enhancing Empowerment and Mood

Strength training, including weightlifting and resistance exercises, is another effective way to reduce PTSX symptoms. Studies have shown that resistance training improves mood, reduces anxiety, and enhances sleep quality. This type of training also builds physical resilience, which can translate into greater emotional confidence and a sense of empowerment. For beginners, incorporating simple bodyweight exercises like squats and push-ups into a weekly routine can provide immediate benefits. Over time, increasing the intensity and incorporating weights can further enhance physical and mental health outcomes.

Psychological and Emotional Benefits of Exercise

Exercise is a proven stress-reliever, particularly for individuals with PTSX who often experience heightened anxiety. Physical activity activates the parasympathetic nervous system, which counters the stress-inducing fight-or-flight response. This physiological shift helps lower cortisol levels and promotes a sense of calm.

Additionally, rhythmic activities like running or swimming have a meditative quality that can soothe an overactive mind. These activities provide a safe outlet for releasing pent-up energy and tension, which are common in PTSX. Over time, the consistent practice of exercise trains the body and mind to respond more adaptively to stressors.

Building a Sense of Control and Agency

Trauma often leaves individuals feeling powerless and disconnected from their sense of control. Exercise offers an opportunity to reclaim that agency. Setting and achieving fitness goals, no matter how small, reinforces self-efficacy and confidence. Whether it's completing a 5K run or mastering a yoga pose, these milestones remind individuals of their resilience and capability.

Moreover, structured physical activities provide a sense of routine and purpose. This consistency can be grounding for those struggling with the unpredictability of PTSX symptoms. Exercise becomes not just a physical activity but a practice of rebuilding trust in oneself.

Promoting Social Connection

Isolation is a common struggle for individuals with PTSX. Group exercise activities like fitness classes, team sports or martial arts training, build social connection and reduce feelings of loneliness. The camaraderie built in these settings creates a sense of belonging and mutual support.

Veteran-specific fitness programs provide safe spaces where participants can share their experiences and encourage each other. These programs often emphasize teamwork, reinforcing the bonds that are so vital for recovery. By engaging with others through exercise, individuals with PTSX can rebuild their social networks and find meaningful connections.

Practical Guidance for Integrating Exercise into Recovery

Common barriers to exercise include lack of motivation, physical limitations, and fear of failure. Addressing these challenges starts with realistic goal-setting. Encouraging small, achievable steps—like a 10-minute walk each day—can build confidence and momentum.

Seeking professional guidance, say, from a trauma-informed fitness trainer or physical therapist, ensures safety and appropriateness. Additionally, finding enjoyable activities increases the likelihood of consistency. Dancing or hiking may feel less like exercise and more like recreation, making it easier to stay committed.

Creating a Personalized Exercise Plan

A well-rounded exercise plan should include aerobic, strength, and flexibility components tailored to individual needs and goals. For beginners, a sample week might include:

Monday: 20 minutes of brisk walking (aerobic).

Wednesday: 15 minutes of yoga (flexibility).

Friday: 10 minutes of bodyweight exercises (strength).

As fitness improves, the duration and intensity can gradually increase. Tracking progress through a journal or app provides motivation and a sense of accomplishment.

Using Technology to Stay Engaged

Fitness apps, wearable devices and online communities offer valuable tools for maintaining motivation. Many apps include guided workouts, progress tracking, and social features that ensure accountability. For individuals with PTSX, apps designed with mindfulness or relaxation components, such as Calm or Headspace, can complement physical activity.

Exercise and Professional Treatment: A Holistic Approach

Exercise enhances the effectiveness of traditional PTSX treatments by creating a more receptive brain state. Aerobic exercise before a therapy session can reduce anxiety, allowing patients to engage more fully. Similarly, yoga's focus on mindfulness complements cognitive therapies by teaching patients to stay present and regulate emotions. All told, exercise is just one way for a person, especially one who's experienced trauma, to take charge of their own life. All you do is get back up and *move*.

Partnering with Healthcare Providers

Collaboration with healthcare providers is key to integrating exercise into a comprehensive treatment plan. Mental health professionals can offer guidance on appropriate activity levels, while fitness trainers with trauma-informed certifications can design safe and effective programs. Open communication ensures that physical activity aligns with broader recovery goals.

Moving Toward Healing Through Movement

Exercise is more than a physical activity, It's a potent form of medicine that nurtures the mind, body and spirit. By enhancing neuroplasticity, reducing inflammation, and building social connections, physical activity addresses the multifaceted challenges of PTSX. Every step, stretch, or breath taken in exercise is a step closer to resilience and healing.

If-Then Guidance

- If you are experiencing heightened anxiety or restlessness as a symptom of PTSX, then incorporate aerobic exercises like walking, running or cycling into your routine. Aerobic activity helps release endorphins, which naturally reduce stress and promote a sense of wellbeing.
- If you struggle with emotional regulation or find it difficult to calm down after triggers, then explore yoga or tai chi. These practices combine movement with breathwork, activating the parasympathetic nervous system to help your body and mind find balance.
- If you are feeling isolated or disconnected due to PTSX, then consider joining a group fitness class or participating in team sports. These activities create a sense of community and belonging that are essential for emotional recovery.

- If you are dealing with hypervigilance or an overactive stress response, then try martial arts or other controlled forms of physical activity. These can teach discipline and body awareness while providing an outlet for pent-up energy.
- If you have difficulty sleeping, which is common in PTSX, then schedule light to moderate exercise earlier in the day. Exercise improves sleep quality by regulating circadian rhythms and reducing nighttime restlessness.
- If chronic pain or physical limitations prevent you from engaging in high-impact activities, then opt for low-impact exercises like swimming, stretching or stationary biking. These activities are gentle on the joints while still improving circulation and mood.
- If you feel overwhelmed by the idea of starting an exercise routine, then begin with short, manageable goals like a 10-minute walk or a few minutes of stretching. Small steps can build confidence and lead to more significant achievements over time.
- If you are managing comorbid conditions such as depression or substance use disorder alongside PTSX, then work with a healthcare provider to design an exercise plan tailored to your needs. Regular physical activity can complement other treatments and enhance overall recovery.

Take the Next Step

- Consult a healthcare provider: Schedule an appointment with your doctor or a physical therapist to assess your current fitness level and determine safe, effective exercises tailored to your abilities and goals.
- Start small: Begin with short, achievable workouts like a 10-minute walk or a few gentle yoga poses, and gradually increase the intensity or duration as your confidence and stamina improve.
- Create a routine: Establish a regular exercise schedule like walking every morning or attending a weekly yoga class, to help make physical activity a consistent part of your day.
- Seek community: Join a fitness group, veteran sports league or exercise class to find camaraderie and support as you work toward

your recovery goals. If necessary, find a workout partner who can push you when you're down or unmotivated.

- Explore variety: Try different forms of exercise: swimming, hiking, dancing or martial arts—to discover what you enjoy and what best supports your healing process.
- Track progress: Keep a journal or use a fitness app to record your activities and note improvements in mood, energy or PTSX symptoms. Seeing your progress can be motivating and affirming.
- Set realistic goals: Aim for attainable milestones: walking a certain number of steps per day or practicing yoga three times a week, and celebrate your achievements along the way.
- Pair exercise with therapy: Collaborate with your mental health provider to integrate physical activity into your broader treatment plan. Discuss how exercise complements other therapies and enhances your recovery journey.
- Celebrate success: Acknowledge and reward your efforts, whether it's treating yourself to new workout gear or simply reflecting on how far you've come. Recognizing your progress reinforces positive habits and encourages continued growth.

Through Their Eyes

"My name is Petty Officer Ryan V., and I've been with the Coast Guard since I was 18. Fourteen years in, I've seen the ocean in ways most people can't imagine—its beauty, its power and its isolation. My job has taken me to places I can't name, patrolling in some of the world's most challenging waters.

"For a long time, I thought I could handle anything. But what I didn't realize was how the stress of those missions was silently building inside me, turning into something I didn't know how to fight.

"Being on a patrol boat is an experience that's hard to explain unless you've lived it. Imagine being in a confined space with the same people, day in and day out, for weeks or even months at a time. You're constantly on alert, working long hours, with little privacy and nowhere to escape. When you're not scanning the horizon for threats, you're dealing with the monotony of routine maintenance and drills. The combination of high stakes and relentless repetition wears you down. On land, you can walk away, find a quiet space, or blow off steam. At sea, there's nowhere to go.

"I started to notice the signs of PTSX after one particularly tough mission. We'd been on patrol for 92 days, intercepting drug runners in a region notorious for its violence. The tension was neverending. Every small boat on the radar was a potential threat. Every boarding could go sideways. When we finally docked, I realized I couldn't relax. My body was still on edge, my mind replaying scenarios over and over. I couldn't sleep, and when I did, the nightmares came. Back on the next patrol, it was even worse. I was irritable, withdrawn, and barely holding it together. My crewmates noticed, but I just brushed it off. 'I'm fine,' I'd say. But I wasn't.

"It was a shipmate who finally pulled me aside. He was older, had been through similar struggles, and he told me straight: "You've got to take care of yourself, man. You can't pour from an empty cup." He suggested I start exercising—not just for fitness, but as a way to manage the stress. At first, I scoffed. When was I supposed to find the time or space on a boat? But he insisted and even offered to join me.

"We started small—push-ups, sit-ups, and resistance bands in the tiny gym area onboard. It wasn't much, but it was something. Soon, I added more: bodyweight circuits, yoga, even shadowboxing. It wasn't just about the physical effort; it became a mental release.

"When I was working out, my focus shifted from the chaos around me to the rhythm of my breath and the burn in my muscles. It gave me a sense of control, something I desperately needed.

"Over time, the benefits became clear. My mood improved, and I started sleeping better. I found myself reconnecting with my crew and feeling more present during the long watches. We've got to look out for each other out there, because the sea doesn't care about your struggles. But with the right tools and support, you can weather the storm and come out stronger on the other side."

—Petty Officer Ryan V., US Coast Guard

10

The Hidden Connection: PTSX and Heavy-Metal Toxicity

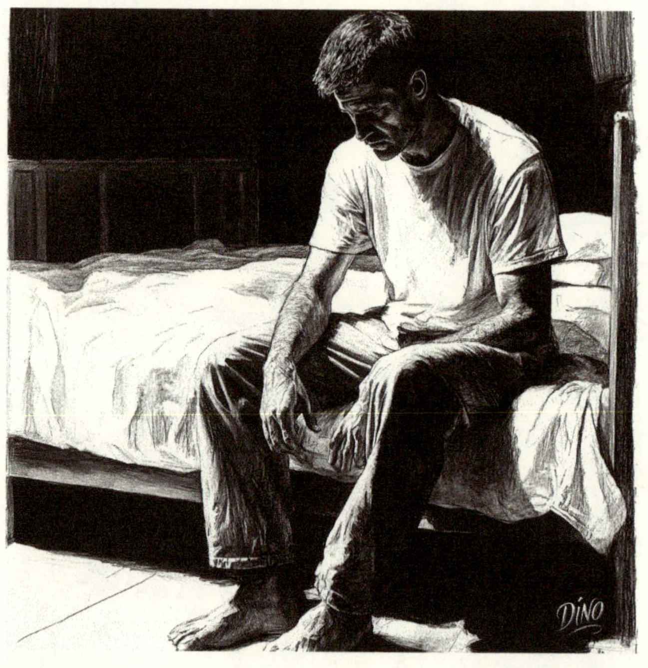

James sat on the edge of his bed, staring at the floor. He couldn't remember the last time he felt like himself. A few years ago, he had been in the best shape of his life—broad shoulders, powerful arms, and lungs that could hold their breath for minutes. Now, though, it didn't matter. Depression had taken hold and wouldn't let go.

A former Coast Guard rescue swimmer, James had spent years pulling people out of chaos. He was the one who stayed calm when everyone else panicked. Now, every day felt like he was drowning.

His doctor had run every test imaginable, but nothing explained it. James ate well, exercised and didn't drink much. The depression shouldn't be there, but it was.

Then, one day, the results came back: heavy metal toxicity. Mercury, likely from years of eating too much fish. It had built up in his body, poisoning his brain. His doctor said the symptoms made sense now—the sluggishness, the brain fog, the weight pressing down on his spirit.

They started chelation therapy, a treatment to flush the metals from his system. At first, James didn't notice much, just more appointments and more waiting. But slowly, things began to shift.

One morning, a few months in, he woke up and realized the heaviness in his chest had lessened. By the time he walked to the gym, he noticed a clarity he hadn't felt in years.

James still had bad days, but he started to feel like himself again. Each week brought a little more light. Standing in front of the mirror after a workout one day, James stared at his reflection. He was back—maybe not entirely, but enough to hope. And for now, that was more than enough.

This chapter features how environmental factors, including toxic exposures, may interact with symptoms of PTSX, and offer new pathways for understanding and addressing injuries and side effects. By expanding the lens beyond traditional psychological and physiological approaches, we gain a richer understanding of the complex interplay of internal and external forces shaping mental health outcomes.

Heavy-metal toxicity refers to the harmful accumulation of metals like lead (Pb), mercury (Hg), cadmium (Cd) and arsenic (As) in the human body. These metals, derived from contaminated water and food, industrial waste, or even common household items, disrupt cellular processes through neurotoxicity and oxidative stress. Unlike acute poisoning, chronic exposure often presents subtly, gradually damaging neural pathways critical for emotional regulation and stress resilience.

Heavy metals can accumulate over time, crossing the blood-brain barrier and influencing key systems associated with mental health, including neurotransmitter balance and stress-response mechanisms. These exposures severely affect populations at risk for PTSX and highlight the need for interdisciplinary approaches to treatment.

Emerging evidence suggests an interplay between PTSX and heavy metal toxicity. Through pathways involving neuroinflammation, oxidative damage and epigenetic changes, heavy metals may amplify the severity of PTSX symptoms.

Overview of Toxic Heavy Metals

Lead (Pb): Found in old paint, contaminated water sources and industrial pollution. Lead exposure often stems from deteriorating infrastructure like old plumbing systems, and disproportionately affects communities with limited access to modern resources. Lead is particularly harmful because its divalent state mimics calcium, interfering with critical processes in bones, nerves and the brain. Even low levels of exposure can result in significant cognitive impairments, especially in children.

Mercury (Hg): Commonly present in seafood, dental amalgams and emissions from industrial processes. Mercury exists in different forms, each with distinct health implications. Methylmercury, found in fish, is a potent neurotoxin that accumulates in the food chain. Elemental mercury, used in some industrial processes, releases vapor that can be inhaled, leading to direct absorption into the central nervous system.

Cadmium (Cd): Inhaled via cigarette smoke or encountered through contaminated soil and batteries. Cadmium exposure often results from agricultural practices that contaminate food crops. This metal accumulates in the kidneys and liver, causing systemic effects that extend to the brain, where it interferes with neurotransmitter function and oxidative balance.

Arsenic (As): A frequent contaminant in water supplies and pesticides. Arsenic exposure is linked to regions with high groundwater contamination, affecting millions worldwide. Chronic exposure to arsenic can lead to changes in skin, cognitive decline, and heightened risks of mental health disorders.

In recent decades, industrialized food production and globalized water supplies have magnified human exposure to these toxic heavy metals. Modern fertilizers, pesticide residues, food packaging, and industrial runoff contribute to a steady rise in cumulative intake, even in populations far removed from direct industrial sites. Processed foods may concentrate trace contaminants, while mass-distribution water systems spread them broadly across communities. The result is a silent but escalating public health threat: persistent, low-level exposure that disproportionately affects vulnerable groups, undermines neurological health, and exacerbates conditions like PTSX by adding an invisible toxic burden to already stressed biological systems.

Hypermasculine silence turns brotherhood into isolation The bravest act may be whispering "I need help" before a pistol in the night becomes the final enemy.

Pathophysiology of Heavy Metal Toxicity

Heavy metals interfere with cellular functions by binding to proteins and enzymes, leading to widespread dysfunction. These metals often accumulate in the brain where they induce neurotoxic effects, oxidative stress and inflammation. Heavy metals' ability to cross the blood-brain barrier is particularly concerning, as it allows them to disrupt delicate neural networks.

Over time, this disruption manifests in a range of symptoms, from subtle cognitive changes to pronounced emotional and behavioral disturbances. By impairing energy production in mitochondria and increasing the production of harmful reactive oxygen species, heavy metals create a cascade of cellular damage that may predispose individuals to neuropsychiatric conditions like PTSX.

Mechanisms Linking PTSX and Heavy Metal Toxicity

Heavy metals stimulate chronic inflammation in the brain by activating microglia, the brain's immune cells. This process leads to the release of pro-inflammatory cytokines like interleukin-6 (IL-6) and tumor necrosis factor-alpha (TNF-alpha).

Chronic neuroinflammation has been identified as a significant contributor to the development and persistence of PTSX, linking environmental toxicity to heightened vulnerability.

Prolonged inflammation damages neural pathways, particularly in areas like the hippocampus and amygdala, which are crucial for memory and emotional regulation. This may explain why individuals exposed to heavy metals often report heightened sensitivity to stress and difficulties in managing trauma-related emotions.

Oxidative Stress

Reactive oxygen species, produced excessively during heavy metal exposure, inflict damage on neurons. This oxidative stress, compounded by mitochondrial dysfunction, accelerates neurodegeneration. The brain's heightened sensitivity to oxidative damage makes it a critical target in individuals with both heavy-metal exposure and PTSX.

Oxidative stress also disrupts the balance of critical antioxidants like glutathione, leaving the brain more vulnerable to external and internal stressors. Over time, this imbalance may lead to structural changes in brain regions associated with decision-making, emotional regulation and memory, compounding the challenges faced by individuals with PTSX.

Dysregulation of the HPA Axis

Heavy metals disrupt this system by altering cortisol levels, leading to either hypercortisolism or hypocortisolism. This disruption compounds the dysregulated stress response already characteristic of PTSX, exacerbating symptoms like hypervigilance and emotional dysregulation. The cumulative stress from both trauma and toxic exposures creates a feedback loop, where the body's inability to properly regulate cortisol levels perpetuates cycles of anxiety, fatigue and emotional instability.

Neurotransmitter Imbalances

Heavy metals interfere with the balance of neurotransmitters: serotonin, dopamine and gamma-aminobutyric acid (GABA). Mercury, for example, depletes serotonin levels, contributing to anxiety and mood instability. These imbalances can intensify PTSX symptoms, including intrusive thoughts, emotional numbing and sleep disturbances. Additionally, changes in dopamine levels may exacerbate symptoms of hyperarousal and impulsivity, while GABA disruption can heighten feelings of tension and restlessness. The combined effects of these neurotransmitter alterations create a storm of psychological and emotional challenges for affected individuals.

Epigenetic Modifications

Heavy metals induce changes in DNA methylation, altering the expression of genes associated with the stress response. These epigenetic modifications may increase susceptibility to PTSX and amplify its severity in affected individuals, creating a legacy of vulnerability that extends across generations. For example, individuals exposed to arsenic in early life may pass on altered stress-response genes to their offspring, perpetuating cycles of trauma and susceptibility. Understanding these epigenetic effects offers valuable insights into how environmental factors can shape long-term mental-health outcomes and emphasizes the need for preventive measures.

Evidence from Research Studies

Results from rodent and other animal studies have provided compelling insights into the impact of heavy metals on stress-related behaviors. For example, exposure to mercury and lead has been shown to increase anxiety-like behaviors and impair memory, with significant changes observed in the hippocampus and amygdala—key brain regions implicated in PTSX.

These studies also reveal that chronic exposure to metals disrupts synaptic plasticity, impairing the brain's ability to adapt to new information or recover from trauma. Such findings underscore the potential for heavy metals to exacerbate vulnerability to stress and trauma- related disorders.

Human Studies

Studies in human populations reveal elevated levels of heavy metals in individuals with PTSX. Veterans exposed to industrial chemicals and ammunition often exhibit higher concentrations of lead and mercury, correlating with increased severity of PTSX symptoms. Similarly, populations residing in polluted environments report higher rates of PTSX and related disorders. These studies highlight the need for targeted interventions in high-risk groups and suggest that addressing heavy metal exposure may alleviate some of the cognitive and emotional burdens associated with PTSX.

Epidemiological Studies

Large-scale epidemiological results confirm a correlation between heavy-metal exposure and mental-health disorders, including PTSX. Notably, communities near industrial sites exhibit a higher prevalence of comorbid conditions like depression and anxiety, which frequently accompany PTSX.

These studies provide valuable context for understanding how environmental factors shape mental health trends across entire populations, emphasizing the importance of policy-driven solutions to reduce exposure.

Case Studies

The results from individually studied cases underscore the profound impact of heavy metal toxicity on mental health. For instance, industrial workers with high arsenic exposure often present with a cluster of symptoms resembling PTSX, including hyperarousal, emotional instability and difficulty concentrating. These individual cases bring a human face to the broader scientific findings, highlighting the urgent need for comprehensive assessments and interventions for those affected by both trauma and toxic exposures.

Populations at Risk

Military environments pose significant risks for heavy metal exposure. Ammunition, explosives and industrial waste are common sources of heavy-metal toxins, compounding the risk of PTSX for servicemembers and veterans even extending after their service. Deployment to regions with poor environmental regulations further increases exposure risks, while the high-stress nature of military life magnifies the effects of toxic exposure. Addressing these compounded risks is essential for improving the mental health outcomes of veterans and active-duty personnel.

Industrial Workers

Workers in mining, manufacturing and smelting industries also face chronic exposure to heavy metals. Over time, this exposure can manifest as cognitive and emotional impairments, increasing susceptibility to PTSX. Occupational safety measures like improved ventilation and personal protective equipment, are critical for reducing these risks. Additionally, routine monitoring of metal levels in high-risk industries can help identify and mitigate long-term health impacts.

Populations in Polluted Environments

Communities near industrial sites or areas with contaminated water supplies experience heightened exposure to heavy metals. Residents in these communities often report higher rates of stress-related disorders, including PTSX. Environmental justice initiatives aimed at reducing pollution and providing access to clean resources are vital for protecting vulnerable communities from the dual burden of toxic exposures and mental health challenges.

Children

Children are particularly vulnerable due to their continuously developing nervous system. Exposure to lead through old paint or contaminated water can result in long-term cognitive and emotional challenges, increasing the risk for PTSX later in life. Early interventions, such as lead testing and nutritional support, can mitigate these risks and improve developmental outcomes.

Clinical Implications

Screening for heavy-metal toxicity in PTSX patients is critical, especially for those with known environmental exposures. Blood, hair and analyses of urine can reveal the presence and extent of heavy metal burden. Early detection allows for timely intervention and treatment.

Detoxification Treatments

Chelation therapy is a cornerstone of treatment, facilitating the removal of heavy metals from the body. Additionally, antioxidants like glutathione and vitamin C are used to counteract oxidative stress. Combining these treatments with lifestyle modifications like avoiding further exposure and adopting a nutrient-rich diet, can enhance recovery and improve quality of life for affected individuals. It doesn't take much to screen for heavy metals, and treating them isn't an issue, either.

Nutritional Interventions

A diet rich in anti-inflammatory and chelating foods—garlic, cilantro and leafy greens—can support detoxification and reduce inflammation. Nutritional counseling is an essential component of holistic care. Supplements like zinc and selenium may also counteract the harmful effects of heavy metals, providing additional protection for the brain and nervous system.

Integrated PTSX Therapies

Combining detoxification protocols with conventional PTSX treatments—for example, psychotherapy and pharmacotherapy—enhances outcomes. Addressing both the mental and environmental dimensions of the condition provides comprehensive relief. Trauma-focused therapies can be paired with detoxification strategies to improve emotional resilience and reduce symptom severity.

Preventive Measures

Reducing heavy-metal exposure is paramount. Implementing stringent environmental regulations, ensuring clean water supplies, and educating communities about the risks of heavy metal toxicity are critical steps toward prevention. Workplace safety measures and public awareness campaigns can further reduce the prevalence of toxic exposures and their associated health impacts.

Challenges and Limitations

The simultaneous presence of multiple risk factors complicates the determination of causality between heavy metal exposure and PTSX. For example, socioeconomic stressors and genetic predispositions often coexist with toxic exposures, making it challenging to isolate specific contributors to mental health outcomes. Future research must address these complexities through comprehensive, multifactorial approaches.

Lack of Longitudinal Studies

Long-term studies are needed to fully understand the trajectory of heavy metal toxicity and its impact on PTSX. Most existing research relies on cross-sectional data, limiting insights into how chronic exposures influence mental health over time. Longitudinal studies could provide valuable information on the progression of symptoms and the effectiveness of interventions.

Variability in Individual Susceptibility

Genetic, epigenetic and lifestyle factors influence individual responses to heavy metal exposure, making generalized conclusions challenging. Personalized medicine approaches, which consider these individual differences, hold promise for developing targeted treatments that address the unique needs of each patient.

Future Directions

Large-scale epidemiological studies assessing the prevalence of heavy metal exposure in PTSX populations will provide valuable insights. By identifying patterns of exposure and their correlation with mental health outcomes, researchers can inform public health strategies and policy decisions.

Mechanistic Studies

Investigating the molecular pathways linking heavy metals to neurobiological changes in PTSX will guide the development of targeted interventions. These studies could uncover new therapeutic targets, paving the way for innovative treatments that address the root causes of symptoms, i.e. at the molecular level. By treating the true cause, rather than symptoms, we can eradicate the issues.

Development of Novel Therapies

Innovative chelation therapies and neuroprotective agents hold promise for mitigating the impact of heavy metal toxicity on PTSX. Advances in drug delivery systems like nanotechnology, could enhance the precision and effectiveness of these treatments, improving outcomes for patients.

Public Health Initiatives

Policies aimed at reducing heavy metal contamination and raising awareness of its mental health impacts are essential. Community-based interventions can empower populations to protect themselves from exposure. For example, educational programs on safe food practices and water purification can significantly reduce individual risk.

Now What?

The relationship between PTSX and heavy-metal toxicity is a compelling example of the interplay between environmental and psychological health. Understanding this connection underscores the importance of comprehensive approaches to diagnosis, treatment and prevention.

By addressing both the physical and emotional dimensions of PTSX, we can pave the way for more effective therapies and improved outcomes. Interdisciplinary research, combined with public-health initiatives, will be crucial in unraveling this complex dynamic and alleviating the silent scars left by trauma and toxicity.

If-Then Guidance

- If you experience symptoms like emotional instability, fatigue, or cognitive fog with no clear cause, then discuss heavy metal toxicity testing with your doctor.
- If you live near industrial areas or consume seafood frequently, then consider regular screening for heavy metals like lead,

mercury, cadmium and arsenic. If you can, move away from affected geographical areas.

- If heavy-metal toxicity is confirmed, then explore chelation therapy to remove these metals from your body under medical supervision.
- If you're struggling with PTSX and suspect environmental factors, then ask your healthcare provider about an integrated treatment plan addressing both trauma and potential toxic exposures.
- If oxidative stress is a concern, then include antioxidant-rich foods like berries, citrus fruits, and green vegetables in your diet to counteract damage.
- If your water supply is potentially contaminated, then use filtration systems certified to remove heavy metals to reduce exposure.
- If you work in high-risk environments, then ensure proper use of personal protective equipment and regular health screenings.
- If prevention is your goal, then focus on creating a toxin-free living environment by avoiding products with harmful chemicals and opting for safer alternatives.

Take the Next Step

- Schedule a comprehensive test: Request blood, urine, or hair analyses from your healthcare provider to detect heavy metal levels in your body.
- Follow a detoxification protocol: If diagnosed with heavy-metal toxicity, adhere to treatments like chelation therapy or supplements recommended by your doctor.
- Revise your diet: Include foods like cilantro, garlic and leafy greens that naturally support detoxification and combat inflammation.
- Switch to low-risk water sources: Use high-quality filters or opt for bottled water certified to remove heavy metals, particularly if you live in areas with known contamination.
- Minimize exposure through awareness: Avoid high-mercury fish such as swordfish and king mackerel, and be cautious with old paint or deteriorating plumbing.
- Incorporate antioxidants: Add supplements like vitamin C and

glutathione to your regimen to protect your brain and nervous system from oxidative stress.

- Educate yourself and others: Learn about the sources of heavy metals in your environment and share this information with your community to promote prevention.
- Adopt an interdisciplinary approach: Work with both medical and mental-health professionals to address the combined effects of PTSX and environmental toxicity for a comprehensive recovery.

Through Their Eyes

"I didn't think much about the headaches at first. Or the way my hands started shaking when I was tired. I chalked it up to stress. A lot of us leave the military carrying more than we came in with. I figured it was the nightmares, the jumpy nerves, the stuff they said could happen after combat. But this wasn't just that. This was something else.

"I'd been out of the Army for six years. I served as a logistics specialist, handling ammunition and gear on bases overseas. It wasn't glamorous, but it mattered. Every round of ammunition, every tank of fuel went through my hands. I took pride in it. I still do.

"But after I got out, things started to fall apart. The headaches got worse, and my memory started slipping. I'd lose track of conversations, forget simple things. It got so bad I couldn't keep a job. My wife said I was 'different.' I didn't know what she meant until I started seeing it too—the irritability, the fog in my head, the feeling that I wasn't me anymore.

"Doctors told me I had depression, maybe some PTSX. They put me on meds, but they didn't help much. Then one day, I saw a neurologist who asked about my military service. When I mentioned working with ammunition and chemicals, her eyes narrowed. 'Have you ever been tested for heavy metals?' she asked.

"A blood test showed elevated levels of lead and mercury. The doctor explained how those metals might have built up in my system over the years. Lead from old ammo storage, mercury from contaminated water supplies—things I hadn't even thought about. She said the toxins could explain my symptoms. I wasn't just depressed. My brain and nervous system were under attack.

"The treatment wasn't easy. Chelation therapy was part of it, pulling the metals out of my system. I started eating differently too—more greens, less seafood. The doctor also gave me supplements to help with oxidative stress.

"It took months, but slowly, I started feeling a difference. The headaches eased. My memory improved. For the first time in years, I could finish a conversation without zoning out. My wife said my temper got better too.

"I'm not saying it's all fixed. The damage heavy metals did to me won't disappear overnight. Some days are still hard, especially when the memories of my time in service mix with the struggles of recovery. But at least now I know what I'm fighting.

"If I could go back, I'd tell the younger version of me to pay attention to what I was being exposed to. The chemicals, the water, even the air in some places—it all adds up. I didn't see it then, but I do now. I'm sharing this because someone out there might be feeling like I did—lost, confused, unsure why their body and mind are betraying them. Get tested. Ask questions. You might find answers you didn't even know you were looking for."

—Rob A., US Army Veteran

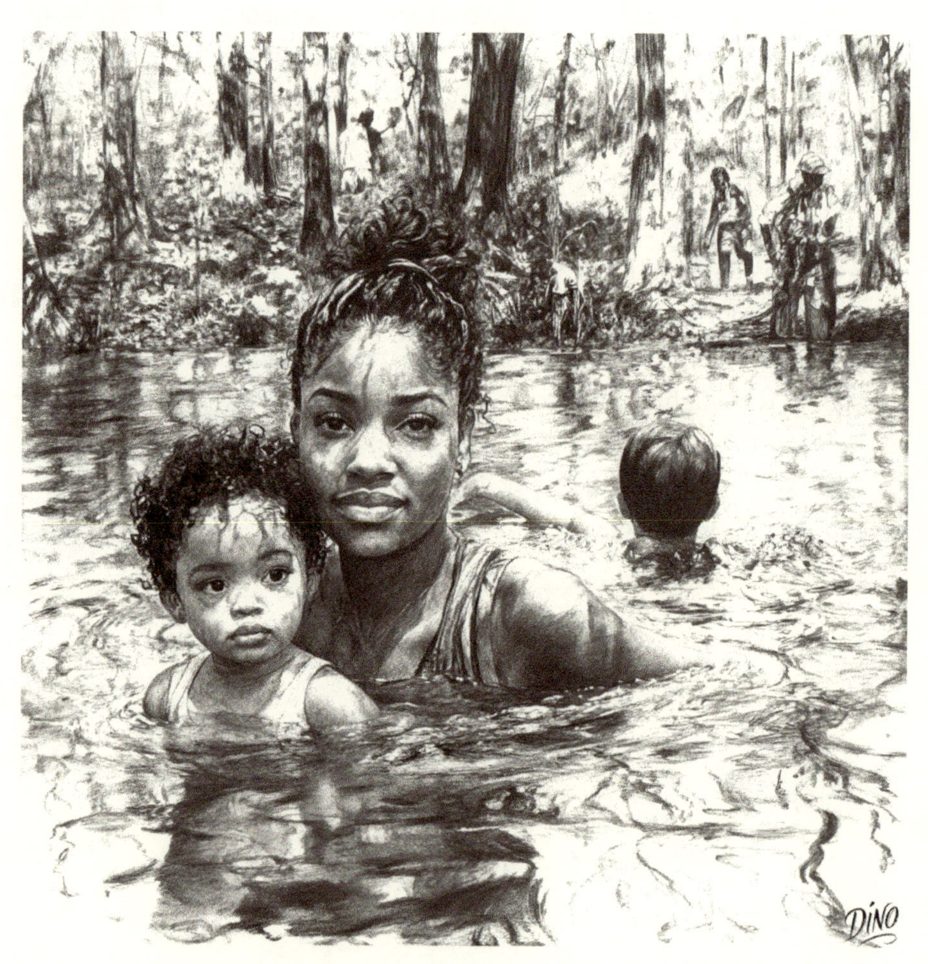
DINO

PART TWO

Challenges and Impacts

11

Challenges Veterans Face in Seeking Proper Treatment

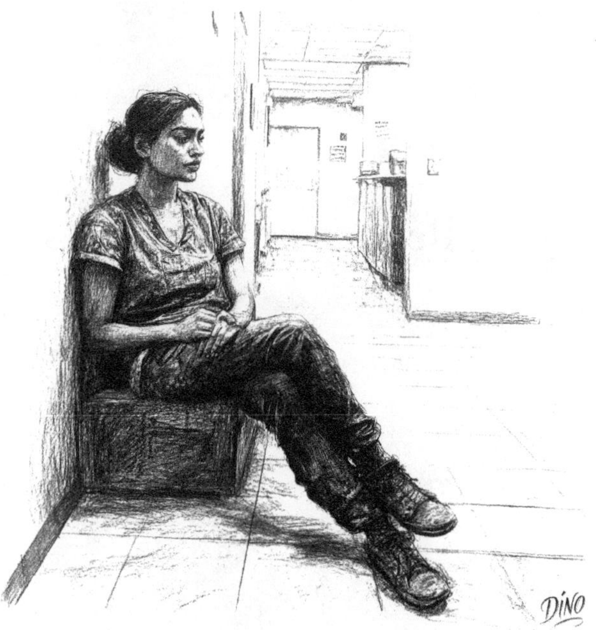

Martina sat in the waiting area of her local VA clinic, tapping her foot against the tiled floor as she tried to steady her nerves. She'd been out of the Army for three months, but the old habits and disciplined demeanor had yet to fade. Deep down, she worried that asking for help meant she was weak—an idea drilled into her by a culture that prized strength above all else.

Across from her sat Omar, a former Marine who wore the same uneasy expression. He confided in her that he still feared what would happen if his old unit found out he was here. Although he was no longer on active duty, just the thought of judgment followed him like a shadow. The idea that a Marine should be able to handle anything on his own still gripped him. They spoke quietly, careful not to draw attention. Martina paused sometimes, her anxiety flaring when she heard the faint hum of overhead lights.

Omar leaned in, recalling how he once tried to report a serious issue but backed off, afraid of reprisals. It made him question whether others had been in the same spot, too scared to speak up. Yet despite the fear, they both had decided to seek help—finally. Martina had learned there were counselors who understood military life, support groups with people who had walked the same path and resources that didn't feel distant or confusing. For the first time in a while, she felt a glimmer of hope.

This chapter examines the barriers veterans face when seeking treatment—from the ingrained military culture of toughness to fears of reprisal and public stigma. Above all, it reminds us that by addressing these challenges head-on, we can create a safer space where veterans like Martina and Omar find the help they deserve.

The Military Culture: Strength, Resilience and Toughness

As stated earlier, the military is built on a foundation of strength, resilience and toughness. These traits are crucial in combat, where the ability to ignore and push through fear, pain and adversity can mean the difference between life and death. However, while these attributes are necessary on the battlefield, they can become obstacles when servicemembers need to seek help for mental health issues. The military culture often creates an environment where psychological struggles are viewed as weaknesses, directly clashing with the ideals of strength and resilience.

As a result, many veterans who experience PTSX or other mental health challenges are reluctant to admit they need help. They fear being judged or ostracized by their peers, who may view them as less capable or even unfit for service.

This pressure to maintain an image of toughness can lead to feelings of shame and guilt, further compounding the mental health struggles veterans face. When individuals who have been trained to prioritize toughness are confronted with the need to seek help, they may feel that doing so undermines their identity as a courageous soldier and a competent human being.

Fear of Reprisal and Ostracism

For some veterans, especially those who have been victims of abuse—whether sexual, physical or psychological—the fear of seeking help is intensified by the possibility of reprisal. The military's hierarchical structure often places those in lower ranks in vulnerable positions, where reporting abuse committed by fellow soldiers, non-commissioned officers (NCOs) or higher-ranking officers may result in retaliation.

> Firearms in the closet, bottles on the shelf, memories in the dark—remove one lethal means and you reopen a pathway to life. Safety planning is strategy, not surrender.

Victims of abuse may also fear involuntary separation from the military, an outcome that can be devastating for individuals whose identity and livelihood are tied to their military service. This also includes students at service academies and ROTC units.

This fear of reprisal creates another layer of stress, further contributing to the onset or exacerbation of PTSX symptoms. Veterans who choose to remain silent about their trauma may feel trapped in a situation where they are unable to seek help without risking their careers, reputations or social standing within the military community. The result is often a vicious cycle, where the fear of being ostracized or punished for seeking help leads to the suppression of symptoms, ultimately worsening the individual's mental health, ultimately causing a severe downward spiral.

The Impact of Emotional Compartmentalization

Veterans face many challenges, including the military's emphasis on emotional and mental compartmentalization. In combat, servicemembers are trained to separate their emotions from the task at hand. This ability to maintain composure under extreme pressure is a crucial survival skill on the battlefield, where hesitation or emotional distraction can lead to fatal consequences.

However, when veterans return to civilian life, compartmentalizing can become a major obstacle to processing and healing from trauma. Many veterans suppress their symptoms for years, believing that they can handle their trauma on their own. This belief often stems from the same cultural values that equate emotional vulnerability with weakness.

Rather than seeking professional help, veterans may attempt to cope by burying their emotions, only to find that the unresolved trauma eventually resurfaces in destructive ways. Whether through substance abuse, aggression or isolation, veterans often find that their coping mechanisms no longer serve them in the long term.

The challenge lies in the fact that veterans are often unaware of the extent to which their mental health has been affected. The training to suppress emotions and focus on mission success can become so deeply ingrained that they may not recognize the signs of PTSX until the symptoms become unmanageable.

By the time veterans realize they need help, the trauma may have already taken a significant toll on their lives, relationships and overall wellbeing.

Stigma in Broader Society

The stigma surrounding PTSX is not confined to the military alone. It extends into society at large. Many people still harbor misconceptions about PTSX, often associating it with violent outbursts, irrational behavior or a loss of control. This misunderstanding can make people hesitant to disclose their condition, fearing that they will be labeled as dangerous or unstable.

In reality, PTSX manifests in a wide range of symptoms, many of which are internal and not immediately visible to others. Veterans with PTSX may experience flashbacks, nightmares, hypervigilance and emotional numbness, among other symptoms. However, because the public perception of PTSX is often distorted by media portrayals and a lack of proper education, veterans keep their struggles hidden.

This societal stigma can create a sense of isolation, who may feel that no one can truly understand what they have been through. This isolation further discourages people from seeking help, as they may believe that their experiences set them apart from the rest of the civilian population. The result is a widening gap between those who suffer in silence and the resources they need to heal.

Breaking the Cycle: Addressing Stigma and Promoting Support

Breaking the stigma surrounding mental health in the military requires a multifaceted approach. First and foremost, the military itself must create a culture that encourages mental-health awareness and support. This can be achieved through leadership initiatives that emphasize the importance of seeking help when needed, without fear of judgment or reprisal. By normalizing mental healthcare as a vital aspect of overall wellbeing, the military can help reduce the stigma that prevents many veterans from seeking treatment.

Additionally, mental healthcare resources need to be more accessible and tailored to the unique needs of veterans. While there are programs in place, such as the VA mental health services, many veterans still face long wait times or logistical challenges in accessing care.

Ensuring that veterans have timely and effective access to mental health support is essential in mitigating the long-term effects of PTSX and other mental health conditions.

Furthermore, society at large must become more educated about PTSX and other mental health issues that affect veterans. Public awareness campaigns, educational programs and media representation can help dispel the misconceptions that contribute to stigma.

When society begins to view mental health struggles as a normal response to extraordinary circumstances rather than a sign of weakness or danger, veterans may feel more comfortable seeking help.

Barriers to Accessing Treatment

Even when veterans are ready to seek help, they often face significant barriers to accessing mental-health services. One of the most prominent challenges is the bureaucratic and logistical complexity of navigating the VA system. Veterans who rely on the VA for healthcare often encounter long wait times, limited availability of mental health professionals and bureaucratic hurdles that delay treatment.

Long Wait Times: Due to the high demand for mental-health services, many veterans face long wait times to see a therapist or psychiatrist. For veterans in crisis, these delays can be detrimental, leading to worsening symptoms or even suicidal thoughts.

Geographical Barriers: Veterans who live in rural or remote areas may have limited access to VA facilities, making it difficult to attend regular therapy sessions. Telehealth services have helped bridge this gap in some cases, but the lack of internet access in certain areas can still be a significant obstacle.

Financial Challenges: While many veterans are eligible for VA benefits, the cost of private mental-health services can be prohibitive for those who do not qualify for full VA coverage. The financial strain of seeking treatment outside the VA system can discourage veterans from pursuing the care they need.

Complexity of the VA System: Navigating the VA system can be a daunting task for veterans, particularly those dealing with mental-health issues. The paperwork, appointments and approvals required to access these services can be overwhelming, leading some veterans to give up on seeking treatment altogether.

Impact on Personal and Professional Life

PTSX affects every aspect of a veteran's life, from their personal relationships to their professional careers. Veterans with untreated PTSX often struggle to maintain steady employment, as symptoms such as irritability, difficulty concentrating and emotional outbursts can interfere with their ability to perform in the workplace. This can lead to financial instability, which in turn exacerbates feelings of stress and anxiety.

On a personal level, PTSX can strain relationships with family members, friends and loved ones. Veterans may become emotionally withdrawn, irritable or prone to angry outbursts, which can create tension and conflict in their relationships. Loved ones may struggle to understand the veteran's behavior, leading to feelings of isolation on both sides.

The emotional toll of PTSX on families is significant, as partners and children may experience secondary trauma from living with a loved one who is suffering from PTSX. Family members often take on the role of caregivers, which can lead to burnout and strained relationships over time.

Veterans' Reluctance to Seek Help

Many veterans view seeking mental-health treatment as a last resort, often waiting until their symptoms have become unbearable. This reluctance to seek help is influenced by a variety of factors, including fear of being seen as weak, concerns about the impact on their military career and mistrust of mental-health professionals and the VA.

For active-duty personnel, there is often a fear that seeking treatment for PTSX will result in negative career consequences. Veterans may worry that disclosing their mental-health struggles will affect their ability to advance in rank or lead to discharge from the military.

This fear can lead to a "suck it up" mentality, where veterans believe they should be able to handle their trauma without assistance. Additionally, some veterans express skepticism or mistrust of mental-health professionals, particularly those who do not have military experience.

Veterans may feel that civilian therapists cannot fully understand the unique challenges of military life and combat, leading to feelings of frustration or disconnection in therapy.

Finding a therapist who is knowledgeable about military culture and PTSX is crucial for establishing trust and creating a safe space for veterans to open up about their experiences.

If-Then Guidance

- If you are a veteran struggling with mental-health issues but hesitant to seek help due to the perception of weakness, then remind yourself that seeking treatment is an act of strength and resilience.
- Overcoming the stigma of mental health is crucial for healing and is just as important as physical recovery after combat.
- If you fear being judged or ostracized by peers for seeking mental-health support, then look for veteran-specific support groups or mental-health services where you can receive care in a safe, understanding, and non-judgmental environment. These groups are designed to assist veterans in seeking care without fear of judgment.
- If you feel shame or guilt about seeking help, then understand that these feelings are common among veterans due to military culture, but they should not prevent you from receiving the treatment you need and deserve. Speak with a therapist or counselor who can help you reframe these emotions and see that taking care of your mental health is a sign of responsibility and courage. Simply put, change the way you think about the situation, then act from this new frame of mind. Release the shame or guilt and adopt a new-found strength. Your personal power will be the fuel that guides you.
- If you are a victim of abuse within the military and fear retaliation for seeking help, then consider reporting the abuse to confidential resources such as the Military Crisis Line or VA services that specialize in supporting survivors. These organizations are structured to protect your privacy and ensure you receive the help you need without facing further harm or reprisal.
- If you are worried that seeking mental healthcare could negatively impact your military career or identity, then remember that early intervention is key to long-term wellbeing. Addressing your healthcare needs now can prevent more serious issues down the road and allow you to continue serving, or transition to civilian life in a healthier state of mind.

- If you are struggling to access care due to concerns about involuntary separation from the military, then explore your legal rights and the options available through military and veteran organizations that advocate for the rights of servicemembers. These groups can help you navigate the process while minimizing the risk of unfair treatment or separation.
- If you are concerned that military culture is preventing you from seeking the healthcare you need, then consider speaking with other veterans who have gone through similar challenges. Their experiences and insights may help you realize that seeking help is not a sign of weakness but rather a necessary step toward recovery and wellbeing.

Take the Next Step

- Acknowledge the Stigma: Recognize the cultural barriers that may be stopping you from seeking help, such as fear of appearing weak. Combat these thoughts by reminding yourself that seeking treatment is a sign of strength. Change the way you look at things. It will change your life for the better.
- Confide in a Trusted Leader: If you're on active duty, consider talking to a trusted superior officer about health concerns. They can provide guidance on how to access treatment without impacting your career.
- Use Confidential Services: Find confidential mental healthcare services offered by the VA or other veteran organizations if privacy is a concern.

Through Their Eyes

"Back when I was in [the service], you didn't talk about needing help—no matter how much the memories weighed you down. We were soldiers, built to endure. Admitting to PTSX or any mental struggle felt like betrayal to everything I'd trained for. But let me tell you—pushing it all down only works for so long. The battlefield changes you, no doubt about it. And just like any other injury, the mind can only take so much before it breaks.

"For years, I thought that asking for help would make me weaker in the eyes of my brothers. The truth is, the strength I found in finally getting help—it's the same strength that got me through the toughest missions. We don't fight alone in war, and we shouldn't fight these battles alone either. If you're struggling, know this: there's no shame in seeking the help you've earned."

—Sergeant John M., US Marine Corps (ret.)

12

Active and Passive Suicide in US Military Personnel and Veterans

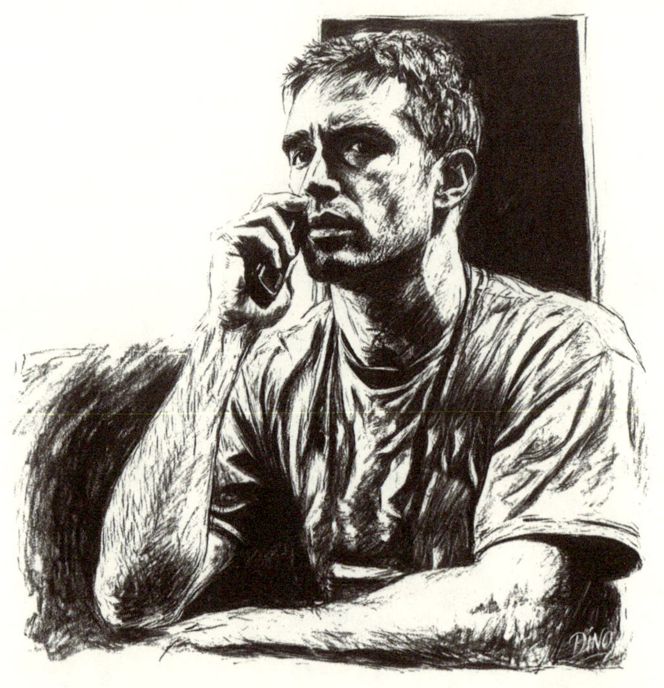

Ricardo stared at the phone in his hand, debating whether to make the call. A former Army medic, he had done three tours in high-conflict zones.

He'd patched up friends in the middle of firefights, telling them, "Hang in there—it'll be okay." But now, back home in his quiet apartment, he wasn't sure he believed his own words anymore. Days slipped by in a fog. Nights became stretches of endless worry that he couldn't outrun.

He avoided family gatherings. His mother called often, leaving voicemails that grew shorter each time. His father left texts like "Checking in, son," which Ricardo never answered. He felt like a burden.

More than once, he thought maybe everyone would be better off if he just disappeared, so he made out a plan to do so, wrote a detailed list of how to do it. He kept the note in a locked box in his garage.

One afternoon, Ricardo found himself at a small veterans' support center. He slumped in a corner chair, waiting for his turn with the intake counselor. Across the room sat Grace, an Air Force veteran he'd never met. She gave him a nod—no words, just a silent, understanding gesture that said, "I've been there too."

When he finally spoke with the counselor, Ricardo surprised himself by admitting he couldn't sleep, and couldn't shake dark thoughts. The counselor listened without judgment. She explained that he wasn't alone, that many veterans faced similar struggles, and that there were ways to find hope: support groups, crisis hotlines, therapy designed specifically for PTSX and depression, and even new treatments offering real promise.

Walking out, Ricardo paused by a bulletin board crowded with phone numbers and flyers. For the first time in weeks, he felt something other than hopelessness—a tiny spark that maybe, just maybe, things could change.

This chapter will explore the many contributing factors to this tragic reality, the mental-health challenges faced by military personnel and veterans, and the current and emerging interventions aimed at prevention. The goal is to shed light on the complexities of both active and passive suicide, while also offering hope through the identification of solutions that can make a real difference.

What is Going On Here!?

Suicide among US military personnel and veterans is a deeply concerning issue, one that impacts not only the individuals directly involved but also their families, communities and the broader society. The gravity of this issue stems from the unique challenges faced by military members, both during active duty and as veterans transitioning back into civilian life. While the nation holds its military in high esteem, the mental-health struggles faced by servicemembers are often less visible, though no less critical. The statistics are staggering. Results from recent studies indicate that military personnel and veterans are at a significantly higher risk of suicide compared to their civilian counterparts.

For example, the *2022 Annual Report* from the Department of Defense (DoD) on suicide shows that the suicide rate among active-duty members was 24.3 per 100,000 in 2021, while the rate for veterans was around 31.6 per 100,000, far exceeding the national average of 14 per 100,000. These statistics do not include passive suicide, which is discussed in detail below.

Moral injury detonates when good people survive bad orders. Only truth-telling in circles of trust can defuse the guilt and let conscience stand at ease.

The Silent Surrender—Confronting Passive Suicide in Our Warriors

Suicide in the active-duty, veteran and first-responder communities is often envisioned as a singular, violent act—a tragic, definitive end. But there is a far more common and insidious killer at work, one that doesn't leave a note or a clear moment of crisis. Passive suicide is a slow, methodical surrender to despair, masked as recklessness, apathy, or neglect. It is death by a thousand cuts, a quiet demolition of the self that is often missed by clinicians and loved ones until it is too late. For every warrior we lose to a recognized suicide, there are others who are simply, quietly, letting go.

This may not be a conscious choice to die, but rather an abandonment of the will to live. It is the diabetic veteran who "forgets" his insulin. It is the retired police officer who drinks himself into liver failure. It is the former Army Ranger who drives his motorcycle at 120 mph on a winding road, not seeking death, but indifferent to its arrival. These are symptoms of a loss of mission and a hollowing out of purpose.

The Anatomy of a Slow Surrender

For warriors and first-responders, life is defined by structure, mission and hypervigilance. The transition away from that high-stakes environment can leave a void that is often filled with self-destructive behaviors. These manifestations of passive suicide generally fall into three categories:

- Physiological Neglect: The body, once a tool for mission accomplishment, becomes an object of neglect. This includes blatant non-compliance with medical treatment for serious conditions like heart disease, diabetes, or cancer. It also encompasses chronic substance abuse where the goal is not a temporary high, but a permanent numbness, regardless of the physical cost. It's a low-grade, long-term poisoning of the self.
- Reckless Indifference: Many veterans and first-responders are "adrenaline-adapted." In the absence of a mission, they may subconsciously seek that same physiological arousal through reckless means. This isn't necessarily thrill-seeking, but a flirtation with oblivion. It manifests as extreme speeding, provoking confrontations, or engaging in dangerous activities without precaution. They aren't trying to die, but they have stopped actively trying to survive.
- The Quiet Retreat: This is the social and emotional component of the surrender. It involves systematically severing protective social bonds, withdrawing from family and friends, and abandoning hobbies and routines. It is a conscious or subconscious dismantling of one's own support system, leaving the individual isolated and adrift. It is the warrior who stops answering the phone, who lets his world shrink to the four walls of his home, effectively "giving up" long before his body does.

The Challenge of "Hidden" Suicides

The concept of passive suicide, also known as "sub-intentional suicide," suggests that the true number of self-inflicted deaths is likely higher. These are deaths that may be officially classified as accidents, natural causes, or undetermined, but are the result of behaviors where the individual was indifferent to their survival. Examples of deaths that could be considered passive suicide include:

- Fatal single-vehicle accidents where the driver was engaging in reckless behavior.
- "Accidental" overdoses from drugs or alcohol where the individual was consistently abusing substances with a disregard for the consequences.
- Deaths from manageable chronic illnesses like diabetes or heart disease, where the individual deliberately neglected their treatment.

Estimating the "Hidden" Number

There is no definitive way to calculate the exact number of passive suicides. However, some researchers and experts have tried to estimate the prevalence of these "hidden" suicides. Some studies suggest that the number of sub-intentional suicides could be equal to or even greater than the number of officially recorded suicides.

Considering this, a conservative estimate could place the number of passive suicides among veterans at a similar rate to active suicides. This would mean an additional 17 to 18 veterans per day could be dying from passive suicide. A more aggressive estimate could put this number even higher.

While a precise figure is unattainable, it is reasonable to estimate that in addition to the 17.6 officially recorded veteran suicides each day, a comparable number of veterans may be dying by passive suicide. This would suggest that the total number of veterans taking their own lives, both actively and passively, could be 35 to 50 per day. It's important to state that this is an *estimate*. The lack of formal tracking for passive suicide means the true number is unknown and likely to remain so.

However, this estimate underscores the gravity of the mental-health crisis facing the veteran community and highlights the need for a broader understanding of suicide that includes these more subtle forms of self-destruction. Regardless of whether the rate is 17 per day or 50 per day, losing an active-duty servicemember or veteran—a loved one, friend or colleague—is devastating and a great loss to all of us.

A Mandate for Healthcare Professionals: From Awareness to Action

Handling passive suicide requires a radical shift in clinical practice, moving from reactive crisis intervention to proactive pattern recognition. The healthcare professional is on the front line of this fight and must adopt a new set of protocols.

Look Beyond the Chart: Clinicians must learn to see the constellation, not just the individual stars. A missed appointment, a refusal to fill a prescription, a high-risk hobby mentioned in passing—viewed in isolation, these are minor issues. Viewed together, they form the clear pattern of a silent surrender.

The central question must shift from "Are you having thoughts of harming yourself?" to "What are you doing to sustain yourself?" Ask the hard questions. Inquiry must be direct and probe for apathy and indifference.

- Instead of: "Are you taking your medication?" Ask: "How important is it to you, on a scale of 1 to 10, to manage your blood pressure right now?"
- Instead of: "Do you have hobbies?" Ask: "What's the most reckless thing you've done in the last month?"

Follow up on mentions of substance use with questions about consequence: "When you drink, are you concerned about what it's doing to your health long-term?"

Reframe Health as a Mission: For a warrior, a mission provides purpose. Clinicians must frame healthcare not as a passive process of receiving treatment, but as an active, honorable mission: the maintenance of their most critical piece of equipment—themselves. Treatment plans become mission objectives. Health metrics become key performance indicators. This reframes the entire dynamic from one of victimhood to one of agency and duty.

Integrate Mental and Physical Health: Passive suicide exists at the deadly intersection of physical and mental health. A primary care physician who notes a pattern of medical self-sabotage must treat it as a mental health emergency and initiate a warm handoff to a psychological health specialist. Likewise, therapists must inquire about their patients' physical health and medical adherence.

The wall between the two disciplines must be torn down; for this population, the mind and body are inextricable casualties of the same war. Confronting passive suicide means recognizing that the deadliest scars of service are often the ones that fester quietly, far from any visible battlefield. It requires us to listen to the silence, to see the patterns in the chaos, and to offer not just a remedy, but a renewed mission: the mission to live.

Risk Factors

Suicide is rarely the result of a single factor and, for military personnel and veterans, a combination of service-related, institutional and psychosocial challenges contribute to this heightened risk. One of the most well-known contributors to suicide risk among military personnel is exposure to combat. The psychological toll of experiencing life-threatening situations, witnessing the death of comrades, and participating in combat can lead to long-lasting mental health issues.

These include PTSX, which is closely linked to suicide risk. PTSX is reported to affect an estimated 10-20% of veterans, particularly those who have experienced combat or other traumatic events during their service. Many professionals feel that the rate is much higher than reported: 50% or more.

Traumatic Brain Injury (TBI) is another significant risk factor. TBIs can occur from exposure to explosions, accidents or direct combat, and have been shown to increase the likelihood of depression, anxiety and suicidal behavior. Veterans with a history of moderate to severe TBI are more than twice as likely to die by suicide compared to those without such injuries. In addition to physical trauma, moral injury—a relatively newer diagnosis—plays a critical role in the mental-health struggles of military personnel.

Moral injury occurs when individuals are involved in, witness or fail to prevent events that transgress deeply held moral beliefs. This can lead to profound feelings of guilt, shame and a loss of meaning, all of which are factors that increase vulnerability to suicide.

Institutional and Cultural Factors

The military culture emphasizes resilience, strength and self-reliance, values that are essential on the battlefield but can be detrimental when it comes to mental health. Stigma surrounding mental healthcare in the military remains a significant barrier to seeking help. Servicemembers often fear that admitting to mental-health struggles could negatively impact their careers or lead to a loss of respect among their peers. The transition from military to civilian life can also be fraught with difficulties.

Many veterans struggle with the loss of identity and purpose after leaving the service, and this can lead to a sense of isolation and hopelessness. Additionally, the structure and camaraderie of military life may be replaced by uncertainty, unemployment or underemployment, all of which can increase stress and the risk of suicidal ideation.

It's often difficult, if not impossible, for a servicemember to find in civilian life the high level of closeness and camaraderie they experienced in the military. Another important factor is the higher rate of firearm ownership among military personnel and veterans. Firearms are the most common method of suicide in this population, accounting for nearly 70% of veteran suicides.

Access to lethal means is a well-established risk factor for suicide, and the widespread availability of firearms in military households significantly raises the danger of impulsive suicide attempts. Those veterans are hypervigilant and feel they must protect their family and themselves. The terrible irony is that the enemy that ends up killing them is the veteran himself.

Psychosocial Factors

Social isolation is a common problem among veterans, particularly those who have retired or separated from the service. Loss of close relationships with fellow servicemembers can lead to feelings of alienation and loneliness. Veterans who struggle to find work or who face financial difficulties are also at higher risk, with unemployment and poverty strongly correlated with increased suicide risk.

Also, family and relationship issues, including divorce or estrangement from loved ones, are often major stressors that contribute to suicidal behavior. Chronic physical pain or disability, common among veterans who have sustained injuries during service, further exacerbates the risk, leading to depression, feelings of helplessness and substance abuse.

Mental Health Challenges and Common Diagnoses

The mental-health diagnoses most commonly associated with suicide in military populations include PTSX, depression and anxiety. These conditions frequently co-occur with other problems, such as substance abuse or physical injuries like TBI, creating complex and multifaceted challenges for both servicemembers and veterans.

Among veterans, PTSX is particularly prevalent, especially for those who served in high-intensity combat roles. The symptoms of PTSX—flashbacks, nightmares, hypervigilance and emotional numbness—are not only distressing but also debilitating, often interfering with the ability to work, maintain relationships, and engage in daily activities.

Depression is another critical factor. The feeling of hopelessness, a core symptom of major depressive disorder, is a strong predictor of suicidal behavior. Depression may develop or worsen following traumatic experiences during service, or as a result of difficulties faced in adjusting to civilian life.

The availability of mental healthcare during active duty varies depending on several factors, including location, rank, and military branch. While the DoD has made some effort to improve mental healthcare for active-duty personnel, including providing access to counseling, screening for PTSX, and offering treatment for substance abuse, significant barriers remain.

Plus, large budget cuts in defense and VA spending have removed many of these programs altogether, leaving active-duty personnel and veterans in the dark. Perhaps worse, the stigma around seeking care, along with concerns about confidentiality and potential career consequences, continues to deter many from accessing the help they need.

Mental Healthcare for Veterans

Early intervention is key to preventing suicide. Ensuring that military personnel and veterans have access to high-quality mental healthcare, both during and after service, is essential. Mental healthcare programs that offer evidence-based treatments, such as cognitive-behavioral therapy and exposure therapy for PTSX, have been shown to significantly reduce symptoms and lower suicide risk.

Veterans, particularly those who rely on the VA for healthcare, often face long wait times and challenges in accessing adequate mental healthcare. Despite the VA's commitment to addressing mental health issues, including PTSX and suicide prevention, systemic issues such as understaffing, budget constraints, and bureaucratic hurdles remain problematic.

In addition, many veterans live in rural areas where access to VA services can be limited. Telehealth options, especially for those with Medicaid, have decreased significantly, so more and more veterans face difficulties in getting timely and appropriate care.

Non-VA options, including community mental healthcare and private care, can help fill the gap. However, depending on one's state of residence and the quality of VA healthcare there, veterans may be unable to see outside providers and also may not have access to telehealth services.

Protective Factors

Despite the numerous risk factors, there are several protective factors that can reduce the likelihood of suicide among military personnel and veterans. One of the most effective protective factors during service is the sense of camaraderie and mutual support within military units. Peer support can help reduce feelings of isolation and offer an outlet for discussing mental health struggles in a non-judgmental environment. Veterans who maintain strong connections with their military peers often report lower levels of depression and suicidal ideation.

A supportive family environment is a crucial buffer against suicide risk. Families can provide emotional and practical support, helping veterans navigate the challenges of post-service life. It is also important that family members receive education and resources to understand the mental-health challenges their loved ones face, enabling them to respond effectively to signs of distress.

Resilience-Building Programs

The military has developed several resilience-building programs aimed at enhancing the psychological wellbeing of its members. These programs focus on equipping servicemembers with coping skills to manage stress, adapt to challenges, and bounce back from adversity. Resilience training, which often includes mindfulness, problem-solving, and emotional regulation techniques, has been integrated into pre-deployment preparation and post-deployment reintegration programs, with promising results in reducing healthcare issues and suicidal behavior.

Special Populations

Certain groups within the military and veteran populations face unique challenges that can further elevate their risk for suicide. Women in the military can experience unique stressors that contribute to their mental-health challenges. Female veterans are more likely than their male counterparts to report sexual trauma during service, a factor closely linked to PTSX, depression and suicidal ideation.

Although female veterans have a lower overall suicide rate than males, they are more likely to attempt suicide, underscoring the importance of targeted prevention efforts for this population. This topic is discussed in depth in a dedicated chapter ahead.

Racial and ethnic minority veterans, as well as LGBTQ+ servicemembers, often face discrimination and minority stress, both during their service and in civilian life. This can exacerbate feelings of isolation, increase mental-health problems, and heighten suicide risk. Suicide-prevention efforts must take into account the unique needs of these populations and provide culturally competent care that addresses their specific challenges.

Aging veterans, particularly those from earlier conflicts such as the Vietnam War and Gulf War, are also at elevated risk for suicide. The loss of physical independence, the onset of chronic health problems, and the deaths of spouses or peers can contribute to feelings of despair in older veterans. Mental-health services for older veterans must include both medical and psychological support to address these multifaceted challenges.

The Role of Firearms

Firearms play a significant role in suicide among military personnel and veterans. As stated previously, approximately 70% of veteran suicides involve firearms, compared to around 50% of suicides in the general population. The lethal nature of firearms means that suicide attempts with guns are far more likely to be fatal than other methods. This makes it critical to address firearm safety as part of suicide-prevention efforts.

Encouraging safe storage of firearms or removing them altogether can reduce the likelihood of impulsive suicide attempts. Several initiatives have been developed to educate veterans and their families about the importance of securing firearms in the home. Programs that provide gun locks, safes, and other tools for limiting access to firearms have been shown to be effective in reducing the risk of suicide.

Unfortunately, the plain fact is, if a veteran wants to take their life, they will. And no amount of preventive measures will stop them. But for the majority of veterans (and civilians), there are excellent ways to prevent suicide, not the least of which is to remove all dangerous weapons from a veteran's home.

One can do this without law enforcement getting involved. Once they are called, a tough situation can escalate to one that goes out of control. Suicidal veterans should be identified as such, then brought into a healthcare facility for evaluation. Family members can play a major role in safe intervention to ensure a veteran does not end up in jail.

VA Suicide Prevention Programs

The VA has developed several suicide prevention programs specifically for veterans, including the Veterans Crisis Line, which provides 24/7 support for veterans in crisis. In addition to crisis intervention, the VA is working to expand access to mental healthcare through the implementation of telehealth services and mobile clinics that can reach veterans in rural areas.

Community-based and non-governmental organizations play a critical role in supporting veterans' mental health. Many of these organizations offer peer-support programs, where veterans can connect with others who understand their experiences. These programs provide a safe space for veterans to talk about their struggles without fear of judgment, and have been shown to significantly reduce feelings of isolation and despair. For those who don't like being around people or groups or crowds, please look into one-on-one care and healing. Even though you may be "different," you still need soul care.

Emerging Treatments and Technologies

Advances in technology are opening up new avenues for suicide prevention. Artificial intelligence (AI) tools are being used to identify veterans at risk of suicide based on patterns in their health data, allowing for earlier intervention.

Innovative treatments, such as psychedelic-assisted therapy and virtual reality-based PTSX treatments, are also being explored as potential solutions to the mental health challenges faced by veterans.

Barriers to Suicide Prevention

Despite the progress being made, several barriers continue to hinder effective suicide prevention efforts for military personnel and veterans. We've said this before and it bears repeating. One of the most significant barriers is the ongoing stigma surrounding mental health in military culture.

The expectation of stoicism and toughness prevents individuals from seeking help, as they fear being perceived as weak or unfit for duty. Efforts to shift this culture are ongoing, but change is slow. Within both the DoD and the VA, there are gaps in care that need to be addressed. These include long wait times for mental healthcare appointments, insufficient staffing, and complex bureaucratic processes that can delay or prevent veterans from receiving the care they need.

Veterans living in rural or remote areas often face difficulties accessing mental-health services due to a lack of providers in their area. While telehealth has helped bridge this gap, not all veterans have reliable internet access or are comfortable using telehealth platforms.

Training Gaps for Healthcare Providers

Another issue is that not all healthcare providers are adequately trained in the unique mental-health challenges faced by military personnel and veterans. This lack of specialized knowledge can lead to misdiagnoses or inappropriate treatment plans, further exacerbating the problem.

The distinct nature of military culture, combined with the complexities of trauma exposure, requires providers to have a deep understanding of conditions like PTSX, traumatic brain injury, moral injury and the impacts of combat stress. Without this knowledge, well-meaning clinicians may fail to recognize the full extent of a veteran's experiences or symptoms.

For example, PTSX symptoms in veterans may differ significantly from those in civilians, often manifesting in hypervigilance, emotional numbing, or intense feelings of guilt related to moral injury. Healthcare providers unfamiliar with military experiences may overlook these nuances, diagnosing veterans with general anxiety or depression without addressing the root cause, leading to treatments that are ineffective or even harmful. What makes it even more challenging is that a veteran may not know the limitations of healthcare workers. So a veteran cannot advocate on their own behalf.

In addition, the stigma within the military surrounding mental health often complicates the treatment process. Veterans may be reluctant to disclose the full scope of their experiences or symptoms, fearing judgment or that their concerns will not be understood. Providers untrained in military mental health may unintentionally reinforce these fears by failing to create an environment where veterans feel safe discussing their experiences.

This can result in fragmented care, where the veteran's mental health deteriorates rather than improves. Moreover, there is often a gap in understanding the interplay between physical and psychological injuries. Many veterans suffer from both TBI and PTSX, and treating one without addressing the other can lead to suboptimal outcomes.

Case Studies and Personal Accounts

Real-life stories from veterans and their families highlight the human impact of the suicide crisis, while also offering hope. Many veterans who have survived suicide attempts describe the importance of having a strong support system, access to mental health care, and the role of peer connections in their recovery. Similarly, family members often emphasize the need for greater awareness and education to recognize the signs of suicide risk. High-profile cases of veteran suicide have also brought greater attention to this issue, prompting public outcry and calls for action. These cases serve as a reminder of the urgent need for comprehensive and effective suicide prevention efforts.

Future Directions Research Needs

Further research is essential to better understand the full scope of the suicide crisis among military personnel and veterans. Suicide is a complex and multifaceted issue, with numerous contributing factors that vary across different subgroups of veterans based on their service experiences, demographics and personal histories.

Longitudinal studies that track mental-health outcomes over time are particularly valuable, as they provide insight into how various risk factors—such as combat exposure, trauma, PTSX, and transitions out of the military—interact over the long term.

These studies can help identify periods of heightened vulnerability for suicide risk, such as during the immediate post-deployment period or after separation from service, allowing for the development of targeted interventions at critical points in veterans' lives. In addition to tracking mental-health outcomes, research focused on the efficacy of different treatment methods is critical for developing more effective prevention strategies.

Current treatments for PTSX, depression and other mental health conditions vary widely in their success rates, and not all veterans respond equally to available therapies. For example, while evidence-based treatments like cognitive-behavioral therapy and exposure therapy are beneficial for many, some veterans may not find relief through these traditional approaches.

Research into alternative therapies—such as ketamine infusions, MDMA-assisted therapy and stellate ganglion block—shows promise, but larger, more comprehensive studies are needed to determine the long-term effectiveness of these emerging treatments, particularly for preventing suicide. And those studies require significant funding, something the pharmaceutical industry is not currently supporting.

Furthermore, research should focus on the role of social determinants of health in veteran suicide. Factors like housing stability, employment, access to healthcare, and social support networks all influence mental health outcomes, yet their specific impacts on suicide risk among veterans are not fully understood.

Studies that examine how these factors interact with mental healthcare could lead to more holistic approaches to care that address not only the psychological aspects of suicide prevention but also the broader social and economic contexts in which veterans live. Finally, greater attention needs to be paid to the experiences of underrepresented groups within the veteran population, including women, LGBTQ+ veterans, and veterans from minority racial or ethnic backgrounds.

These groups may face unique stressors that elevate their suicide risk, but they are often underrepresented in research. Ensuring that future studies include diverse populations is key to developing prevention strategies that are inclusive and effective for all veterans.

Policy Recommendations

Legislative reforms are needed to ensure that veterans receive timely and appropriate care. Currently, many veterans face significant delays in accessing mental-health services, and these gaps in care can have life-threatening consequences, especially for those at risk of suicide. Increased funding for the VA is essential to address these issues.

Additional resources are needed to hire more mental-health professionals, reduce patient wait times, and enhance the VA's capacity to serve the growing number of veterans in need of care. More than ever, these issues must be addressed, as the number of veterans entering the VA healthcare system is larger than ever before. What's more, cuts to VA funding loom large and threaten to undermine even current VA research and treatment programs, especially those for suicide. The question then becomes: what are we willing to do to prevent active and passive suicide?

Telehealth has already proven to be an effective tool for connecting veterans with healthcare providers, and additional support for these programs would significantly enhance care delivery in underserved areas. Improving coordination between the DoD and the VA is also crucial to ensure continuity of care during the transition from active duty to civilian life.

Patients fall through the cracks during this critical period, particularly as they navigate the complexities of leaving the military healthcare system and entering the VA system. Legislative reforms should focus on creating a seamless handoff of medical records, ensuring that veterans do not experience gaps in mental healthcare when transitioning from military to civilian life.

Many veterans struggle to access the benefits and services they are entitled to due to complex, time-consuming application processes. Simplifying these procedures and providing more proactive support to veterans navigating the VA system would help ensure they receive the care they need in a timely manner.

Moreover, expanding eligibility for mental-health services to veterans who may not meet strict service-related criteria would ensure that more individuals receive help, particularly those who may have been dishonorably discharged due to untreated mental-health issues.

Overall, legislative reforms must prioritize the mental health and wellbeing of veterans by increasing resources, expanding access to care, improving coordination between military and civilian health systems, and simplifying access to services. Such measures are essential to providing veterans with the timely, comprehensive care they deserve.

Expanding Community-Based Support

Veteran peer networks and family support systems are an important part of the solution to addressing the mental healthcare challenges faced by military personnel and veterans. These networks offer a unique form of support, as they are built on shared experiences, mutual understanding, and trust. Veterans often feel more comfortable opening up to fellow veterans who have gone through similar hardships, including combat exposure, post-deployment struggles, and the difficulties of transitioning back to civilian life.

The sense of camaraderie that develops in these peer networks can be a lifeline for veterans who may feel isolated or misunderstood in traditional healthcare settings. By expanding community-based mental healthcare and providing more resources for peer-support programs, veterans can receive the care they need even outside of clinical environments. Peer-support activities, which are typically run by veterans for veterans, offer an informal yet effective means of addressing mental-health concerns.

These programs can take various forms, including group therapy sessions, one-on-one mentorship, or even online forums where veterans can connect and share their experiences. Peer support is not meant to replace professional care but to complement it by offering a safe and relatable environment where veterans can feel heard and understood. Often, veterans in these groups are referred to healthcare professionals.

Family support systems are equally vital. Family members, often the first to notice signs of mental health distress, play a critical role in encouraging veterans to seek help and providing ongoing emotional support. Expanding resources for families, such as education on the signs of PTSX and depression, coping strategies, and access to family counseling, can significantly improve outcomes for veterans. When families are empowered with the right tools and knowledge, they are better equipped to support their loved ones through the recovery process.

Community-based mental healthcare and peer networks also help bridge gaps in care, particularly for veterans who may have limited access to VA services or prefer to seek support outside of formal healthcare institutions. For example, veterans in rural or underserved areas may find it difficult to travel to VA facilities for regular appointments, but peer-support groups within their communities can provide accessible and immediate assistance.

By creating strong local networks, communities can offer veterans a sense of belonging and purpose, which are critical in combating feelings of isolation, depression and suicidal ideation. Moreover, peer-support programs can be especially effective for veterans who are hesitant to engage with traditional mental-health services due to stigma or mistrust of the healthcare system.

The informal nature of peer-led programs can break down these barriers, making it easier for veterans to seek help without fear of judgment. These programs also offer a degree of flexibility that traditional healthcare settings may lack, allowing veterans to access support in a manner that aligns with their comfort levels and schedules.

So by expanding community-based mental healthcare and increasing resources for both peer and family support systems, we can create a more comprehensive and inclusive approach to veteran mental healthcare. These efforts not only complement traditional healthcare but also provide accessible, relatable, and effective avenues for veterans to receive the support they need, ultimately contributing to better mental-health outcomes and a stronger sense of community among veterans and their families.

A holistic approach to suicide prevention recognizes that mental health is influenced by multiple factors, including physical health, social support and a sense of purpose. Programs that address all aspects of veterans' wellbeing—mental, physical and spiritual—are more likely to be successful in reducing suicide rates.

Suicide Among Special Operations Warriors: A Hidden Struggle

The warriors of United States Special Operations Forces (SOF)—Special Forces (Green Berets), Navy SEALs, Army Rangers, Air Force Pararescue Jumpers, and Combat Controllers and other elite units—are widely regarded as the epitome of strength, resilience and valor. Trained to operate in the most hostile environments and to engage in missions that often defy the limits of human endurance, these operators are the very embodiment of courage under fire.

Yet, beneath the surface of their unparalleled bravery lies a grave and often unspoken reality, the alarming rates of suicide among members of the special-operations community. Unlike their counterparts in conventional forces, special-operations warriors face unique stressors that compound the typical challenges of military service. The high demands placed upon these individuals, combined with the psychological toll of repeated and extended deployments and very high operational tempo, often result in profound mental and emotional strain.

These operators are trained to adapt, survive and excel in environments of chaos and danger, the very skills that make us formidable in combat become liabilities when we transition back to civilian life or even during periods of downtime between missions. How does one go from hunting down bad guys thousands of miles from loved ones to shopping for sundries at your local store?

The Burden of Expectations and Hypermasculinity

One of the defining characteristics of special-operations soldiers is their unwavering commitment to the mission, their team and their country. This sense of duty, while admirable, can sometimes transform into an immense psychological burden.

The expectation to perform at an elite level, to never falter, and to continually meet the rigorous demands of their role creates an environment where seeking help is perceived as a sign of weakness. In a culture that values stoicism and resilience, many warriors internalize their struggles rather than seek assistance. What they must learn in civilian life is that they are still a part of a highly functioning team. Just different.

This hypermasculine ethos—an intrinsic part of the special-operations identity—often inhibits open discussions about mental health. While the bonds forged between teammates in the field are strong, admitting vulnerability can be seen as a betrayal of the very identity that these warriors have cultivated over years of intense training and operational experience.

For many, the idea of reaching out for help or showing signs of emotional distress feels tantamount to failing their team, their country and, most of all, themselves. This perceived failure can, tragically, lead to feelings of isolation and hopelessness—two of the most dangerous precursors to suicide. Again, special-operations warriors must recognize and transition to a new team. A team dedicated to caring for and healing them.

Repeated Exposure to Trauma

Combat exposure and the high-risk nature of their missions further compound the issue. Special operations missions are often clandestine, operating in environments where death, injury and violence are everyday occurrences. Unlike conventional soldiers, who may experience intervals of relative safety, special-operations forces engage in a sustained and relentless pattern of deployment.

These frequent missions place warriors in life-threatening situations more often, with minimal recovery time in between. This constant exposure to traumatic events—whether the loss of a fellow operator, moral injuries sustained from actions taken during operations, or the inherent violence of their missions—creates a unique psychological toll that becomes a very real physical problem, that must be cared for an healed.

The human mind can only endure so much trauma before the effects begin to manifest, often in the form of PTSX, depression or anxiety. For many special operations warriors, the cumulative effect of these repeated traumas eventually becomes unbearable.

The Challenges of Reintegrating into Civilian Life

For those who manage to complete their service, the transition from the battlefield to civilian life poses yet another monumental challenge. After years of operating in high-adrenaline, high-stakes environments, many special operations warriors struggle with the comparatively mundane nature of civilian life. Perhaps worst of all, they have lost a close-knit family, their team and its individuals.

The sense of purpose, camaraderie and adrenaline-fueled combat that once defined their existence is suddenly gone, leaving a void that many find difficult to fill. Moreover, the skills that made them effective in combat—hypervigilance, aggression, emotional detachment—are often maladaptive in civilian settings.

This can lead to a deep sense of disconnection from society and even from loved ones. Feelings of purposelessness, combined with the weight of unresolved trauma, can create the conditions for severe depression and suicidal ideation. Tragically, many special-operations warriors feel that their only way to escape the psychological pain is through taking their own life, a sad fact that's demonstrated in the statistics of suicide.

Breaking the Silence

Addressing suicide within the special operations community requires a profound cultural shift. While there have been recent efforts to destigmatize mental-health struggles within the military, much work remains to be done, particularly within elite units. The key to reducing suicide rates among special operations warriors lies in creating an environment where seeking help is not viewed as weakness, but as an act of courage—one that is just as heroic as any act on the battlefield.

Equally important is providing targeted mental-health resources specifically designed for the unique experiences of special-operations personnel. These warriors need access to trauma-informed care that acknowledges the distinct psychological toll of their service. Initiatives like peer-support programs, where veterans of special operations can openly discuss their struggles with those who have walked the same path, are essential in breaking the cycle of silence and despair.

Ultimately, saving the lives of special operations warriors requires more than just addressing mental health at an individual level—it requires a collective commitment to changing the narrative around mental health in this storied and honored community. Only by doing so can we hope to stem the tide of suicide that continues to claim the lives of these extraordinary individuals.

Cutting-Edge Treatments for PTSX and Suicidal Behavior in Special Operations Warriors

In recent years, advances in mental-health treatment have begun to offer new hope for special-operations warriors grappling with PTSX and suicidal behavior. Traditional therapies, while effective for some, often fall short in addressing the unique and complex trauma endured by these elite soldiers. As a result, innovative and cutting-edge treatments are emerging to meet the specific needs of this population, focusing on both the physiological and psychological aspects of trauma.

Neurofeedback and Brain Stimulation Therapies

A promising area of treatment is the use of neurofeedback and brain stimulation therapies. Transcranial Magnetic Stimulation (TMS) and Deep Brain Stimulation (DBS) are non-invasive techniques that use electromagnetic fields to target specific areas of the brain associated with mood regulation and trauma processing.

These therapies have shown promising results in treating PTSX by rewiring neural pathways and restoring balance to the brain's activity. For veterans suffering from severe depression or suicidal thoughts, brain stimulation offers a breakthrough when traditional therapies or medications have failed to provide relief.

Psychedelic-Assisted Therapy

Another innovative approach that has gained traction is the use of psychedelic-assisted therapy, particularly with substances like MDMA (commonly known as Ecstasy) and psilocybin (the active ingredient in magic mushrooms). In clinical settings, these substances are administered under the guidance of trained therapists, allowing individuals to process deeply buried trauma.

For special-operations warriors, who often have difficulty accessing and confronting the full emotional weight of their experiences, these therapies offer a controlled environment to unpack their psychological burdens. Early clinical trials have shown significant reductions in PTSX symptoms and suicidal ideation, marking a promising step forward.

Integrative Approaches: Mind-Body Healing

Finally, integrative approaches like yoga, mindfulness and trauma-informed therapies continue to play an important role in the healing process. These practices help regulate the nervous system, promote emotional resilience, and restore a warrior's connection to their body, offering a holistic pathway to recovery.

Combining these therapies with cutting-edge medical interventions provides a comprehensive approach that addresses both the physical and emotional scars carried by these courageous individuals. These advances are not just treatments but lifelines, offering special-operations warriors a renewed sense of hope and the possibility of healing from the invisible wounds of war.

In addition to neurofeedback, brain stimulation and psychedelic-assisted therapies, other groundbreaking treatments are proving to be particularly effective for special-operations warriors facing PTSX and suicidal behavior. These innovative approaches target the neurological and physiological roots of trauma, offering rapid and sometimes life-saving results.

Ketamine Infusion Therapy

One treatment making waves in mental healthcare is ketamine infusion therapy. Originally developed as an anesthetic, ketamine has shown remarkable efficacy in treating severe depression and PTSX, particularly for individuals resistant to traditional medications. Ketamine works by modulating the brain's glutamate system, which is associated with synaptic plasticity and neural communication.

In contrast to standard antidepressants, which can take weeks or months to have an effect, ketamine often provides relief from suicidal thoughts and severe depression within hours of treatment. For special-operations warriors experiencing the overwhelming weight of combat trauma and emotional pain, this rapid response can be a critical intervention, reducing the risk of suicide in acute situations.

Dr. Eugene Lipov and Stellate Ganglion Block (SGB)

Another cutting-edge treatment gaining traction is stellate ganglion block (SGB), a procedure originally used to treat chronic pain. The stellate ganglia are two collections of nerve bundles on either side of the neck. They play a crucial role in regulating the body's fight-or-flight response, often over-active in individuals with PTSX.

By injecting a local anesthetic into each nerve cluster, SGB can reset a particular part of the sympathetic nervous system, dramatically reducing symptoms of hypervigilance, anxiety and trauma responses. This relatively simple, non-invasive procedure has been shown to provide immediate and long-lasting relief for many special-operations warriors, helping them regain control over their mental and emotional responses.

Unfortunately, not all military personnel and veterans respond to SGB. Twenty percent do not. Also, not all have access to this treatment via the military or VA. You can pay out of pocket for SGB, about $3,000 for Dual Sympathetic Reset (an advanced form of SGB), i.e. injections on both sides of the neck. We recommend Dr. Lipov at the Stella Clinic outside Chicago. He developed the procedure and has trained many other physicians across the country. We discuss Dr. Lipov and SGB in depth, in laters chapters.

Eye Movement Desensitization and Reprocessing (EMDR)

Another promising treatment, Eye Movement Desensitization and Reprocessing (EMDR), is widely used to address trauma by helping individuals reprocess distressing memories in a controlled manner. Special-operations warriors who have experienced repeated traumatic events can benefit from EMDR's ability to desensitize them to traumatic memories and alter how these memories are stored in the brain. Over time, this therapy reduces the emotional intensity associated with combat-related trauma, enabling warriors to lead more functional and peaceful lives.

Dr. Mark Gordon's Brain Rescue Therapy

Rather than treating the symptoms of PTSX and other maladies, Dr. Mark Gordon, an expert in neuroendocrinology, targets the molecular basis of these insults, using tried and true methods. His Brain Rescue 3 regimen of various amino acids, nootropics and nutrients have produced astounding results in people with TBI. Combined with other regimens, like hyperbaric oxygen therapy, Dr. Gordon's program provides even greater success rates among those worst affected by TBI.

Comprehensive Care and a Holistic Approach

These cutting-edge treatments, when combined with traditional therapies like cognitive-behavioral therapy and trauma-informed care, create a comprehensive approach that addresses the full spectrum of PTSX and suicidal behavior. Moreover, peer-support programs, where special-operations warriors can speak openly with others who have shared similar experiences, provide a crucial layer of emotional reinforcement. As these treatments become more widely available, they offer hope that special-operations veterans can heal from the invisible wounds of combat.

The integration of therapies such as ketamine infusions, SGB and EMDR, alongside novel approaches like psychedelic-assisted therapies, represents a significant shift in how the mental health of these brave individuals is addressed. This shift has the potential to reduce the devastating toll of PTSX and suicide among these warriors.

US Military Efforts for Active-Duty Special Operations Warriors

The US military has implemented several programs tailored to the needs of active-duty special-operations personnel, with a focus on both prevention and treatment. Acknowledging the need for mental healthcare that is specific to the experiences of elite forces, the military has integrated mental-health resources directly into special-operations units, ensuring that help is readily available in an environment that is familiar and trusted by the warriors.

One of the primary initiatives is embedding mental healthcare professionals in special-operations units to provide immediate care and confidential counseling. These professionals build rapport with the soldiers and can offer timely interventions to mitigate the early onset of PTSX symptoms and other mental-health issues.

This is particularly important for active-duty special-operations warriors, who often avoid seeking help due to the stigma of mental health struggles within military culture.

Additionally, the military has begun to implement cutting-edge medical treatments like ketamine infusions and SGB, as part of their mental healthcare offerings for special-operations personnel. These therapies, previously mentioned for their effectiveness in treating PTSX and suicidal behavior, are becoming more widely available within military treatment facilities. Active-duty warriors can receive these treatments while continuing their service, providing an immediate intervention for those struggling with severe symptoms.

The VA and Special Operations Veterans

For veterans who have left active-duty service, the VA plays a critical role in addressing the long-term mental health challenges associated with PTSX and suicidal behavior. The VA has made efforts to expand its range of mental healthcare services for veterans, including those from special operations backgrounds.

One of the primary strategies employed by the VA is the Veterans Crisis Line, a 24/7 service that provides immediate support for veterans experiencing suicidal ideation. Specially trained responders, many of whom are veterans themselves, offer counseling and crisis intervention services tailored to the unique needs of those who have served in special-operations roles.

This crisis line is a key component in the VA's broader suicide-prevention strategy, which aims to reduce the alarming rates of veteran suicide, particularly among those who have experienced multiple deployments or intense combat situations.

For ongoing treatment, the VA has expanded access to evidence-based therapies, including Cognitive Behavioral Therapy, Prolonged Exposure Therapy, and Eye Movement Desensitization and Reprocessing. These therapies are particularly effective in treating the emotional and cognitive aspects of PTSX, helping veterans process traumatic memories and reduce the symptoms that often lead to depression and suicidal behavior.

The VA's National Center for PTSX (https://www.ptsd.va.gov) has been at the forefront of developing these therapies and training VA clinicians nationwide to provide specialized care for veterans. In addition to traditional therapies, the VA is increasingly adopting innovative treatments like TMS and psychedelic-assisted therapies such as MDMA therapy.

The VA is also collaborating with research institutions to further study the effects of these cutting-edge treatments, ensuring that veterans have access to the most effective care available. Furthermore, the VA offers Vet Centers, which are community-based counseling centers specifically designed for combat veterans and their families. These centers provide confidential, no-cost mental healthcare services to help veterans transition from military to civilian life. For special-operations veterans who often experience difficulty adjusting to life after the military, Vet Centers offer a safe space to discuss their unique challenges without fear of judgment or stigma.

Finally, the VA is also using telehealth services to reach veterans in remote areas or those who may be hesitant to seek in-person treatment. This approach is particularly beneficial for special-operations veterans, who may feel more comfortable engaging in therapy from the privacy of their own homes. Through telehealth, veterans can access counseling, therapy and medication-management services, making it easier for them to receive the help they need, no matter where they are located.

If-Then Guidance

- If you or someone you know is experiencing thoughts of suicide, then seek immediate help through available resources such as the Veterans Crisis Line (1-800-273-8255, Press 1) or speak to a healthcare professional. Reaching out for support is a crucial first step in preventing a crisis.
- If you are a veteran or active-duty servicemember struggling with mental-health challenges, such as PTSX, depression or anxiety, then consider seeking mental-health treatment early. Proactive treatment, such as counseling or therapy, can help address these issues before they worsen, and may reduce the risk of suicidal thoughts or behaviors.
- If you are transitioning from military to civilian life and feeling overwhelmed by the challenges of reintegration, then reach out to veteran support organizations that offer programs specifically tailored to help with this difficult transition. Reintegration stress is a known risk factor for mental-health struggles and suicide, so accessing these resources early can make a significant difference.
- If you have noticed behavioral changes in a fellow servicemember or veteran—such as isolation, increased anger or expressions of hopelessness—then take these signs seriously and encourage them to seek professional help. Or do an intervention on their behalf. Suicide prevention often begins with recognizing warning signs and offering support to those at risk.
- If you are concerned about the stigma surrounding mental healthcare treatment in the military or veteran communities, then remember that seeking help is a sign of strength, not weakness. The more

veterans and servicemembers openly address mental health concerns, the more we can reduce the stigma and encourage others to seek the care they need.

- If you are involved in veteran advocacy or healthcare, then focus on promoting emerging interventions for suicide prevention, such as peer-support programs, mindfulness-based therapies, or newer treatments like ketamine infusion or psychedelic-assisted therapy. These emerging treatments hold promise in addressing the mental-health struggles unique to veterans.
- If you feel a sense of hopelessness due to the rising rates of suicide among veterans, then look for stories of hope and recovery from those who have faced similar struggles. Many veterans have found healing and meaning through treatment, community support and advocacy, proving that recovery is possible.

Take the Next Step

- Recognize Warning Signs: Be aware of warning signs such as feelings of hopelessness, withdrawing from others, or thoughts of harming yourself. If you're experiencing these, reach out immediately.
- Call the Veterans Crisis Line: Dial 988 and press 1, or text 838255 for confidential support if you're feeling overwhelmed or in crisis. Also contact http://VeteransCrisisLine.net. Trained responders are available 24/7.
- Build Your Support System: Identify a few trusted people you can turn to when you're feeling down. Whether it's a family member, friend or counselor, having someone to talk to can save lives.
- Contact Dr. Mark Gordon at The Millennium Health Centers and schedule an appointment to discuss your issues. They offer generous veterans discounts: https://tbihelpnow.org/service.

Through Their Eyes

"I remember the weight of it all—coming home, but never really leaving the battlefield behind. You try to push through, just like you were trained to, but there comes a point when even that isn't enough. It wasn't the bullets or bombs that nearly took me out—it was the silence, the feeling that no one could possibly understand.

"You feel like a burden, like there's no escape from the guilt or the pain. I lost a friend to suicide, then another, and I thought, 'Maybe that's the only way to end it.' But here's the thing: you don't have to face this alone. The real strength comes in reaching out, not in suffering in silence. I know, because I almost didn't make that call.

"But I did, and I'm still here. That silence I talked about—it can haunt you at odd hours, like when you're driving or just trying to sit down to dinner. Everything looks normal on the surface, but inside, it's like you're still scanning the horizon for threats, waiting for the worst.

"Some nights, I'd wake up drenched in sweat, heart pounding, sure I heard an explosion that never happened. Other times, I'd replay a friend's last words, fixating on the idea that I could have done something different, said something more. It's a guilt that doesn't fade when the uniform comes off.

"Then there are the triggers you never expect: the smell of diesel, fireworks on the Fourth of July, even a TV commercial showing a desert landscape. That's the hardest part—how everyday moments can flip a switch in your mind and throw you back into combat mode. You try to rationalize it, remind yourself you're home, you're safe, but the mind doesn't always listen. It's exhausting to keep it all locked up, pretending you're fine just because you're in civilian clothes now.

"Yet, there's hope in admitting you can't fight this battle solo. I had to learn the hard way that real courage means picking up the phone, showing up at the counselor's office, or telling a buddy, 'I need help.' Over time, I found that talking to people who genuinely understand—other vets, therapists trained in trauma—can make all the difference. You start to realize your story isn't shameful. It's a testament to what you've endured and survived."

—Specialist Michael T., US Army Veteran

13

PTSX: The Toll on Relationships and the Path to Recovery

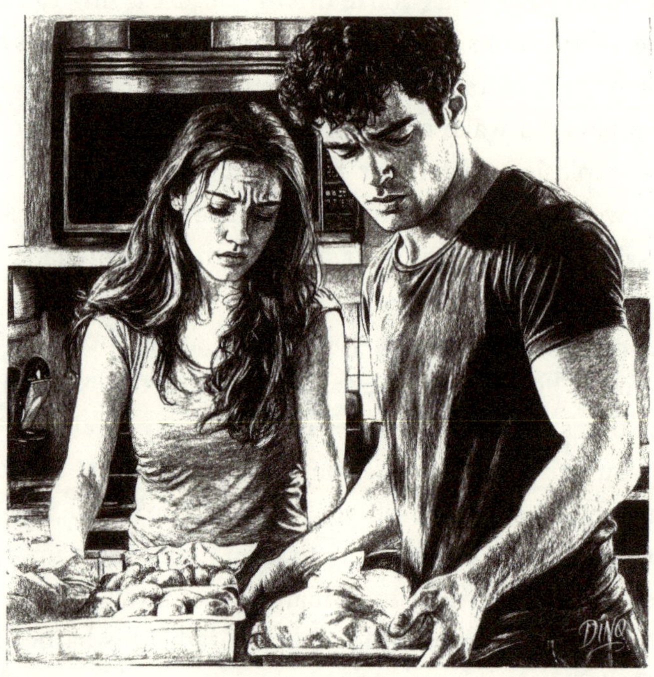

The house felt different since David got back from his last deployment. He was quieter, more on edge. Little things—a dropped fork, a door closing too hard—could set him off. His wife Tara tiptoed around him, trying to gauge his mood. Their teenage son Luis used to talk nonstop about school and soccer, but now he barely said a word at the dinner table. Their daughter Mia kept asking why Dad never smiled anymore.

One Saturday, David came home from grocery shopping, hands shaking as he recounted how someone's car backfiring nearly made him drop to the ground. Tara placed a hand on his shoulder, but he shrugged her off, retreating to the bedroom without a word. The tension weighed heavily on everyone. Mia texted her friends, embarrassed to invite them over. Luis stayed out late, not wanting to see his dad so distant.

A few weeks later, Tara found a flyer about a family-support group for military and veteran families dealing with PTSX. She convinced David to try it out together. It wasn't easy—sitting in a circle, listening to other families describe the same anger, nightmares, and withdrawn silence that had consumed their homes. But hearing those stories gave them hope they weren't alone.

Families serve too—marriages buckle, children flinch, siblings mourn. Healing belongs in living rooms as much as clinics, because trauma is contagious. So are healing and restoration.

In the sessions, they learned basic tools: how to communicate when emotions flare up, how to recognize triggers before they boil over, and how to give each other space to process feelings. They had good days and bad, but Tara noticed changes: David apologizing after snapping at Luis, and Mia smiling when her dad asked about her day. Slowly, the family felt less like scattered pieces and more like a team again.

This chapter dives into the impact PTSX has on families and highlights how support, empathy, and shared coping strategies can pave the way for true healing. PTSX is often regarded as a personal battle fought by those who have endured the horrors of war.

However, the reality is that the impact of PTSX extends far beyond the individual suffering from the condition. It reverberates through families, friends and social networks, often reshaping the dynamics of relationships and placing significant emotional, psychological, and even financial strain on those closest to the veteran or active-duty service member.

While the military culture instills values such as strength, resilience, and independence, the effects of PTSX can create a paradox for veterans and their families. It also discusses the deep social and familial impacts of PTSX, examining how spouses, children, friends and the broader social network are affected. It will also explore how family based interventions and therapies can play a pivotal role in the recovery process, offering hope for healing and reconnection.

The Emotional and Psychological Toll on Spouses

Spouses of veterans with PTSX often bear the brunt of the emotional and psychological strain. The trauma experienced by the veteran can disrupt the intimacy and communication that are vital for maintaining a healthy relationship. PTSX can manifest in behaviors like emotional numbing, irritability, hypervigilance and withdrawal, all of which can create emotional distance between the veteran and a spouse. The inability to emotionally connect, coupled with the veteran's avoidance of situations that trigger traumatic memories, can leave the spouse feeling isolated, unsupported and helpless.

Many veterans with PTSX experience emotional numbing, which may result in a lack of affection or difficulty expressing love and care. This can cause their spouse to feel rejected or unloved, leading to frustration and resentment. Moreover, veterans may experience irritability and outbursts of anger, often triggered by seemingly minor events. Spouses may feel as though they are walking on eggshells, constantly trying to avoid situations that could provoke their partner's anger.

Over time, this chronic state of emotional tension can lead to burnout, depression, and anxiety in the spouse. Additionally, the unpredictability of PTSX symptoms like flashbacks or nightmares can disrupt daily routines and interfere with social activities. Spouses may find themselves taking on additional responsibilities, such as managing household tasks or caring for children, without the emotional support of their partner. The emotional and physical exhaustion from this additional caregiving burden further strains the relationship.

Impact on Relationship Dynamics

The relationship dynamics between spouses can also shift as a result of PTSX. In some cases, the spouse may assume a caregiver role, focusing on managing the veteran's symptoms and needs.

This caregiver dynamic can disrupt the balance of power in the relationship and diminish the sense of equality and partnership that is essential for healthy marriages. Furthermore, the spouse may struggle with their own needs for emotional support, as they prioritize their partner's mental health over their own wellbeing.

The Impact on Children: Navigating a Fragile Environment

Children of veterans with PTSX face unique challenges that can profoundly affect their emotional and psychological development. Growing up in a household where PTSX is present exposes children to high levels of stress, anxiety and unpredictability. Veterans may experience mood swings, outbursts of anger or emotional withdrawal, leaving children confused or frightened by their parent's behavior. One of the most significant challenges for children is the inconsistency in their parent's emotional availability. Veterans with PTSX may have difficulty maintaining stable relationships with their children due to emotional numbing or avoidance behaviors.

A parent with PTSX may withdraw from family activities like attending school events or playing with their children, leading to feelings of abandonment or neglect in the child. Over time, children may internalize these experiences, believing that their parent's distance is a reflection of their own worth or desirability.

Effects on Emotional Development

Children of veterans with PTSX may develop heightened sensitivity to emotional cues, constantly monitoring their parent's mood to avoid triggering an outburst or episode. This hypervigilance can create a state of chronic anxiety in the child, affecting their ability to relax or feel safe in their own home. In some cases, children may develop symptoms of anxiety, depression, or behavioral problems as a result of the stress and instability in the household.

In addition, children struggle to understand why their parent behaves differently from other parents. They may feel embarrassed or ashamed to invite friends over or discuss their home life, further isolating them from their social peers. The lack of a stable emotional connection with a parent can also lead to difficulties forming healthy attachments in their own relationships later in life.

In some cases, children may take on a caregiving role, becoming responsible for managing their parent's emotional state or avoiding triggering situations. This role reversal, known as "parentification," can place an undue emotional burden on the child, forcing them to grow up too quickly and neglect their own emotional needs.

The Social Isolation of Veterans and Families

The social isolation caused by PTSX can be especially damaging because it deprives the family of critical social support. Friends and extended family members may not fully understand the challenges the veteran is facing, and as a result, they may distance themselves or offer well-meaning but unhelpful advice. Without a strong support network, the family may struggle to cope with the emotional toll of PTSX, leading to further strain on relationships within the household.

Financial Strain and Its Impact on Relationships

PTSX can also create significant financial strain for veterans and their families. Veterans with PTSX may have difficulty maintaining steady employment due to the severity of their symptoms. Frequent absenteeism, inability to concentrate, or conflicts with coworkers can jeopardize their job security. In some cases, veterans may be unable to work at all, leading to a loss of income and financial instability.

For families that rely on the veteran's income, this financial strain can exacerbate existing emotional and psychological stress. Spouses may need to take on additional employment or work longer hours to make up for the lost income, which can further disrupt family dynamics and create additional stress for the spouse. The financial burden of medical expenses, therapy and medication for PTSX treatment can also strain the family's resources, forcing difficult decisions about budgeting and prioritizing care.

Impact on Marital Satisfaction

Financial strain is a well-known contributor to marital dissatisfaction, and in families where PTSX is present, the combination of emotional and financial stress can be overwhelming. Spouses may feel resentful or frustrated by the veteran's inability to contribute financially, while veterans may feel guilty or ashamed of their inability to support their family. These feelings of resentment and guilt can create a cycle of blame and defensiveness, further damaging the relationship and creating devastating impacts that may last years.

Family-Based Interventions: A Path to Healing

While the impact of PTSX on family dynamics can be profound, family-based interventions and therapies offer a path to healing and recovery. Research has shown that involving family members in the treatment process can improve outcomes for both the veteran and their loved ones.

Couples Therapy and Communication Training

One effective approach is couples therapy, which focuses on improving communication, understanding and emotional intimacy between the veteran and their spouse. Couples therapy can help spouses better understand the nature of PTSX and how it affects their partner's behavior. It can also provide a safe space for both partners to express their feelings, frustrations, and needs, creating greater empathy and emotional connection.

Family Therapy

Family therapy is another valuable tool for addressing the impact of PTSX on the entire family unit. In family therapy, all members of the household participate in sessions to explore how PTSX has affected their relationships and to develop strategies for coping with the challenges they face. Family therapy can help children express their feelings and fears, reduce the emotional burden on the spouse, and create a more supportive and understanding home environment for everyone. Healing begins with good communication.

Support Groups

Support groups for spouses and children of veterans with PTSX can also provide a crucial outlet for emotional support. These groups offer a space for family members to connect with others who are facing similar challenges, share their experiences, and learn coping strategies. For children, support groups can reduce feelings of isolation and help them develop resilience in the face of their parent's PTSX.

Moving Forward: Building Resilience and Reconnection

While the toll of PTSX on families is sometimes devastating, there is hope for healing and recovery. By recognizing the impact of PTSX on family relationships and seeking help through family-based interventions, veterans and their loved ones can rebuild emotional connections, strengthen their bonds, and create a more supportive home environment.

The journey to recovery may be long and difficult, but with the right tools and support, families can emerge stronger and more resilient. As awareness of PTSX and its impact on families grows, so too does the availability of resources and support for veterans and their loved ones.

By addressing the emotional, psychological, and financial challenges of PTSX as a family unit, veterans can find the strength to move forward and rebuild their lives, while families can rediscover the love, trust and connection that are essential for healing.

This chapter has taken a deep dive into the various aspects of PTSX's impact on military and veteran families, shedding light on the emotional, psychological, and financial toll it takes on relationships. Family-based interventions and therapies offer hope for healing, emphasizing the importance of communication, support and resilience in the recovery process. With the right resources and support, families affected by PTSX can find ways to navigate these challenges together, ultimately emerging stronger and more connected.

If-Then Guidance

- If you are a spouse of a veteran with PTSX and are feeling isolated or emotionally disconnected from your partner, then consider seeking couples therapy or counseling. Therapy can help rebuild communication and emotional intimacy, giving both of you a safe space to express your feelings and needs.

- If you are a child of a parent with PTSX and are struggling with anxiety or confusion about your parent's behavior, then reach out to a family therapist or a support group for children of veterans. Speaking to a counselor can help you understand your parent's challenges while also addressing your own emotional needs.
- If you notice that your loved one with PTSX is withdrawing from family activities or showing signs of irritability and hypervigilance, then create an open, non-judgmental environment for communication. Encouraging them to talk about their feelings and offering gentle support can help bridge the emotional gap caused by PTSX.
- If you are feeling overwhelmed by the financial burden of managing a household with a veteran suffering from PTSX, then consider reaching out to veteran support services, which can provide financial counseling or resources for caregivers. Spouses should not feel alone in managing these responsibilities, and there may be assistance available.
- If your family is socially isolated due to PTSX-related withdrawal from social gatherings and activities, then take gradual steps to reintroduce social engagement. Start with smaller gatherings or encourage participation in veteran-specific community events where your loved one can feel more comfortable.
- If you or a family member are experiencing burnout or emotional fatigue from caring for a loved one with PTSX, then seek respite care or professional support. Taking breaks from caregiving duties is essential for maintaining your own mental health and can improve your ability to support your loved one in the long term.
- If your family is struggling to cope with the ongoing stress and unpredictability of PTSX symptoms, then explore family therapy as a solution. Family therapy can help all members understand the condition better and work together to create a more supportive, understanding environment.

- If you are a friend or extended family member of someone with PTSX and feel unsure how to offer support, then educate yourself about PTSX and approach your loved one with empathy and patience. Your understanding and support can be crucial in helping them feel less isolated and more connected to their social circle.
- If you are witnessing emotional and behavioral changes in your family dynamics due to PTSX, then communicate with your family members about creating a plan for mutual support. Family-based interventions like stress-management workshops or support groups can provide guidance and coping strategies for everyone involved.

Take the Next Step

- Schedule an appointment with a couples counselor to create a safe space for rebuilding communication and emotional intimacy in your relationship.
- Find a local or online support group specifically for spouses or children of veterans to connect with others who understand your challenges and can offer practical coping strategies.
- Initiate a calm, non-confrontational family meeting to open a dialogue about how PTSX is affecting everyone and to establish a unified goal of healing together.
- Create a new, simple family ritual, such as a weekly game night, a shared meal without distractions, or a Saturday morning walk, to build a sense of safety, predictability, and connection.
- Contact a family therapist experienced with military families to help your children express their feelings and to provide the entire family with tools for creating a more supportive home environment.
- As a spouse or partner, schedule a medical check-up for yourself and protect time for your own hobbies and rest to prevent caregiver burnout and maintain your own health.
- Work together as a family to create a written plan for what to do when PTSX symptoms flare up, so that everyone feels prepared

and knows how to support one another constructively.

- If you are a friend or extended family member, educate yourself on the specifics of PTSX so you can offer informed, empathetic support rather than generic advice.
- Contact veteran support services to inquire about financial counseling or resources for caregivers if the financial strain of PTSX is impacting your family.

Through Their Eyes

"When John came home from his deployment, I thought the hardest part was over. But that's when the real battle started—not just for him, but for all of us. He wasn't the same man he was when he left. The little things set him off, and he started pulling away from me and the kids.

He stopped showing up for the things that used to matter to him—like our son's football games or family dinners. At night, the nightmares would jolt him awake, and he'd be drenched in sweat, yelling things I didn't understand. I tried to comfort him, but he'd push me away. It wasn't long before I started feeling more like a caregiver than a wife. I couldn't reach him, and the emotional distance between us was so thick, it felt like we were living in separate worlds under the same roof.

"Our children were confused. They'd ask me, 'Why is Dad so angry?' or 'Why doesn't he come to my games anymore?' It broke my heart. I tried to explain it wasn't their fault, but they felt the change just as much as I did. My oldest son even started acting out, picking fights at school, maybe because he didn't know how to handle everything going on at home. I felt so alone. Friends didn't understand, and it was hard to explain why we didn't go out to family gatherings or why John never wanted to leave the house.

"I started pulling away from everyone too. But one night, after a particularly bad episode, I realized I couldn't do it on my own anymore. We needed help—he needed help, and so did I.

"We started couples therapy, and for the first time in months, I felt like I wasn't carrying everything by myself. The therapist helped me understand what John was going through and how PTSX was affecting our family. And it wasn't just about him getting better. We needed to heal together. We learned how to communicate again, how to handle the tough moments without shutting down.

"It took time, but we started to find our way back to each other. John is working through his trauma, and we're figuring out what our 'new normal' looks like. The kids are in therapy too, learning how to cope with the changes and express their own feelings.

"We've joined a support group for families of veterans with PTSX, and it's been a lifeline for me. Knowing there are other families going through the same thing has given me strength on the days when it feels overwhelming.

"I won't say it's easy, because it isn't. But we're not giving up on each other. We're finding a new way to live, to be a family. And that's worth fighting for."

—Sarah, wife of a US Marine Corps Veteran

14

An Open Letter to the President of the United States and Members of Congress

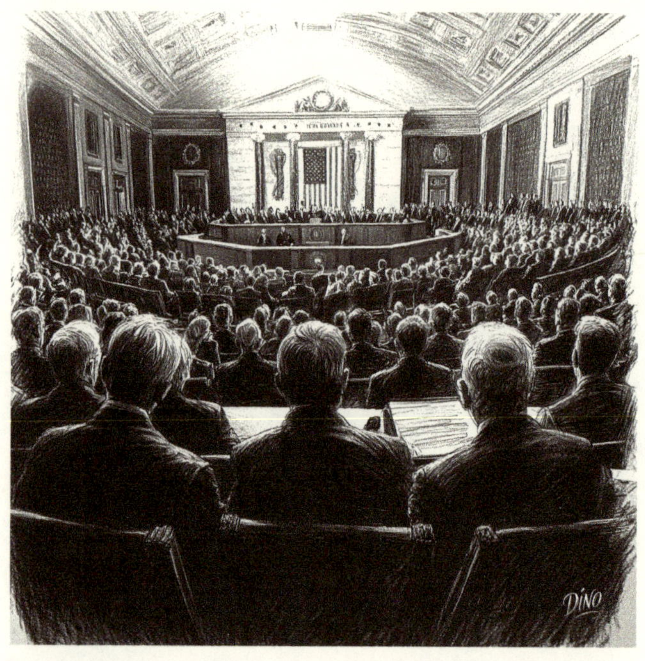

Jackson stood outside the Capitol dome, the morning sun gleaming off white marble pillars. He clutched a worn folder of medical documents, letters from fellow veterans, and a trembling hope that someone—anyone—would listen. Twelve years in uniform had taken him across seas and deserts, forging lifelong bonds and invisible wounds. Now he was here, in this place of grandeur and legislation, determined to speak for those too weary to speak for themselves.

Inside, corridors buzzed with swift-footed staffers, their conversations mingling with echoes of brisk footsteps. Jackson found the hearing room, heart pounding. He recalled the shattered eyes of a friend back home—a Marine stuck in a cycle of nightmares and pills. Another buddy, Army, who turned to alcohol to numb a pain no prescription could touch. Jackson had read every study he could about new therapies: stellate ganglion block, ketamine infusions, even the controversial MDMA sessions. He believed they could help.

Standing before a panel of suited lawmakers, Jackson began reading from his folder: statistics, testimonies, pleas. He held up a photograph of his friend, now gone—another life lost to the silent war of PTSX. "We can do better," he said, voice trembling. "Our veterans deserve more than waitlists and outdated meds. They need real help—emerging treatments that show promise and dignity."

> Entrenched bureaucracy should never be deadlier than actual combat. Navigate the VA with good intel, persistence and allies with expertise to battle VA's dedicated lawyers and legal teams. Fight hard for your benefits and don't give up. In the end, your fight will return those stolen nights of sleep and hardship.

A hush settled in the chamber. He saw sympathy in some eyes, skepticism in others. But Jackson pressed on, reminding them that bills, budgets and bureaucracies held lives in the balance. Finishing, he handed each member a copy of his appeal, calling for comprehensive support—research funding, legislative action, and a shift away from stigma toward holistic care.

Leaving the room, Jackson felt relief. He might've only planted a seed, but sometimes, a single seed changes everything. This was his mission: to ensure no soldier's silent scars went unheard.

Subject: An Urgent Appeal to Support Comprehensive PTSX Therapies for Our Active-Duty Military Personnel and Veterans

Dear Mr. President, Honorable Members of Congress and Esteemed Senators,

As citizens of this great nation, we are bound by a collective responsibility to honor and care for those who have selflessly served in our armed forces. Our military active-duty members and veterans have stood on the front lines, facing unimaginable horrors to safeguard the freedoms we cherish. Yet, upon their return, many are left to grapple with the silent scars of war—Post-Traumatic Stress Injuries (PTSX)—often without adequate support or resources.

The Silent Scars of Combat

PTSX is not a condition that can be healed with time alone. It is a profound psychological injury that affects the very core of an individual's being. In another chapter, we delve into how exposure to life-threatening situations, witnessing the loss of comrades, and the constant hyper-vigilance required in combat zones contribute to long-lasting mental health issues. These experiences alter brain chemistry and neural pathways, making it incredibly challenging for veterans to reintegrate into civilian life.

Consider the story of Sergeant Michael Thompson [A pseudonym.], a decorated combat veteran who served multiple tours overseas. Upon returning home, he struggled with nightmares, flashbacks and severe anxiety. Traditional therapies offered little relief. Far too depressed to ask for help, he took his own life at age 27. Michael's story is not unique. It represents thousands who suffer in silence due to the stigma associated with mental health and the lack of effective treatment options.

Barriers to Seeking Help

In the chapter "Challenges Veterans Face in Seeking Proper Treatment," we outline the systemic obstacles that prevent veterans from accessing care. Long wait times at VA facilities, bureaucratic red tape, and a shortage of mental-health professionals skilled in treating combat-related PTSX are just a few of the hurdles. Additionally, the stigma surrounding mental health in military culture often discourages individuals from seeking help, fearing it may be perceived as a sign of weakness or impact their careers.

The Dual Diagnosis Dilemma

Complicating matters further is the prevalence of substance abuse among veterans with PTSX. "Navigating Dual Diagnosis: PTSX and Substance Abuse in Veterans" highlights how many turn to alcohol or drugs as a coping mechanism, leading to a dangerous cycle that exacerbates their mental-health issues. Without integrated treatment plans that address both PTSX and substance abuse, recovery remains elusive.

A Growing Crisis: Suicide Among Veterans

Perhaps the most alarming consequence of inadequate support is the rising rate of suicide among veterans. "Suicide in US Military Personnel and Veterans: Risk Factors, Prevention and Hope" presents sobering statistics: an estimated 30 veterans die by suicide each day. The figure is perhaps more each day, as many deaths are not recorded accurately as suicides. This is a national tragedy that demands immediate attention. Behind each statistic is a life lost, a family shattered and a community in mourning.

Emerging Therapies Offer Hope

Traditional treatments like Cognitive Behavioral Therapy (CBT) and medication have been beneficial for some but fall short for many others. Recognizing this, researchers and clinicians are exploring innovative therapies that show promise. In "A Shift in Treatment Paradigms: From Conventional to Emerging Approaches," we discuss the potential of treatments such as Eye Movement Desensitization and Reprocessing, virtual reality exposure therapy, and neurofeedback.

The Promise of Psychedelic-Assisted Therapies

One of the most groundbreaking areas of research is detailed in "Comparative Efficacy of Psychedelic and Hallucinogenic-Assisted

Therapies." Substances like MDMA (commonly known as Ecstasy) and psilocybin (the active compound in magic mushrooms) have demonstrated remarkable results in clinical trials.

For instance, a recent study reported that 68% of participants no longer met the criteria for PTSX after MDMA-assisted therapy. These treatments work by enhancing the therapeutic process, allowing individuals to process traumatic memories without being overwhelmed by fear or anxiety.

Cannabinoids in PTSX Treatment

Similarly, "Integration of Cannabinoids in Conventional PTSX Treatment" explores how medical cannabis can alleviate symptoms like insomnia, nightmares, and anxiety. While federal regulations have hindered extensive research, preliminary studies and anecdotal evidence suggest significant benefits.

Veterans like Corporal Sarah Martinez (another pseudonym), who struggled with insomnia and hyperarousal, found relief through regulated cannabinoid use, enabling her to resume a semblance of normal life. Eventually, she weaned herself off cannabinoids altogether.

Direct-Stimulation Techniques and Medical Interventions

Advancements in medical technology offer additional avenues for treatment. One chapter discusses methods like Transcranial Magnetic Stimulation and Deep Brain Stimulation, which have shown efficacy in modulating neural activity associated with PTSX symptoms. Furthermore, "Stellate Ganglion Block and Veterans: Five Case Studies" presents compelling evidence of how a simple injection can provide immediate and lasting relief from anxiety and hyperarousal symptoms.

Ketamine and MDMA: Fast-Acting Solutions

In the chapter "Ketamine Infusion Therapy: Outcomes and Best Practices," we examine how low-dose ketamine infusions can rapidly reduce depressive symptoms and suicidal ideation, offering a critical window for further therapeutic intervention. Additionally, "Mechanisms of MDMA-Assisted Therapy" underscores the sustained benefits observed in patients, with many reporting improved relationships, emotional regulation, and quality of life years after treatment.

Ethical Considerations and Regulatory Challenges

While these emerging therapies offer hope, they are not without controversy. The chapter "Ethical Considerations in Hallucinogenic and Psychedelic Substances Treatments" emphasizes the need for rigorous clinical trials, informed consent, and adherence to medical ethics to ensure patient safety. "Navigating Federal Regulatory Challenges" outlines the obstacles posed by current drug classifications, which restrict research and access to these potentially life-saving treatments.

Calls to Action

Given the urgency and magnitude of this issue, we respectfully and firmly call upon you to take the following actions:

<u>Increase Funding for Research and Treatment</u>: Allocate substantial federal funding specifically for PTSX research, focusing on emerging therapies highlighted in this letter. This includes supporting clinical trials and expanding access to treatments that have demonstrated efficacy.

<u>Legislative Reform</u>: Enact legislation to reclassify certain controlled substances like MDMA and psilocybin for medical use under strict guidelines, as has been done in countries like Canada and Israel. This will facilitate research and allow for compassionate use in cases where traditional treatments have failed.

<u>Streamline Access to Care</u>: Reduce bureaucratic barriers within the Department of Veterans Affairs. Implement policies that expedite the approval process for treatment plans, and ensure that veterans are not subjected to excessive wait times.

<u>Expand Training for Healthcare Professionals</u>: As discussed in "Training and Education for Healthcare Professionals," invest in programs that train clinicians in administering these emerging therapies safely and effectively.

<u>Promote Holistic and Alternative Therapies</u>: Recognize and fund holistic approaches like those in "Animal-Assisted Interventions: Healing Through Human-Animal Bonds." These therapies provide

additional avenues for healing that resonate with many veterans.

Support Community-Based Programs: Enhance support for local organizations as detailed in "Community-Based Support Systems for Veterans," which play a crucial role in reintegration and ongoing support.

Address the Needs of Underrepresented Groups: Pay special attention to the unique challenges faced by female veterans and those from minority backgrounds, as outlined in "PTSX in Female Military Personnel and Veterans: Unique Challenges and Approaches."

Tackle Restrictive Practices: Take a stand against exploitative practices that prioritize profit over the wellbeing of our veterans. Ensure medications are affordable and that pharmaceutical companies are held accountable.

Restoring Faith and Upholding Honor

Our nation prides itself on being a global leader, yet we lag in providing adequate healthcare for those who have sacrificed the most. This discrepancy not only tarnishes our international standing but erodes trust within our own borders. By implementing these actions, we can begin to restore faith in our institutions and reaffirm our commitment to those who have served.

Personalizing the Crisis

Allow me to share the journey of Patrick O'Neill, as chronicled in "Patrick's Saga: A Journey Through Battle and Healing." Patrick returned from deployment haunted by the atrocities he witnessed.

Traditional therapy offered little solace. It was only after participating in a program that combined MDMA-assisted therapy with mindfulness practices that he began to heal. Today, Patrick is an advocate for veteran mental health, but his path to recovery was fraught with unnecessary obstacles that could have been mitigated with better policies and support.

The Toll on Families

PTSX doesn't just affect the individual, it also reverberates through families and communities. "PTSX: The Toll on Relationships and the Path to Recovery" illustrates how spouses, children and loved ones bear the emotional burden. Marriages dissolve, parent-child relationships strain, and support networks crumble under the weight of untreated PTSX.

Harnessing Emerging Technologies

Innovation is at the heart of American progress. "Exploring the Role of Emerging Technologies in PTSX Treatment" discusses how artificial intelligence, virtual reality and biofeedback devices are being leveraged to create personalized treatment plans and immersive therapy environments. These technologies have the potential to revolutionize mental health care but require investment and regulatory support to reach their full potential.

A Vision for the Future

Looking ahead, "Future Trends in PTSX Care: The Next Decade" envisions a future where mental healthcare is proactive, personalized, and accessible. By embracing interdisciplinary approaches and building collaboration among government agencies, private sector innovators and healthcare providers, we can make this vision a reality.

Spiritual and Cultural Dimensions of Healing

Healing is not solely a medical process but also a spiritual and cultural journey. "Spirituality and Faith in the Healing Process" emphasizes the importance of acknowledging and integrating a veteran's belief systems into their recovery plan. This holistic approach has been shown to enhance treatment outcomes and provide a deeper sense of peace and purpose.

Provide Significant Funding to Study the Molecular Basis of PTSX

The final chapters cover what is perhaps the most important information in the book: the underlying causes of PTSX, TBI and other trauma-related issues. We must fully integrate psychiatry, psychology and other disciplines with neurobiology and biophysics, molecular biology and physics and chemistry. We know that PTSX isn't just "all in your head." It has a firm molecular basis that must be studied so effective treatments can be administered.

Taking Action Now is a Moral Imperative

This is more than a policy issue. There is a moral imperative. The practice of sending our citizens into harm's way without a robust plan for their return is untenable and unconscionable. We have the knowledge, resources and capability to enact meaningful change. What is required now is the political will and commitment to do so.

By addressing the needs outlined in this letter, you will be taking definitive steps toward rectifying long-standing injustices and setting a precedent for how this nation honors its heroes. The eyes of the nation—and indeed, the world—are upon you. Let us seize this moment to lead with compassion, integrity and courage.

We stand ready to support these initiatives and work collaboratively to ensure their success. Our veterans deserve nothing less.

Thank you.

15

Relief From Traditional Treatment Approaches

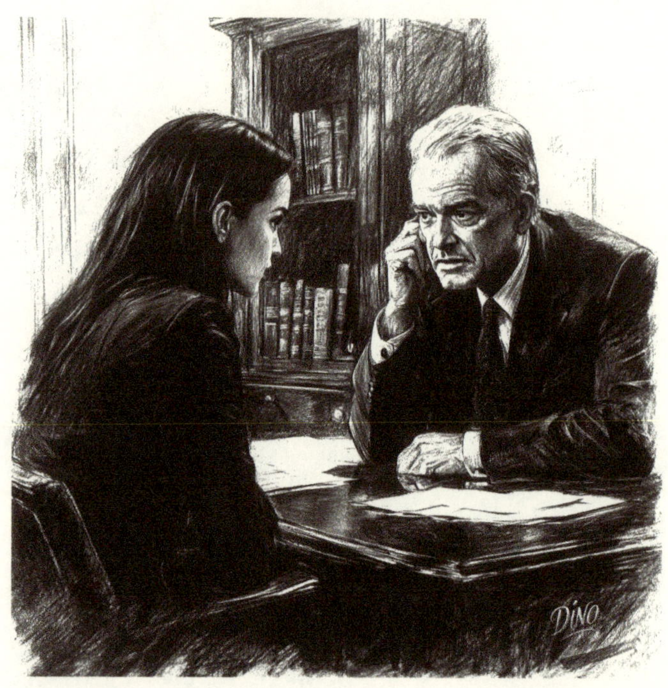

Alicia pushed open the heavy wooden doors of her congressman's district office, the sound echoing like the finality of the choice she'd made. She was tired of seeing her fellow veterans struggle to access the kind of care that had turned her life around—alternative treatments like MDMA-assisted therapy and stellate ganglion block—only to be told it wasn't "standard" or that the treatment hadn't "been approved." After all she had endured in uniform, the thought that profit might stand between her comrades and their healing enraged her.

She took a seat in the modest waiting area, clutching a folder filled with case studies, personal testimonies, and scientific articles. Her heart thumped with a mix of nerves and resolve. She recalled nights in the barracks where fellow servicemembers whispered about off-label solutions that truly worked. Moreover, about the point of view of certain pharmaceutical reps who claimed only conventional meds were legitimate. Those stories reminded her: the system needed change.

A legislative aide finally appeared, greeting her with a polite but guarded smile. Alicia's voice shook at first as she explained how the US pharamceutical industry's control was stifling innovative treatments for PTSX. But the more she spoke—about the promising outcomes she'd witnessed, about the veterans who'd found genuine relief through therapies outside the mainstream—the steadier her words became. The aide's expression shifted from mere courtesy to active listening.

The landscape of mental healthcare for military personnel and veterans is at a critical inflection point. While established, evidence-based treatments remain the bedrock of care, a growing body of research into innovative therapies—from psychedelic-assisted psychotherapy to advanced neuromodulation—offers new hope for those with treatment-resistant PTSX. However, the integration of these novel approaches into mainstream practice is often slowed by a complex web of systemic, regulatory, and industrial factors.

This chapter examines the forces that shape the standard of care within military and VA healthcare systems. It explores how the established paradigms of drug development and medical education can create barriers to the adoption of new, non-pharmacological, or off-patent treatments. By understanding these dynamics, advocates, clinicians, and policymakers can work together to foster a more agile, inclusive, and effective system of healing for those who have served.

The Role of the Pharmaceutical Industry in Shaping Treatment Standards

The pharmaceutical industry plays an indispensable role in modern medicine, investing billions of dollars in the research and development of life-saving medications. For post-traumatic stress injury (PTSX), pharmacological interventions, particularly Selective Serotonin Reuptake

Inhibitors (SSRIs), have become a first-line treatment, providing crucial symptom relief for many veterans. This therapeutic standard is the result of decades of clinical trials, regulatory approvals, and educational outreach funded and conducted by pharmaceutical manufacturers.

By contacting members of Congress, sharing data-driven research, and elevating the personal stories of those who have found healing through innovative means, we can build the momentum needed for meaningful reform.

This system, while productive, has economic and structural realities that influence the broader therapeutic landscape:

- Focus on Patentable Molecules: The research and development model is built around the creation of new, patentable drugs, which allows companies to recoup the immense costs of clinical trials. This naturally prioritizes novel pharmacological solutions over other types of interventions, such as non-patentable compounds (like psilocybin), therapeutic techniques, or medical devices. This economic imperative also fosters a cycle of "evergreening," where minor molecular tweaks to existing, highly profitable drugs are prioritized over the high-risk, high-cost development of entirely new classes of medication. The result is incremental innovation rather than paradigm-shifting breakthroughs, leaving significant gaps in care for those who do not respond to standard treatments.
- Influence on Medical Education and Research: The industry is a primary source of funding for medical research and continuing medical education for physicians. While governed by strict ethical guidelines, this funding inevitably shapes the focus of scientific inquiry and clinical training. For decades, this has

centered on a neurotransmitter-based model of mental health, reducing complex conditions like PTSX to presumed imbalances in chemicals like serotonin. This focus, while valuable, has created a powerful, self-perpetuating research loop that often overlooks other critical biological pathways.

- Marketing and Clinical Guidelines: Pharmaceutical companies engage in extensive marketing to healthcare providers and contribute to the development of clinical practice guidelines. This ensures that practitioners are well-informed about the latest approved medications, but it can also result in a slower adoption of non-pharmacological or less-marketed therapies.

These factors have collectively created a healthcare environment where pharmaceutical solutions are often the most visible, accessible, and well-understood treatment option for PTSX. While these medications are a vital part of the toolkit, this paradigm creates systemic inertia that slows the integration of other promising, evidence-based therapies.

The Consequence: Neurobiological Blind Spots

The persistent focus on neurotransmitter-based solutions has inadvertently overshadowed other critical areas of PTSX pathophysiology. Emerging evidence reveals that the biological aftermath of trauma extends far beyond serotonin levels, deeply impacting the brain's inflammatory state, mitochondrial function, and resilience to oxidative stress.

Chronic psychological trauma triggers a cascade of physiological events, including a persistent state of systemic inflammation. This "neuroinflammation" is not merely a symptom but a destructive force that can damage neural circuits. At the same time, the immense energetic demand of hypervigilance and stress taxes mitochondria—the cellular powerhouses—leading to dysfunction. This, in turn, generates excessive reactive oxygen species, creating a state of severe oxidative stress. This stress depletes the brain's master antioxidant, glutathione, leaving neurons vulnerable to damage and disrupting the delicate processes of memory consolidation and fear extinction.

This explains why SSRIs, which do not directly address these foundational issues, provide only partial relief for so many. Therapies targeting these neglected pathways, from interventions that boost glutathione (like its precursor N-acetylcysteine) to techniques that resolve neuroinflammation, hold immense promise. Yet, because many of these solutions involve non-patentable compounds or lifestyle modifications, they lack the commercial engine needed to propel them through clinical trials and into mainstream practice, leaving them on the periphery of standard care.

The Challenge of Integrating Novel and Alternative Therapies

For veterans and clinicians seeking to explore treatments beyond the conventional, the path is often impeded by significant barriers. Therapies such as MDMA-assisted psychotherapy, cannabinoid-based treatments, and Stellate Ganglion Block (SGB) face a unique set of challenges on the road to widespread adoption.

- Regulatory Hurdles: Many promising psychedelic substances are classified as Schedule I drugs by the DEA, which imposes severe restrictions on research and clinical use. While the FDA has granted "Breakthrough Therapy" status to MDMA and psilocybin, navigating the multi-phase clinical trial process is a slow and expensive undertaking, especially for non-profit sponsors who lack the vast resources of large pharmaceutical firms.
- Educational and Institutional Gaps: Most medical schools and residency programs do not include comprehensive training on emerging therapies like psychedelic medicine or the endocannabinoid system. As a result, many mental health professionals lack the understanding and confidence to discuss or recommend these options, even as patient interest grows.
- Stigma and Historical Bias: Decades of social and political messaging have created a powerful stigma around substances like cannabis and psychedelics. This bias can influence perceptions among clinicians, administrators, and policymakers, making them hesitant to embrace therapies that challenge long-held conventions, despite emerging scientific evidence.

A Call for an Evolved and Integrated System of Care

Addressing the complex, multifaceted nature of PTSX requires a healthcare model that is equally multifaceted. The goal is not to abandon effective, established treatments, but to build a more inclusive framework that evaluates all potential therapies on their scientific merit and clinical outcomes. Such a system would:

- Prioritize Patient-Centered Outcomes: Shift the focus from a one-size-fits-all approach to personalized care. This includes adopting biomarker-guided treatment strategies, where objective biological data—such as markers for inflammation or oxidative stress—are used to tailor interventions. This moves beyond treating symptoms to correcting the underlying neurobiological disruptions unique to each veteran, increasing the likelihood of a successful and lasting recovery.
- Reform Regulatory Pathways: Create streamlined regulatory pathways for therapies that do not fit the traditional pharmaceutical model, facilitating research and compassionate use for non-patentable substances and novel medical devices.
- Expand Professional Education: Mandate and fund continuing education for VA and military healthcare professionals on the science, ethics, and application of emerging therapies.
- Fund Independent Research: Increase federal funding for independent research into non-pharmacological and integrative treatments, ensuring that the evidence base is not solely driven by commercial interests.

Advocacy and the Path Forward

Effecting this change requires a concerted effort from all stakeholders. Veterans and their families, clinicians, researchers, and policymakers must unite to advocate for a more balanced and forward-thinking healthcare system.

By contacting members of Congress, sharing data-driven research, and elevating the personal stories of those who have found healing through innovative means, we can build the momentum needed for meaningful reform. Our military personnel and veterans deserve access to every safe and effective tool available in the fight against the invisible wounds of their service. By fostering an environment that champions scientific innovation, clinical courage, and systemic flexibility, we can honor their sacrifice by providing a standard of care that is as resilient and adaptable as they are.

If-Then Guidance

- If you are unfamiliar with current lobbying efforts, then consider joining veteran advocacy groups or organizations like the Veterans of Foreign Wars or the American Legion, which regularly advocate for veterans' healthcare rights. Beyond national groups, look for grassroots organizations specifically focused on expanding access to novel therapies. These groups can provide information on how you can get involved in lobbying for better access to PTSX treatments.
- If you feel current approaches limit your access to treatments, then you might want to support policies and initiatives aimed not just at reforming drug pricing, but at fundamentally shifting research priorities. Advocate for specific legislation that mandates increased VA and Department of Defense funding for research into non-patentable therapies, nutritional neuroscience, and innovative medical devices. Research nonprofit groups that focus on healthcare reform and join their efforts to pressure Congress for changes that benefit veterans.
- If you have personally benefited from an alternative therapy, then your story is the single most powerful tool for change. Lawmakers and policymakers respond to compelling, real-world evidence. Frame your experience not just as a personal victory, but as a data point proving that other pathways to healing exist and deserve to be explored. Contact advocacy groups and offer to provide testimony; your lived experience can dismantle stigma and inertia far more effectively than a clinical abstract.
- If you are not involved in advocacy but would like to be, then you can start by signing petitions and attending town halls to make your voice heard. When you contact your local representatives, go

beyond a form letter. Request a brief meeting with their district staffer who handles veterans' affairs. A face-to-face conversation, even a brief one, builds a foundation of trust and demonstrates your commitment. Networking takes time: people need to meet you in person and see your passion, then they will trust you and your word.Many advocacy organizations provide templates and tools to make lobbying easier for veterans who want to take part.

- If you would consider supporting efforts to reduce the influence of pharmaceutical companies, then you should research groups focused on healthcare reform or speak with your healthcare provider about how the pharmaceutical industry impacts your treatment options. Engaging with these groups can help amplify your concerns about veteran healthcare.

Take the Next Step

- Get Involved in Advocacy: Join veteran advocacy groups working to reduce the negative influence of pharmaceutical companies on PTSX treatment options.
- Contact Your Representatives: Write to your Congressional representatives about the importance of affordable, accessible and effective treatments for PTSX.
- Spread Awareness: Use your voice to raise awareness about the need for veterans to have access to diverse, non-pharmaceutical treatment options.

Through Their Eyes

"As a US Coast Guard helicopter pilot, I've been through more rescue missions than I can count. From harrowing storms to life-threatening situations, the stress of my job was always part of the deal. But what they don't tell you is how those experiences pile up over the years, how the things you've seen and felt out there on the water don't just fade away when you're back on land.

"PTSX crept into my life long after my hardest missions were behind me. Sleepless nights, constant anxiety, flashbacks—it was like I couldn't shut off the noise in my head. When I went to the VA for help, the first thing they did was hand me a prescription. Then another. Soon enough, I was on a cocktail of medications that dulled my senses but didn't really get to the root of the problem. I was tired all the time, detached from my family, and just going through the motions. Sure, the meds took the edge off, but I never felt like I was actually healing—just managing.

"I started hearing about other treatments that were showing real promise for guys like me—veterans who had seen and done things they couldn't easily forget. Ketamine infusions, MDMA-assisted therapy, even cannabinoids. There were stories of other veterans turning their lives around with these alternative therapies, finally finding the relief they needed to get back to living, not just surviving.

"I brought these options up to my doctors at the VA, but all I got was pushback. It wasn't that they didn't think these treatments could help—it was clear they just weren't allowed to offer them. BigPharma has such a tight hold on the system that anything outside their realm of conventional drugs seems off-limits.

"This was frustrating, but it also opened my eyes. Why should veterans be stuck with outdated treatments when there are new, effective therapies out there? It felt like the pharmaceutical industry was standing in the way of real solutions, more interested in pushing their pills than in letting us explore alternatives that might actually heal the trauma. The deeper I looked into it, the clearer it became: this was a fight worth taking on.

"I started advocating for change. I wasn't alone—other Coasties and veterans from every branch were seeing the same thing. We've fought our battles in service, and now we're fighting another one at home: the battle for better access to innovative PTSX treatments. I joined forces with veteran advocacy groups to lobby Congress and push for legislation that would force the VA to consider treatments like MDMA, ketamine and cannabinoids as part of their options.

"It's not an easy road. BigPharma has deep pockets and a strong presence in Washington, constantly lobbying to maintain their control over us. But our stories—the stories of veterans who've found relief through these alternative therapies—are powerful. When I tell lawmakers about the impact of these treatments on the lives of veterans who were out of options, it's hard to ignore. This isn't just about us asking for something different. This is about survival and quality of life. BigPharma is standing in the way of progress.

"The VA can't offer these alternative therapies because the pharmaceutical companies have built a system that prioritizes profit over our wellbeing. But we can change that by putting pressure on Congress to act. Our goal is to open up access to these treatments so that other veterans don't have to fight the same battles just to get the care they deserve.

"For me, it's simple: I'm doing this not just for myself, but for every Coastie, every veteran, and every servicemember out there who deserves more than a prescription pad. We need a system that works for us, not for the drug companies. It's time for all of us to help give the VA the freedom to provide the treatments that actually work."

—Evan W., US Coast Guard (ret.)

16

FAQs, SAQs and NAQs

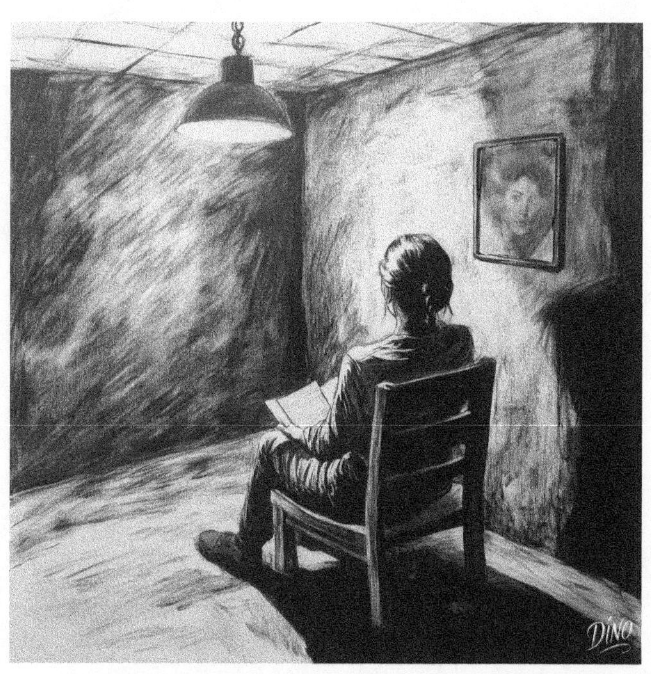

Sergeant Isabella Grant sat in her small barracks room, the hum of the overhead fluorescent light her only companion. She'd been wrestling with relentless nightmares and unexplainable bouts of rage for months—maybe years. Flipping through an old notebook, she recalled the half-remembered hints of "PTSX," a term she'd heard in passing but never fully understood. Then, late one night, she stumbled across a newly released booklet, FAQs, SAQs and NAQs About PTSX. At first glance, it looked like just another list of generic questions. But as she skimmed the 100+ entries, something clicked.

There were the usual suspects: "What is PTSX?" and "How is it diagnosed?" But then came the SAQs—"Seldomly Asked Questions" that dove deeper. One asked about moral injury and shattered values in combat. Another probed how migraines or chronic pain could stem from trauma. She felt her pulse quicken. These were the very issues she'd tried to articulate to her chain of command but could never quite phrase properly.

Then there were the NAQs—almost never-asked queries. One question asked, "How do I make peace with surviving when others didn't?" Another confronted the guilt and shame tied to moral compromises. Tears stung her eyes reading them. It was all there—like someone had finally recognized the realities she and her battle-worn buddies lived with every day.

As she read on, Isabella felt a wave of relief. Here was a resource that not only named her struggles but also offered direction. Each answer pointed toward new therapies, potential support groups, or ways to discuss these topics with family. That night, finally she didn't sleep in dread. She slept in hope.

This chapter compiles frequently asked, seldomly asked, and almost-never-asked questions about PTSX. By addressing common and overlooked issues in equal measure, it provides veterans—and anyone touched by trauma—with a clear, structured guide to recognizing symptoms, seeking help, and finding a path toward genuine healing.

We all know FAQs. They're the questions frequently asked by curious people. SAQs are those seldomly asked but probably should be. NAQs are those almost if not ever (read: never) asked but definitely should be.

1. What is PTSX?

PTSX is a series of physical and mental-health injuries triggered by experiencing or witnessing traumatic events. Symptoms include flashbacks, nightmares, severe anxiety, and uncontrollable thoughts about the trauma, significantly affecting daily functioning.

2. How prevalent is PTSX among veterans?

According to US government statistics, PTSX affects approximately 11-20% of veterans from recent conflicts, like Iraq and Afghanistan, with

Vietnam veterans showing even higher rates. Combat exposure and other stressors during military service increase the risk. We believe at least 50% of all veterans suffer from some form of PTSX, mostly untreated.

3. What causes PTSX in military personnel?

PTSX in military personnel is often caused by combat exposure, witnessing death, personal injury, or experiencing threats to one's safety. Non-combat-related traumas like military sexual trauma also contribute.

4. What are the common symptoms of PTSX?

Symptoms include intrusive memories, avoidance of trauma reminders, negative changes in mood and thoughts, hyperarousal, and exaggerated startle responses. Physical symptoms like sleep disturbances and irritability are also common.

5. How is PTSX diagnosed?

PTSX is diagnosed through a combination of clinical interviews and assessments by mental health professionals. The diagnosis is based on the presence of specific symptoms for at least one month following the traumatic event.

6. What is complex PTSX (C-PTSX), and how does it differ from PTSX?

Complex PTSX results from prolonged, repeated trauma, often in situations where escape is impossible, such as military captivity. It includes additional symptoms like emotional dysregulation, difficulty maintaining relationships, and a sense of permanent damage.

7. Why is PTSX often misunderstood or overlooked?

PTSX symptoms can be invisible and misinterpreted as normal reactions to stress. Misconceptions about mental illness and the stigma attached to seeking help often prevent individuals from addressing their condition. This is just one reason why we feel more than 50% of veterans suffer from PTSX.

8. What factors increase the risk of developing PTSX?

Factors include the intensity and duration of trauma, previous mental health issues, lack of social support, and a family history of psychological disorders. Personal resilience and coping strategies can mitigate risk.

9. Can PTSX be prevented?

While it can't always be prevented, early intervention, access to mental health care, and resilience-building programs can reduce the risk of developing PTSX after trauma.

10. What treatments are available for PTSX?

Treatments include psychotherapy (Cognitive Behavioral Therapy, Eye Movement Desensitization and Reprocessing), medication (antidepressants like SSRIs), and holistic approaches (mindfulness, yoga, and acupuncture). Many veterans benefit from a combination of therapies.

11. How does Cognitive Behavioral Therapy work for PTSX?

CBT helps veterans identify and reframe negative thoughts and behaviors related to their trauma. This therapy enables them to process traumatic memories and develop healthier coping mechanisms.

12. What is Eye Movement Desensitization and Reprocessing therapy?

EMDR involves recalling distressing events while focusing on external stimuli like guided eye movements. This helps veterans reprocess traumatic memories, reducing their emotional impact.

13. What medications are commonly prescribed for PTSX?

SSRIs (Selective Serotonin Reuptake Inhibitors) like sertraline and paroxetine are commonly prescribed. Other medications, such as prazosin, are used to address specific symptoms like nightmares and insomnia.

14. What is trauma-informed care, and why is it important?

Trauma-informed care is an approach that recognizes the prevalence of trauma and its impact on individuals. It ensures a safe, supportive, and non-retraumatizing environment during treatment.

15. What is dual diagnosis in PTSX and substance abuse?

Dual diagnosis refers to having both PTSX and a substance-use disorder, which often occur together. Veterans may self-medicate with drugs or alcohol to cope with PTSX symptoms, complicating treatment.

16. Why do veterans with PTSX often turn to substance abuse?

Veterans may use substances to manage PTSX symptoms like anxiety, depression and insomnia. Over time, this can lead to addiction, creating a cycle that worsens both conditions.

17. What are the signs of dual diagnosis in veterans?

Substance dependence, increased PTSX symptoms after using drugs or alcohol, withdrawal from social support, and failure to seek treatment.

18. What is integrated treatment for PTSX and substance abuse?

Integrated treatment addresses both PTSX and substance abuse simultaneously using trauma-informed care, therapy (CBT, EMDR), and medication. This approach helps veterans manage both conditions effectively.

19. What are the risk factors for suicide in veterans with PTSX?

Risk factors include combat exposure, substance abuse, social isolation, feelings of hopelessness and access to firearms. Lack of mental health support exacerbates these risks.

20. How can veterans access suicide prevention resources?

Veterans can contact the Veterans Crisis Line, access VA mental health services, or seek peer-support groups. VA programs focus on early intervention and providing personalized care plans.

21. What are some protective factors against suicide in veterans?

Strong social connections, access to mental healthcare, participation in resilience-building programs, and avoiding substance abuse are key protective factors. Reducing access to lethal means, like firearms, also helps.

22. What is the role of family support in PTSX recovery?

Family support provides emotional stability, reduces isolation, and encourages veterans to seek and stick with treatment. Family members can also help identify signs of relapse or suicidal behavior.

23. What are family-based interventions for veterans with PTSX?

Interventions include family therapy, couples counseling, and psychoeducation, helping family members understand PTSX and develop healthy communication strategies. This strengthens relationships and aids in a veteran's recovery.

24. What is the role of a service animal in PTSX treatment?

Service animals, particularly dogs, provide emotional support, interrupt anxiety attacks, and offer companionship. They can also perform tasks like waking veterans from nightmares and offering a calming presence.

25. How can veterans apply for a PTSX service dog?

Veterans must submit an application to organizations like K9s for Warriors or Patriot PAWS, often requiring medical documentation of PTSX. Approved applicants are matched with trained dogs and undergo training together.

26. How do PTSX service dogs help reduce symptoms?

PTSX service dogs help reduce anxiety, provide comfort during flashbacks, and offer a sense of security. They can also perform specific tasks to help veterans manage symptoms like hypervigilance and panic attacks.

27. What is the importance of sleep hygiene for veterans with PTSX?

Good sleep habits help reduce insomnia, nightmares, and hyperarousal commonly experienced by veterans with PTSX. Consistent sleep routines, limiting caffeine, and creating a restful environment can improve sleep quality.

28. How can veterans address PTSX-related nightmares?

Medications like Prazosin, therapy (CBT for Insomnia or Imagery Rehearsal Therapy), and good sleep practices can reduce PTSX-related nightmares. Creating a calming pre-sleep routine is also helpful.

29. What is neurofeedback therapy, and how does it help with PTSX?

Neurofeedback monitors brain activity and trains veterans to regulate their emotional responses by creating new neural patterns. It is effective in reducing hyperarousal and emotional dysregulation in PTSX.

30. What is Ketamine infusion therapy for PTSX?

Ketamine, administered through IV infusion, has been shown to rapidly reduce symptoms of severe depression and PTSX, especially suicidal thoughts. It influences neurotransmitters like glutamate, promoting rapid mood improvement.

31. What is Stellate Ganglion Block (SGB) therapy, and how does it help with PTSX?

SGB is an injection that blocks nerve signals from the sympathetic nervous system, reducing the "fight or flight" response associated with PTSX. It is used to alleviate anxiety, hypervigilance and insomnia.

32. What are the ethical considerations of using psychedelics to treat PTSX?

Ethical concerns include ensuring informed consent, patient safety, and appropriate cultural sensitivity during treatment. Psychedelics are still experimental and should be administered under controlled, professional conditions.

33. What is MDMA-assisted therapy for PTSX?

MDMA is used in therapeutic settings to help veterans process trauma by reducing fear responses. Early studies show promising results in decreasing PTSX symptoms over time.

34. How does PTSX affect military spouses and children?

PTSX can cause emotional distance, increased anger and unpredictability, negatively affecting family dynamics. Children may experience anxiety, behavioral issues and emotional withdrawal due to the veteran's symptoms.

35. What resources exist for military families dealing with PTSX?

Resources include family therapy, support groups, psychoeducation programs and VA-sponsored services. Many organizations also provide specific programs for military spouses and children.

36. What is trauma-focused CBT, and how does it differ from standard CBT?

A specialized form of CBT designed to help individuals process and cope with trauma. It incorporates trauma narratives and works on reducing the impact of negative emotions tied to traumatic memories.

37. How can veterans overcome the stigma of seeking mental health care?

Education about PTSX as a medical condition, normalizing therapy in military culture, and peer support can help reduce stigma. Open discussions about mental health challenges also contribute to reducing fear of judgment.

38. Why do some veterans with PTSX delay seeking treatment?

Veterans may delay seeking treatment due to stigma, fear of appearing weak, lack of awareness about available resources, or emotional avoidance. Many veterans feel a strong cultural pressure to appear resilient.

39. What is the relationship between PTSX and traumatic brain injury (TBI)?

PTSX and TBI often co-occur in military personnel, particularly after blast-related injuries. Both conditions share symptoms like irritability, cognitive difficulties and mood disturbances, complicating diagnosis and treatment.

40. What is the role of mindfulness in treating PTSX?

Mindfulness helps veterans focus on the present moment, reducing anxiety and intrusive thoughts. It encourages acceptance and non-judgmental awareness of thoughts, which helps veterans regulate their emotions.

41. How does group therapy help veterans with PTSX?

Group therapy provides veterans with a supportive environment where they can share their experiences and learn from others facing similar challenges. It helps reduce isolation and encourages personal growth through shared healing.

42. What are equine-assisted therapies, and how do they help veterans?

Equine-assisted therapies involve working with horses to build trust, communication and emotional awareness. Veterans often benefit from the calming presence of horses, which helps them reconnect with their emotions and reduce stress.

43. What is polyvagal theory, and how does it relate to PTSX treatment?

Polyvagal theory explains how the vagus nerve regulates the body's response to stress and trauma. Treatment focuses on stimulating the vagus nerve to promote a sense of safety and calm.

44. How can spirituality support PTSX recovery?

Spirituality, whether through organized religion or personal practices, provides veterans with a sense of purpose, community and inner peace. Many veterans find solace in faith-based practices or secular spirituality, which helps with emotional healing.

45. What role does faith-based counseling play in PTSX treatment?

Faith-based counseling integrates spiritual beliefs with therapeutic techniques and assists veterans process trauma while strengthening their faith. It can offer hope, purpose and community support during recovery.

46. What is post-traumatic growth (PTG), and how does it benefit veterans?

PTG refers to the positive psychological changes that result from struggling with trauma, such as increased resilience, a stronger sense of purpose, and deeper relationships. Veterans who experience PTG may feel stronger and more capable than before.

47. How can veterans access emerging therapies for PTSX?

Veterans can access emerging therapies like MDMA, ketamine and neurofeedback through clinical trials, specialized clinics and research programs. The VA is gradually integrating some of these treatments into its care network.

48. What is Virtual Reality (VR) therapy, and how is it used for PTSX?

VR therapy involves exposing veterans to virtual environments that simulate trauma-related scenarios in a controlled setting. This helps them process and desensitize themselves to their traumatic memories.

49. How does VA disability compensation work for PTSX?

Veterans can apply for VA disability benefits based on the severity of their PTSX symptoms. Compensation is determined by the level of impairment in daily functioning and the impact on employability.

50. What are common barriers veterans face in accessing mental health care?

Barriers include stigma, long wait times, lack of nearby facilities, and limited awareness of available services. Veterans in rural areas may face additional challenges related to distance and transportation.

51. What are the benefits of peer support for veterans with PTSX?

Peer support groups provide veterans with a sense of community, shared understanding and validation of their experiences. Peers can offer practical advice, encouragement and emotional support.

52. How does PTSX affect employment opportunities for veterans?

PTSX can impair concentration, memory and emotional regulation, making it difficult to maintain employment. However, workplace accommodations and supportive employers can help veterans succeed.

53. What are some strategies for managing PTSX in the workplace?

Veterans can request accommodations like flexible hours, private workspaces and time off for therapy. Mindfulness techniques and stress management strategies can also help veterans cope with triggers in the workplace.

54. How can employers support veterans with PTSX?

Employers can provide reasonable accommodations, create a supportive work environment, and offer access to mental health resources. Education about PTSX helps reduce stigma in the workplace.

55. What is moral injury, and how does it differ from PTSX?

Moral injury occurs when a veteran's values or beliefs are violated during combat or military service, leading to guilt, shame or spiritual distress. Unlike PTSX, it is not always related to fear or trauma.

56. What treatments are available for moral injury?

Treatments for moral injury focus on reconciliation, forgiveness and rebuilding a sense of moral integrity. Faith-based counseling, group therapy and narrative therapies are often used.

57. What role does exercise play in managing PTSX symptoms?

Regular physical activity helps reduce anxiety, improve mood, and enhance overall wellbeing in veterans with PTSX. Exercise releases endorphins, which can counteract the effects of stress and depression.

58. What are the long-term effects of untreated PTSX?

Untreated PTSX can lead to chronic depression, anxiety, substance abuse, relationship problems and an increased risk of suicide. It can also affect physical health, leading to issues like heart disease and chronic pain.

59. Can veterans with PTSX fully recover?

While many veterans do not "cure" PTSX, they can manage their symptoms effectively through therapy, treatment, medication and support. With the right treatment, veterans can lead fulfilling, productive lives.

60. How does PTSX affect physical health?

PTSX is linked to increased risk of cardiovascular disease, chronic pain, immune system dysfunction, and gastrointestinal problems. Stress hormones and chronic hyperarousal contribute to these physical health issues.

61. What is imagery rehearsal therapy (IRT), and how does it help with PTSX nightmares?

IRT involves rehearsing and rewriting traumatic nightmares with more positive, non-threatening outcomes. It helps veterans reduce the frequency and intensity of nightmares.

62. What is prolonged exposure therapy (PE), and how does it help with PTSX?

PE involves confronting trauma-related memories and situations in a controlled, therapeutic setting. It helps veterans reduce avoidance behaviors and gradually desensitize themselves to trauma triggers.

63. What is the relationship between PTSX and depression?

Many veterans with PTSX also experience depression, with overlapping symptoms like sadness, hopelessness, and lack of interest in activities. Depression can exacerbate PTSX symptoms and vice versa.

64. What is the VA Mission Act, and how does it benefit veterans with PTSX?

The VA Mission Act expands access to community-based care for veterans, allowing them to seek treatment outside of VA facilities. This helps veterans in rural areas or those facing long wait times for VA services.

65. What is the difference between PTSX and Acute Stress Disorder (ASD)?

ASD occurs in the first few weeks after a traumatic event and includes symptoms similar to PTSX. If symptoms persist for longer than one month, the diagnosis may change to PTSX.

66. How can veterans find PTSX support groups?

Veterans can find support groups through the VA, local mental health organizations, or online platforms. Many groups are tailored to specific populations, like combat veterans or those with dual diagnoses.

67. How does the VA rate PTSX for disability compensation?

The VA rates PTSX on a scale of 0 to 100% based on the severity of symptoms and their impact on the veteran's life and employability. Higher ratings correspond to more severe symptoms and greater functional impairment.

68. What is Moral Reconation Therapy (MRT), and how does it help veterans with PTSX?

MRT is a cognitive-behavioral therapy designed to help individuals make more rational decisions and build moral reasoning. It is often used in group settings to help veterans overcome maladaptive behaviors related to trauma. It differs from cognitive behavioral therapy in that it deals with the morals of a veteran's thoughts, actions and behaviors.

The term "reconation," coined in 1974, refers to the part of your mind that deals with your will and motivation to act. While cognition is about thinking and affect is about feeling, conation is all about doing. It's the conscious, intentional part of you that decides to move forward. It's the source of your personal drive, your perseverance, and your ability to turn a goal—like healing—into a reality. It is the power behind every purposeful step you take.

Cognition: This is our thinking part—our thoughts, memories and beliefs.

Affect: This is our feeling part—our emotions, moods and gut reactions.

Conation: This is our doing part. It's the internal drive, the willpower, that pushes us to act on our thoughts and feelings. It's the force that turns the desire to heal into the first step of a journey. Conation is the bridge from intention to action.

69. How does acupuncture help with PTSX symptoms?

Acupuncture stimulates specific points on the body to reduce stress, anxiety and chronic pain associated with PTSX. It promotes relaxation and helps regulate the nervous system.

70. What is the role of forgiveness in PTSX recovery?

Forgiveness, whether of oneself or others, can help veterans process guilt and shame associated with trauma. It is often explored in therapy as a way to promote healing and reduce emotional burden.

71. How does the VA's Whole Health approach support PTSX recovery?

The VA's Whole Health approach focuses on personalized care that integrates traditional treatments with complementary therapies like mindfulness, yoga and nutrition, addressing the mind, body and spirit.

72. What is the connection between PTSX and chronic pain?

PTSX and chronic pain often co-occur, with each condition worsening the other. Trauma can heighten pain sensitivity, and chronic pain can trigger PTSX symptoms.

73. What is Acceptance and Commitment Therapy (ACT), and how does it help with PTSX?

ACT helps veterans accept difficult emotions rather than trying to eliminate them. It focuses on increasing psychological flexibility and living a values-based life, even with PTSX symptoms.

74. How do psychedelics like psilocybin help treat PTSX?

Psilocybin, in controlled settings, has been shown to promote emotional openness and help veterans process trauma. Research is still ongoing, but early studies show promising results in reducing PTSX symptoms.

75. What is the role of storytelling in PTSX treatment?

Storytelling allows veterans to express their trauma narratives, helping them process and make sense of their experiences. It can be therapeutic in both individual and group settings.

76. What is Transcranial Magnetic Stimulation (TMS), and how does it help with PTSX?

TMS uses magnetic pulses to stimulate areas of the brain involved in mood regulation. It has shown promise in reducing symptoms of PTSX, especially in veterans with treatment-resistant depression.

77. What is the impact of PTSX on social relationships?

PTSX can lead to social withdrawal, irritability, and emotional numbness, straining relationships with family, friends and colleagues. Veterans may struggle to maintain connections due to their symptoms.

78. How does the Veterans Crisis Line help veterans with PTSX?

The Veterans Crisis Line provides 24/7 support for veterans in crisis, offering immediate assistance and connecting them with local resources. It helps prevent suicide and offers guidance on managing PTSX symptoms.

79. What is the relationship between PTSX and anger-management issues?

Veterans with PTSX often struggle with irritability, frustration and uncontrolled anger. Therapy and anger management techniques can help veterans regulate these emotions and prevent outbursts.

80. How does PTSX affect a veteran's ability to parent?

PTSX can impact a veteran's emotional availability, patience and ability to engage with their children. Family therapy and parenting support programs help veterans manage these challenges.

81. What is the connection between PTSX and hypervigilance?

Hypervigilance, or constantly being on high alert for danger, is a common symptom of PTSX. Veterans may struggle to relax or feel safe, even in non-threatening environments.

82. What role does art therapy play in PTSX treatment?

Art therapy allows veterans to express and process their trauma in a non-verbal, creative way. It can help reduce anxiety and create emotional healing.

83. How does PTSX affect a veteran's sense of identity?

PTSX can alter a veteran's sense of self, leading to feelings of disconnection from their pre-trauma identity. Therapy helps veterans rebuild their identity and find new meaning in their lives.

84. What is the role of gratitude practices in PTSX recovery?

Practicing gratitude helps veterans shift their focus from negative experiences to positive aspects of their lives. It can improve mood and build a sense of wellbeing.

85. How does PTSX affect veterans' ability to experience joy?

PTSX can cause emotional numbness, making it difficult for veterans to feel joy or pleasure. Therapy and mindfulness practices help veterans reconnect with positive emotions.

86. What is the role of community in PTSX recovery?

A supportive community of peers and healers provides veterans with a sense of belonging, reducing isolation and promoting healing.

87. How does PTSX affect financial stability?

Veterans with PTSX may struggle to maintain steady employment, leading to financial difficulties. Access to VA benefits, financial counseling and workplace accommodations can help mitigate these challenges.

88. What is the connection between PTSX and feelings of guilt?

Veterans with PTSX often experience survivor's guilt or guilt over actions taken during combat. Therapy helps veterans process these feelings and reduce their emotional burden.

89. How can veterans rebuild trust after experiencing trauma?

Rebuilding trust takes time and often requires therapy to address feelings of betrayal or fear. Group therapy and peer support can also help veterans regain trust in others.

90. What is the role of humor in PTSX recovery?

Humor can be a powerful coping mechanism, helping veterans reduce stress and build emotional resilience. Laughter therapy and positive social interactions can lighten the emotional load.

91. How does PTSX affect decision-making abilities?

PTSX can impair concentration, memory and emotional regulation, making it difficult to make decisions. Therapy and cognitive rehabilitation can help veterans regain clarity and focus.

92. What is the connection between PTSX and intrusive thoughts?

Intrusive thoughts are unwanted, distressing memories or images related to trauma. Therapy like CBT and mindfulness help veterans manage these thoughts and reduce their impact.

93. How does PTSX affect sleep patterns?

Veterans with PTSX often experience insomnia, nightmares and disrupted sleep cycles. Sleep hygiene practices and therapy for sleep disorders can improve sleep quality.

94. What is moral injury, and how is it treated?

Moral injury refers to the deep emotional and spiritual distress caused by actions that go against one's values. Treatment focuses on forgiveness, reconciliation and rebuilding moral integrity.

95. How does PTSX affect veterans' perception of safety?

Veterans with PTSX may feel constantly threatened, even in safe environments. Therapy helps veterans reframe their thoughts and reduce hypervigilance.

96. What role does hope play in PTSX recovery?

Hope is essential in maintaining motivation for treatment and building resilience. Veterans who cultivate hope through therapy, community and spiritual practices are more likely to experience positive outcomes.

97. How does PTSX affect emotional regulation?

Veterans with PTSX may experience intense emotional swings, from anger to numbness. Therapy, mindfulness and emotional regulation techniques help veterans manage these fluctuations.

98. What is the connection between PTSX and dissociation?

Dissociation occurs when a veteran disconnects from their thoughts, feelings or surroundings as a defense mechanism against trauma. Therapy helps veterans stay grounded and reduce dissociative episodes.

99. How does PTSX affect veterans' relationships with authority figures?

Veterans with PTSX may struggle with trust and respect for authority figures, especially if they experienced betrayal or abuse in the military. Therapy helps veterans rebuild these relationships.

100. What is the future of PTSX treatment?

Emerging treatments like gene therapy, personalized medicine, and advanced neurostimulation offer hope for more effective, individualized PTSX care. Research continues to explore new therapies and technologies to improve recovery outcomes for veterans.

101. How can veterans advocate for their mental health rights?

Joining veteran advocacy organizations, sharing their experiences with policymakers, and lobbying for improved access to care. Participating in public awareness campaigns and educating others about PTSX.

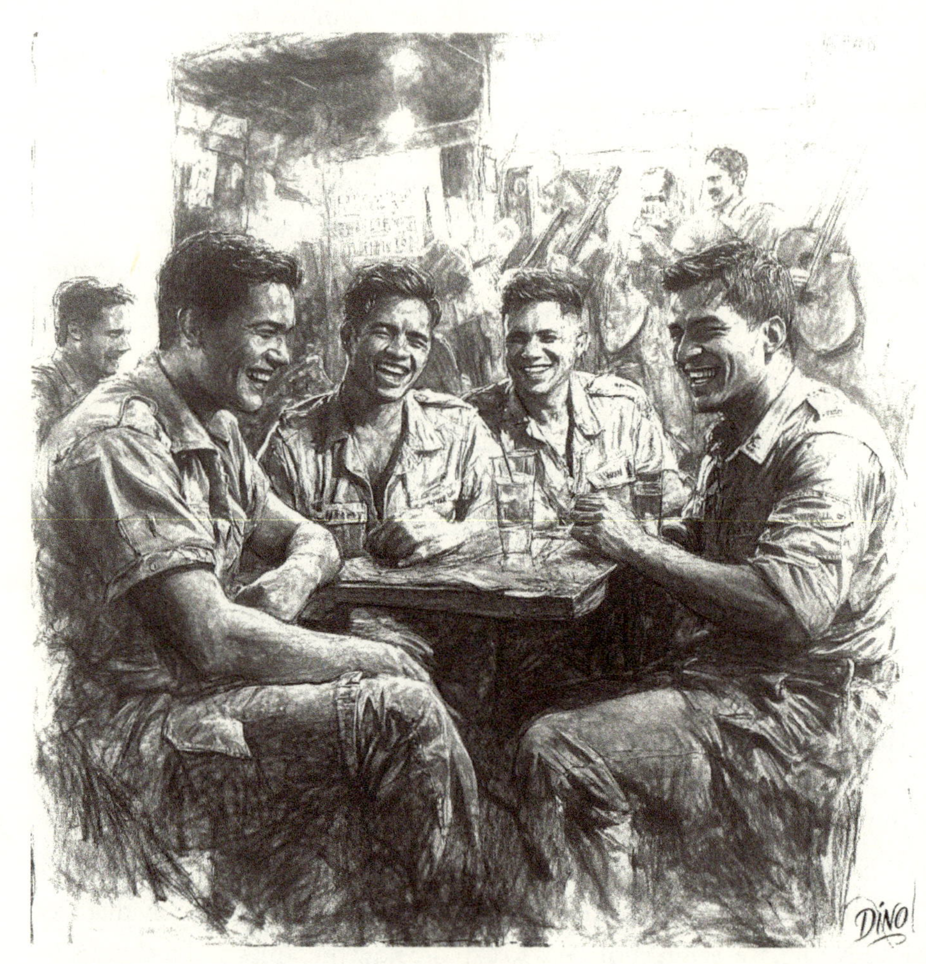
DINO

PART THREE

Therapies and Treatments

17

A Shift in Treatment Paradigms: From Conventional to Emerging Approaches

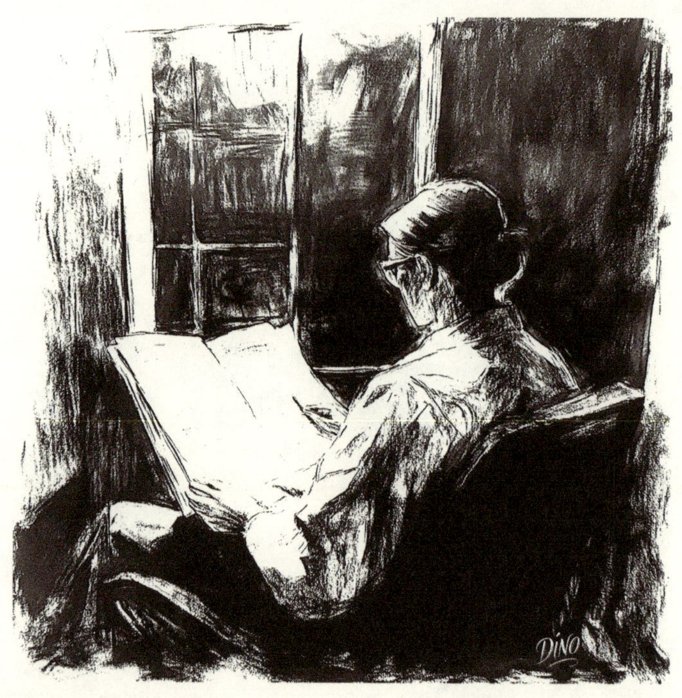

Margo flipped through an old medical journal she found in her grandfather's attic, its pages yellowed and brittle. She was researching PTSX for a paper, but as she read about treatments from decades ago, she realized how little had changed in the mainstream approach—most of it drug-based, with the same laundry list of side effects.

That evening, she spoke with her friend Carlos, a Marine veteran who had been through multiple rounds of medication to manage his PTSX. "Nothing really helped me feel whole," he admitted. "It just dulled things, but the nightmares and tension never went away." His doctor had finally mentioned newer therapies—like neurofeedback and even the possibility of psychedelic-assisted sessions. Carlos was skeptical but intrigued. It was the first time anyone had offered options beyond the usual pills.

Margo found herself drawn to these emerging approaches, too. She discovered stories of veterans who tried MDMA-assisted therapy and felt genuine breakthroughs in processing traumatic memories. She read about mindfulness programs that focused on the body's nervous system, not just prescribing more pills. And she learned how the old "Rockefeller model" of medicine, with its heavy emphasis on pharmaceuticals, had overshadowed countless other ways to heal.

Over a video call, Carlos told her about a local pilot program he was entering—one that combined talk therapy, physical exercise and neurofeedback to help veterans reconnect with themselves. "It feels like someone finally sees there's more to me than my diagnosis," he said.

> Aging Vietnam vets teach us that longevity amplifies unhealed injury. Late-life loneliness is treatable when community is prescribed alongside good care and treatment.

In this chapter, we'll dive into the historical forces that shaped our current system and examine why newer, more holistic options are now coming to the forefront. It's about finding real hope by embracing every proven path to healing.

As we have explored earlier, the treatment of PTSX, particularly in military personnel and veterans, has undergone significant evolution over the decades, especially the past few years. From the early understanding of shell shock to the more nuanced approaches seen today, mental healthcare has advanced dramatically, driven by scientific inquiry, research and the need to provide veterans with comprehensive care. However, understanding the evolution of PTSX treatments—and mental healthcare as a whole—requires that we place it within the broader historical context of sound medical practice in the United States. There is a significant, often overlooked, chapter in medical history that shaped not only how we treat mental-health conditions today but also how the entire medical industry operates.

To appreciate how therapies for PTSX are now emerging and why some of these groundbreaking approaches took so long to gain traction, we need to take a step back and examine the origins of the American medical establishment and the influence of key figures like John D. Rockefeller.

This is a transition between our focus on PTSX treatments and the broader historical forces that have shaped the medical landscape in the US, directly impacting the types of treatments that are available to veterans today. Before we can change the way medicine is practiced in the US, we must first understand how it was originally designed.

The Dominance of Conventional Medicine and Its Origins

To understand the current state of PTSX treatments and methods of healing, we must recognize how the medical field itself has been shaped by powerful financial and industrial interests. In the early 20th century, the rise of modern medicine as we know it today—often referred to as "conventional," "allopathic" or "Western" medicine—was not solely driven by scientific breakthroughs. It was largely shaped by significant economic forces, most notably the influence of oil magnate John D. Rockefeller.

Prior to the 1900s, the medical field in the US was quite diverse. There were multiple approaches to healthcare, including herbalism, homeopathy, naturopathy and chiropractic practices. Many of these methods had been developed over centuries, in many different countries, incorporating both indigenous and folk practices as well as European and Asian medical traditions. People had the liberty to choose among a variety of treatments, and medicine was more pluralistic than it is today.

However, this changed dramatically in the early 20th century when John D. Rockefeller identified an opportunity to shape the medical industry. Along with some others, Rockefeller, who had already monopolized the oil industry, saw the burgeoning pharmaceutical industry as a new frontier. With the discovery that many pharmaceutical products could be derived from petrochemicals— chemicals derived from oil—he realized that gaining control over medicine could be both incredibly profitable and strategically advantageous.

Rockefeller's influence over the medical industry was consolidated through his funding of medical schools and research institutions, which would go on to form the foundation of modern medicine. Since no one else could counter his moves or match his money, his actions began a shift in focus from holistic and natural therapies to a system dominated by pharmaceutical interventions.

This standardization of medicine, though it brought many advances, also created a system where the emphasis on pharmaceutical interventions overshadowed other treatment modalities. The long-term effect of Rockefeller's influence can still be felt today. The dominance of drug-based treatments over more holistic or non-pharmaceutical approaches remains entrenched in the medical establishment, with significant implications for how mental health and PTSX are treated.

The Long-Term Effects on Mental-Health Treatment

The Rockefeller-driven shift toward allopathic (treatment of disease by modern "conventional" means instead of homeopathic methods), pharmaceutical-focused medicine had profound consequences for mental healthcare, particularly for conditions like PTSX. Early mental healthcare was diverse, incorporating various therapeutic techniques that focused on the mind-body connection, as well as more natural remedies.

However, as pharmaceutical companies gained power, the medical field began to heavily push its drug-based treatments for mental-health disorders, even though many had significant side effects, and still do to this day. Worse, perhaps, many of these treatments remain largely ineffective, if not detrimental to patients.

For PTSX, the emphasis on medication as a primary treatment option can be traced back to this period. Antidepressants, antipsychotics and anxiolytics (treatment that reduces anxiety) have become central to the treatment of PTSX, with pharmaceutical companies playing a significant role in the development and marketing of these drugs, and lobbying Congress to force their use throughout the healthcare industry.

While medications can sometimes provide relief for some veterans, the focus on drug therapy has often sidelined other potentially more effective or complementary therapies like cognitive behavioral therapy, eye movement desensitization and reprocessing, or more holistic approaches like mindfulness and meditation.

It's important to recognize that the dominance of pharmaceuticals in mental healthcare is not simply a matter of scientific consensus. It is also the result of decades of industrial influence and the prioritization of profit-driven medicine.

This historical context helps explain, in part, why emerging therapies for PTSX, such as psychedelic-assisted therapy, neurofeedback and virtual reality, have taken so long to gain mainstream recognition and acceptance.

Resurgence of Alternative and Emerging Therapies

As awareness of PTSX grows, so too does recognition of the limitations of conventional, pharmaceutical-driven medicine. For years, the treatment of PTSX in veterans and military personnel has centered on prescription medications, particularly antidepressants and anti-anxiety drugs.

While these treatments have provided temporary relief for some, they have not been universally effective, and the side effects associated with long-term medication use can be substantial, including suicide. In response, both veterans and mental healthcare professionals are increasingly advocating for a more holistic approach to treating trauma—one that integrates traditional therapies with newer, innovative methods.

This resurgence of interest in alternative and emerging therapies for PTSX reflects a broader rethinking of how trauma should be treated, moving beyond the pharmaceutical model to encompass a broader understanding of health and healing.

Treatments like MDMA-assisted psychotherapy, psilocybin therapy and neurofeedback are gaining traction as promising alternatives to conventional drug-based treatments. These therapies aim to address not only the mind, but also the body and spirit, offering a more integrated, whole-person approach to care.

Limitations of Conventional Treatments

Pharmaceutical treatments for PTSX, including selective serotonin reuptake inhibitors (SSRIs), benzodiazepines and other psychotropic medications, have long been the cornerstone of mental healthcare for veterans. While these medications can be helpful in temporarily managing symptoms like anxiety, depression and insomnia, they fail to address the root causes of trauma. i.e at the molecular level.

Moreover, the side effects of these medications—including fatigue, weight gain, sexual dysfunction and cognitive impairment—can negatively impact a veteran's quality of life, not the least of which sometimes leads to suicide.

In addition, medications do not work for everyone. Many veterans find that while medication may help to manage some symptoms of PTSX, it does not facilitate the deep healing necessary for long-term recovery. Veterans who have tried traditional pharmaceutical treatments often report feelings of emotional numbness or disconnection, as if the medication merely masks their trauma rather than helping them process and overcome it.

This growing recognition of the limitations of conventional treatments has fueled interest in alternative approaches that offer more comprehensive and sustainable paths to healing.

A Return to Holistic Health

This movement toward holistic health recognizes that mental health is not solely a matter of brain chemistry. Instead, it encompasses the entire person—mind, body and spirit. By integrating traditional therapeutic approaches with emerging treatments, mental healthcare professionals can offer veterans a more comprehensive and individualized path to healing.

The resurgence of alternative and emerging therapies for PTSX offers new hope for veterans and military personnel who have struggled to find relief through conventional treatments. MDMA-assisted psychotherapy, psilocybin therapy and neurofeedback are just a few examples of the innovative approaches proving to be effective treatments for trauma. These therapies represent a shift toward a more holistic, integrated view of health. One that recognizes the importance of healing the whole person and not focusing on treating only the symptoms with drugs.

As the field of mental healthcare continues to evolve, it is essential that we expand the range of treatment options available to veterans. By embracing alternative therapies alongside conventional treatments that actually work, we can better support the diverse needs of those who have served and ensure that they receive the care they deserve.

By thoroughly integrating innovative treatments like psychedelic therapy, neurofeedback and holistic approaches, we can offer veterans a broader range of options to heal from PTSX, and not just treat the symptoms.

If-Then Guidance

- If you feel that conventional PTSX treatments, such as pharmaceuticals or Cognitive Behavioral Therapy, have not been effective for you, then consider exploring emerging approaches like psychedelic-assisted therapy, neurostimulation or holistic treatments. These alternatives may offer new pathways for healing, especially for those who have not found success with traditional methods.
- If you are concerned about the dominance of pharmaceutical-based treatments in PTSX care, then discuss with your healthcare provider the possibility of integrating more holistic or non-pharmaceutical therapies, such as mindfulness, acupuncture, or herbal treatments. These approaches, which predate the modern medical system influenced by financial interests, may complement conventional treatments and provide a more comprehensive approach to care.
- If you are skeptical of emerging therapies due to their experimental nature, then research the scientific evidence and ongoing clinical trials supporting these treatments. Many of these new approaches are being studied rigorously, and their effectiveness may be backed

by modern research, even though they are not yet as widely accepted as conventional treatments.

- If you feel overwhelmed by the limited treatment options currently offered by the mainstream medical system, then consider seeking care from practitioners who offer integrative or functional medicine approaches. These providers often combine the best of conventional medicine with alternative therapies, offering a broader range of treatments tailored to individual needs.
- If you are concerned about the historical influence of economic and industrial forces shaping today's PTSX treatments, then look into emerging treatments that prioritize patient wellbeing over profit.
- These treatments, such as psychedelic therapy or cannabinoid use, are often supported by non-profit research organizations and advocacy groups aiming to offer natural, patient-centered solutions.
- If you have been relying solely on pharmaceutical treatments for PTSX, then talk to your healthcare provider about incorporating non-pharmaceutical interventions. Combining treatments like therapy, physical activity, and natural or holistic approaches may enhance the effectiveness of your overall treatment plan, while reducing dependence on medications.

Take the Next Step

- Educate Yourself on Emerging Therapies: Research innovative PTSX treatments such as MDMA-assisted therapy or neurofeedback. Look for clinical trials through the VA or veteran organizations.
- Consult Your Healthcare Provider: Ask your VA or civilian doctor about emerging therapies that could complement your current treatment.
- Stay Open to New Approaches: If traditional therapies haven't worked for you, consider trying an alternative therapy. Many veterans have found success with non-conventional treatments.

Through Their Eyes

"When I first started treatment, it was all about medications. I was handed pills—one for anxiety, another for depression, something else to help me sleep. Then I heard about new therapies, things I'd never even considered—like MDMA-assisted therapy or stellate ganglion block. I was skeptical at first.

But something changed when I tried them. These emerging treatments opened a door I didn't even know existed. If you're like I was—thinking there's no way out—trust me, it's worth exploring what's out there. The future of PTSX treatment is more than just managing symptoms. It's about getting your life back."

—Captain Ryan W., US Air Force

18

Somatic Psychology in PTSX Treatment

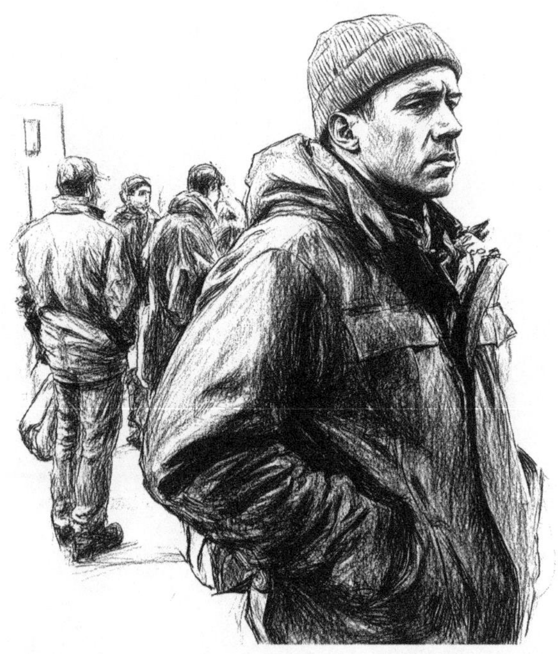

Raúl stepped out of the crowded VA lobby into the crisp morning air, his shoulders tight and his breath shallow. He'd been battling persistent flashbacks and nightmares ever since he left the Marines, but talking about them in group therapy always left him feeling raw and exposed. He kept thinking: *There's gotta be another way.*

A friend from his old unit mentioned somatic psychology—an approach that focuses on how trauma can linger in the body, not just the mind. Skeptical but curious, Raúl attended a small workshop at a local veterans' resource center. There, he met a somatic therapist who asked him not about what happened overseas, but how his body reacted whenever fear or memories struck.

At first, Raúl was surprised. No one had asked him to notice his breath, his racing heart, or the tension in his legs before. The exercises were simple—grounding through his feet, gentle stretching, and paying attention to tingles or tightness. A few sessions in, he felt moments of calm he hadn't experienced in years. He realized that trauma wasn't just stuck in his head. It showed up as constant readiness for a threat that was no longer there.

As the weeks passed, Raúl began to pair these body-centered techniques with regular counseling. When he felt himself shutting down in talk therapy, he'd pause and do a quick scan of his shoulders and chest, letting the tension ease before continuing. His nightmares softened, and the stress headaches he'd been fighting slowly faded. More than anything, he felt a newfound sense of control—over his body and his reactions.

Raúl learned that PTSX is an enduring challenge faced by many veterans and active-duty military personnel, impacting not only mental health but also physical wellbeing. Historically, treatments have focused primarily on cognitive and pharmacological therapies, aiming to address the psychological aftermath of trauma.

His therapist told him about the growing recognition of the profound connection between the mind and body that has led to the emergence of somatic psychology as a valuable tool in PTSX treatment. Somatic (refers to the body) psychology acknowledges that trauma is stored not just in the brain but also in the body, and it emphasizes the importance of treating both the mental and physical effects of trauma to achieve holistic healing.

This chapter explores somatic psychology, its principles, and its specific relevance to active-duty military personnel and veterans. We will examine how somatic interventions can complement traditional therapies, addressing the unique needs of those who have served in high-stress environments. Please keep in mind that the underlying features of psychology and psychiatry are actually *physical*: atoms, molecules, tissues, organs, biochemical reactions and cascades. All physical.

Understanding Somatic Psychology

Somatic psychology is a therapeutic approach that focuses on the integration of the mind and body in the treatment of trauma. It is based on the premise that trauma is not only a cognitive or emotional experience but also a physical one. Traumatic experiences often leave an imprint on the body, manifesting as chronic pain, tension or other somatic symptoms.

Direct-stimulation techniques silence limbic alarms in minutes, reminding warriors that their nervous systems are rewirable, rebootable and worthy of upgrade and repair.

These physical manifestations are frequently linked to the nervous system's response to trauma— specifically, the fight, flight or freeze response that becomes dysregulated in individuals suffering from PTSX. FYI, stellate ganglion block therapy directly addressed this issue by resetting the body's fight-or-flight response.

For veterans and active-duty personnel who often endure intense physical and psychological stress, the body can become a repository for unresolved trauma. Military training conditions individuals to be hyper-aware of their surroundings and to maintain a heightened state of readiness, which can make it difficult to "turn off" the body's stress response even after returning to civilian life.

Over time, this persistent state of arousal can lead to a range of physical symptoms, including sleep disturbances, chronic muscle tension, headaches and gastrointestinal issues. Somatic psychology seeks to address these physical symptoms by working with the body, helping individuals regulate their nervous system and release stored trauma.

The Body's Role in Trauma

To understand the relevance of somatic psychology for military personnel, it is essential to recognize how the body reacts to traumatic events. When faced with a threat, the body activates the sympathetic nervous system, triggering the fight-or-flight response.

This response is a survival mechanism designed to help humans respond quickly to danger. However, when the threat is overwhelming or prolonged, as it often is in combat situations, the body may also enter a freeze state, where the individual becomes immobilized and unable to respond appropriately.

For many veterans, the body remains "stuck" in a state of hypervigilance or dissociation long after the traumatic event has passed. This can result in a range of physical and emotional symptoms, including anxiety, depression, nightmares and difficulty regulating emotions. The body's inability to return to a state of calm and safety perpetuates the cycle of trauma, contributing to the development and persistence of PTSX.

Somatic psychology recognizes that the physical body plays a central role in trauma recovery. By helping individuals reconnect with their bodily sensations and release physical tension, somatic therapies aim to restore balance to the nervous system and facilitate healing. This is particularly important for veterans who may struggle to articulate their trauma in words, or who may have difficulty accessing traditional talk therapies due to the intensity of their experiences.

Somatic Therapy Techniques for PTSX

There are several somatic therapy techniques that have shown to be effective in treating PTSX, especially for individuals with military backgrounds. These techniques focus on body awareness, movement, and regulating the nervous system. Below are a few key approaches used in somatic psychology.

Somatic Experiencing (SE)

SE is a trauma-focused therapy developed by Dr. Peter Levine. It is based on the observation that animals in the wild, despite being regularly exposed to life-threatening situations, do not develop PTSX. Levine hypothesized that this is because animals naturally release the energy generated by the fight-or-flight response through physical movement, such as shaking or trembling, after the threat has passed.

In humans, however, this energy often becomes "trapped" in the body, contributing to the symptoms of PTSX. SE focuses on helping individuals become more aware of their bodily sensations and guiding them through the gradual release of this stored energy. And also doing moderate to intense workouts on a rowing machine, treadmill, stationary bike or lifting weights.

Unlike traditional talk therapy, SE does not require individuals to relive or recount traumatic events in detail. Instead, it encourages them to notice physical sensations associated with the trauma, such as tension or heat, and to work through these sensations in a safe and controlled manner. For veterans who may find it difficult or overwhelming to talk about their trauma, SE provides an alternative pathway to healing. By focusing on the body rather than solely on cognitive processing, SE allows veterans to address the physical manifestations of their trauma and gradually return to a state of equilibrium.

Sensorimotor Psychotherapy (SP)

This approach combines cognitive and somatic approaches to trauma treatment. Developed by Dr. Pat Ogden (PhD), this therapy focuses on how traumatic experiences are stored in the body and how these experiences can influence emotions, thoughts and behaviors. SP helps individuals develop greater awareness of their physical responses to trauma like posture, breathing patterns and muscle tension, and teaches them how to modulate their reactions to these responses.

The therapy involves a combination of body-centered techniques, mindfulness and traditional talk therapy. Veterans are encouraged to pay attention to their bodily sensations and movements while discussing traumatic memories. This dual focus on the mind and body helps to integrate the physical and emotional aspects of trauma, facilitating a more comprehensive healing process.

One of the key benefits of SP is that it helps veterans develop a greater sense of control over their bodies. Many veterans with PTSX feel disconnected from their physical selves or experience dissociation, where they feel detached from their bodies. By helping individuals become more attuned to their physical sensations, SP creates a sense of grounding and embodiment, which is beneficial intense combat situations.

Trauma Release Exercises (TRE)

TRE is a somatic approach that focuses on using the body's natural shaking or trembling response to release trauma. Developed by Dr. David Berceli, TRE consists of a series of simple physical exercises that aim to activate the body's innate tremor mechanism. These tremors are believed to help release deep muscular tension and stored trauma, allowing the nervous system to "relax."

TRE is based on the understanding that the body instinctively responds to trauma by tensing muscles, particularly in the core, legs, and back. Over time, this tension can become chronic, contributing to physical pain and emotional distress. By engaging in specific exercises that activate tremors, veterans can release this tension and promote relaxation.

One of the advantages of TRE is that it can be practiced independently, giving veterans a tool to manage their symptoms outside of a clinical setting. For veterans who may not have easy access to regular therapy sessions, TRE offers a self-directed approach to trauma recovery that can be used as needed.

The Role of the Nervous System in Healing

Somatic psychology places a strong emphasis on understanding and regulating the nervous system. Many veterans with PTSX experience dysregulation of their autonomic nervous system, which includes both the sympathetic nervous system (turns on fight/flight actions) and the parasympathetic nervous system (turns off fight/flight), which can result in hyperarousal (a constant state of alertness) or hypoarousal (numbness or dissociation). Both of these states can interfere with daily functioning and prevent individuals from fully engaging in their lives.

Somatic therapies help veterans learn to regulate their nervous system by teaching them how to move between states of activation and relaxation. This process, known as pendulation, involves gradually increasing the individual's tolerance for discomfort or distress. It assists them in regulating their parasympathetic nervous system and thus returning to a state of calm.

By learning to move smoothly between these states, veterans can build resilience and develop greater control over their emotional and physical responses to stress. The DoD should mandate this for military personnel. It doesn't take much, especially considering how costly it is to care and treat veterans for PTSX.

Breathing exercises, grounding techniques and mindfulness practices are often incorporated into somatic therapy sessions to help veterans develop skills for self-regulation. These practices can be particularly helpful in moments of high stress, such as during flashbacks or panic attacks, by providing veterans with practical tools to calm their nervous system and regain control.

The Relevance of Somatic Psychology for Military Personnel

Veterans and active-duty military personnel face unique challenges in their trauma recovery. The nature of military training and combat often conditions individuals to suppress or ignore physical and emotional pain to remain focused on the mission. While this adaptive strategy may be necessary in the field, it can lead to long-term physical and psychological consequences if left unaddressed.

Somatic psychology study and training should be taught during basic training, starting on Day One, then introduced often throughout training over the few months trainees are present.

This therapy is particularly well-suited to the needs of veterans because it offers a way to address trauma without requiring individuals to verbalize or relive their experiences. Many veterans find it difficult to talk about their trauma, either because the memories are too painful or because they have been conditioned to avoid discussing their emotions.

Somatic therapy allows veterans to work through their trauma on a physical level, bypassing the need for extensive verbal engagement and processing. Additionally, somatic therapies can help veterans reconnect with their bodies and regain a sense of control. Many veterans with PTSX feel disconnected from their physical selves or experience chronic pain and discomfort. By focusing on bodily sensations and movement, somatic therapies help veterans re-establish a positive relationship with their bodies, empowering them during the healing process.

Integrating Somatic Psychology with Conventional Treatments

Somatic psychology is not meant to replace other effective treatments for PTSX, such as cognitive-behavioral therapy or medication. Rather, it can be integrated with these treatments to provide a more holistic approach to healing.

Veterans who participate in somatic therapy alongside traditional therapies often report improved outcomes, including reduced physical symptoms, greater emotional regulation, and enhanced overall wellbeing. For example, somatic therapy can be used in conjunction with Eye movement desensitization and reprocessing, a widely used trauma therapy that incorporates elements of body awareness.

If-Then Guidance

- If you experience chronic physical symptoms like muscle tension, headaches or gastrointestinal issues alongside your PTSX, then consider exploring somatic therapies like SE or TRE exercises. These therapies can help release the physical tension stored in your body and alleviate the somatic symptoms associated with trauma.
- If you find it difficult or overwhelming to talk about your traumatic experiences, then somatic therapy may provide an alternative pathway to healing. Somatic approaches focus on bodily sensations rather than verbal processing, making them a good option for veterans who are uncomfortable with traditional talk therapy.
- If you feel disconnected from your body or experience episodes of dissociation, then somatic therapies such as SP can help you reconnect with your physical self and regain a sense of control. These therapies work to ground you in the present moment by increasing awareness of bodily sensations.

- If you have already tried conventional PTSX treatments but continue to struggle with emotional regulation or hypervigilance, then integrating somatic therapies into your treatment plan could help. Somatic approaches can complement existing therapies by addressing the physical aspects of trauma to better regulate your nervous system.

Take the Next Step

- Research somatic therapy options. Look into these different somatic therapy approaches. Reading about how these therapies work will help you understand which ones might be most suitable for your needs. Many resources are available online, or you can ask your healthcare provider for recommendations.
- Consult with a therapist who specializes in somatic approaches. Find a therapist trained in somatic psychology and experienced in working with veterans or military personnel. Organizations like the Somatic Experiencing Trauma Institute or the Sensorimotor Psychotherapy Institute provide directories of certified practitioners. You can also inquire at your local VA hospital or clinic to see if somatic therapies are available.
- Begin incorporating somatic practices into your daily routine. Even if you're not ready to commit to formal therapy, you can start with simple techniques like mindful breathing, body scanning or gentle movement exercises. These practices help you reconnect with your body and manage stress and can serve as a foundation for deeper somatic work if you pursue therapy later.
- Evaluate your progress as you engage in somatic therapy or integrate somatic practices. Take time to reflect on any changes in your physical or emotional symptoms. Ask yourself if you feel more in control of your body or if you are better able to regulate your emotions. Monitoring your progress will help determine if this approach is right for you and if further adjustments to your treatment plan are needed.
- Consider connecting with a support network. Healing from trauma often requires support from others who understand what

you're going through. You might join a veteran's support group or an online community focused on PTSX recovery. Sharing your experiences can provide valuable encouragement and accountability as you take steps toward healing.

Through Their Eyes

"For years, the roar of jet engines and the adrenaline of the skies were my world. I flew countless missions, each one pushing the boundaries of fear and courage. From the cockpit, I faced dangers that few can imagine, navigating hostile territories and making split-second decisions that weighed life and death in the balance.

"When I returned home, I expected to hang up my flight suit and seamlessly transition back into civilian life. But the battles didn't end when I left the aircraft carrier—they merely shifted fronts. The enemy was now invisible, waging war inside me.

"Sleep became a battleground of its own, haunted by nightmares that pulled me back into the cockpit, reliving moments of terror. Sudden noises would send jolts through my body, my heart pounding as if I were back in the skies evading enemy fire.

"I felt disconnected—from my family, my friends, even from myself. The man in the mirror wore my face, but behind the eyes was a stranger. Traditional talk therapy felt like an uphill climb. Words seemed inadequate to express the turmoil within. How could I articulate the weight of responsibility, the split-second decisions that haunted me, or the comrades I lost along the way?

"Medication dulled the edges but left me feeling numb, a shadow of who I once was. I began to believe that perhaps this was my new normal—a life spent navigating an internal storm with no clear horizon in sight. It reminds us of a movie with Jack Nicholson, in which he played a crazy guy who offended just about everyone he met. In a scene near the end, he looks around and says, 'Maybe this is as good as it gets.'

"Then, a fellow veteran told me about somatic psychology. He spoke of it not as a cure-all but as a different approach—one that didn't rely solely on words. Skeptical yet desperate, I decided to give it a try. That's how I found myself sitting across from Dr. Evans, a therapist specializing in somatic experiencing. From the very beginning, our sessions were unlike anything I'd encountered. Instead of pressing me to recount painful memories, Dr. Evans asked me to focus on what I was feeling in my body at that very moment.

"'Notice any sensations, okay?' she asked. 'There's no right or wrong—just observe.'

"At first, it felt strange. I was accustomed to pushing through discomfort, not dwelling on it. But as I sat there, I became aware of the tension in my shoulders, the tightness in my jaw, the way my foot tapped restlessly on the floor. We explored these sensations together. She guided me to breathe deeply, to allow myself to feel without judgment. When memories surfaced, she helped me stay grounded in the present, reminding me that I was safe.

"One session stands out vividly. I felt a knot in my stomach—a familiar discomfort that I'd long ignored. As we focused on it, images flashed in my mind: the glare of warning lights in the cockpit, the sound of alarms blaring, the suffocating grip of fear as I navigated a malfunctioning aircraft.

"My body began to tremble. Embarrassed, I tried to suppress it, but Dr. Evans encouraged me to let it happen. 'Your body is releasing stored energy,' she explained. 'It's okay. Let it move through you.'

"I shook uncontrollably for what felt like an eternity. When it finally subsided, I was exhausted but strangely lighter. I felt a heavy weight I'd been unconsciously carrying had begun to lift.

"Over the following weeks, we continued this work. I learned to recognize when my body was entering a state of hyperarousal and how to bring myself back to equilibrium. Simple practices—deep breathing, grounding exercises, mindful movement—became tools I could rely on.

"I started to feel a reconnection between my mind and body. The constant tension eased, the nightmares became less frequent and intense. I found moments of peace where there had only been chaos.

"One afternoon, while walking in a park, I paused to feel the sun on my face and the breeze against my skin. It was a simple pleasure, but one I'd been oblivious to for so long. Tears welled in my eyes—not from sorrow, but from a profound sense of gratitude. I was beginning to reclaim parts of myself that I thought were lost forever.

"Somatic psychology didn't erase my experiences, nor did it promise a complete end to my struggles. But it offered a path to healing that honored the complexities of trauma stored within my body. It acknowledged that some wounds run deeper than words can reach and that sometimes, the body speaks a language all its own.

"To my fellow servicemen and women, I share my story in hopes that it might resonate with you. If you've felt trapped, disconnected or overwhelmed by invisible battles, know that there are avenues beyond traditional therapies. Somatic psychology may provide the bridge you need to reconnect with yourself.

"Healing is not a sign of weakness, nor is seeking help a form of surrendering who you are inside. It is an act of courage—a mission to reclaim your life. We trained to be resilient in the face of adversity, to adapt and overcome. This is just another challenge, one that you don't have to face alone.

"Today, I'm not the same person I was before my service, but that's okay. I've come to accept that healing is a journey, not a destination. There are still days when the shadows creep in, but now I have the tools to navigate them. I can find calm in the storm.

"If you're reading this and see parts of yourself in my story, I encourage you to reach out, to explore the possibilities that somatic therapy might offer. Your body holds not just the silent scars of the past but also the key to your healing. Listen to it. Honor it. Give yourself the grace to heal.

"In solidarity,"

—Lt. Cmdr. James M., US Navy (ret.)

19

Integration of Cannabinoids in Conventional PTSX Treatment

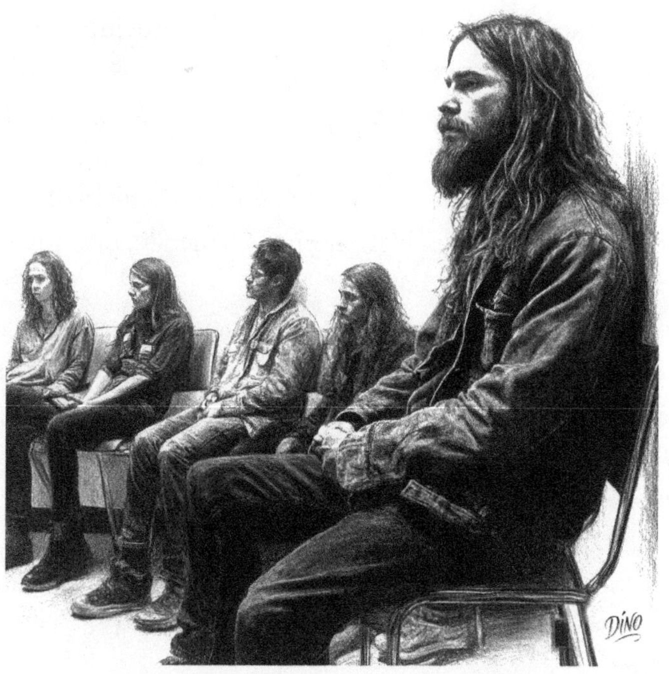

After years of restless nights and anxious days, Kevin, a former Army medic, found himself in a small clinic waiting room, contemplating a new possibility—cannabinoid therapy. He'd gone through talk therapy and tried traditional medications, but nothing seemed to bring lasting relief. A friend had mentioned cannabinoids and how it might ease the racing heart and constant worry he couldn't shake. So here he was, unsure but hopeful.

The clinic staff explained how cannabis-derived compounds could interact with the body's own endocannabinoid system—a set of receptors found everywhere from brain tissue to immune cells. Kevin learned how certain cannabinoids, like cannabidiol (CBD), might help calm his hypervigilance and improve sleep quality. They also talked him through potential side effects and legal considerations. It felt both reassuring and eye-opening: there was a real science behind what he'd once dismissed as just "weed."

In the weeks that followed, Kevin began a carefully monitored regimen. No overnight miracles, but he noticed gradual changes—a little less dread when stepping out of the house, fewer jolts awake at 3 a.m. Over time, the therapy blended neatly with his existing routine: he still did occasional talk therapy sessions, and his therapist found it easier to work through deep-seated triggers when Kevin's anxiety was more manageable.

This chapter delves into that same process: how cannabinoids fit into a broader, conventional PTSX treatment plan. From reviewing the latest studies on CBD's impact on sleep and anxiety, to understanding best practices for safe use, we'll explore the genuine promise (and real limitations) of integrating cannabis-based therapies for veterans seeking new paths to healing.

Cannabinoids: An Overview

Cannabinoids, a diverse group of chemical compounds found in the *Cannabis sativa* plant, have emerged as a focal point in the exploration of innovative treatments for various mental-health conditions, including PTSX. Understanding the nuanced mechanisms through which cannabinoids interact with the human brain is crucial for mental-health professionals working with military personnel and veterans.

These compounds, particularly the psychoactive tetrahydrocannabinol (THC) and non-psychoactive CBD, have shown promise not only in alleviating symptoms of PTSX but also in enhancing the overall wellness of individuals navigating the complexities of trauma recovery. As we delve into this overview, we highlight the significance of cannabinoids in contemporary therapeutic protocols. Our brain and body have an endocannabinoid system (ECS) that can be modulated by external (phyto)cannabinoids. We have specialized receptors on neurons in the central nervous system and also outside the CNS in just about every type of cell, i.e. bone, fat, immune, muscle, etc.

The ECS plays a pivotal role in modulating emotional responses and stress-related behaviors. This biological system consists of cannabinoid receptors, endogenous cannabinoids and enzymes that regulate their synthesis and degradation. Promising research results suggest that the ECS is involved in the physiological processes and behaviors associated with stress responses, making it a vital area of study for veterans suffering from the impacts of trauma.

By leveraging cannabinoids to positively influence the ECS, mental healthcare professionals can potentially create resilience in veterans, helping them reclaim their lives from the debilitating effects of PTSX.

Recent studies have illuminated the potential benefits of cannabinoids in conjunction with traditional PTSX treatments. While conventional therapies, including cognitive behavioral therapy and exposure therapy, have been effective for many, they do not work universally. Cannabinoids could serve as an adjunct to these therapies, enhancing their efficacy and providing a more comprehensive approach to healing.

For example, CBD has been associated with reducing anxiety and improving sleep quality, two critical areas often affected in those with PTSX. By integrating cannabinoids into treatment protocols, healthcare professionals may be able to offer a more tailored and effective therapeutic experience for veterans.

However, the integration of cannabinoids into PTSX treatment protocols is not without its challenges. A thorough understanding of the legal landscape, various state regulations and the need for further research on long-term effects and potential side effects is essential.

Healthcare professionals must also consider the ethical implications of prescribing cannabinoids, ensuring that informed consent is obtained and that patients are fully aware of the potential risks and benefits. As the research evolves, it is vital for practitioners to stay informed and engaged in the discussion surrounding cannabinoids, ensuring that their implementation is grounded in scientific evidence and ethical practice.

Guidelines for Incorporating Cannabinoids into Treatment

Incorporating CBDs into treatment protocols for PTSX among military personnel and veterans represents a frontier of therapeutic potential that warrants consideration and strategic implementation. Recent advancements in neurobiology have illuminated the intricate ways in which cannabinoids interact with the endocannabinoid system, which plays a crucial role in regulating mood, stress responses and emotional processing. It's imperative to understand the guidelines that will facilitate the responsible integration of cannabinoids into existing treatment frameworks.

First and foremost, a comprehensive assessment of the individual's medical history and current mental health is essential. This includes evaluating any co-occurring disorders, current medications and previous treatment responses.

By employing a personalized approach, professionals can tailor cannabinoid therapies to suit the unique needs of each veteran or servicemember, ensuring that the treatment is both safe and effective. Open communication with patients about their expectations and concerns regarding cannabinoid use creates trust and empowers them in their healing journey.

Education is a cornerstone of implementing cannabinoid therapies. Professionals must be well versed in the various forms of cannabinoids, their mechanisms of action and potential side effects. This knowledge not only enhances the therapeutic alliance but also equips them to provide accurate information to patients, demystifying the treatment process.

Collaborative discussions about the benefits and limitations of cannabinoid integration can help patients make informed decisions, thereby promoting adherence to treatment and improving outcomes.

Moreover, establishing a multidisciplinary approach can significantly strengthen the incorporation of cannabinoids into treatment plans. Coordination among researchers, physicians, psychiatrists, psychologists, addiction specialists and primary-care providers and nurses allows for a holistic view of the patient's health.

This collaboration can lead to innovative treatment strategies that combine cannabinoids with evidence-based therapies, such as cognitive-behavioral therapy or exposure therapy. Such integrative models can enhance overall treatment efficacy, addressing the multifaceted nature of PTSX and promoting sustained recovery.

Now that cannabis pharmacies dot the country, one can easily self-medicate without first getting a baseline blood chemistry and health study. We recommend discussing your CBD treatment plan with an expert in the field, preferably a board-certified endocrinologist who understands the neurochemistry of CBD.

If-Then Guidance

- If you are not familiar with cannabinoid-based treatments for PTSX, then research how cannabinoids may help manage symptoms such as anxiety, sleep disturbances, or hypervigilance. You can also consult with a healthcare provider who is knowledgeable about cannabinoid therapy to understand its potential benefits and risks in relation to PTSX.
- If you are interested in exploring cannabinoid therapy but live in an area where it is not yet legal or regulated, then consider speaking with your healthcare provider about alternative treatments or legal options. You might also stay informed about changes in legislation that could make cannabinoid therapy more accessible in your region.
- If you have used cannabinoids for PTSX and found them helpful, then discuss with your healthcare provider how to safely incorporate these products into your long-term treatment plan. It's important to use cannabinoid therapies under medical supervision, especially if you are also using other medications or treatments.
- If you are worried about the potential side effects or risks associated with cannabinoid use (e.g., dependency, cognitive effects), then seek detailed guidance from a healthcare professional who specializes in cannabinoid therapies. They can help you weigh the risks and benefits and explore the safest way to proceed with treatment.
- If cost or access to high-quality cannabinoid products is a barrier

for you, then look for programs or dispensaries that offer discounts to veterans. Some states also have medical marijuana programs that may offer financial assistance, and there may be research studies you can join that provide access to these treatments.
- If you are concerned about a possible stigma associated with cannabinoid therapy, then talk to your healthcare provider or fellow veterans who have used these treatments. Education and open conversations can help reduce stigma, and hearing from others who have had positive experiences may provide reassurance.

Take the Next Step

- Explore Cannabinoid Treatments: Research how cannabinoids like CBD or medical marijuana are being used to manage PTSX symptoms. Learn about their legal status and availability in your state, county, city or local area.
- Consult a Medical Professional: If you're interested in using cannabinoids, talk to your VA doctor or a licensed provider to see if this treatment could be a safe addition to your current plan.
- Look for Veteran-Specific Programs: Check for veteran-focused programs that integrate medical cannabis or CBD into treatment plans for PTSX.

Through Their Eyes

"I was skeptical about trying cannabis to help with my PTSX. After years of dealing with the constant anxiety, the sleepless nights and the flashbacks that never seemed to end, I had tried everything else—medications, therapy, but nothing really stuck. The side effects from the medications were rough, and I never felt fully present.

"A friend of mine, another veteran, mentioned that he had been using CBD and THC to manage his symptoms, and it got me thinking that maybe it was time to try something different.

"At first, it felt strange. I mean, I grew up hearing all about the dangers of marijuana, so the idea that it could help me with my mental health seemed almost contradictory. But I did my research, spoke to a doctor who specializes in cannabinoid therapies, and decided to give it a go. I started with CBD—no THC at first, because I didn't want to feel 'high.' I just wanted to see if it could help me feel a little more balanced.

"The first thing I noticed was the change in my sleep. For the first time in months, I slept through the night. It wasn't perfect, but it was better than the usual tossing and turning, waking up drenched in sweat from my nightmares. It was like my mind could finally relax, just for a little bit. And during the day, I felt more calm. The anxiety that usually sat like a weight on my chest felt lighter, more manageable. After a few weeks, I talked to my doctor again, and we adjusted the dosage. I added a bit of THC for the nights when my anxiety was worse. It helped ease my mind without making me feel out of control or 'stoned.' It was a relief to know there was something natural I could turn to that didn't have the side effects of the other medications I'd been on.

"One thing that really made a difference was having a doctor who understood the neurobiology of it all—how the cannabinoids were interacting with my brain, why they were helping with my PTSX symptoms. It wasn't just about masking the pain. It was about healing. I wasn't just treating the symptoms, I was addressing the underlying issues, helping my brain find its balance again.

"PTSX is still a small part of my life, but with cannabis, I've found a way to live with it in a way that feels manageable. I can be more present with my family, I can engage in conversations without feeling overwhelmed by stress or hypervigilance. It's given me back a sense of control I hadn't felt in a long time.

"Cannabis isn't for everyone, and it's not the only thing that's helped me. Therapy, support from my family, and staying connected with other veterans have all played a part. But having this tool in my toolbox, something natural that helps me feel like myself again, has made all the difference."

— Tom, US Army Veteran

20

Ketamine Infusion Therapy: Outcomes and Best Practices

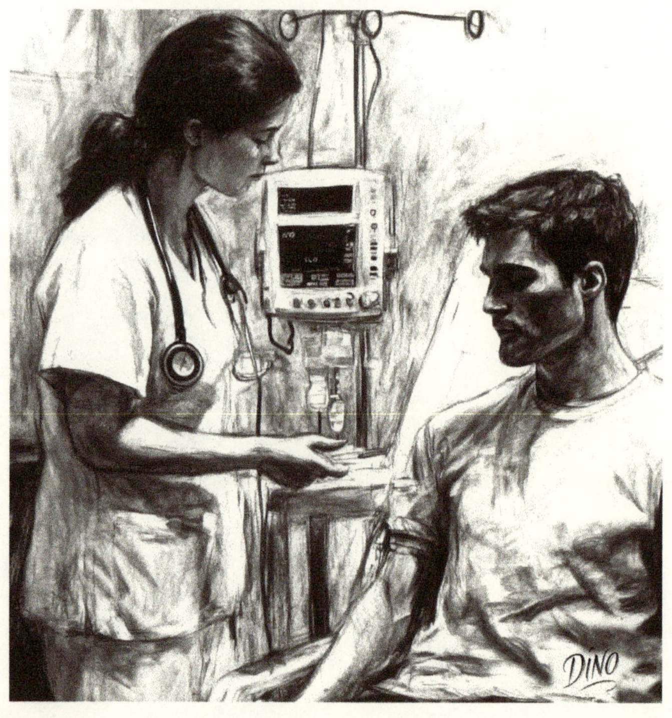

Matthew had tried talk therapy and medications, but the shadow of his deployments still haunted him at home. Day after day, he battled a crushing sense of dread and recurring nightmares. Finally, his doctor suggested something new: ketamine infusion therapy. Matthew felt apprehensive—ketamine had always sounded experimental—but after endless nights of wakefulness and worry, he was ready for a different road.

On the day of his first infusion, he settled into a quiet room, an IV line placed in his arm. The nurse explained every step, reassuring him that he'd be closely monitored. Almost immediately, he sensed a deep calm replacing his usual tension. By the end of the session, Matthew noticed his thoughts felt clearer, less weighed down by the same old loop of traumatic memories.

In the weeks that followed, his improvements held steady. No, ketamine wasn't a "miracle cure." He still had work to do—his therapist helped him process those battlefield memories now that his mind was more flexible. But he felt newly motivated, able to catch his breath and see future possibilities instead of unrelenting fear.

By weaving in real-world testimonials—like Matthew's—we see how this promising therapy can fit into a broader treatment plan, offering renewed hope for those who've carried heavy burdens far too long.

This chapter details that shift: how ketamine, through its unique mechanisms in the brain, can reduce chronic stress reactions and help veterans move forward. We'll explore recommended dosing protocols, discuss the importance of trained medical oversight and highlight the long-term monitoring needed to sustain meaningful change.

Mechanisms of Ketamine in PTSX Treatments

The exploration of ketamine as a treatment for PTSX marks a pivotal moment in mental health care, particularly for military personnel and veterans who often face unique challenges in recovery. Traditional therapeutic approaches, while effective for some, frequently fall short for those suffering from the severe and persistent symptoms of PTSX.

Ketamine, a dissociative anesthetic with rapid-acting antidepressant properties, presents a groundbreaking alternative by offering a new avenue for healing. Understanding the neurobiological mechanisms through which ketamine operates can illuminate its potential to transform treatment protocols and enhance the lives of those who have bravely served.

Ketamine's action on the brain is primarily mediated through its antagonistic effect on the N-methyl-D-aspartate (NMDA) receptor, which plays a crucial role in synaptic plasticity and memory formation. In PTSX patients, the dysregulation of glutamate—an excitatory neurotransmitter—can lead to maladaptive neural circuits associated with fear and anxiety. By inhibiting these NMDA receptors, ketamine effectively reduces hyperactivity in the amygdala, the brain's fear center, allowing for a recalibration of emotional responses. This mechanism not only alleviates acute symptoms but also creates an environment conducive to therapeutic interventions, encouraging veterans to engage in trauma-focused therapy with a renewed sense of hope.

Furthermore, ketamine's influence extends beyond NMDA receptor antagonism. It stimulates the release of brain-derived neurotrophic factor (BDNF), a protein integral to the growth and survival of neurons. Increased levels of BDNF promote neurogenesis and synaptic connectivity, critical factors for recovery in individuals with PTSX.

Ketamine cracks open the locked room of despair long enough for therapy to walk in and switch on the light.

In practical terms, this means that after a ketamine infusion, a veteran may experience enhanced cognitive flexibility and emotional resilience, which are essential for processing traumatic memories and integrating therapeutic insights. The rapid onset of these effects can be particularly beneficial for military personnel who require immediate relief from debilitating symptoms.

Ketamine also presents a unique opportunity for personalized treatment. Given its different effects on individuals, mental-health professionals can tailor dosages and delivery methods like intravenous infusions or intranasal administration to meet the specific needs of each veteran. This flexibility is crucial in addressing the diverse manifestations of PTSX, allowing for a more nuanced and responsive approach to care.

Moreover, the integration of ketamine therapy into existing treatment frameworks can facilitate a comprehensive strategy that includes psychotherapy, community support and lifestyle changes, ultimately enhancing long-term outcomes. As the field of PTSX treatment evolves, the mechanisms of ketamine offer hope for veterans grappling with the aftermath of their experiences. By harnessing the power of this innovative therapy, mental health professionals can significantly improve the quality of life for those who have served.

Developing Safe Protocols for Administration

In the development of PTSX treatments for military personnel and veterans, the establishment of well-defined protocols for administration is paramount. These protocols serve as a framework that ensures consistency, safety and efficacy in delivering innovative therapeutic modalities. Protocols also demand that practitioners have a thorough understanding of neurochemistry and molecular biology, and collaborate with other healthcare professionals to ensure safe administration of ketamine.

By integrating ketamine into the treatment spectrum, mental-health professionals can provide tailored interventions that resonate with the unique experiences of veterans. The importance of these protocols lies not only in their ability to standardize care but also in their capacity to create an environment of healing that is grounded in empathy and understanding. Again, implementing these protocols requires a comprehensive understanding of the neurobiological and molecular mechanisms underlying PTSX.

Establishing partnerships between VA and civilian mental health services can enhance accessibility and provide veterans with a continuum of care that meets their diverse needs.

Long-Term Efficacy and Patient Monitoring

Long-term efficacy and patient monitoring are critical components in developing ketamine treatment for military personnel and veterans. It is essential to establish robust frameworks for assessing the long-term impact on mental health. These frameworks not only help gauge the sustainability of therapeutic benefits but also ensure that we remain vigilant in monitoring potential side effects or complications that may arise over time. By prioritizing these elements, we can enhance our commitment to the wellbeing of those who have bravely served our nation. The molecular mechanisms underlying PTSX necessitate a nuanced understanding of how various treatments influence brain function and emotional regulation over the long term.

Moving Testimonials and Stories

The journey of healing from PTSX is deeply personal and often fraught with challenges, yet the stories of those who have navigated this path can inspire hope and resilience. For military personnel and veterans, the effects of trauma can be profound.

One veteran shared, "After years of struggling with the weight of my experiences, I found solace in ketamine infusion therapy. It didn't just alleviate my symptoms, but opened a door to a new way of living. I can now engage with my family and enjoy moments that once felt out of reach."

Such testimonials underscore the transformative potential of alternative therapies and the importance of integrating these approaches into conventional treatment protocols.

Right now, ketamine therapy is in the wild, wild west phase, with production labs producing pills of various concentrations, although they should be the same concentration per batch. Some companies now offer at-home self-injections of ketamine. We recommend seeing a board-certified anesthesiologist who's an expert in ketamine neurobiology before experimenting with these protocols. Also, the administration of ketamine by an unlicensed and untrained person has the potential to create an unpleasant, if not dangerous, dissociative experience and also the potential for abuse.

In the end, it distills down to this: you must learn about ketamine and its effects, and do in-depth research on its mechanisms of action, so you may predict your outcomes. Doing your own research on physicians is an important point, too. Thankfully, doctors who administer ketamine have their health grades posted on the web. Start with the highest-ranked doctors and interview them. It's also a good idea to have a series of questions in mind when you interview a doctor.

If-Then Guidance

- If you are unfamiliar with ketamine infusion therapy as a treatment for PTSX, then consider researching reliable sources such as clinical studies or consulting with a mental health professional who specializes in emerging therapies. Learning more about how ketamine works, its success rates, and its risks can help you decide if it's worth exploring further.
- If you are interested in ketamine infusion therapy but unsure if it's appropriate for you, then schedule a consultation with a psychiatrist or medical professional who offers this treatment. They can evaluate your specific case and determine if you are a suitable candidate based on your PTSX symptoms and history of treatment resistance.
- If you have already undergone ketamine infusion therapy and found it beneficial, then discuss with your healthcare provider how to maintain these results long term. You may need to incorporate ongoing maintenance sessions or combine ketamine therapy with traditional treatments like therapy for sustained relief.
- If you are worried about potential side effects or risks of ketamine therapy, then ask your healthcare provider for a detailed explanation of the possible outcomes, both short- and long-term. Understanding the risks will allow you to weigh the pros and cons of the treatment and make an informed decision.
- If you are struggling to access ketamine therapy due to cost or insurance limitations, then explore financial assistance programs or clinical trials that offer subsidized treatments. Some clinics may also offer payment plans or sliding scale fees to make the treatment more affordable.

Take the Next Step

- Research Ketamine Therapy: Learn how ketamine works as a fast-acting antidepressant and its effectiveness in treating severe PTSX symptoms.
- Find a Reputable Clinic: If ketamine therapy interests you, locate a clinic experienced in administering ketamine for PTSX. Make

sure the clinic has a proven track record and proper medical oversight.

- Talk to a Provider: Ask your mental-health provider if ketamine therapy is appropriate for you, especially if you have not responded to other treatments.

Through Their Eyes

"I've been through a lot of treatments for PTSX over the years. Therapy, medications—you name it, I've probably tried it. Nothing really stuck. The nightmares, the hypervigilance, the feeling of being on edge every minute of the day—it was all still there, no matter what I did. Then I heard about ketamine. At first, I was hesitant. The idea of using something that sounded like a party drug to treat PTSX seemed strange, but I was desperate, and the research seemed promising.

"The first session was surreal. The doctor explained how ketamine works, how it helps rewire the brain by blocking the NMDA receptors tied to trauma and anxiety. I went into the infusion room, feeling nervous but hopeful. I knew that a board-certified anesthesiologist would be administering the drug.

"As the ketamine started to take effect, it was like the walls I'd built around my trauma began to dissolve. I didn't feel detached or numb. Instead, I felt like I was floating above everything, able to look at my memories from a distance. I saw the trauma without being swallowed by it. For the first time, I wasn't overwhelmed by fear or pain. The effects lasted long after the session.

"Over the next few days, I noticed that the weight I'd been carrying—the constant dread, the anger—it wasn't as heavy. It wasn't gone, but it was lighter, manageable. I found myself able to talk about things in therapy that I had always avoided. The nightmares were less frequent, and for the first time in years, I had a real night's sleep.

"Each session since then has brought me more clarity and more relief. It's not just that the ketamine lifts the fog of PTSX for a while. It's that it opens up a space where healing can actually happen. It's hard to explain, but it feels like my brain is learning to function again without being stuck in survival mode.

"I still do therapy, and I've had to go back for more ketamine sessions to keep the progress going, but I can honestly say it's been a game-changer. Ketamine didn't just treat the symptoms of my PTSX. It gave me the chance to heal in ways I didn't think were possible. For anyone who's struggling and feels like they've hit a wall with other treatments, I'd say this is worth looking into. It's not a miracle, but it's the closest thing I've found to one."

—Mark, US Army Veteran

21

Mechanisms of MDMA-Assisted Therapy

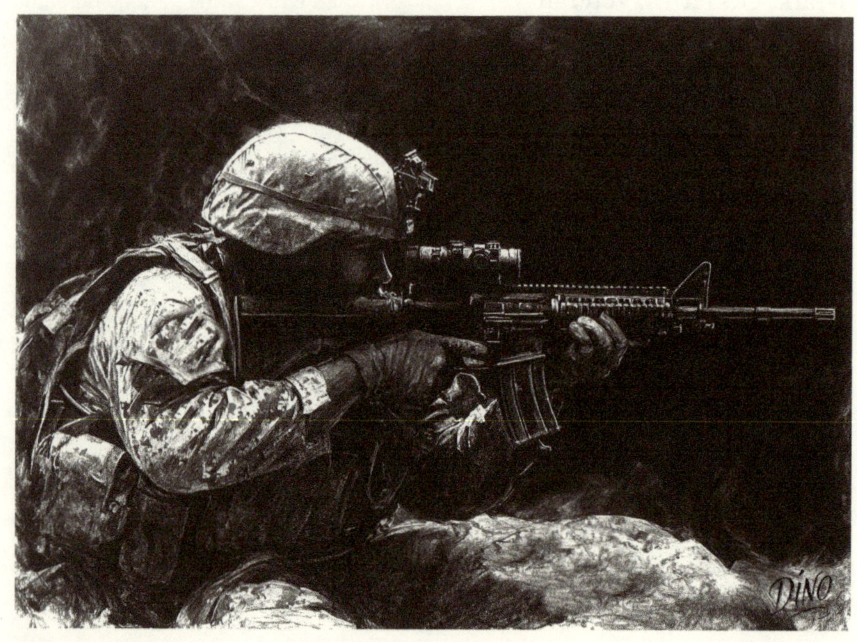

David never imagined he'd be back in a small therapy room, facing the harsh memories of a distant battlefield. But here he was, committing to a treatment that had once been unthinkable—MDMA-assisted therapy. He'd diligently read all the studies and heard other veterans describe breakthroughs they'd not found in traditional talk therapy. Still, part of him wondered if it was all just hype.

When the session began, David felt a warmth and clarity flood through him—a gentle spotlight illuminating the darkest corners of his mind. Past events that usually triggered fear or shame felt more approachable. With his therapist's guidance, he revisited his most painful memories, this time without the overwhelming grip of terror. In those moments, he felt compassion toward himself, something he'd never experienced before. Over subsequent sessions, David noticed changes that stretched beyond the clinic walls. He slept deeper, woke up without the usual tightness in his chest and found it easier to connect with his family. His wife, who had watched him struggle to put words to his anxieties for years, marveled at how he now opened up about what he'd seen overseas. It wasn't a quick fix—he still had rough nights and times of doubt—but the fear no longer felt insurmountable.

This chapter dives into stories like David's, revealing how MDMA-assisted therapy can create long-lasting shifts in how veterans process traumatic memories. We'll explore the science behind MDMA's effects on the brain, how structured sessions help veterans confront what haunts them, and why community support remains vital long after the therapy ends.

As real-life accounts show, this emerging approach can lead to more resilient coping, deeper emotional connections and a renewed sense of possibility—even in the aftermath of life's most harrowing experiences. Remember: PTSX is not simply "all in your head." There's a very real physical (molecular) basis for all you sense and feel.

MDMA and Its Therapeutic Potential

MDMA, commonly known as "Ecstasy," has emerged as a powerful ally in the quest to heal the deep-seated wounds of post-traumatic stress disorder among military personnel and veterans. This psychedelic compound, originally synthesized in the early 20th century, has shown promising therapeutic potential in recent clinical trials, revealing its ability to facilitate profound emotional breakthroughs and enhance the healing process.

The neurobiological mechanisms underpinning MDMA's efficacy in treating PTSX are fascinating. Research indicates that MDMA acts on the brain's serotonin system, promoting the release of neurotransmitters that enhance mood and emotional resilience. This chemical cocktail not only creates feelings of safety and trust, but also allows individuals to confront and process traumatic memories with greater clarity and less emotional distress. For military personnel who have experienced the chaos of combat, this ability to revisit traumatic events in a supportive environment can be transformative, facilitating a journey from survival to healing.

As we explore the comparative efficacy of psychedelic-assisted therapies, MDMA stands out for its unique capacity to promote therapeutic alliance and emotional connection between the therapist and the patient. The structured, supportive environment of MDMA-assisted therapy creates a space where veterans can share their experiences without fear of judgment.

> MDMA-assisted sessions teach the amygdala to unclench while empathy floods the room—chemistry in service of connection, not escape.

This connection is vital, as it helps to dismantle the isolation that often accompanies PTSX. By integrating MDMA into treatment protocols, mental-health professionals can empower veterans to reclaim their personal narratives, creating resilience and a renewed sense of agency over their lives. However, introduction of MDMA into PTSX treatment protocols calls for careful consideration of ethical implications and best practices.

Mental-health professionals must be equipped with the knowledge and skills to navigate the complexities of psychedelic-assisted therapies. This includes understanding the potential benefits and risks, ensuring informed consent and recognizing the importance of community-based support systems for veterans undergoing alternative therapies. Research results indicate that veterans who engage with peer-support groups and community resources demonstrate greater resilience and improved mental health outcomes.

Case Studies Highlighting Success

Case studies serve as powerful illustrations of how innovative treatments can transform the lives of military personnel and veterans grappling with PTSX. The stories that emerge from these studies not only highlight the efficacy of alternative therapies but also underscore the importance of a holistic approach to mental health care. Each case exemplifies the potential for recovery and resilience, offering hope and inspiration for mental health professionals navigating the complexities of PTSX treatment.

One remarkable case involves a veteran who participated in a groundbreaking MDMA-assisted therapy program. After years of struggling with debilitating flashbacks and anxiety, this individual found relief through a carefully structured therapeutic environment that combined the empathogenic effects of MDMA with guided psychotherapy. The results were profound: not only did the veteran experience a significant reduction in PTSX symptoms, but he also reported enhanced emotional connection with loved ones, creating a sense of community and belonging that had long been absent. This case exemplifies the transformative potential of integrating psychedelics into conventional treatment protocols.

As we continue to explore and validate alternative therapies, it is crucial to remain committed to ethical considerations and community-based support systems that ensure veterans receive comprehensive and compassionate care. The journey toward healing is multifaceted and by learning from these success stories, we can create a culture of resilience and recovery in the military community.

If-Then Guidance

- If you have undergone MDMA-assisted therapy and experienced long-lasting relief from PTSX symptoms, then consider discussing this success with your healthcare provider to assess how you can maintain or continue improving your mental health. It may also be helpful to connect with others who are considering this treatment, sharing your experience through support groups or advocacy platforms.

- If you did not experience sustained relief or your symptoms returned after MDMA-assisted therapy, then it's important to revisit your treatment plan with a mental-health professional. There may be additional therapies, like cognitive behavioral therapy or stellate ganglion block, that could complement MDMA therapy or provide further relief.
- If you are concerned about the potential long-term impacts of MDMA-assisted therapy on your mental or physical health, then consult your healthcare provider to discuss any ongoing symptoms or side effects. Regular follow-up appointments can help monitor your health and address any concerns that may arise from the treatment.
- If you have experienced significant improvements from MDMA-assisted therapy, then you might consider maintaining lifestyle practices that support your mental health, such as mindfulness, exercise and therapy. This holistic approach can help sustain the positive effects of the therapy over time.
- If you are considering undergoing MDMA-assisted therapy but are unsure about its long-term effects, then research peer-reviewed studies and clinical trial outcomes to gain a better understanding of the therapy's potential risks and benefits. Discuss these findings with your healthcare provider to make an informed decision about whether this treatment is right for you.

Take the Next Step

- Learn About MDMA-Assisted Therapy: Read how MDMA can facilitate emotional openness during therapy and reduce PTSX symptoms. The Multidisciplinary Association for Psychedelic Studies (MAPS) is best known for sponsoring clinical trials investigating MDMA-assisted psychotherapy as a potential treatment for PTSX.
- Explore Legal Pathways: MDMA is currently in Phase 3 clinical trials but could soon be an approved treatment. Keep an eye on changes in its legal status and availability for veterans.
- Consider Participation in a Trial: Check clinicaltrials.gov or

other resources for MDMA therapy trials focused on PTSX, and discuss your eligibility with a doctor.

Through Their Eyes

"For years after I left the Army, I was stuck in survival mode. No matter how much I tried to push forward, the memories of what I had seen and done followed me everywhere. Traditional therapy helped to a degree, but it always felt like there was something missing—like no matter how many sessions I went through, I couldn't get past the walls I had built around myself. Then I heard about MDMA-assisted therapy, and though it seemed unconventional, I was willing to try anything at that point. The therapy itself was nothing like what I expected. MDMA didn't numb me or make me feel disconnected—instead, it opened me up in ways I never thought possible.

"With my therapist there to guide me, I was able to look at the trauma and understand it, without being overwhelmed by fear or pain. It was like I could finally see the trauma clearly and, in doing so, it lost its power over me. What made the biggest difference, though, was the emotional connection I felt during the sessions. It wasn't just about revisiting the past—it was about feeling understood, a sense of trust and connection stayed with me long after the therapy was over. I felt safe.

"Since completing the MDMA sessions, my life has transformed. MDMA has given me the tools to work through my trauma in a way that traditional therapy never could. I still have tough days, but I no longer feel trapped by my past. I can finally breathe again, and that sense of relief is something I never thought I'd experience."

—Brad, US Army Veteran

22

Comparative Efficacy of Psychedelic- and Hallucinogenic-Assisted Therapies

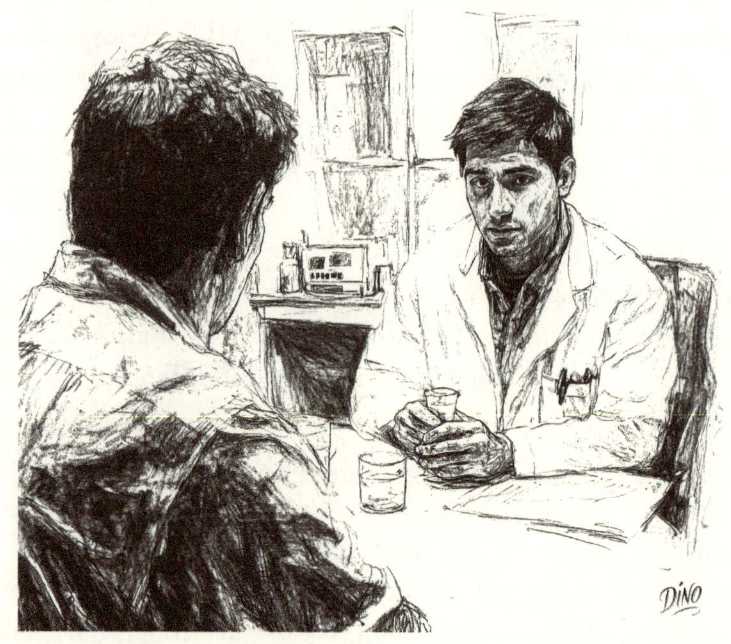

Daniel remembered the cool desert air of the night, where he'd once stood watch on a foreign base, counting every breath to keep calm. Those days felt half a lifetime away now that he was back home, fighting a different battle: the relentless flashbacks and surges of anxiety that came with PTSX. Traditional therapy helped, but only so much. It wasn't until he heard about a study using psychedelics—psilocybin, MDMA—that his mind sparked with cautious curiosity.

Sitting in a small clinic room, Daniel felt nervous yet oddly hopeful. He'd read that these substances could open new pathways in the brain, almost like rewriting a story you'd told yourself for too long. Under careful supervision, he tried a guided session with a low dose of psilocybin, the active ingredient in "magic mushrooms." It was unlike anything he'd experienced—colors felt more vivid, memories somehow gentler. Most important, he sensed a door creaking open to parts of himself he'd locked away.

In the following days, Daniel noticed a subtle shift. Nightmares came, but they didn't clamp down on him as tightly. He felt he could stand back, observe them and let them pass. His therapist explained how psychedelics might jumpstart the brain's healing processes, allowing a sense of calm or insight that traditional methods couldn't always reach. Some veterans tried MDMA for the same reason, reporting breakthroughs in trust and self-acceptance. Others used cannabinoids to tame anxiety and sleep issues.

It wasn't a miracle cure—Daniel still had tough nights. But each hurdle felt a bit more manageable. The research showed promise, and the clinic's supportive environment helped anchor him.

This chapter explores these emerging, neurochemistry-altering therapies—how they compare, why they work, and how they might lead veterans like Daniel closer to the steady ground they've been seeking all along.

Overview of Hallucinogenic and Psychedelic Substances

The exploration of hallucinogenic and psychedelic substances (HPS) within the context of PTSX treatment for military personnel and veterans represents a transformative frontier in mental healthcare. These substances, once shrouded in stigma and misunderstanding, are emerging as powerful tools in the therapeutic arsenal against the debilitating effects of traumatic experiences.

As research results are published, it is becoming increasingly clear that HPS can facilitate profound psychological insights but also catalyze neurobiological changes that hold promise for healing deep-seated trauma. Understanding these substances and their mechanisms paves the way for innovative treatment protocols that can offer hope to those who have served. Psychedelics like psilocybin, MDMA and ayahuasca have demonstrated the potential to alter perception and consciousness, allowing individuals to confront painful memories and emotions in a safe and supportive environment. These substances can promote neuroplasticity, creating new connections in the brain that may help rewire maladaptive thought patterns commonly associated with PTSX.

Psychedelic ethics start with consent, set and setting. Visions without guardrails can wound as deeply as war.

Artificial thoughts and experiences from hallucinogens can be dangerous, and can have long-lasting negative consequences. Scientists calls these "side effects." LSD is now prepared in lower concentrations that make its effects manageable. The VA has yet to prioritize experimenting with LSD for PTSX treatments.

By engaging with these profound experiences, veterans can gain new perspectives on their trauma, often leading to emotional release and a sense of catharsis. The integration of these drug-assisted experiences into therapeutic frameworks is crucial for maximizing benefits and ensuring that healing is not only profound but also sustainable.

Moreover, the comparative efficacy of psychedelic-assisted therapies is being scrutinized in clinical settings, revealing encouraging outcomes for veterans who engage with these approaches. Initial studies indicate that veterans receiving MDMA-assisted therapy report significant reductions in PTSX symptoms, with many experiencing improvements that persist long after the treatment sessions have concluded.

This is particularly compelling given the chronic nature of PTSX and the often-limited effectiveness of conventional treatments. As mental-health practitioners, understanding the nuances of these therapies—including dosage, setting and integration techniques—will be vital in optimizing treatment outcomes for military personnel and veterans.

In addition to psychedelics, the integration of cannabinoids into conventional PTSX treatment protocols continues to gain traction.

Cannabinoids have been shown to alleviate anxiety and promote relaxation, which can be particularly beneficial for veterans grappling with the hyperarousal and intrusive memories characteristic of PTSX.

As the legal landscape surrounding cannabis continues to evolve, there is a unique opportunity for mental health professionals to explore its potential alongside traditional therapies, creating a holistic approach that addresses the multifaceted nature of trauma. It's essential to consider the ethical implications and community support systems associated with alternative therapies for PTSX. As we venture into this new territory, ongoing training and education for mental-health professionals will be paramount. This ensures that practitioners are equipped with the knowledge and skills necessary to navigate the complexities of HPS treatment while prioritizing patient safety and welfare.

Research Findings on Veterans and HPS

Results from recent studies have demonstrated that veterans often respond differently to treatment modalities compared to the civilian population. This underscores the importance of tailored approaches, particularly when integrating psychedelic-assisted therapies such as MDMA and psilocybin into PTSX treatment protocols.

Research has shown that these substances can facilitate profound emotional processing, enabling veterans to confront trauma in a safe, supportive environment. The neurobiological underpinnings of these therapies reveal a potential for rewiring maladaptive neural pathways, leading to lasting improvements in mental health and wellbeing.

Stimulation techniques like SGB and Ketamine Infusion Therapy have also shown promise in alleviating the debilitating symptoms of PTSX. Clinical outcomes suggest that these interventions can prompt rapid relief where traditional therapies may have faltered. By initiating discussions around best practices and outcomes, healthcare practitioners can cultivate a comprehensive understanding of these techniques, empowering them to make informed decisions that prioritize the health and safety of veterans.

Finally, the importance of community-based support systems cannot be overstated. As veterans navigate their healing journeys, the integration of peer support and shared experiences can enhance the effectiveness of alternative therapies. Success stories from veterans who have undergone innovative treatments inspire hope and create a culture of resilience within military communities.

The commitment to training and education for mental-health professionals on these alternative therapies will ensure that they are equipped to guide veterans toward the healing they deserve, ultimately transforming the landscape of PTSX treatment.

Mechanisms of Action: How HPS Agents Facilitate Healing

Psychedelic-assisted therapies like those incorporating MDMA and psilocybin, have shown remarkable efficacy in treating PTSX by promoting neuroplasticity and emotional processing. These substances interact with serotonin receptors, particularly the 5-HT2A receptor, which plays a crucial role in mood regulation and emotional response.

By altering the brain's chemistry, psychedelics help patients confront traumatic memories in a safe context, ultimately leading to a profound reconnection with their emotions. This reconnection is vital for veterans who often struggle with emotional numbing, allowing them to process their experiences and integrate them into a coherent narrative that creates healing.

As veterans experience a reduction in their physiological symptoms, they are often better equipped to participate in psychotherapy and other healing modalities, thereby accelerating their recovery journey. Remember: behavioral therapy changes chemistry, and that new chemistry enhances subsequent behavioral therapy. The cycle continues to build on itself and so improves overall chemistry and behavior.

As we elevate the standard of care for those who have served, understanding the mechanisms of action behind HPS agents asssist us in developing new pathways of healing and resilience for our veterans.

If-Then Guidance

- If you are unfamiliar with psychedelic and hallucinogenic-assisted therapies (such as MDMA, psilocybin, or LSD) for PTSX, then consider researching these treatments or speaking with a healthcare provider who specializes in emerging therapies. These treatments are currently being studied for their efficacy in reducing PTSX symptoms, and understanding the latest research can help you determine if they might be a viable option for you. To date, Oregon and Colorado have legalized psilocybin as a therapeutic agent, though federally it is still a controlled substance and thus remains illegal to use in therapy.

- If you are interested in trying psychedelic-assisted therapy but are unsure of its legality or accessibility, then consult your healthcare provider or local veterans' support organizations to learn about ongoing clinical trials. These therapies are often available through controlled research settings where you can receive supervised care.
- If you have already tried psychedelic or hallucinogenic therapies and found them to be effective, then discuss with your provider how to integrate the benefits of the therapy into your long-term treatment plan. They may recommend follow-up therapies or additional treatments to sustain your progress.
- If you are concerned about the potential risks or psychological effects of psychedelic therapy, then speak to a qualified healthcare professional to explore these concerns in-depth. They can explain the safety protocols used in clinical settings and help you assess whether the potential benefits outweigh the risks for your specific situation.
- If you are interested in exploring psychedelic therapy but concerned about the stigma or skepticism surrounding it, then consider joining a support group or online forum where veterans who have undergone this therapy share their experiences. Hearing from others can help you gain a clearer perspective on the outcomes and alleviate concerns about societal perceptions.
- If you are facing challenges in accessing psychedelic-assisted therapy due to costs or insurance coverage, then explore research programs or nonprofit organizations that may offer financial assistance. Many clinical trials provide treatment at little or no cost to participants, and advocacy groups may help you navigate potential cost barriers.

Take the Next Step

- Educate Yourself: Research the potential benefits and risks of psychedelic-assisted therapies like MDMA and psilocybin. Start by reading reputable studies and veteran testimonials.
- Check for Clinical Trials: Look for clinical trials focused on veterans and psychedelic therapy. Many are in experimental phases but may offer new treatment options.
- Visit ClinicalTrials.gov, a database maintained by the US National Library of Medicine. Enter keywords like "PTSD" or "Post-Traumatic Stress Disorder" in the search bar (the term PTSX is, for the first time, presented in this book and has yet to be adopted by healthcare professionals). Use filters like recruiting status, location, age group, or study phase to narrow your search.
- Contact the National Institute of Mental Health (NIMH). Visit their Clinical Trials webpage for ongoing studies or call their information line.
- If you are a veteran, the Department of Veterans Affairs offers PTSD research and clinical trials. Visit the VA's Research and Development page: https://www.research.va.gov.
- Reach out to Universities and Medical Centers. Many universities and hospitals run PTSD research programs. Check the research pages of institutions like Stanford University, Harvard or local medical schools.
- Organizations like the PTSD Foundation of America or the National Center for PTSD provide resources and may list trials
- Ask your VA healthcare provider or mental healthcare specialist for recommendations or referrals to clinical trials.

Tips for Participating in a Clinical Trial:

Understand the Purpose: Know the trial's goals and how it relates to PTSD

Inquire About Risks and Benefits: Ask about the potential risks and expected outcomes.

Review Eligibility: Ensure you meet the criteria (e.g. age, diagnosis)

Ask About Costs: Clarify whether there are any costs or if the trial covers all expenses. If not, ask whether anyone can pay the costs. Some private organizations provide these services to veterans and qualified civilians free of charge.

Discuss Options with a Provider: Ask your healthcare provider if these therapies might be appropriate for you and if there are legal, supervised programs available in your area.

Through Their Eyes

"I had tried just about everything—therapy, medication, you name it. After years of struggling with PTSX, it felt like I was still trapped in my own mind, reliving the worst moments over and over. Every time I thought I had found something that worked, the relief would be temporary. I didn't know what else I could do.

"Then I heard about psychedelic-assisted therapy. To be honest, I was skeptical at first. I had spent my entire life following orders, keeping everything under control. The idea of using something like MDMA to treat PTSX seemed way out of left field. I was willing to try anything.

"My first session was nothing like I expected. I wasn't 'tripping' or lost in a dreamland like you might imagine with drugs. Instead, it was like the walls I had built around my trauma started to come down, but in a way that felt safe. I could actually look at my memories—memories I had spent years trying to bury—and I didn't feel overwhelmed by them. I saw them dispassionately as I would a movie. I knew the violence in the movie couldn't harm me. It was all show.

"During those hours, I confronted things I hadn't been able to talk about since I came back from deployment. But it wasn't just about talking or thinking. I could feel myself processing it on a deeper level, like my brain was rewiring the way I related to those memories. It was hard work, but it wasn't like the therapy sessions I had done before, where I would just go home and feel drained afterward. This felt different—like something was finally shifting inside me.

"In the weeks and months that followed, I realized I wasn't reacting the same way to my triggers. The flashbacks weren't gone, but they didn't control me in the same way anymore. It was like I had more space to breathe, more room to think. I wasn't just managing my symptoms anymore. I was actually starting to heal. What surprised me the most was how the therapy kept working even after the sessions. My therapist explained that the MDMA had helped my brain connect in new ways—something called neuroplasticity—and that those changes didn't just go away once the drug wore off. I felt calmer, more at peace with my past. And for the first time, I wasn't terrified of my future, because I learned to live in the present.

"I never thought I'd say this, but I'm living proof that psychedelic therapy works. It's not a magic fix, but it's a powerful tool. It gave me the breakthrough I needed when nothing else seemed to help. Now, I'm not just surviving—I'm actually starting to live again."

—Emma, US Marine Corps Veteran

23

Dr. Eugene Lipov: Stellate Ganglion Block and Dual Sympathetic Reset

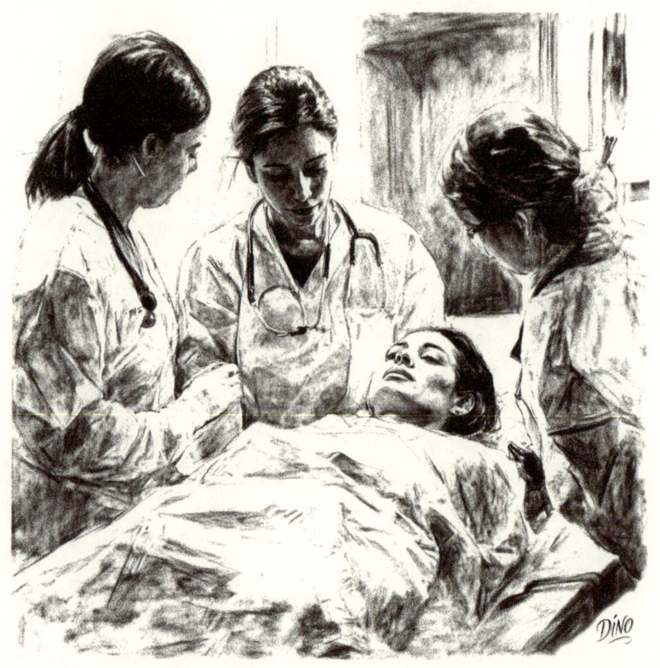

Leila always felt a knot in her stomach, a low-grade alert that never let her relax. Since coming home from her last deployment, she'd tried group therapy, medication and meditation apps—all provided some help, but the anxiety lingered like a shadow. Then she heard about a treatment called stellate ganglion block, or SGB, pioneered by an anesthesiologist and researcher, Dr. Eugene Lipov, outside Chicago. It sounded almost too good to be true—a quick procedure that could calm the body's relentless "fight-or-flight" state.

Traveling to Dr. Lipov's Westmont, Illinois clinic, The Stella Center, Leila found herself face-to-face with a calm, reassuring physician. He explained how injecting a local anesthetic into a cluster of nerves in her neck could "reset" her overactive stress response. The idea was simple: if the nervous system could relax, so could the rest of her.

She went through with it, feeling that familiar tightness rise as the doctor prepped the injection site. But within hours, Leila noticed a subtle shift—an uncoiling in her chest, a softening of the constant tension in her shoulders. That night, she slept more peacefully than she had in years. Over the next week, each day felt a bit lighter. Her mind still held the memories, but the overwhelming grip they had on her body loosened.

> One stellate ganglion injection granted me more peace than nearly 20 years of pills. Relief this dramatic demands fast-track policy, not red-tape purgatory.

When she returned for a follow-up, they talked about Dual Sympathetic Reset (DSR), a more comprehensive version of SGB that targets both sides of the neck, administered on two separate days. She learned that for some people, a second injection could deepen or extend the relief. For her, the single treatment made all the difference. Leila felt energized to continue therapy, to focus on regaining parts of herself she thought were lost.

This chapter unpacks that journey—how SGB quiets the overactive alarm systems in the body, how Dr. Lipov's pioneering work has transformed PTSX treatment and why it's giving veterans like Leila fresh hope for recovery. It also explores how SGB works, the science behind its effectiveness, the different variations of the technique—including Dual Sympathetic Reset—and why it is changing the landscape of PTSX treatment for veterans. Please note this chapter is not meant as a promotional piece for Dr. Lipov. His work in SGB therapy is presented here objectively. If SGB is right for you, please consult Dr. Lipov. Also note that he has trained many physicians on SGB therapy.

Understanding Stellate Ganglion Block and Dual-Sympathetic Reset Treatments

In the quest to find effective treatments for PTSX, a promising and relatively new approach has emerged that is making waves in the field of trauma therapy. SGB is an innovative procedure that offers a groundbreaking method for treating the physiological roots of PTSX, anxiety and depression. It offers hope to military personnel and veterans who have long struggled with the effects of trauma. SGB's unique ability to address both the physical and psychological symptoms of PTSX has made it one of the most exciting developments in trauma care.

Understanding Anxiety Disorders

Anxiety disorders are a group of mental-health conditions characterized by persistent and overwhelming worry, fear or nervousness. Unlike everyday stress, anxiety disorders create intense feelings of dread that are difficult to control and can last for long periods. These disorders, such as Generalized Anxiety Disorder (GAD), Social Anxiety Disorder, Panic Disorder and specific phobias, can significantly impair daily functioning, relationships and overall wellbeing.

While traditional treatments like medication and therapy have been the primary methods of managing anxiety disorders, there is a growing interest in more innovative approaches like SGB for treating anxiety, particularly in veterans and military personnel who have experienced trauma.

Anxiety manifests in various forms, including social anxiety disorder, separation anxiety, phobias and the most common type, GAD. Each of these can cause significant symptoms that affect day-to-day life: trouble sleeping, difficulty concentrating, or experiencing overwhelming panic episodes.

While treatments like cognitive-behavioral therapy and exposure therapy are often effective, they require significant time, effort and significant patient commitment. Veterans and trauma survivors may face additional hurdles in seeking traditional therapies due to the nature of their experiences and the stigma surrounding mental health in military culture. For some, alternative treatments like the SGB are a breakthrough in alleviating symptoms where conventional methods may fall short.

Symptoms of Anxiety

The symptoms of anxiety can manifest in various ways. The following are eight of the most common signs that someone may be experiencing an anxiety disorder:

1. Restlessness: This refers to the inability to relax or sit still, a feeling of being perpetually "on edge."
2. Impending Doom or Worry: A pervasive sense of danger or dread that something bad is about to happen, often without any real cause.
3. Panic Episodes: Sudden surges of overwhelming fear or discomfort, often accompanied by physical symptoms like chest pain, dizziness and difficulty breathing.
4. Difficulty Concentrating: Anxiety can interfere with one's ability to focus on tasks or think clearly.
5. Fatigue: Chronic anxiety can lead to exhaustion, both mental and physical, even after minimal exertion.
6. Trouble Sleeping: Anxiety often disrupts sleep patterns, causing difficulty falling asleep or staying asleep due to racing thoughts.
7. Obsessions/Compulsions: These may resemble symptoms of Obsessive-Compulsive Disorder, where persistent thoughts or behaviors emerge as a coping mechanism for anxiety.
8. Agitation: A constant state of irritability or nervous excitement that can escalate into aggressive behavior if left untreated.

While many people may experience some of these symptoms without having a formal anxiety diagnosis, chronic and persistent symptoms significantly affect daily life. For those, particularly veterans and individuals suffering from PTSX, anxiety is often one aspect of a more complex mental-health picture, which requires targeted, effective treatments.

Causes and Risk Factors for Anxiety Disorders

Anxiety disorders can arise from a combination of genetic, environmental and psychological factors. Some individuals may have a family history of anxiety, making them more genetically predisposed to developing the condition. Traumatic events, ongoing stress, or significant life changes can also trigger or worsen anxiety.

Additionally, certain personality traits like perfectionism or pessimism can make individuals more vulnerable to developing anxiety disorders. Physical health issues and substance use can further exacerbate the problem, leading to a cycle of distress that becomes increasingly difficult to manage without proper treatment.

Traditional Treatments and Their Limitations

Conventional treatments for anxiety typically involve medication, such as antidepressants or benzodiazepines and psychotherapy. While these treatments can be effective, they often come with drawbacks. Medications can have side effects such as drowsiness, weight gain, or dependency and they do not always address the underlying causes of anxiety. Psychotherapy, while beneficial, requires a long-term commitment and it may not work for everyone, especially for those with trauma-related anxiety.

For veterans and military personnel, these treatments may feel insufficient or slow. Many struggle with the lingering effects of trauma, which can complicate their ability to benefit fully from traditional methods. As awareness grows about the limitations of these treatments, alternative approaches like SGB are gaining recognition for their ability to offer rapid and effective relief from anxiety symptoms, particularly in cases related to trauma and PTSX.

What Is Stellate Ganglion Block?

SGB is an innovative treatment that has emerged as a promising solution for veterans and others suffering from trauma-related anxiety and PTSX. The stellate ganglia are bundles of nerves located on both sides of the neck. They are part of the sympathetic nervous system, the part of the body responsible for the “fight or flight” response to stress.

In cases of chronic anxiety and PTSX, the sympathetic nervous system, which turns on the "fight or flight" response, can become overactive, leading to persistent feelings of fear, hypervigilance and anxiety. If it is turned on too long, it can lead to heightened anxiety, depression and other PTSX issues.

SGB involves the injection of a local anesthetic into the stellate ganglion on one side of the neck to "reset" the sympathetic nervous system. By temporarily blocking nerve transmission, the treatment reduces the activity of the fight-or-flight response, allowing the patient to experience a reduction in anxiety symptoms. The procedure is typically performed by a trained healthcare professional and can take as little as five to ten minutes.

SGB has been used to treat chronic pain conditions, but in recent years, it has gained attention for its ability to alleviate symptoms of PTSX and anxiety. While the exact mechanisms are still being studied, the procedure's ability to calm an overactive sympathetic nervous system provides immediate relief for many patients, particularly those who have not responded to traditional treatments. For most, the relief is felt within a few hours.

The Science Behind SGB and Anxiety Treatment

Several studies have shown that SGB can be highly effective in reducing anxiety and PTSX symptoms. One key aspect of SGB's success is its ability to provide rapid relief compared to conventional treatments, which may take weeks or even years to show effects.

In clinical trials, SGB has been linked to improvements in core PTSX and anxiety symptoms, such as reduced hyperarousal, better emotional regulation and an improved ability to engage in daily activities without overwhelming fear or dread.

In 2020, a clinical trial specifically evaluating the impact of SGB on PTSX and anxiety revealed a significant reduction in symptoms. Veterans who received SGB treatment reported improvements across all core measures, including the PTSX Checklist (PCL-5), Patient Health Questionnaire (PHQ-9) and Generalized Anxiety Disorder 7-Item Scale (GAD-7). These improvements were not only immediate but long-lasting, demonstrating that SGB can offer enduring relief for individuals struggling with trauma-related anxiety.

In 2023, another study focusing on dual-level stellate ganglion block, or Dual Sympathetic Reset, an advanced form of SGB with injections on both sides of the neck within a 24-hour period, found that patients experienced a 50% reduction in anxiety symptoms as measured by GAD-7 scores. This case series involving 285 patients confirmed that SGB is not just a temporary fix, but an effective treatment for significantly reducing the emotional and physical toll of anxiety disorders.

SGB as Part of a Holistic Treatment Plan

While SGB is a powerful tool for alleviating anxiety and PTSX symptoms, it is most effective when used as part of a comprehensive treatment plan. For many individuals, SGB can serve as a starting point for reducing the intensity of symptoms, which can then make other therapeutic approaches, such as psychotherapy or cognitive-behavioral therapy, more accessible and effective.

Professionals often recommend that patients who undergo SGB continue to engage in therapy and other supportive treatments to address the psychological aspects of trauma. By combining SGB with psychotherapy, mindfulness practices and other holistic interventions, patients can achieve a more complete and lasting recovery from the effects of anxiety and PTSX.

SGB is an innovative and promising treatment for individuals suffering from anxiety disorders and PTSX. By targeting the sympathetic nervous system, SGB offers rapid and long-lasting relief from symptoms that have often proven resistant to conventional therapies. For veterans and trauma survivors, this treatment provides a path to recovery that emphasizes the importance of both physiological and psychological healing.

As awareness of SGB and its effectiveness continues to grow, it is becoming an increasingly valuable tool in the mental-health field. Whether used as a standalone treatment or in conjunction with other therapies, SGB offers hope and healing to those who have long struggled with the debilitating effects of these conditions.

Motivation of a Pioneer

Dr. Eugene Lipov is internationally recognized as a leading expert in the treatment of PTSX symptoms. A true pioneer in SGB for post-traumatic stress disorder, Dr. Lipov's expertise is deeply personal. His childhood, marked by his father's struggles with PTSX and his mother's tragic battle with depression, has given him a profound understanding of the devastating impact trauma can have on individuals and their families. This personal experience has driven his lifelong mission to provide relief and restore hope to those suffering from PTSX.

In 2006, Dr. Lipov revolutionized the use of SGB for the treatment of PTSX. Initially approved by the US Food and Drug Administration (FDA) in the 1950s to treat certain types of pain and circulatory issues, the SGB procedure was not widely known for its potential in trauma treatment. Historically used for pain relief, especially in cases of menopause symptoms, cancer-related hot flashes, and shingles, Dr. Lipov's research brought new attention to its ability to alleviate symptoms of PTSX.

Through his work, he discovered that administering injections into both stellate ganglia could yield even more significant relief, a breakthrough that led to the development of his advanced protocol, Dual Sympathetic Reset.

While the use of nerve blocks in pain management is well established, Dr. Lipov's innovation was in recognizing the potential of SGB to address PTSX, fundamentally changing the way trauma is understood and treated. As a board-certified anesthesiologist and researcher, Dr. Lipov identified the critical role of the sympathetic nervous system, particularly the stellate ganglion, in the manifestation of PTSX symptoms.

His research demonstrated that PTSX is not solely a psychological condition but one with deep neurochemical roots. By targeting these roots, SGB offers a direct and rapid intervention to alter the brain's response to trauma, unlike traditional therapies, which often require longer periods to produce results.

Dr. Lipov's contributions have been instrumental in promoting SGB as an effective treatment for veterans, military personnel and others suffering from PTSX. Through extensive clinical trials, case studies and continued research, he and his colleagues have shown that SGB can dramatically reduce symptoms of hypervigilance, anxiety, panic attacks, depression and intrusive thoughts.

In recognition of his groundbreaking work, Dr. Lipov has testified before the US House Committee on Veterans' Affairs (2010) on PTSX treatment. His collaborations with neuroscientists have solidified his reputation as the foremost authority on the physiology of stellate ganglion block in treating PTSX. His research has been widely published in prestigious journals such as *Biological Psychiatry*, *Current Psychiatry*, *Military Medicine*, *Pain Research & Treatment*, *Psychiatric Annals*, and *The Lancet*. Please see the References chapter at the end of the book for citations to his articles and papers.

His work has also garnered significant media attention, with features in the *Wall Street Journal*, *Los Angeles Times*, *Chicago Tribune*, *USA Today*, and appearances on ABC, NBC, WGN, and many more. Dr. Eugene Lipov's dedication to advancing PTSX treatment continues to offer new hope to those affected by trauma, reshaping the way the medical community approaches mental health and trauma recovery.

How SGB Heals

PTSX often leaves individuals in a constant state of fight-or-flight, a response governed by the sympathetic nervous system. This heightened state of arousal can lead to symptoms like anxiety, irritability, sleep disturbances and an exaggerated startle response. SGB calms the overstimulated sympathetic nervous system, effectively "resetting" it to a more balanced state. Here's how it happens:

Calming the Overactive Amygdala: The amygdala is the part of the brain responsible for processing fear and emotional responses. In people with PTSX, the amygdala is often hyperactive, leading to heightened anxiety and emotional reactivity. By blocking a stellate ganglion, SGB helps to reduce the excessive stimulation of the amygdala, allowing individuals to experience a reduction in fear and anxiety.

Reducing Hypervigilance and Anxiety: One of the hallmarks of PTSX is the feeling of constant alertness or hypervigilance, where individuals feel as though they are always on guard for potential threats.

This state of hyperarousal is driven by the sympathetic nervous system, which is responsible for the body's fight-or-flight response. SGB helps "reset" this system by blocking the signals that trigger excessive alertness and anxiety, allowing individuals to feel more relaxed and at ease in their environments.

Improving Sleep and Reducing Nightmares: Many veterans with PTSX suffer from insomnia, nightmares and restless sleep due to their heightened state of alertness. SGB has been shown to improve sleep quality by reducing the stress signals that interfere with rest. This can lead to fewer nightmares and more restorative sleep, which is crucial for overall mental health and recovery from trauma.

Enhancing Emotional Regulation: Trauma can impair an individual's ability to regulate emotions, often leading to mood swings, irritability and outbursts of anger or sadness. By reducing the activity of the sympathetic nervous system, SGB helps individuals regain control over their emotional responses. This allows them to process and manage their emotions more effectively, leading to improved relationships and overall quality of life.

Restoring Cognitive Function: PTSX can cause cognitive disruptions, including difficulty concentrating, memory problems and impaired decision-making. SGB has been reported to improve cognitive function by allowing the brain to operate without the constant interference of stress-related signals. Veterans who undergo SGB often report feeling sharper, more focused and better able to engage in everyday tasks.

Different Types of SGB and the Dual Sympathetic Reset (DSR)

The standard SGB involves injecting a local anesthetic into the stellate ganglion on one side of the neck, typically the right side. This is because the right stellate ganglion is more closely associated with the fight-or-flight response and blocking it can produce significant reductions in PTSX symptoms. In some cases, a second injection may be administered on the left side if further symptom relief is needed.

This standard approach is highly effective for many individuals and can provide relief for weeks to months, with some patients experiencing long-term benefits. However, some veterans may require a more comprehensive intervention, especially if their symptoms are severe or if they have not responded fully to the standard SGB.

Dual Sympathetic Reset (DSR)

DSR is an enhanced version of the SGB procedure that targets both sides of the neck. This improved procedure is a more complete reset of the sympathetic nervous system. In DSR, the clinician performs SGB on both the right and left sides of the neck, ensuring that both hemispheres of the sympathetic nervous system are treated. The rationale behind DSR is that treating both sides of the stellate ganglion creates a more comprehensive reset of the body's stress response system, leading to deeper and longer-lasting symptom relief. DSR works well in treating veterans with severe PTSX or those not responding standard SGB.

Repetition of SGB for Long-Term Relief

Some veterans may require repeat SGB procedures to maintain symptom relief over time. While the initial effects of SGB can be profound, the body's nervous system may eventually revert to its previous state of hyperarousal. By repeating the procedure, clinicians can help patients maintain the benefits of SGB for longer periods, allowing them to engage more fully in other forms of therapy and recovery.

SGB vs. Traditional Treatments for PTSX

Traditional treatments for PTSX like cognitive behavioral therapy, eye movement desensitization and reprocessing and medications like antidepressants and anxiolytics, often require months or even years to produce significant results. While these therapies can be effective for many individuals, they focus primarily on addressing the psychological and behavioral symptoms of PTSX rather than its physiological roots.

SGB, on the other hand, works directly on the neurobiological mechanisms that contribute to PTSX, offering faster relief from symptoms. Many veterans who have undergone SGB report feeling immediate improvements in their mood, anxiety levels and ability to function. This immediate effect makes SGB a powerful tool for veterans who need rapid symptom relief, especially those who may be at risk of self-harm or suicidal thoughts.

Moreover, SGB can be used in conjunction with other therapies. By reducing the physiological symptoms of PTSX, SGB can make veterans more receptive to talk therapy and trauma processing, allowing them to engage more fully in their treatment and recovery.

If-Then Guidance

- If you experience persistent anxiety, hypervigilance, or intrusive thoughts, then consider discussing Stellate Ganglion Block (SGB) with your doctor as a treatment option. Dr. Eugene Lipov: 1 E Oak Hill Dr., Ste 100. Westmont, IL 60559; (855) 519-2122; https://stellamentalhealth.com.
- If traditional therapies for PTSX, such as talk therapy or medication, have not provided sufficient relief, then ask about innovative treatments like SGB or Dual Sympathetic Reset (DSR). Dr. Lipov at The Stella Center specializes in both.
- If you are a veteran or trauma survivor struggling with heightened fight-or-flight responses, then SGB may help to "reset" your nervous system and reduce these symptoms.
- If sleep disturbances and nightmares are affecting your daily life, then SGB could improve your sleep quality by calming your overactive sympathetic nervous system.
- If you have difficulty regulating emotions, leading to mood swings or irritability, then SGB might provide the emotional stability needed to regain control over your responses.
- If you feel stuck in your recovery journey, unable to engage fully in traditional therapies, then SGB may reduce your symptoms enough to make other treatments more effective.
- If you experience cognitive difficulties like trouble concentrating or making decisions, then SGB could improve mental clarity by decreasing stress-related interference.
- If you are skeptical about new treatments, then consider reviewing clinical studies showing SGB's rapid and lasting effects on PTSX and anxiety symptoms.

- If you worry about the invasiveness of the procedure, then know that SGB is minimally invasive, takes only minutes, and often delivers relief within hours.
- If you are looking for a holistic approach to healing, then combine SGB with psychotherapy, mindfulness, or other supportive treatments for comprehensive recovery.

Take the Next Step

- Consult with a healthcare provider experienced in trauma care to determine if SGB is appropriate for your symptoms and history.
- Research clinics or specialists, such as those trained in Dr. Eugene Lipov's protocols, who can provide high-quality SGB treatment.
- Prepare for your initial consultation by documenting your symptoms, treatment history, and any triggers that exacerbate your anxiety or PTSX.
- Explore insurance coverage or financial assistance options, as SGB may not yet be fully covered by all providers.
- If recommended for SGB, ensure the procedure is performed by a licensed and experienced clinician to minimize risks and maximize effectiveness.
- After undergoing SGB, maintain a journal to track symptom changes, sleep patterns, and emotional shifts to share with your healthcare team.
- Schedule follow-up appointments to assess the need for additional treatments or DSR for enhanced symptom relief.
- Support your recovery with a balanced lifestyle, incorporating exercise, healthy eating, and practices like mindfulness to complement SGB's benefits.
- Engage in psychotherapy or support groups post-SGB to address the psychological aspects of trauma and build coping mechanisms for the future.
- Advocate for awareness of SGB among fellow veterans or trauma survivors, sharing your experience to help others explore this transformative treatment.

Through Their Eyes

"I spent twenty-two years in the Teams. I was a sniper. My job was to make sure my guys made it out alive. I've taken lives—more than forty combatants in Iraq and Afghanistan. I don't keep a tally for pride. It's just fact. Those decisions, those shots, saved my brothers. But they left a mark on me.

"The worst of it wasn't the killing. It was the day I got hit. We were patrolling through a Taliban-held village in Afghanistan, a routine operation. I stepped on what turned out to be a pressure plate IED. I'll never forget the sound. It wasn't a boom. More like the earth just cracked open beneath me. I went down hard. Shrapnel tore through my leg and back. My team got me out, but I knew I'd never be the same.

"The physical wounds healed, but the nightmares didn't. The dreams were vivid, violent, relentless. I'd wake up in a cold sweat, heart pounding, reaching for a weapon that wasn't there. Even awake, I'd feel that old hypervigilance, my body ready to fight or flee at every little noise.

"I tried therapy, medications, even meditation. Nothing worked. The VA said I had PTSD. A buddy of mine called it PTSX—post-traumatic stress injury. It felt like an injury, like something deep inside me had been broken. After years of struggling, I was losing hope.

"Then one of my old teammates called me up. He'd been through some of the same hell and told me about Dr. Eugene Lipov and something called the stellate ganglion block. He swore it saved his life. I didn't buy it at first. A shot in the neck to fix your brain? Sounded like snake oil. But my buddies dragged me to the Stella Center in Chicago.

"Dr. Lipov's team was professional but relaxed, like they knew how to talk to guys like me. They explained how PTSX screws with the sympathetic nervous system, locking it into fight-or-flight mode. SGB was supposed to "reset" that system. They recommended the Dual Sympathetic Reset, which meant two injections, one on each side of my neck over two days. I'll admit, I was skeptical. But I was also desperate.

"The first injection was quick, just a few minutes. They numbed the area, guided a needle into my neck using ultrasound, and injected a local anesthetic into the stellate ganglion—a bundle of nerves that controls the body's stress response. The sensation was strange, like a warm wave washing over me. By the time I walked out, I felt *lighter*. That night, in the hotel room by the clinic, I slept for ten straight hours, something I hadn't done in years. No nightmares, no jolting awake at every creak of the floor as a stumbled about. I almost didn't believe it.

"The second injection the next day deepened the effect. It was like a fog had lifted from my mind. The constant edge, that hypervigilance, was just gone. For the first time in a long time, I could exhale comfortably.

"The transformation wasn't just physical. It was emotional. I started seeing the world differently—less as a battlefield, more as a place to live. That's when I met Sarah. She was a nurse at a nearby clinic in Chicago, and a Licensed Clinical Social Worker who worked with veterans. She understood PTSX better than anyone I'd ever met.

"Sarah didn't see me as broken. She saw me as someone worth saving. She helped me navigate what came next—therapy, building routines, and finding purpose outside of the Teams. We fell in love, and for the first time in years, I felt like I had a future.

"Now, I channel my energy into triathlons and Ironman competitions. Training keeps me sharp, keeps my edge, but it's also my way of proving to myself that I'm still strong, still capable. The old Derrick didn't disappear. He just learned how to live with the scars.

"I tell this story because I know there are others like me out there—guys who feel like they've tried everything and nothing works. That was me but no more. There's hope. SGB didn't erase my past but it gave me hope for the future."

—Master Chief Derrick P., US Navy (ret.)

24

Stellate Ganglion Block and Polyvagal Theory

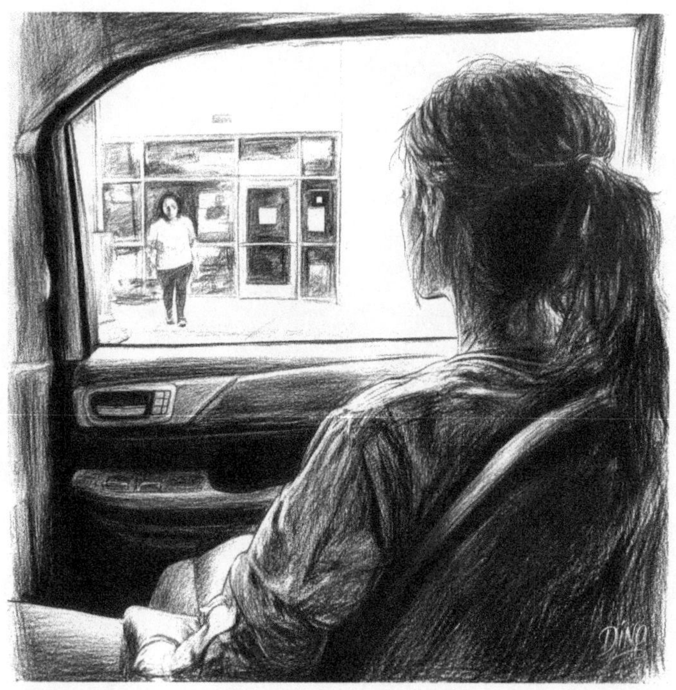

Carolina sat in her car outside the clinic, the hum of the engine reminding her of the ever-present tension she felt in her chest. She'd heard about stellate ganglion block from a fellow veteran who said it eased his constant fight-or-flight sensation. Curious and exhausted, Carolina signed up for a consultation.

Inside, the physician showed her a simple diagram: a tiny bundle of nerves in the neck—part of the system that flips the body into high alert. Block those signals, he explained, and the body could ease out of survival mode. Carolina listened with guarded hope. Years of hypervigilance had left her weary, unable to shake the sense of threat that never truly faded.

After the procedure, she noticed something odd: she could breathe more fully, without the usual tightness. Over the following days, she felt a shift—her shoulders didn't climb to her ears every time a door slammed. It was as if her nervous system finally caught a break, allowing space for calm moments.

When she told her trauma counselor about it, he mentioned Polyvagal Theory—how our nervous system has layers of response. "When your sympathetic system isn't always on," he said, "it's easier to settle into the parasympathetic, that place of safety and social connection." Carolina felt relief flood through her. For the first time in ages, normal everyday life felt less like a battleground.

This chapter explores the connection between Stellate Ganglion Block (SGB) and Polyvagal Theory—how blocking those overactive "fight-or-flight" nerves can help restore balance, helping patients like Carolina move from constant alert into a more peaceful state. By understanding both the medical procedure and the underlying science of how our bodies detect safety and threat, we glimpse a powerful new approach to healing trauma.

SGB, when examined through the lens of Polyvagal Theory, becomes particularly interesting due to its impact on the body's stress response mechanisms. The stellate ganglion is part of the sympathetic chain, which is responsible for activating the body's "fight or flight" response. By blocking these ganglia, the procedure essentially reduces the hyperactivation of the sympathetic nervous system (SNS). This can lead to a decrease in symptoms of anxiety, hyperarousal and other stress-related disorders.

Polyvagal Theory, developed by Dr. Stephen Porges, focuses on the interplay between different branches of the autonomic nervous system: the parasympathetic system (which includes the vagus nerve) and the sympathetic system (of which stellate ganglia are a part).

By integrating the concept of SGB into Polyvagal Theory, we gain a deeper insight into how altering the function of the sympathetic nervous system can promote greater autonomic balance and healing in individuals with stress or trauma-related disorders.

Restoring Balance in the Autonomic Nervous System

According to Polyvagal Theory, the autonomic nervous system operates hierarchically, with the ventral vagal complex (VVC) allowing social engagement and safety, the sympathetic system activating during stress (fight/flight), and the dorsal vagal complex (DVC) triggering shutdown responses during extreme threat.

In patients with PTSX or anxiety, the SNS can remain chronically overactive, making it difficult to engage the VVC and return to a state of social connection and calmness. By reducing sympathetic activity through SGB, the procedure may help patients more easily access their parasympathetic "rest and digest" state, enabling better emotional regulation.

Facilitating the Ventral Vagal State

Polyvagal Theory emphasizes the importance of the ventral vagal system in promoting social engagement and feelings of safety. By calming the SNS through a stellate ganglion block, the ventral vagal system may become more active, allowing individuals to experience increased relaxation, improved social interactions, and reduced defensive states (fight, flight or freeze). SGB can thus support individuals in moving out of the survival mode driven by sympathetic dominance and into a more connected, regulated state.

Potential for Trauma Treatment

One of the more promising applications of SGB, particularly when viewed through the Polyvagal lens, is its potential to help individuals with trauma histories. Trauma often locks people in a heightened sympathetic state (fight or flight) or a dorsal vagal state (shutdown or dissociation).

SGB may help reduce the sympathetic arousal, which in turn could create an environment where the body and mind can more easily access the social engagement system. This has profound implications for trauma recovery, as it can break the cycle of chronic autonomic dysregulation.

Neuroception and Threat Detection

A critical aspect of Polyvagal Theory is "neuroception," or the nervous system's unconscious detection of safety or threat. Neuroception is a term coined by Dr. Stephen Porges as part of his Polyvagal Theory to describe the unconscious process by which the nervous system detects environmental and interpersonal cues of safety, danger or life-threatening conditions.

Unlike "perception," which is conscious, neuroception occurs below the level of conscious awareness and triggers physiological responses, either promoting social engagement (when safety is detected) or defensive behaviors (when danger or threat is detected).

Trauma survivors often experience distorted neuroception, perceiving danger in safe situations, which keeps their SNS abnormally active. By blocking the stellate ganglion, SGB may help recalibrate this process, enabling individuals to experience greater safety and reducing their chronic hyperarousal.

Key Aspects of Neuroception

Unconscious Detection of Safety or Threat: Neuroception operates as a subconscious surveillance system, continuously scanning the environment for signs of safety or danger. This process is driven primarily by the vagus nerve, which plays a crucial role in the body's response to stress and social engagement.

Influence on Behavior and Physiology: When the neuroception system detects cues of safety (calm voice, friendly facial expressions or non-threatening body language), it activates the ventral vagal system of the parasympathetic nervous system.

This promotes relaxation, social interaction, and a sense of calm. Conversely, when neuroception detects danger (such as a loud noise or threatening posture), it can activate the sympathetic nervous system (leading to fight-or-flight behaviors) or the dorsal vagal system (leading to shutdown or dissociation).

Errors in Neuroception: In cases of trauma, PTSX, or chronic stress, the neuroceptive system may become distorted, leading to inappropriate or exaggerated threat responses. For example, individuals with trauma histories may perceive benign social situations as dangerous, which can lead to hypervigilance, anxiety or withdrawal. Conversely, people with impaired neuroception might fail to detect actual threats, leading to inappropriate risk-taking.

Social Engagement System: Neuroception is deeply tied to the social engagement system, a concept within Polyvagal Theory that highlights how the ventral vagal system regulates facial expressions, vocal intonation and hearing, allowing individuals to connect with others.

When neuroception detects safety, it enables social bonding and prosocial behavior, enhancing interpersonal relationships. This might allow them to be more present in social situations and enhance their ability to engage with others.

Therapeutic Implications and Future Directions

The integration of SGB into therapeutic approaches based on Polyvagal Theory holds significant promise for treating disorders related to autonomic dysregulation: PTSX, anxiety and trauma. While SGB offers a medical intervention targeting the sympathetic nervous system, Polyvagal-informed therapies like somatic experiencing or EMDR work with the body's autonomic responses to restore a sense of safety. Combining these approaches could lead to more comprehensive and effective treatment plans.

Short-Term Relief of Symptoms

SGB provides immediate, though temporary, relief by calming the overactive sympathetic system. This can allow patients to engage more fully in trauma-focused therapies, where they can learn to regulate their autonomic responses long-term.

Integration with Polyvagal Theory-Based Therapies

By addressing the physiological aspects of trauma through SGB, patients may be better able to participate in therapies that focus on enhancing vagal tone (the activity of the vagus nerve) and creating a more resilient autonomic response to stress. And incorporating SGB into the framework of Polyvagal Theory, we can better understand how medical interventions targeting the autonomic nervous system can support emotional regulation and healing. SGB offers a promising avenue for treating sympathetic overactivation, which is often present in conditions like PTSX and chronic anxiety.

When combined with polyvagal-informed therapies, SGB has the potential to enhance the balance between the parasympathetic and sympathetic systems, facilitating recovery from trauma and promoting greater wellbeing.

If-Then Guidance

- If you are a veteran or individual suffering from PTSX or trauma-related anxiety, then consider learning about SGB to “reset” the overactive sympathetic nervous system that perpetuates anxiety and hyperarousal symptoms.
- If you are experiencing core PTSX symptoms like hypervigilance, insomnia and intrusive thoughts, then note that SGB has been effective in reducing these symptoms by calming the sympathetic nervous system.
- If you are considering SGB as part of your treatment plan, then combine it with psychotherapy or cognitive behavioral therapy to address the psychological aspects of trauma, enhancing the overall efficacy of the treatment.
- If you have undergone SGB but continue to experience symptoms, then ask your healthcare provider about Dual Sympathetic Reset (DSR), an advanced form of SGB that targets both sides of the neck and thus the sympathetic nervous system for more comprehensive relief.
- If you are concerned about the long-term effects of SGB, then be aware that while SGB offers immediate relief, some individuals may require repeat treatments over time to maintain symptom control. Results vary among patients, so please be patient.
- If you are exploring cutting-edge approaches to PTSX, then review how SGB’s integration with Polyvagal Theory highlights its role in balancing the autonomic nervous system, promoting emotional regulation, and reducing hypervigilance and anxiety.

Take the Next Step

- Understand Direct-Stimulation Therapies: Learn about techniques like SGB and how it works in treating PTSX.
- Consult a Specialist: Ask your doctor if this treatment is appropriate for your symptoms and if they are offered in your area. The VA is beginning to incorporate some of these therapies.
- Consider Alternative Therapies: If you've tried traditional therapies without success, explore whether direct-stimulation treatments could be an option to break through stubborn symptoms.

Through Their Eyes

"I've tried a lot of different treatments for my PTSX over the years. Medications, therapy, even some experimental stuff. But nothing really seemed to get to the root of the problem—until I heard about stellate ganglion block. A buddy of mine, another vet, told me about it. He said it was like flipping a switch, taking him from a constant state of fear and anxiety to a place where he could finally relax for the first time in years. At first, I was skeptical, but when you've been dealing with PTSX as long as I have, you're willing to try anything that offers hope.

"The first time I went in for the procedure, I was a little nervous. I mean, they were injecting something into my neck. But the doctor explained how it worked—how the stellate ganglion is part of the system that keeps you in 'fight-or-flight' mode, and how this block can reset that system. The procedure itself was quick, just a few minutes, and I didn't feel much at all.

"Then, almost immediately, it was like a weight had been lifted off my chest. For the first time in a long time, I wasn't on edge. I wasn't scanning the room for threats or waiting for something bad to happen. I could breathe. That night, I slept without waking up from nightmares, and in the days that followed, I felt more in control of my emotions. The constant hypervigilance that was a part of my life for years was gone.

"I know SGB isn't a cure-all. I still go to therapy and learn about polyvagal therapy. I still have some tough days once in a while, but now I can actually engage in the work I'm doing in therapy. My mind isn't hijacked by anxiety anymore. It's like my brain has the space to process things, to really start healing. It's hard to put into words, but it's like I can be present in my life again. I can be there for my family, for my friends, and even for myself.

"I've had to go back for a second SGB treatment after six months, but it was just as effective the second time. I'd recommend SGB to any veteran struggling with PTSX, especially if you feel like nothing else has worked. It's not just about numbing the symptoms. It's about resetting something deep inside that's been stuck in overdrive for too long. The therapy also helps because I can talk about my thoughts as they change in front of me."

—Jake, US Marine Corps Veteran

25

Stellate Ganglion Block and Veterans: Four Case Studies

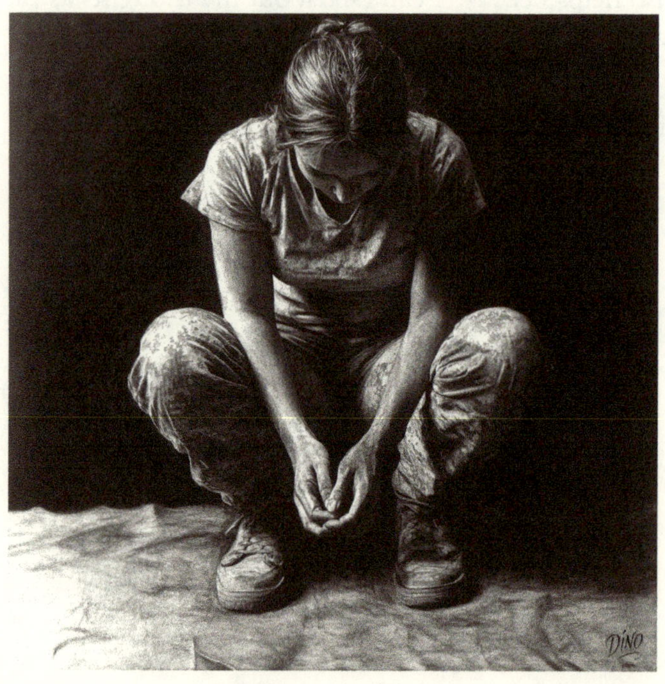

After years of struggling with nightmares and anxiety, John found himself in a sterile waiting room, pinning his last hope on something called Stellate Ganglion Block. A fellow veteran had told him how SGB gave him immediate relief from flashbacks. Skeptical but desperate, he decided it was worth a shot. The moment the anesthetic hit, he felt something shift inside—like a weight lifting off his chest. Within a week, the nightmares that used to jolt him awake every night began to fade.

He wasn't alone. On the other side of town, Maria, once known for her fiery temper, tried SGB to reclaim her life from bouts of rage and constant tension. After just one procedure, she noticed that loud noises no longer triggered panic. Gradually, she laughed with her kids again, something she hadn't done in years.

James was different. He'd slipped into a deep depression and battled suicidal thoughts nearly every day. SGB offered him a mental "reset," giving him enough stability to finally see a path forward—one that didn't revolve around despair. Meanwhile, Alan, who'd felt forever trapped in combat mode, discovered how SGB allowed him to function without scanning every corner for threats. He found a job, enrolled in college and began piecing a future together.

All four veterans shared one thing in common: after endless cycles of therapy and medication, SGB was the game-changer. For many it was the missing piece—a direct way to calm an overactive nervous system and open the door to a life not dictated by trauma. These examples highlight the efficacy of SGB in reducing PTSX symptoms, improving quality of life and restoring emotional balance in veterans who had previously struggled with traditional forms of therapy.

Case Study 1: Rapid Relief from Nightmares, Hypervigilance

Background: John, a 35-year-old US Army veteran, served multiple deployments in Iraq and Afghanistan. After his final tour, he returned home plagued by nightmares, hypervigilance and extreme anxiety. He would wake up multiple times a night drenched in sweat, convinced that he was still in combat. John struggled to maintain relationships and had difficulty focusing on work, leading to job loss. Traditional PTSX therapies, including Cognitive Behavioral Therapy (CBT) and medications, offered minimal relief and he grew increasingly frustrated.

Treatment: John underwent the Stellate Ganglion Block procedure after hearing about its success in treating PTSX. The SGB was administered on the right side of his neck, targeting the overstimulated sympathetic nervous system.

Outcome: Within hours of the procedure, John reported feeling a sense of calm that he hadn't experienced in years. The constant hypervigilance, which had made daily activities stressful, diminished significantly. His nightmares also became less frequent and within the first week, he reported sleeping through the night without waking in panic.

For John, SGB provided immediate relief from the chronic anxiety that had dominated his life. Over the next several months, he continued to engage in therapy but found that SGB had significantly enhanced his ability to process his trauma and live with a greater sense of normalcy.

Case Study 2: A Veteran's Path to Rebuilding Relationships

Background: Maria, a 30-year-old former Marine, returned from her deployment in Afghanistan with PTSX symptoms that manifested in severe emotional outbursts, irritability and difficulty connecting with loved ones. She was particularly sensitive to loud noises, which triggered panic attacks.

Maria's condition strained her marriage and she felt increasingly distant from her children. While medications such as antidepressants and anti-anxiety drugs helped take the edge off her symptoms, they didn't address the root cause of her heightened stress response. She sought a more holistic solution.

Treatment: Maria decided to try the Stellate Ganglion Block after reading about its success in calming the overactive sympathetic nervous system in veterans. She underwent the SGB procedure on both sides of her neck (Dual Sympathetic Reset).

Outcome: The results were profound. Maria felt an immediate reduction in her emotional reactivity. She reported that loud noises no longer triggered the same intense fear or panic. Within a week, her family noticed a significant change in her demeanor. She was more relaxed, able to communicate more effectively and less prone to angry outbursts. Over time, Maria and her husband began to rebuild their relationship and she felt more connected to her children. For Maria, SGB allowed her to reclaim her role as a mother and partner, giving her the emotional stability she needed to heal.

Case Study 3: Overcoming Depression and Suicidal Thoughts

Background: James, a 42-year-old Navy veteran, was haunted by guilt and depression after witnessing the death of several fellow servicemen during his deployment. For years, he suffered from intense feelings of worthlessness and hopelessness, often contemplating suicide.

He had been hospitalized twice for suicide attempts and had tried multiple forms of therapy, including medication and intensive inpatient programs, but nothing provided lasting relief. His doctors suggested he try the Stellate Ganglion Block as a potential solution to alleviate the intense anxiety and depression he experienced daily.

Treatment: James underwent the SGB procedure targeting the right side of his stellate ganglion. Given the severity of his symptoms, his medical team also considered administering a second SGB to enhance the effects.

Outcome: Almost immediately after the procedure, James reported a marked reduction in his anxiety and the sense of impending doom that had overshadowed his thoughts for years. His feelings of depression began to lift within days and for the first time, he was able to imagine a future without constant psychological pain.

Over the next several weeks, James continued his therapy, but the SGB procedure had created a foundation of emotional stability that allowed him to more effectively process his trauma. Six months after the procedure, James was no longer experiencing suicidal thoughts and his quality of life had improved dramatically. He credits the SGB with saving his life.

Case Study 4: Returning to Civilian Life After Combat Trauma

Background: Alan, a 29-year-old Army Ranger, had experienced significant trauma during combat missions in Afghanistan, where he witnessed the deaths of multiple comrades and civilians. Upon returning home, Alan was unable to reintegrate into civilian life.

He constantly felt as though he was still in a combat zone, his mind hyper-focused on potential threats. Alan experienced flashbacks and panic attacks regularly, making it impossible for him to hold down a job or engage in social activities. His PTSX left him isolated and struggling with depression.

Treatment: After several unsuccessful attempts to manage his PTSX through medication and talk therapy, Alan's therapist recommended the Stellate Ganglion Block. He received the procedure on his right side and reported feeling a significant reduction in his anxiety and hypervigilance.

Outcome: Alan noticed an immediate reduction in his flashbacks and anxiety. The constant feeling of being "on edge" disappeared and he found himself able to relax in situations that previously would have caused intense distress. Over the following months, Alan was able to return to work and even enrolled in college courses.

SGB allowed him to break free from the grip of his combat trauma and re-engage with civilian life. He continues to receive therapy, but the SGB has given him a new foundation of calm that has enabled him to rebuild his future.

A Powerful New Tool

SGB has proven to be a powerful and transformative tool for veterans struggling with PTSX. In these four case studies, veterans reported immediate and long-lasting relief from symptoms like anxiety, hypervigilance, nightmares, depression and emotional outbursts. For many, SGB provided the breakthrough they needed to regain control over their lives and begin the healing process. In the very least, SGB allowed for a new beginning in each of their lives.

As research and clinical experience with SGB continue to grow, this treatment holds great promise for the military and veterans communities, offering hope and healing to those who have long struggled with the invisible wounds of war.

If you're a veteran struggling with PTSX, anxiety, or depression, you may be wondering if SGB is the right treatment for you. While SGB is not a cure for PTSX, it offers a powerful tool to help manage the symptoms that make everyday life difficult. For many veterans, the relief provided by SGB allows them to re-engage in their lives, whether that means returning to work, improving relationships, or simply finding peace.

The procedure is safe, minimally invasive and has been shown to provide relief for a wide range of trauma-related conditions. If traditional treatments have not worked for you, or if you need faster relief from the debilitating symptoms of PTSX, SGB could be a valuable part of your treatment plan.

A New Path to Healing

For many veterans, the battle with PTSX continues long after they leave the battlefield. However, treatments like Stellate Ganglion Block offer new hope. With the pioneering work of Dr. Eugene Lipov and the development of advanced techniques like Dual Sympathetic Reset, SGB is proving to be one of the most promising treatments available for trauma-related conditions.

By addressing the neurophysiological mechanism of PTSX, SGB provides veterans with a faster path to relief, allowing them to reclaim their lives from the grip of trauma. As research continues to support the efficacy of SGB, more veterans will have access to this groundbreaking therapy, offering a new way forward in the treatment of PTSX.

26

Ethical Considerations in Hallucinogenic and Psychedelic Substances Treatments

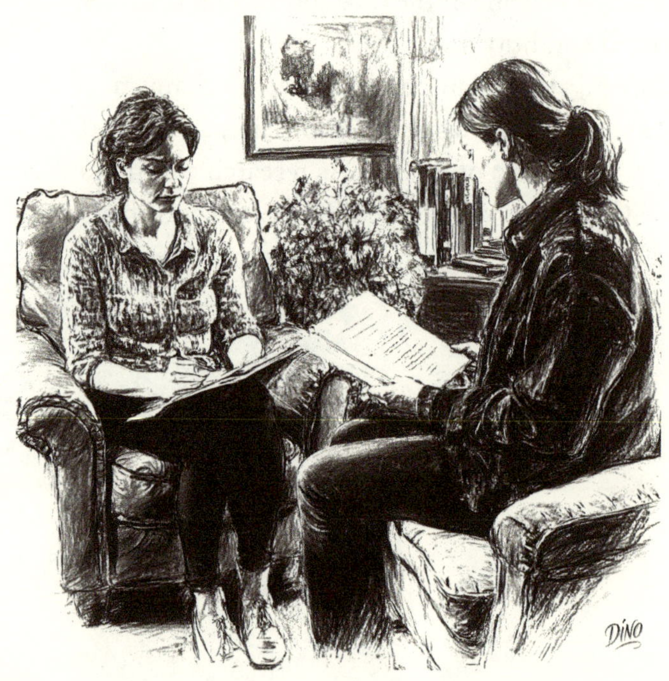

Monique sat with her counselor, reviewing a lengthy consent form detailing a new therapy she was considering—a guided session using a low dose of psilocybin. She had a list of questions she'd jotted down: potential side effects, how long the effects might last, what kind of emotional space she'd be in.

The counselor answered each one without rushing her, stressing that Monique was in the driver's seat. If she decided to back out, no one would push her forward. That sense of choice calmed her nerves more than she expected. In the waiting area, she met Elena, another veteran who came from a strong cultural background that emphasized caution toward any mind-altering substance. Elena shared how she'd initially felt uneasy about the idea of psychedelics.

"Where I'm from, spirituality and healing are deeply intertwined, but drugs are viewed with suspicion." The clinicians had honored her perspective, encouraging her to talk with family members and consult a traditional healer before deciding. She appreciated how nobody dismissed her beliefs as irrelevant—rather, they saw it as part of her overall healing journey.

They both sat in a small group session later that day, hearing from others who had tried or were about to try alternative therapies like cannabis or psilocybin. The staff facilitated respectful conversations—no judgment, no sales pitch. Just candid discussions about what might help and where each person stood. For Monique, seeing how seriously the team took consent and inclusivity made her decision easier. She felt valued not just as a patient but as a person bringing her own culture, history and concerns to the table.

That evening, she decided to proceed. Knowing she had the freedom to change her mind, to ask questions, and to integrate her own values into the treatment plan gave her a sense of agency she hadn't felt in years. And in that moment, she realized healing wasn't just about the therapy itself—it was about having a voice in every step along the way.

This chapter deals with informed consent, a cornerstone of ethical medical practice, especially in the context of treating complex conditions like PTSX among military personnel and veterans. It transcends mere legal obligation. It embodies the principles of respect for patient autonomy, self-determination and partnership in the therapeutic process.

Informed Consent and Patient Autonomy

For mental-health professionals working within the VA system, understanding the nuances of informed consent is essential, particularly as innovative treatments like psychedelic-assisted therapies, cannabinoids and advanced neurostimulation techniques become increasingly integrated into PTSX treatment protocols. By creating an environment where patients feel empowered to make informed choices about their care, therapeutic outcomes are honored. Patient autonomy is paramount in the healing journey and it is critical that veterans and active-duty personnel understand their treatment options, including the risks and benefits of emerging therapies.

Informed consent is not merely a one-time event but an ongoing dialogue that respects the evolving nature of the patient's understanding and comfort level with their treatment plan. The integration of alternative therapies into the conventional treatment landscape raises important ethical considerations regarding informed consent.

In the case of psychedelics and cannabinoids, where research is still evolving, it is crucial to equip veterans with comprehensive knowledge that encompasses both the potential benefits and the uncertainties. Simply put, these therapies and treatments are not for everyone, and sometimes things go wrong.

This transparency not only creates trust but also encourages a culture of shared decision-making, where veterans feel valued as partners in their healing process. Mental-health practitioners must prioritize education and training in these areas, ensuring that they can provide accurate, up-to-date information that supports informed decision-making.

Building community-based support systems further enhances informed consent and patient autonomy. Veterans often find solace and strength in shared experiences, and peer support can be instrumental in navigating the complexities of treatment options.

By creating environments where veterans can openly discuss their concerns and experiences with alternative therapies, we empower them to make informed choices that resonate with their personal values and healing journeys. This community-driven approach not only enriches the informed consent process but also cultivates a sense of belonging and support that is vital for recovery.

The journey of healing is deeply personal and every veteran and patient deserve the opportunity to engage actively in that journey, making choices that reflect their needs, hopes and aspirations. Together, we can create a future where informed consent is not just a procedural formality but a dynamic, integral part of the therapeutic landscape for those who have bravely served our country.

Cultural Sensitivity and Inclusivity

Cultural sensitivity and inclusivity are critically important in the treatment of military personnel and veterans grappling with PTSX. Understanding the diverse backgrounds and unique experiences of servicemembers is essential for mental health professionals tasked with providing effective care. Military personnel come from various cultural, ethnic and socio-economic backgrounds, each with its own set of values, beliefs and coping mechanisms.

Creating an environment of respect and understanding ensures that professionals build a therapeutic space where veterans feel safe to express their emotions and share their stories. This sensitivity not only facilitates trust but also enhances the efficacy of treatment approaches, including innovative therapies such as psychedelic-assisted treatments and cannabinoid integration.

Incorporating cultural competence into PTSX treatment requires ongoing education and training for mental-health professionals. It is vital that practitioners are equipped with the knowledge and skills to recognize and address the cultural factors influencing a veteran's mental health. This can be achieved through workshops, seminars and community engagement initiatives that emphasize the importance of inclusivity in therapy.

By understanding cultural contexts surrounding trauma and healing, professionals can tailor their approaches to resonate with the individual experiences of veterans. Such efforts can significantly improve the outcomes of treatments like ketamine infusion therapy or stellate ganglion block, as they align therapeutic techniques with the patient's cultural and personal context.

Inclusivity also extends to the integration of community-based support systems, which play a crucial role in the recovery journey. Veterans often find solace and understanding within their communities, making it essential for mental-health practitioners to collaborate with local organizations, peer support groups and veteran service organizations.

By creating a network of support that respects and honors the diverse backgrounds of veterans, healthcare professionals can enhance the efficacy of alternative therapies. Success stories from the field, showcasing the positive impact of inclusive practices, can inspire others to adopt similar approaches, ultimately leading to a more supportive environment for all veterans.

Open dialogue about the potential benefits and risks associated with therapies like MDMA-assisted treatment can empower veterans to make informed choices that align with their cultural values. By prioritizing ethical practices and cultural understanding, professionals can create a therapeutic alliance that supports veterans in their healing journeys.

Ultimately, embracing cultural sensitivity and inclusivity can transform the landscape of PTSX treatment for military personnel and veterans. By recognizing and valuing the unique experiences that each individual brings to therapy, mental-health professionals can create a more compassionate and effective treatment environment.

If-Then Guidance

- If you have ethical concerns about using psychedelics or experimental treatments for PTSX, then it's important to have an open discussion with your healthcare provider about these concerns. They can provide information on the safety protocols, scientific evidence, and ethical frameworks in place for these treatments. This can help you make an informed decision and feel more comfortable with your options.
- If you are uncertain about the long-term effects of experimental treatments, then consider seeking out peer-reviewed studies and consulting with professionals who specialize in these therapies. Understanding the potential risks and benefits, as well as the current research, can help alleviate concerns and guide you toward a decision that aligns with your values.
- If you are uncomfortable with the lack of regulation or the experimental nature of certain PTSX treatments, then it may be worth exploring more established and regulated therapies. While experimental treatments may offer hope, you may feel more secure with treatments that have undergone extensive clinical testing and have a longer history of use in PTSX care.
- If you believe that personal autonomy in treatment decisions is

crucial, then ensure you are fully informed about your options, including both traditional and experimental therapies. Speak with multiple providers, if necessary, to explore all perspectives and make sure that your choices align with your personal beliefs and healthcare goals.

- If you feel that the experimental nature of some treatments raises ethical questions, then consider discussing these concerns with a bioethicist or a mental health professional with experience in clinical research ethics. They can help you better understand the ethical oversight of these therapies and how patients' rights and safety are protected in the process.

Take the Next Step

- Understand the Ethics: Reflect on the importance of informed consent, safety and cultural sensitivity when considering psychedelic or hallucinogenic treatments.
- Ask the Right Questions: If you're considering HPS treatments, ensure that the facility you work with prioritizes ethical considerations and provides clear information on risks and benefits.
- Participate in Discussions: Engage with veteran groups or mental-health forums that discuss the ethical aspects of these treatments, helping shape future care models.

Through Their Eyes

"The informed consent process wasn't just a form I signed. It was an ongoing agreement between me and my providers. After each session, I met with my therapist to talk about how I was feeling and whether I wanted to continue. I was in control the entire time, and that made a world of difference.

"When I first heard about MDMA-assisted therapy, I didn't know what to think. After years of service and carrying the weight of PTSX, I was desperate for relief but hesitant about something that felt so experimental. I'd always been a believer in science and trusted medicine, but MDMA? It seemed like a drug from my past, not a solution for my future. Still, traditional therapies hadn't gotten me the results I needed. So, when my doctor brought it up, I felt I had to learn more.

"The process wasn't just about whether or not MDMA could help me. It was about understanding the risks, the science, and how the therapy would actually work. I remember sitting down with my therapist. We talked about the potential benefits, sure, but also the uncertainties. Would it be safe for me?

"Would it really help me confront my trauma in ways other treatments hadn't? It wasn't an easy decision, but I felt respected throughout the process. I wasn't just a patient. I was part of the team making this choice.

"What really helped was being part of a group of veterans who had either gone through MDMA therapy or were considering it. Hearing their stories—both successes and challenges—gave me perspective. It made me realize I wasn't alone in my concerns, and the decision wasn't about one size fits all. Everyone was in a different place, and that was okay. Eventually, I decided to move forward with the treatment. The treatment is still ongoing. Time will tell."

—Andrew, US Army Veteran

27

Navigating Federal Regulatory Challenges

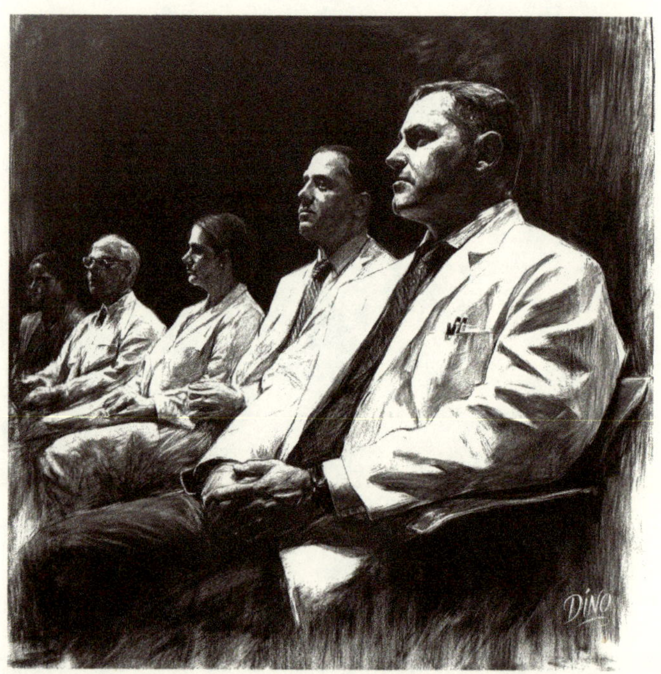

Mason shuffled through the VA lobby, a folder of papers tucked under his arm—the latest research on psychedelic-assisted therapies. He'd spent months reading about how MDMA or psilocybin could transform the lives of veterans with severe PTSX. But the whisper around every corner was the same: "Federal regulations are no joke. Getting these treatments approved is an uphill battle."

Later that week, he sat in a cramped conference room alongside fellow clinicians, a visiting legal advisor, and a few veterans who'd volunteered to share their experiences. Each story highlighted the pressing need for new avenues of care. Yet each time someone mentioned ketamine,

MDMA, or cannabis, the legal advisor reminded them, "Until it's federally recognized, there's only so much we can do. I'm sorry but that's the reality at this point. In the future, we hope it won't be this difficult."

One vet, Kelly, spoke of traveling out of state—nearly across the country—for a single, experimental treatment. "I got more relief from that session than I did from five years of pills and therapy," she said, voice trembling with equal parts gratitude and frustration. Everyone in the room felt the weight of her words. They knew there were answers out there—but red tape stood in the way.

Mason left the meeting both motivated and overwhelmed. He realized that steering through the DEA and FDA regulations wasn't just a bureaucratic exercise. It was a mission for patient wellbeing. He got in touch with local veteran advocacy groups, merging their passion with his clinical expertise. Step by step, they drafted letters to lawmakers, shared patient success stories, and pushed for expanded research trials.

This chapter examines the maze of federal regulations shaping PTSX treatment, how practitioners and advocates like Mason and Kelly navigate it, and what it takes to ensure innovative therapies reach those who need them. Though the path is far from simple, each step forward can help break down barriers— offering veterans and civilian patients a real chance at relief, rather than a lifetime spent waiting for red tape to clear.

Know Your Adversary

Navigating the intricate landscape of federal regulations is crucial for advancing innovative PTSX treatments for military personnel and veterans. It's imperative that mental-health professionals, dedicated to the wellbeing of those who have served, understand these regulatory challenges, which are key to implementing effective therapies that incorporate emerging neurobiological insights.

One of the primary challenges facing the integration of emerging therapies is the stringent regulatory framework established by federal agencies, particularly the DEA and the FDA. These agencies govern the use of substances like MDMA, ketamine and cannabinoids, which have shown promise in treating PTSX but remain tightly controlled. A practical strategy for veterans and civilian patients seeking novel treatments is to stay abreast of clinical trials and investigational programs that offer legal avenues for using Schedule I substances. The FDA's Expanded Access program (sometimes called "compassionate use") can grant permission for patients with serious conditions to receive investigational drugs outside of clinical trials, provided certain criteria are met.

Regulatory gridlock costs innocent lives. Science is ready, veterans are waiting.Congress must move like seasoned combat medics, not lazy auditors that drag their feet.

In the case of MDMA and psilocybin, both substances have been awarded Breakthrough Therapy status by the FDA, indicating strong preliminary evidence of efficacy and speeding up some aspects of the review process.

Collaborating with reputable research organizations and nonprofits, such as the Multidisciplinary Association for Psychedelic Studies (MAPS), provides access to updates on current trials and regulatory developments. Veterans' advocacy groups absolutely must maintain close communication with these organizations, helping their members enroll in approved protocols or pilot studies.

Such participation not only offers potential relief but also contributes valuable data that may accelerate federal acceptance of these therapies. On the legal front, patients and providers must remain vigilant about both federal and state regulations. Cannabis, for instance, may be legal under certain state statutes yet still face federal restrictions.

Consulting legal counsel experienced in health and drug policy can clarify permissible treatment pathways, especially when navigating cross-state differences. Forming coalitions with medical professionals, patient advocacy groups and policymakers amplifies the collective voice.

Develop a Solid Network of Friends and Colleagues

Navigating these regulations requires a strategic approach that balances the urgency of patient needs with compliance to ensure safety and efficacy. By creating collaborative relationships with regulatory bodies, mental-health professionals can advocate for research and trials that demonstrate the effectiveness of these treatments, paving the way for greater accessibility for veterans.

Moreover, the ethical considerations surrounding the use of psychedelics and alternative therapies cannot be overlooked. As practitioners, it is essential to engage in ongoing dialogue about the moral implications of utilizing these substances in clinical settings. This includes addressing concerns surrounding informed consent, potential for misuse and the long-term effects on mental health.

By developing robust ethical frameworks, healthcare practitioners can ensure that innovative therapies are administered responsibly and with respect for the autonomy and dignity of each veteran. This commitment to ethical practice not only safeguards patients but also enhances the credibility of alternative treatments within the broader healthcare community.

Community-based support systems play a vital role in navigating these federal regulatory challenges. Engaging with local organizations, veterans' groups and advocacy networks can create a supportive environment for sharing knowledge and resources. These collaborations can amplify the voices of mental-healthcare professionals, advocating for policy changes that prioritize the mental health needs of veterans.

Don't Give Up!

Ultimately, the road to effectively navigating federal regulatory challenges in PTSX treatment is paved with determination, advocacy and a commitment to innovation. Healthcare professionals must embrace this path to educate themselves, engage in advocacy and collaborate with others in the field.

By staying informed about regulatory changes, actively participating in research and supporting ethical practices, they can ensure that the most effective and compassionate treatments reach those who need them most. Together, all of us can create a future where military personnel, veterans and civilian patients receive the comprehensive care they deserve, empowering them to reclaim their lives and thrive in their post-service journeys.

If-Then Guidance

- If you have faced challenges accessing treatments due to federal regulations, then consider exploring clinical trials or advocacy groups that work to expand access to these therapies. Clinical trials often provide early access to experimental treatments under controlled conditions, and advocacy efforts can help push for legislative changes that may open up new treatment options.
- If you are not fully aware of the legal limitations on experimental treatments, then it might be beneficial to research the current status of these therapies in your state and at the federal level. Understanding the legal landscape can help you make informed decisions about which treatment options are available to you and what steps you may need to take to access them.
- If regulatory approval is important in your treatment decisions, then consider discussing alternative or experimental treatments with your healthcare provider. They can provide guidance on the safety, legality, and availability of these treatments, as well as help you find approved therapies that meet your needs while staying within the bounds of regulatory standards.
- If you have encountered delays due to regulatory barriers, then you might want to seek out specialized providers or clinics that offer emerging treatments like ketamine or psychedelic therapy through legal avenues. Additionally, staying informed about changes in legislation could help you access these treatments more easily in the future.

Take the Next Step

- Stay Informed on Legislation: Keep up with changes in regulations surrounding PTSX treatments, such as access to cannabinoids, psychedelics, or emerging therapies.

- Engage in Advocacy: Join veteran advocacy groups working to improve access to PTSX treatments. Your voice can help push legislation that makes alternative therapies more accessible to veterans.
- Consult a Legal Expert: If you're considering a treatment that's in a legal gray area, such as cannabis or MDMA, seek legal guidance before proceeding.

Through Their Eyes

"At first, I was confused. I had read about how MDMA could help veterans with PTSX, yet it was still illegal outside of clinical trials. The same with cannabis—legal in some states, but not others, and federally prohibited. It felt like I was hitting a wall, not because of a lack of hope for recovery, but because the system wasn't built to help me access these treatments.

"Talking with my healthcare provider helped. He explained that while these treatments are showing promise, federal regulations from agencies like the DEA and FDA were making it difficult to expand their availability. It wasn't just about me and what I needed. A whole system had to change.

"So, I joined a group of veterans who were advocating for these treatments. We spoke to lawmakers, shared our stories, and tried to make a case for why expanding access to therapies like MDMA or cannabinoids is critical. The experience gave me a sense of purpose—it wasn't just about my healing anymore, but about helping others in the same situation.

"Despite the setbacks, I haven't given up. I've participated in clinical trials and stayed connected to advocacy efforts, knowing that change is coming. It may be slow, but with every step forward, I feel a little closer to the treatment we all deserve."

—Lucas, US Marine Corps Veteran

28

Massed Prolonged Exposure Therapy

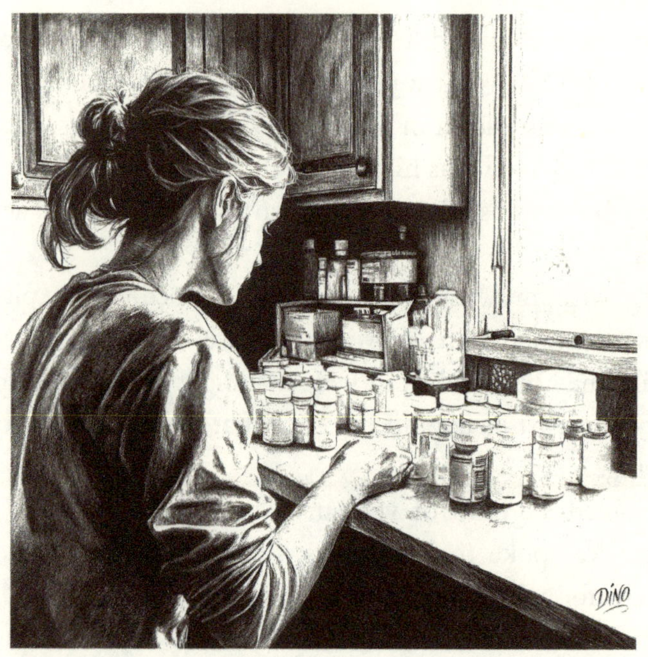

Annabelle stared at the rows of medication bottles lined up on her kitchen counter—reminders of years spent tackling her unrelenting flashbacks and anxiety. She used to believe that traditional talk therapy and a steady prescription routine were her only way forward. Yet deep down, she couldn't shake the feeling that something was missing.

That hint of possibility led her to try a new PTSX support group. In the meeting room's comfortable chairs, she listened as other veterans shared surprising success stories: one found relief through ketamine sessions that loosened the tight grip of repressed memories. Another praised a nerve-block procedure that quickly dialed down hypervigilance. A few spoke with excitement about MDMA-assisted therapy, describing it as the key that finally unlocked their trauma's emotional core. Someone else mentioned "massed prolonged exposure therapy," something she'd never heard of before. All of a sudden, she felt a glimmer of hope. Could all these therapies coexist with her long-standing cognitive behavioral work? She decided to find out, bringing the question to her usual counselor.

Together, they sketched a broad plan—incorporating both the steady framework of traditional methods and the potent effects of newer, alternative paths. She started small: gradually adding gentle body-based exercises and mindfulness sessions, learning how physical tension fed her anxious mind. Then she explored the possibility of a ketamine infusion, carefully weighing pros and cons alongside her healthcare team.

Within months, the synergy became clear. Each technique complemented the others, reinforcing what she learned in therapy. Annabelle discovered a renewed sense of control—not from a single "miracle cure," but from a combination of approaches that addressed every layer of her distress.

This chapter introduces Massed Prolonged Exposure (Massed PE), a time-efficient and highly effective adaptation of traditional exposure therapy designed for military personnel and veterans facing logistical constraints. By condensing multiple sessions into a shorter timeframe, Massed PE helps individuals rapidly confront and process traumatic memories, leading to significant and lasting reductions in PTSX symptoms. It explores the therapy's advantages, challenges and its powerful synergy when integrated with other innovative treatments for a truly holistic approach to healing.

Clinical Applications for Military Personnel and Veterans

The neurobiological understanding of PTSX has significantly advanced, particularly in the context of military personnel and veterans. As we delve into clinical applications, it becomes evident that tailored approaches can lead to remarkable healing journeys for those who have bravely served.

The integration of innovative therapies, such as psychedelic-assisted treatments and cannabinoid therapies, represents a paradigm shift in our understanding of mental healthcare. These approaches not only address the symptoms of PTSX but also tap into the underlying neurobiological mechanisms, creating a more profound and lasting recovery.

Psychedelic-assisted therapies, including MDMA and psilocybin, have shown great promise in recent studies, revealing their potential to facilitate emotional processing and enhance therapeutic engagement. For veterans grappling with the profound effects of trauma, these substances can serve as catalysts for healing, allowing individuals to confront their experiences within a supportive therapeutic framework.

The long-term effects of MDMA-assisted therapy are particularly encouraging, demonstrating significant reductions in PTSX symptoms and creating a renewed sense of hope and connection among participants. This approach represents a beacon of possibility for veterans who may have exhausted conventional treatment options without finding relief.

In addition to psychedelics, the integration of cannabinoids into traditional PTSX treatment protocols offers another avenue for healing. Cannabinoids have been shown to modulate anxiety and improve sleep, two critical factors in the recovery process for veterans.

As we explore the efficacy of these alternative therapies, it is crucial to establish evidence-based guidelines that ensure safe and effective implementation. This involves not only rigorous clinical trials but also the development of comprehensive training programs for mental health professionals, enabling them to navigate the complexities of these treatments with confidence and compassion.

Stimulation techniques like stellate ganglion block have emerged as innovative interventions for trauma recovery. This technique has provided rapid relief to many veterans suffering from PTSX symptoms, showcasing the potential for immediate improvement in quality of life.

By understanding and harnessing these neurobiological mechanisms, mental health professionals can offer more effective, multi-faceted treatment options that cater to individual needs. The incorporation of these techniques within a broader treatment framework can significantly enhance the healing journey of military personnel and veterans.

Ultimately, the success stories emerging from the application of these alternative therapies illuminate a path forward for the military, veteran and civilian mental-health communities. Community-based support systems are essential in creating an environment where veterans can share their experiences and successes, creating a sense of belonging and understanding.

By prioritizing education and collaboration among mental-health professionals, we can cultivate a culture of innovation that champions the healing potential of our military personnel and veterans.

Integrating Traditional and Alternative Behavioral Approaches

Integrating traditional and alternative approaches in the treatment of PTSX for military personnel and veterans represents a promising frontier in mental health care. As the understanding of neurobiological mechanisms behind trauma evolves, it becomes increasingly evident that a multifaceted treatment strategy can be more effective than relying solely on conventional methods.

This integration is not merely about combining therapies. It's about creating a holistic framework that respects the unique experiences of our servicemembers while leveraging the latest scientific advancements. By embracing both traditional therapies and innovative alternatives, we can pave the way for more comprehensive healing journeys.

Traditional approaches such as cognitive behavioral therapy (CBT) and exposure therapy have long been the cornerstone of PTSX treatment. These methods provide invaluable tools for understanding and processing trauma. However, many veterans have reported limited success with these conventional techniques alone.

This is where alternative treatments, including psychedelic-assisted therapies, cannabinoid integration and massed prolonged exposure therapy, offer new possibilities.

Since we have discussed the other therapies in detail elsewhere, we will now focus on massed prolonged exposure therapy.

Massed Prolonged Exposure Therapy: A Time-Efficient Approach to PTSX Treatment

Massed PE has emerged as a promising approach for treating PTSX, particularly among veterans, active military personnel, and individuals exposed to trauma. It is an adaptation of the traditional Prolonged Exposure (PE) therapy, which is a well-established and evidence-based treatment for PTSX. Massed PE condenses the therapeutic process into a shorter timeframe, with multiple sessions held in a compressed period—often over a few days or weeks—rather than being spread out over months.

This accelerated format is designed to offer quicker relief while maintaining the core principles of PE, making it an appealing option for military personnel who face logistical or time constraints.

Understanding Prolonged Exposure Therapy

To fully appreciate the value of Massed PE, it's essential to first understand Prolonged Exposure therapy in its traditional form. PE is based on the principles of exposure therapy, a psychological treatment method where individuals are gradually exposed to trauma-related stimuli under controlled and safe conditions. The goal is to help individuals confront and process their traumatic memories rather than avoid them, which can perpetuate PTSX symptoms.

PE typically involves four main components:

Imaginal Exposure: The individual repeatedly recounts their traumatic experiences in vivid detail during therapy sessions, helping them process the trauma and reduce its emotional intensity.

In Vivo Exposure: The individual is gradually exposed to real-world situations that they have been avoiding due to trauma-related fear or anxiety, reinforcing the idea that these situations are not dangerous.

Psychoeducation: The therapist educates the individual about PTSX, its symptoms, and the mechanisms behind exposure therapy.

Breathing Retraining: Relaxation techniques are taught to help manage anxiety and stress responses.

Prolonged Exposure therapy is considered one of the most effective behavioral treatments for PTSX, particularly for individuals who have experienced combat-related trauma, sexual assault or other life-threatening events. However, the traditional PE format often involves one session per week over the course of 8 to 12 weeks, which can be a challenge for certain populations, particularly military personnel who may have limited availability due to deployments or other responsibilities.

The Emergence of Massed Prolonged Exposure Therapy

Massed Prolonged Exposure Therapy was developed to address some of the practical limitations of the traditional PE model. In the massed format, multiple PE sessions are conducted within a short period, sometimes with multiple sessions per day over the course of just a few days or weeks.

This condensed approach was initially developed to better accommodate military personnel, who may have limited time for therapy before deployment or during transitions between duty and civilian life. The idea was that if the same therapeutic benefits of traditional PE could be achieved more quickly, it would allow individuals to receive treatment without extended interruptions to their duties or lives.

The principles of Massed PE are the same as traditional PE: patients engage in imaginal and in vivo exposure exercises, learning to confront their traumatic memories and gradually reduce their fear and avoidance. However, by condensing these sessions into a shorter time frame, patients undergo more intense, focused exposure to trauma-related stimuli, which some research suggests may facilitate faster habituation to the distressing memories and situations.

Effectiveness of Massed PE

Studies have demonstrated that Massed PE is highly effective in reducing PTSX symptoms, and it has been found to be just as effective as traditional PE in terms of treatment outcomes. One of the most important findings in recent research is that Massed PE allows for rapid reduction in symptoms, often within a matter of days or weeks, rather than months. This is especially important for military personnel or veterans who may need to see quicker improvements in order to return to duty or successfully reintegrate into civilian life. Veterans who undergo Massed PE often report significant reductions in intrusive thoughts, nightmares, hypervigilance and avoidance behaviors—the hallmark symptoms of PTSX.

Additionally, Massed PE has been shown to have long-term benefits. Follow-up studies have indicated that individuals who complete Massed PE maintain their symptom reductions for months or even years after treatment. This durability of effect is critical for ensuring that PTSX sufferers do not experience a relapse of symptoms after their treatment concludes.

Advantages of Massed PE for Military Personnel and Veterans

Massed PE offers several distinct advantages for military personnel and veterans. One of the primary benefits is its time efficiency. Military personnel often have demanding schedules, and the traditional weekly therapy model may not be feasible for those preparing for deployment or transitioning out of active duty. Compressing therapy into a shorter timeframe, Massed PE provides the flexibility needed to fit into these schedules.

Another advantage is that Massed PE can help reduce dropout rates. One of the challenges in PTSX treatment is the high dropout rate, particularly in therapies that require long-term engagement. Some individuals, especially those in high-stress professions like the military, may struggle to commit to months of weekly therapy sessions. Massed PE, by contrast, allows patients to complete their treatment in a condensed period, reducing the likelihood that they will drop out before completing the therapy.

Furthermore, the intensity of the exposure in Massed PE may be beneficial for some individuals. By engaging in multiple therapy sessions over a short period, patients may experience faster habituation to their traumatic memories and fears.

This accelerated process can lead to quicker symptom relief, which is particularly important for those who need to return to duty or move on with their lives as soon as possible. And when Massed PE is combined with other therapies like stellate ganglion block the results are even better and longer lasting.

Challenges and Considerations

While Massed PE has many advantages, it is not without its challenges. One of the main concerns is whether the intensity of the therapy may be overwhelming for some individuals. PTSX treatment, by its nature, involves confronting distressing memories and emotions, and undergoing multiple therapy sessions in a short period could potentially lead to emotional exhaustion or heightened distress in some patients. Therapists need to carefully monitor patients' reactions to the therapy and ensure that they are able to tolerate the intense exposure without becoming overwhelmed. Cannabinoids and stellate ganglion block can allow patients to participate in Massed PE in a calmer state.

Another consideration is the availability of trained therapists. Massed PE requires therapists to be available for multiple sessions within a condensed timeframe, which may not be feasible in all treatment settings. Additionally, therapists must be highly skilled in managing the intense emotional reactions that can arise during the therapy, especially when sessions are held back-to-back.

Finally, more research is needed to determine which patients are most likely to benefit from Massed PE. While the therapy has been shown to be effective for many individuals, it may not be the best option for everyone. Some patients may benefit more from the slower, more gradual approach of traditional PE, particularly if they have complex trauma histories or comorbid mental health conditions such as depression or substance-use disorders.

As the evidence base for Massed PE grows, future research will likely focus on further refining the treatment and determining how to best tailor it to individual patients. One area of interest is whether combining Massed PE with other treatments like pharmacotherapy or innovative approaches like MDMA-assisted therapy, could enhance its effectiveness. Additionally, more research is needed to explore the neurobiological mechanisms behind Massed PE, such as how it affects brain circuits related to fear and trauma processing.

There is also growing interest in using digital tools to enhance Massed PE. Virtual reality (VR) exposure therapy, for example, has shown promise in delivering immersive exposure to trauma-related stimuli in a controlled and safe environment. By combining VR with Massed PE, therapists may be able to offer even more effective and engaging treatment options for PTSX sufferers.

What's In Store for the Future?

Mental-health professionals must understand that the synergy between these techniques and traditional methods positions them to create tailored, individualized treatment plans. The goal is to create resilience and promote healing by addressing both the mind and body, drawing from the strengths of each approach.

Ethical considerations play a crucial role in this integrative model. As science and medicine explore the use of psychedelics and other alternative therapies, it's essential to prioritize the safety and wellbeing of veterans and civilian patients. Healthcare professionals must be well-versed in the nuances of these treatments, ensuring informed consent and a robust understanding of potential risks and benefits.

Training and education in these emerging therapies will empower practitioners to make informed decisions, enhancing the quality of care provided to military personnel and veterans. This commitment to ethical practice will not only build trust but also support the broader acceptance of alternative therapies in the military and veteran communities.

Ultimately, the success of integrating traditional and alternative approaches relies heavily on community-based support systems. Veterans often find strength in shared experiences and creating environments where they can connect with peers undergoing similar healing journeys can amplify the impact of treatment. By building supportive networks that encourage dialogue and shared learning, we create a culture of resilience and hope.

If-Then Guidance

- If you are not aware of emerging PTSX treatments, then consider following organizations like the National Center for PTSD or reputable medical journals for updates on the latest advancements. Keeping informed can empower you to make more knowledgeable treatment decisions in the future.

- If you are open to new treatments, then consult with your healthcare provider about ongoing clinical trials or newer therapies that might benefit you. Being proactive about emerging options could give you access to treatments before they become widely available.
- If you do not follow research closely, then try subscribing to newsletters from veteran organizations, or follow mental health advocacy groups that provide updates on research. This can make it easier to stay informed about the latest treatment options for PTSX.
- If you believe in the role of technology in PTSX care, then explore innovative tools like mobile apps (e.g., PTSX Coach) or virtual reality therapy, which are already being used as supplementary treatment methods. Talk with your healthcare provider about how these innovations might be integrated into your current treatment plan.

Take the Next Step

- Research Cutting-Edge Treatments: Stay informed about the latest research and advancements in PTSX treatment, including new therapies being tested or approved, especially including massed prolonged exposure therapy.
- Discuss Emerging Therapies: Have a conversation with your healthcare provider about integrating cutting-edge treatments into your care plan.
- Join a Clinical Trial: If you're interested in exploring new treatments, check for clinical trials that may offer access to innovative therapies for veterans.

Through Their Eyes

"As an Army Special Forces medic, I was trained to respond to crises, to keep a cool head in the chaos of battle, and to patch up wounds no matter how deep. But what they don't teach you is how to treat the invisible injuries you take home—the trauma that sinks in long after the firefights are over, and the adrenaline fades.

"After years of deployments, I found myself in a constant state of hypervigilance, battling flashbacks, insomnia, and a gnawing sense of guilt that I couldn't shake. Despite my medical training, I didn't know how to fix what was broken inside me. I'd patched up soldiers, saved lives, but couldn't figure out how to save my own.

"Like so many veterans, when I returned home, the first response was medication and therapy. I was prescribed antidepressants, anti-anxiety meds, and sleep aids—anything to dull the sharp edges of my PTSX. And while they took the edge off, they also left me numb, disconnected, and distant from my family. The therapy sessions helped to an extent, but talking about my experiences wasn't enough. There was always a barrier between me and healing—a part of the trauma that I couldn't reach, no matter how hard I tried.

"Then I started hearing about alternative treatments—psychedelic-assisted therapy, ketamine infusions, stellate ganglion block. These treatments weren't just buzzwords—they were being used by fellow veterans, and the results were hard to ignore. A few of the guys I served with had tried MDMA-assisted therapy and told me how, for the first time, they could actually process their trauma without feeling overwhelmed by it. Another tried ketamine therapy and found a way out of the depression that had been changing him for years.

"As a medic, I've always been skeptical of anything that wasn't backed by science. But when I started digging into the research on these therapies, and also this new one, massed prolonged exposure therapy, I was blown away by what I found. There's hard science behind these treatments. It was about creating a space where veterans could finally confront their trauma in a meaningful way.

"Massed PE therapy changed the game for me. Instead of months of weekly sessions, I dedicated a few intense weeks to confronting my memories head-on. Each day, I replayed those harrowing moments: the incoming fire, the frantic rush to stop bleeding, the cries for help I couldn't ignore. It was brutal, but my therapist guided me through imaginal exposure, ensuring I revisited every detail until its grip on me began to loosen. Because sessions were compressed, the emotional roller coaster was steep. Some days, I'd leave exhausted, convinced I couldn't return.

"Yet the rapid pace also forced me to stay focused on healing. I leaned on breathing techniques and, when cleared by my healthcare team, a stellate ganglion block to calm my nerves. This combination made it possible to persevere through each session without quitting. By the end of those weeks, I noticed my nightmares losing their intensity. For the first time since returning stateside, I felt grounded—able to face each day as it came. Massed PE didn't erase the scars, but it gave me the tools and courage to move forward, finally free from trauma's stranglehold."

—Jason, US Army Special Forces Medic Veteran

29

Hyperbaric Oxygen Therapy in Treating PTSX

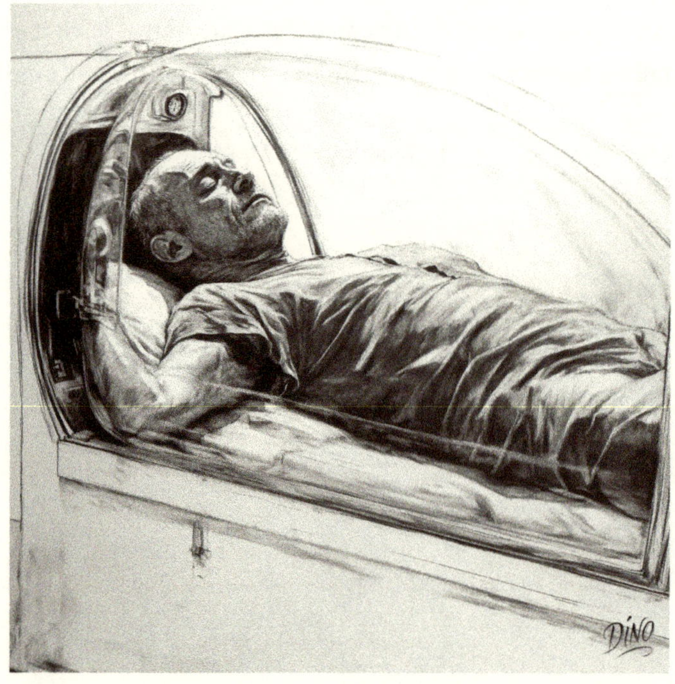

Tommy never imagined he'd be lying in a pressurized chamber, sipping cool air that felt oddly dense. Yet there he was, eyes closed, letting the low hum of machinery cradle him into a calm he hadn't felt in years. It wasn't a spa trip or some experimental fad—this was hyperbaric oxygen therapy (HOT), and he'd arrived after hearing how oxygen, given at high pressure, might mend old wounds that seemed impossible to heal.

For Tommy, the baggage of traumatic memories had anchored his nights in restless sleep and his days in constant worry. Standard treatments helped, sure—but after a while, he wondered if there was more out there. He found stories of veterans swearing by HOT, describing how intense oxygen infusions eased both physical pains and the relentless mental weight. Most nights, he'd catch himself scrolling through their testimonies, thinking, "Could that be me someday?"

Stepping into the chamber for his first session felt surreal, like entering a quiet, futuristic pod. The pressure built slowly, making his ears pop—like heading up a mountain or descending in a plane or into the depths on scuba. But instead of anxiety, he felt a gentle wave of relief. Over the next weeks, session by session, he noticed changes he couldn't dismiss: calmer mornings, a subtle lightness in his step, improved focus during conversations. Even his blood pressure dropped.

Soon, Tommy found himself recommending HOT to friends dealing with lingering traumas. It wasn't a magic fix—nothing is—but for him, it was a breakthrough. Like a deep breath he hadn't taken in years.

This chapter shines a light on that same possibility: how HOT, once reserved for divers and unusual cases, might just be a critical puzzle piece for those wrestling with PTSX. By boosting oxygen concentration to compromised areas of the body and brain, HOT can spark real, tangible improvements—proving that sometimes, a fresh dose of air is exactly what the soul needs.

HOT might sound a little futuristic, but it's actually a well-established medical treatment that's been making waves in the world of healing—and it's not just for divers anymore. Originally used to treat decompression sickness, HOT has evolved into a therapeutic option for many conditions, including some of the toughest cases of post-traumatic stress experience, or PTSX. Let's take a closer look at what HOT is and why it might just be the breath of fresh air—literally—that many people need.

What is HOT?

At its core, hyperbaric oxygen therapy involves breathing 100% oxygen while inside a pressurized chamber noramlly at 2 atmospheres. This unique environment allows the body to breathe in and absorb oxygen at much higher levels than normal. Imagine giving your body an oxygen supercharge, flooding your bloodstream, tissues and cells with this essential element to accelerate healing. HOT began as a treatment for divers suffering from decompression sickness, also known as "the bends," and has since expanded into a wide range of medical uses. It's been used to help people recover from carbon monoxide poisoning, severe infections, and even slow-healing wounds. Over time, researchers began to notice its potential for brain health and emotional wellbeing, paving the way for its application in conditions like PTSX.

Hyperbaric oxygen therapy pushes pressurized hope deep into tissue starved for second chances.

Why Consider HOT for PTSX?

So why are we talking about HOT in a book about PTSX? The answer lies in the growing search for therapies that can go beyond traditional treatments. For many people, especially veterans and others who've experienced severe trauma, the standard approaches like medication and talk therapy may not be enough. That's where HOT comes in, and it can be used in combination with other treatments and therapies.

Recent research has shown that HOT can be a game-changer for people living with PTSX. Unlike traditional therapies, which often focus on managing symptoms, HOT works at a deep subcellular level to promote healing. By increasing oxygen delivery to the brain, it can help repair damage, reduce inflammation, and create the conditions for emotional recovery.

Another exciting aspect of HOT is its potential to complement other treatments. For example, combining HOT with therapies like cognitive processing therapy has shown promising results in clinical studies. This synergy can provide a more holistic approach to healing.

The Connection Between Oxygen and Brain Health

To understand why HOT might work for PTSX, it's important to know a bit about the role of oxygen in the body—and specifically in the brain. Oxygen isn't just something we breathe. It's also a critical "fuel" for our cells. When oxygen levels are optimized, the body and brain can heal and function more effectively.

Trauma, whether physical or emotional, can wreak havoc on the brain. It can cause inflammation, disrupt blood flow, and even damage neural connections. HOT addresses these issues by delivering a concentrated dose of oxygen directly to the brain and other affected areas. This helps reduce inflammation, repair damaged tissues, and promote neuroplasticity—the brain's ability to adapt and form new connections.

The implications of this are huge. For someone with PTSX, it could mean fewer intrusive thoughts, better emotional regulation, and an overall improvement in quality of life. It's not magic, but it's a scientifically backed way to give the brain the support it needs to recover.

How HOT Works: The Science Simplified

HOT might seem mysterious, but the process is surprisingly straightforward. Imagine stepping into a chamber that looks a bit like a futuristic pod. Once inside, the chamber is sealed, and the air pressure increases to approximately two atmospheres, i.e. much higher than what we experience at sea level.

As this happens, you're breathing in pure oxygen—not the 21% oxygen we're used to, but 100%. This combination of increased pressure and pure oxygen creates the perfect environment for your body to absorb more oxygen than it ever could under normal circumstances.

A typical HOT session lasts anywhere from 60 to 90 minutes. Patients often describe it as peaceful— some even use the time to relax, meditate, or catch up on their favorite podcast. The increased pressure helps dissolve oxygen into the plasma of your blood, allowing it to travel deeper into tissues and areas that might not be receiving optimal blood flow. This is particularly beneficial for healing wounds, reducing inflammation and repairing damaged cells.

The key mechanisms of HOT's effectiveness lie in its ability to supercharge the body with oxygen. More oxygen means enhanced energy production in cells, faster repair of damaged tissues, and reduced inflammation. For individuals dealing with PTSX, these benefits translate into better overall physical and mental health, creating a foundation for recovery.

HOT and Brain Healing

The brain is one of the most oxygen-hungry organs in the body. It's no wonder that when the brain doesn't get enough oxygen, it struggles to function optimally. This is where HOT can make a significant difference.

One of the most exciting areas of research is HOT's ability to promote neurogenesis—the creation of new neurons. After trauma, whether physical or emotional, the brain often suffers damage that can lead to symptoms like memory issues, difficulty concentrating and emotional instability. By flooding the brain with oxygen, HOT stimulates the growth of new neurons and strengthens connections between existing ones. Neuroplasticity helps the brain adapt and recover from the effects of trauma.

HOT also improves blood flow to the brain. Better circulation means that the brain receives not just oxygen but also essential nutrients needed for healing. Studies have shown that this can lead to improved cognitive function, reduced symptoms of anxiety and depression and enhanced emotional regulation—all critical factors for individuals managing PTSX.

Another major benefit of HOT is its ability to reduce oxidative stress and neuroinflammation. Trauma can trigger an overactive immune response in the brain, leading to inflammation that disrupts normal functioning. By delivering high levels of oxygen, HOT helps calm this response, allowing the brain to heal without the interference of chronic inflammation.

HOT and the Body's Healing Systems

While much of the focus on HOT is on the brain, its benefits extend to the entire body. Oxygen is a universal healer, and when the body receives it in abundance, every system can function more effectively.

HOT supports healing by boosting the immune system. The increased oxygen levels enhance the activity of white blood cells, which are essential for fighting infections and repairing tissue damage. This is particularly helpful for individuals with PTSX who may have underlying physical injuries or a weakened immune response due to chronic stress.

Neuroinflammation and, outside the CNS, inflammation are areas where HOT shines. Chronic inflammation is a common issue in individuals with PTSX and can contribute to both physical and mental health challenges. HOT's ability to reduce inflammation at the cellular level helps alleviate pain, improve mobility and support overall recovery. This is especially valuable for veterans and others who may be dealing with injuries alongside their PTSX.

Beyond these specific benefits, HOT also promotes a general sense of wellbeing. Many patients report feeling more energized, less fatigued, and better able to cope with stress after completing a series of HOT sessions. This holistic improvement can be the first step toward a more comprehensive healing journey, addressing not just the symptoms of PTSX but the underlying physical and emotional toll it takes.

HOT for PTSX: What the Research Says

HOT has been the subject of numerous studies, and the growing body of evidence points to its potential as a transformative treatment for individuals with PTSX. Researchers have conducted systematic reviews and meta-analyses that consolidate findings from controlled trials. These studies highlight the ability of HOT to improve symptoms, enhance cognitive function, and reduce the emotional toll of trauma.

Researchers are studying how to optimize HOT protocols for combat-related PTSX. A recent study reviewed protocols specifically designed for veterans and active-duty servicemembers. These protocols include adjustments to pressure levels and session frequencies to cater to the unique needs of this population. Results have been promising, demonstrating significant improvements in symptom management and overall quality of life.

HOT and Symptoms of PTSX

For those living with PTSX, the symptoms can feel overwhelming. Hyperarousal, flashbacks and intrusive thoughts often dominate daily life. Research shows that HOT can help reduce these symptoms by addressing the underlying physiological issues contributing to them. By improving oxygen delivery to the brain, HOT calms overactive areas of the brain responsible for these symptoms, helping individuals regain a sense of control.

Mood and emotional regulation are other areas where HOT has shown promise. Many individuals with PTSX struggle with feelings of anger, sadness or numbness. HOT supports the brain's natural ability to regulate emotions by promoting neuroplasticity and reducing inflammation. This leads to improved mood stability and a greater capacity to cope with stress.

HOT as a Complementary Therapy

One of the most exciting aspects of HOT is its ability to work alongside other treatments. Recent studies have explored the combination of HOT with cognitive processing therapy (CPT). The results suggest a synergistic effect, where HOT enhances the effectiveness of CPT by creating a calmer, more receptive brain state. This combination allows patients to process trauma more effectively and achieve better outcomes.

HOT also pairs well with other approaches, including medications and mindfulness practices. By addressing the physical and emotional effects of trauma, HOT provides a solid foundation for these therapies to work more effectively. The holistic nature of this approach ensures that patients receive comprehensive care tailored to their unique needs.

Military Applications of HOT

The use of HOT for veterans is more than theoretical. It's backed by compelling evidence and real-life success stories. Case studies of veterans who have undergone HOT highlight significant improvements in their symptoms, including reduced anxiety, fewer flashbacks and a greater sense of emotional stability.

For many, HOT has been the turning point in their recovery journey. Multicenter trials targeting treatment-resistant PTSX have further validated the efficacy of HOT in military contexts. Research has demonstrated that even for individuals who have not responded to conventional therapies, HOT can provide meaningful relief. By addressing the physical underpinnings of PTSX, such as brain inflammation and impaired oxygen flow, HOT creates the conditions necessary for emotional healing.

Accessibility is a key consideration when it comes to implementing HOT in military healthcare systems. Efforts are underway to integrate HOT into VA hospitals and clinics, making it more accessible to those who need it most. Advocacy from veterans themselves has played a crucial role in driving these changes, as their firsthand accounts of HOT's benefits inspire others to consider this innovative therapy.

Addressing the Stigma

One of the challenges in promoting HOT for veterans is overcoming the stigma associated with seeking treatment. For many service members, acknowledging the need for help can feel like admitting weakness. It's crucial to reframe the narrative around HOT, emphasizing that it's a medical treatment aimed at healing the body and mind—no different from addressing a physical injury.

Success stories are a powerful tool in reducing this stigma. When veterans share their experiences with HOT, they not only validate the therapy's effectiveness but also normalize its use. Hearing about a fellow servicemember's journey can inspire hope and encourage others to explore HOT as a viable option for their recovery.

HOT Beyond the Military: Civilian Applications

While much of the discussion around, and research on, HOT focuses on military populations, its potential extends far beyond the battlefield. In civilian contexts, PTSX can arise from a variety of life-altering events, including abuse, accidents and natural disasters. Firefighters, in particular, suffer some of the worst PTSX, especially during fire season. What we've seen recently is nothing short of devastating. And our brave firefighters have suffered as much as those who lost homes and businesses. These experiences can leave lasting scars, both emotional and physical, that disrupt daily life. HOT provides a path to healing that addresses the root causes of these challenges.

Research has demonstrated HOT's effectiveness across broader populations. Studies on civilians dealing with trauma have shown reductions in symptoms like hyperarousal, anxiety and emotional numbness. By improving oxygen delivery and reducing inflammation, HOT creates the ideal conditions for the brain and body to recover. These findings are encouraging for anyone seeking relief from the burdens of PTSX.

HOT has proven especially helpful for individuals who have experienced ongoing or complex trauma. In cases where traditional therapy may take longer to yield results, HOT's physiological benefits can create a solid foundation for healing. By addressing both the physical and emotional aftermath of trauma, it empowers individuals to reclaim their lives more fully.

HOT for Related Conditions

The benefits of HOT don't stop at PTSX. This therapy has shown promise for several related conditions that often overlap with trauma, offering a comprehensive approach to recovery.

Anxiety: For individuals struggling with anxiety, HOT provides a calming effect that supports emotional regulation. By improving oxygen flow to the brain, it helps balance neurotransmitter production, maintenance, release and uptake, reducing the intensity of anxious thoughts and feelings. The relaxation experienced during HOT sessions also allows the body and mind to reset, making it easier to manage stressors outside the chamber.

Depression: Depression often accompanies PTSX, creating a heavy emotional burden. HOT enhances mood by reducing inflammation and increasing energy levels. Many patients report feeling less fatigued and more hopeful after completing HOT sessions. The treatment's ability to alleviate the physical sensations of depression—such as low energy and brain fog—can also make engaging in therapy or other interventions more effective.

Traumatic Brain Injuries (TBIs): TBIs are a common comorbidity with PTSX, particularly among athletes, accident survivors and veterans. HOT's ability to repair brain tissue and reduce neuroinflammation makes it an invaluable tool for addressing these overlapping symptoms, promoting cognitive and emotional recovery. Improvements in memory, focus, and overall cognitive clarity have been noted in individuals undergoing HOT for TBI recovery.

Practical Considerations for HOT

Safety is a top priority in HOT, and the procedure is generally considered safe for most individuals. However, as with any medical treatment, there are potential side effects. The most common include mild ear pressure, temporary fatigue or lightheadedness, which usually resolve quickly after a session.

To minimize risks, HOT is administered under the supervision of trained medical professionals. Safety protocols include thorough health assessments before treatment, monitoring during sessions, and ensuring that the pressure settings are appropriate for the individual's condition. Contraindications like certain lung conditions or untreated sinus infections, are carefully screened to ensure patient safety.

Finding a Provider

Choosing the right provider is an essential step in starting HOT. Look for licensed clinics with certified hyperbaric technicians and medical oversight. Reading reviews and asking for recommendations from trusted sources can also help identify reputable facilities. Before committing to a clinic, consider asking the following questions:

- What certifications and training do the staff hold?
- How is patient safety monitored during sessions?
- What is the recommended treatment plan for my condition?
- Are there any contraindications I should be aware of?
- How much does it cost?
- Will insurance fully cover it?

Personal Stories and Testimonials

Veterans who have experienced transformation through HOT often describe the therapy as life-changing. For instance, one Marine Corps veteran suffering from severe PTSX after multiple combat tours shared how HOT gave him his life back. Struggling with hypervigilance, insomnia, and emotional numbness, he found that after 30 sessions of HOT, his symptoms significantly improved. He reported sleeping peacefully for the first time in years and reconnecting with his family in ways he hadn't thought possible.

Another Army veteran who had been resistant to traditional therapy and medication turned to HOT as a last resort. The results were profound. His debilitating anxiety subsided, and the flashbacks that once dominated his days were reduced to fleeting memories. These stories underscore the unique ability of HOT to address both the physical and emotional wounds of war.

Civilian Success Stories

Civilians have also found immense relief through HOT. A middle-aged woman who survived a devastating car accident struggled with PTSX symptoms for years, including panic attacks and a constant sense of dread. After undergoing HOT, she experienced a significant reduction in her anxiety and regained the confidence to drive again.

Another inspiring story comes from a young man who suffered abuse during his childhood. For years, he battled depression and intrusive thoughts that impacted his ability to maintain relationships and hold a steady job. HOT not only alleviated his depressive symptoms but also gave him the mental clarity to pursue therapy more effectively. Today, he describes himself as finally feeling free from the weight of his past.

The Future of HOT for PTSX

HOT holds incredible promise for individuals living with PTSX, but it is not without its obstacles. One of the biggest hurdles is access. Many individuals who might benefit from HOT live far from clinics offering this therapy, particularly in rural or underserved areas. The costs associated with treatment can also be prohibitive, as insurance coverage for HOT remains limited. This financial burden often deters those who need it most.

Another significant challenge is the lack of standardized protocols. While research supports the efficacy of HOT, the optimal pressure levels, session durations, and treatment frequencies for PTSX are still under development. Variability in protocols across clinics can lead to inconsistent outcomes, undermining the therapy's credibility. More research is needed to establish evidence-based guidelines that practitioners can universally adopt. Finally, awareness is a persistent issue. Many individuals, including healthcare providers, remain unaware of HOT as a treatment option for PTSX. Lack of awareness prevents patients from exploring a potentially life-changing therapy.

Promising Advances

Despite these challenges, the future of HOT for PTSX is bright, thanks to ongoing advancements in technology and research. Emerging technologies are making HOT more effective and affordable. For example, portable hyperbaric chambers are now available for home use, for a unit that administers 100% oxygen at 1.2 atmospheres. These innovations have the potential to reduce costs, expand access and increase convenience for patients. The downside is that some patients report that 1.2 atmospheres is not enough to stimulate healing in tissues in the way that forty, 90-minute treatments at 2.0 atmospheres promotes healing.

Simultaneously, researchers are conducting robust studies to refine HOT protocols. By identifying the ideal pressure levels, oxygen concentrations, and treatment schedules, these studies aim to maximize the therapy's efficacy. Some trials are also exploring HOT in combination with other treatments, such as psychotherapy or pharmacotherapy, to uncover synergistic effects that enhance overall outcomes.

Additionally, efforts to use artificial intelligence (AI) in tailoring HOT treatments are gaining traction. AI-driven models could analyze individual patient data to recommend personalized treatment plans, improving both effectiveness and patient satisfaction.

Advocacy for HOT

Advocacy plays a critical role in overcoming the barriers to HOT. Policymakers must be encouraged to expand insurance coverage for this therapy. Including HOT in government healthcare programs like Medicare and Medicaid would make it more accessible to a broader population. Advocacy groups, veteran organizations and patient testimonials can help build the case for this inclusion.

Increasing public awareness is equally important. Educational campaigns highlighting the benefits of HOT for PTSX can inspire individuals to explore this therapy and prompt healthcare providers to recommend it. Success stories, whether shared through media outlets or community events, have the power to humanize the science and reach those in need. Collaborations among researchers, clinicians and patient advocates can accelerate progress in these areas.

Where To Now?

HOT is more than just a medical intervention. It's an encouraging treatment for individuals living with the profound effects of PTSX. By delivering oxygen to areas of the brain and body that need it most, HOT addresses the physical and emotional toll of trauma in a way that few other therapies can. From veterans reclaiming their lives after combat to civilians overcoming the weight of personal tragedies, the stories of transformation fueled by HOT are both inspiring and validating.

These personal accounts, combined with a growing body of scientific research, underscore the therapy's potential to revolutionize how we approach trauma recovery. Yet, the journey toward making HOT universally accessible is far from over. Challenges related to cost, access and standardization remain, but promising advancements in technology and advocacy offer a path forward. With continued effort, HOT can become a cornerstone of trauma care, available to all who need it.

As we look to the future, one thing is clear: the potential of HOT is immense. For those grappling with PTSX, exploring this therapy could be a life-changing step toward healing. For clinicians and advocates, supporting the integration of HOT into mainstream care represents an opportunity to transform countless lives.

If-Then Guidance

- If you or someone you know is living with PTSX and traditional treatments have fallen short, then consider exploring HOT as an innovative therapy that addresses the physiological roots of trauma. HOT works by delivering high levels of oxygen under pressure, promoting brain and body healing at a subcellular level.

It has shown promise in reducing symptoms like hyperarousal, anxiety and intrusive thoughts while enhancing emotional regulation and cognitive function.

- If accessing HOT seems challenging due to geographic or financial barriers, then investigate emerging technologies such as portable hyperbaric chambers or seek financial assistance programs offered by advocacy groups. Efforts are underway to make HOT more affordable and accessible, with potential coverage expansions through Medicare and Medicaid as awareness grows.
- If you are unsure about the safety of HOT, then rest assured that this therapy is generally safe when administered under professional supervision. Discuss potential contraindications with a healthcare provider, and look for certified clinics with a track record of patient safety.
- If you are considering combining HOT with other treatments, then consult with your therapist or doctor about its compatibility with cognitive processing therapy or medications. Research results suggest that HOT enhances the effectiveness of other interventions, creating a synergistic approach to healing.
- If you are a veteran struggling with the dual burdens of physical injuries and PTSX, then take heart in the growing body of evidence showing HOT's transformative effects for servicemembers. Results from trials reveal significant improvements in symptoms and quality of life for veterans who have undergone HOT.
- If you are a civilian dealing with PTSX caused by abuse, accidents or natural disasters, then know that HOT is not just for military populations—it has helped countless civilians recover and reclaim their lives. Its benefits extend to conditions like anxiety, depression and traumatic brain injuries, making it a versatile therapy for overlapping challenges.
- If awareness about HOT feels limited in your community, then advocate for broader educational campaigns and share success stories to inspire others. Public testimonials both from veterans and civilians can demystify HOT and highlight its potential for those still seeking effective care.

- If you are looking for hope and a way forward, then remember that HOT represents not only a cutting-edge therapy but also the future of trauma recovery. With ongoing advancements in technology, research and advocacy, the barriers to accessing HOT are slowly diminishing, ensuring that its benefits reach all who need them.

Take the Next Step

- If you're considering HOT as a path to healing, there are several actionable steps you can take to move forward with confidence.
- Begin by educating yourself thoroughly about HOT. Read up on its benefits, challenges and the science behind how it works, particularly for those living with PTSX. Knowledge is empowering and will help you make informed decisions.
- Seek out qualified providers in your area. Look for clinics with licensed practitioners and certified hyperbaric technicians. Don't hesitate to ask about their protocols, safety measures and experience treating PTSX. Verifying their credentials will give you peace of mind as you start this journey.
- Consult with your healthcare team about incorporating HOT into your treatment plan. Share what you've learned and discuss how HOT might complement other therapies you're currently undergoing. Their guidance can ensure that HOT aligns with your overall recovery goals.
- If access to HOT is a concern due to cost or location, explore alternative options like portable hyperbaric chambers or financial aid programs. Advocacy groups and community organizations may provide resources to help bridge these gaps.
- Engage with others who have benefited from HOT. Reach out to support groups or online forums where veterans, civilians and patients share their experiences. Their stories can provide inspiration and practical insights into what to expect.
- Finally, consider becoming an advocate for HOT. Share your journey and raise awareness about its potential to transform lives. Whether through personal testimonials, community outreach, or

discussions with policymakers, your voice can help make HOT more accessible to those in need.

Through Their Eyes

"For two decades, I lived in a constant state of survival. As a pararescue jumper in the US Air Force, my job was to go into the most dangerous situations and save lives. Afghanistan, Iraq—I saw more combat than I care to remember. And while I was good at saving others, I couldn't save myself from the invisible wounds I carried home.

"PTSD—what I now know as PTSX—became my constant shadow. It robbed me of sleep, peace and connection with my family. Nightmares resulted in sleepless nights. Simple triggers would send me back to the battlefield in my mind. For 20 years, I tried everything: medications, therapy, just toughing it out. Nothing worked. I was trapped. Then I discovered something that changed everything: hyperbaric oxygen therapy and stellate ganglion block. These treatments gave me a second chance at life. HOT was the first step. At first, I didn't know what to expect—breathing pure oxygen in a pressurized chamber sounded more like science fiction than therapy.

"But after the first few sessions, I started noticing small changes. My mind felt clearer. My vision changed back to an old prescription from 10 years ago! The weight in my chest started to lift. Over time, I realized I wasn't just managing my symptoms. I was actually healing and I could feel the effects. The oxygen helped repair my brain on a level I didn't even know was possible. It was like my body was finally getting the support it needed to recover from decades of trauma. Stellate ganglion block came next, and it was just as transformative. The procedure was quick, but its impact was profound.

For the first time in years, I felt like my nervous system wasn't in overdrive. That constant fight-or-flight feeling was gone. I could breathe deeply, think clearly and truly relax. Together, HOT and stellate ganglion block created a foundation for real healing—not just band-aid fixes but deep, lasting change.

"Now that I'm retired, I meet with a Licensed Clinical Social Worker once a month—not because I'm struggling, but because I've learned the value of staying proactive about my mental health. I'm back with my wife, my kids, and even my grandkids. I'm present for them in a way I never was before. I wake up every day grateful, not just for surviving but for living fully.

"I want you to know there is a way forward. HOT and stellate ganglion block gave me my life back, and they just might do the same for you. It's not about being tough enough to handle it alone. Healing isn't about toughness. Look at it like finding the right tools and being brave enough to use them. You deserve a second chance, just like I got."

—Chief Master Sergeant Albert R., USAF (ret.)

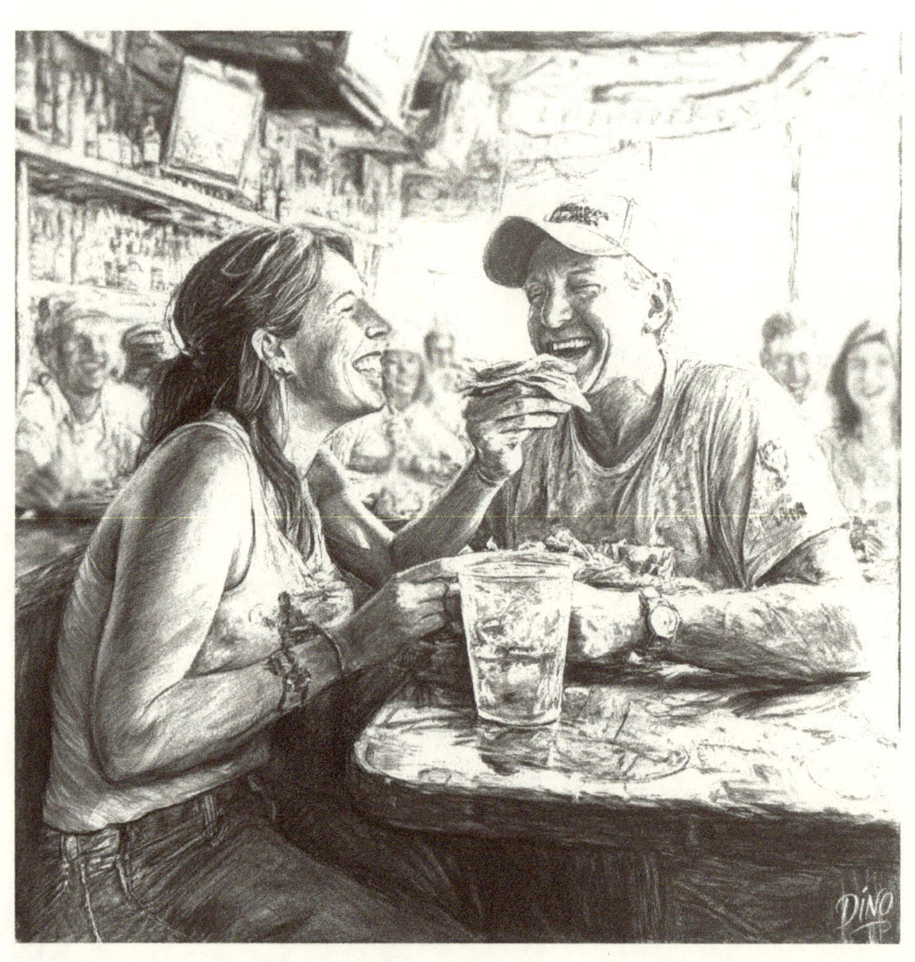
DINO

PART FOUR

Foundational Healing Approaches

30

Trauma-Informed Care Models: Building a Foundation for Comprehensive Healing

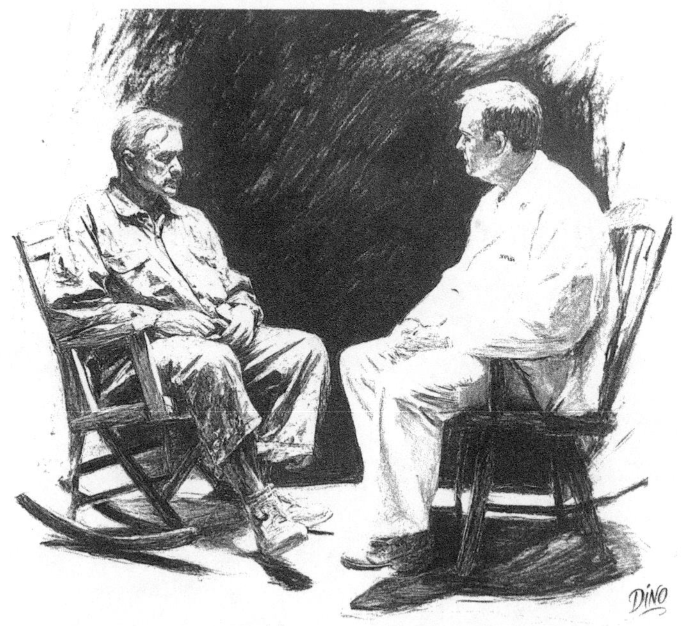

The room was silent except for the rhythmic creak of a rocking chair. James, the therapist, sat across from a man who had seen wars and battles that stretched across decades, both on foreign soil and within his own mind. The veteran's eyes were sharp, darting to every corner of the room, scanning for threats that weren't there.

James leaned forward, his voice low but steady. "You're safe here," he said. "No one's coming for you. Not anymore."

The veteran's shoulders relaxed just a fraction, but that was enough. It was the beginning. Trust wasn't given easily in these spaces. It had to be earned, brick by brick, word by word. Trauma had built walls around the man, high and unyielding. His therapist didn't rush to scale them or smash through with platitudes. Instead, he offered choices. "Would you rather start with art or equine therapy?" The healing wasn't in a single word or session. It was in the layers: safety, trust, empowerment. It was in understanding that trauma didn't have to define the future.

This chapter discusses trauma-informed care, a framework that transforms treatment into a partnership of healing, understanding, and humanity. It's a promise that every veteran deserves: the chance to heal with dignity.

For military personnel and veterans living with PTSX, the road to healing can feel like navigating uncharted territory. Combat, loss, and sacrifice leave invisible scars, and finding the right treatment can be overwhelming.

Trauma-informed care offers a path forward, one that acknowledges the depth and complexity of trauma while creating an environment of safety, trust, and empowerment. By integrating trauma-informed principles into every aspect of care, we can create a foundation for comprehensive healing that addresses the unique needs of those who have served.

This type of care isn't a single treatment or protocol—it's a framework that informs how care is delivered. It ensures that the systems, professionals and treatments involved in PTSX recovery are designed with a deep understanding of trauma's impact on the mind, body and soul. This approach transforms traditional care into something holistic and profoundly human.

The Key Principles of Trauma-Informed Care

Trauma-informed care operates on a set of principles designed to create a supportive and healing environment for individuals affected by trauma. These principles guide every interaction, ensuring that care is sensitive, respectful and effective.

<u>Safety</u>: The cornerstone of trauma-informed care is creating a sense of physical and emotional safety. For veterans, this might mean reducing sensory triggers in treatment settings or establishing predictable routines that build trust.

Trustworthiness and Transparency: Building trust is essential for effective care. Trauma-informed practices prioritize honesty, clear communication and consistency, ensuring that veterans feel respected and valued.

Peer Support: Veterans often find comfort and understanding in the company of others who have shared similar experiences. Peer support builds connection, reduces isolation, and promotes healing.

Collaboration and Mutuality: Trauma-informed care emphasizes partnership. Veterans are not passive recipients of treatment but active participants in their recovery journey. Collaborative care empowers individuals and respects their autonomy.

Empowerment, Voice and Choice: Empowering veterans means recognizing their strengths and giving them control over their healing process. Trauma-informed care offers choices and honors the individual's unique needs and preferences.

Cultural, Historical and Gender Sensitivity: Recognizing the diverse experiences of veterans, trauma-informed care respects and integrates cultural, historical and gender considerations into treatment plans.

Implementation in Veteran-Specific Healthcare Settings

Adopting trauma-informed care in veteran-specific settings requires intentional design and continuous commitment:

Physical Environment: Treatment spaces are designed to minimize stress and triggers. For instance, soft lighting, comfortable seating and calming decor can create a sense of safety and calm.

Staff Training: All personnel, from clinicians to administrative staff, are trained in trauma awareness and sensitivity. This training helps ensure that every interaction is supportive and respectful.

Screening and Assessment: Trauma-informed care incorporates comprehensive assessments that go beyond symptoms to explore the individual's history, strengths and goals. These assessments are conducted in a way that minimizes re-traumatization.

Personalized Care Plans: Each veteran's journey is unique. Care plans are tailored to address individual needs, preferences and cultural contexts, ensuring that treatments are relevant and effective.

Support Systems: Veterans are connected with peer groups, family counseling and community resources that provide ongoing support and encouragement.

Enhancing the Effectiveness of Therapies

Trauma-informed care doesn't replace existing therapies, and it enhances them by providing a foundation that amplifies their impact. Below are examples of how this approach integrates with key therapies:

Psychedelic-Assisted Therapies: Psychedelics like MDMA and psilocybin are showing promise for treating PTSX. Trauma-informed care ensures that these therapies are delivered in safe, controlled environments with skilled practitioners who prioritize emotional and psychological safety.

Somatic Therapies: Somatic practices like body-based mindfulness and movement therapies, benefit from trauma-informed approaches that emphasize gentle, non-invasive techniques. This sensitivity helps veterans reconnect with their bodies without feeling overwhelmed.

Hyperbaric Oxygen Therapy (HOT): By integrating trauma-informed care, HOT sessions can be structured to reduce anxiety and enhance comfort, ensuring that veterans feel supported throughout the process.

Traditional Talk Therapies: Trauma-informed care enhances the therapeutic alliance between veterans and therapists, thus building trust and openness that are essential for effective talk therapy.

Cannabinoid Integration: Trauma-informed care ensures that cannabinoid therapies are introduced in a way that emphasizes education and informed consent. By creating a safe, stigma-free environment, veterans can explore the potential benefits of cannabinoids for anxiety, sleep disturbances and pain management.

Stellate Ganglion Block (SGB): For veterans considering SGB as a treatment for severe PTSX symptoms, trauma-informed care ensures that the procedure is explained thoroughly, and veterans are supported throughout the process. Follow-up care integrates emotional and psychological support to maximize the benefits of this cutting-edge therapy.

Animal-Assisted Interventions: Trauma-informed care enhances the effectiveness of human-animal bonds by ensuring that veterans feel comfortable and safe during interactions with therapy animals. Programs are tailored to individual needs, building trust and emotional resilience.

Spiritual and Faith-Based Therapies: Trauma-informed care integrates spirituality in a way that honors individual beliefs and preferences. Veterans are encouraged to explore spiritual practices or traditions that resonate with them, creating a sense of purpose and connection.

Post-Traumatic Growth (PTG) Programs: By focusing on empowerment and resilience, trauma-informed care amplifies the benefits of PTG programs. Veterans are supported in reframing their experiences and discovering newfound strengths.

Emerging Technologies: Virtual-reality therapy, biofeedback and AI-driven tools are increasingly used in PTSX treatment. Trauma-informed care ensures these technologies are introduced thoughtfully, with clear communication about their purpose and benefits, reducing anxiety and building trust. Most people are not familiar with these advanced technologies so it's imperative that they understand how important tech is to their long-term care and healing.

Case Studies: Trauma-Informed Care in Action

Case Study 1: Rebuilding Trust Through Peer Support

Mark, a combat veteran, struggled with severe hypervigilance and mistrust. After joining a trauma-informed peer support group, he began to share his experiences in a safe and understanding environment. The group's facilitator, a fellow veteran trained in trauma-informed practices, created an atmosphere of empathy and connection.

Over time, Mark's trust in others grew, allowing him to engage more fully in therapy and rebuild relationships outside the group. During one group session, Mark shared a deeply personal story about his time in combat. The group responded with compassion, which helped him feel less alone. As his confidence grew, he began volunteering to help other veterans, finding purpose and solidarity in giving back. This new sense of belonging and contribution became a cornerstone of his recovery.

Case Study 2: Tailoring Treatment for Cultural Sensitivity

Melissa, a Latina veteran, faced unique cultural barriers in seeking care. Her trauma-informed therapist incorporated elements of her heritage into treatment, such as traditional healing rituals and family involvement. This culturally attuned approach made her feel seen and respected, enabling her to engage more deeply in therapy.

Recognizing her strong connection to her family, the therapist invited her mother and sister to participate in certain sessions, building a supportive network. Additionally, the therapist used storytelling—a cherished tradition in Melissa's culture—to help her process traumatic events. By framing her healing journey within the context of her cultural values, she found strength in her identity and felt empowered to confront her trauma. Over time, she became an advocate for other Latina veterans, helping to bridge the gap between cultural barriers and mental health care.

Case Study 3: Empowerment Through Choice

James, an Iraq War veteran, felt powerless and disconnected from his care team. A trauma-informed approach transformed his experience by involving him in every decision about his treatment plan. He was given options like choosing between group therapy and one-on-one sessions, which restored his sense of control and dignity. James' therapist also introduced him to several therapeutic modalities, including art therapy, mindfulness meditation and equine therapy.

Encouraged to explore these options, James discovered that working with horses helped him feel calm and connected. This choice-driven approach not only reduced his anxiety but also reignited his confidence. By actively participating in his recovery, James began to trust the process and take ownership of his healing. His newfound sense of agency inspired him to mentor younger veterans, demonstrating the power of choice in trauma recovery.

The Broader Impact of Trauma-Informed Care

The benefits of trauma-informed care extend beyond individual veterans to families, communities, and the healthcare system as a whole.

By addressing trauma at its roots and building resilience, this approach:

Reduces Stigma: Trauma-informed practices normalize the experience of trauma, reducing shame and encouraging more veterans to seek help.

Improves Outcomes: Veterans receiving trauma-informed care are more likely to complete treatment and experience lasting recovery.

Strengthens Families: By involving loved ones in the healing process, trauma-informed care supports better relationships and family dynamics.

Transforms Systems: Trauma-informed care can inspire systemic changes that make healthcare settings more compassionate and effective for all patients.

Trauma-Informed Care is More Than a Framework

It's a commitment to understanding and honoring the human experience of trauma. For veterans and civilian patients navigating the complexities of PTSX, this approach offers a foundation of safety, trust and empowerment that makes healing possible. By adopting trauma-informed principles in every aspect of care, we can build a system that not only treats symptoms but also creates resilience, connection and hope. For the brave individuals who have served, this comprehensive, compassionate approach is nothing less than they deserve.

If-Then Guidance

- If a veteran feels overwhelmed by traditional talk therapy, then consider somatic therapies. Trauma-informed care ensures these approaches are gentle and non-invasive, helping veterans reconnect with their bodies without feeling triggered or retraumatized.
- If a veteran is struggling with severe flashbacks or intrusive thoughts, then explore psychedelic-assisted therapies. Under trauma-informed care, psychedelics like MDMA are administered in a controlled environment, ensuring safety and emotional support throughout the process.
- If a veteran is hesitant to engage with formal therapy, then peer support groups can be an excellent starting point. Trauma-informed care ensures these groups are facilitated by trained peers, creating trust and connection in a non-threatening environment.

- If a veteran experiences chronic physical symptoms alongside PTSX, then integrate hyperbaric oxygen therapy (HOT) into their treatment plan. Trauma-informed care creates a calming atmosphere for HOT sessions, reducing stress and ensuring the veteran feels supported.
- If a veteran struggles with insomnia or chronic pain, then cannabinoid therapies may provide relief. Trauma-informed care ensures that these treatments are introduced with clear education and informed consent, minimizing stigma and maximizing comfort.
- If a veteran finds traditional therapy culturally irrelevant, then explore culturally tailored interventions. Trauma-informed care ensures that cultural, historical and gender sensitivities are respected, making the therapy more meaningful and impactful.
- If a veteran is exploring cutting-edge treatments, then consider introducing emerging technologies like virtual reality therapy. Trauma-informed care ensures these tools are used thoughtfully, reducing anxiety and emphasizing transparency about their purpose and benefits.
- If a veteran is resistant to structured therapy, then animal-assisted interventions may help. Trauma-informed care facilitates safe, meaningful interactions with therapy animals, building trust and emotional connection in a low-pressure setting.

Take the Next Step

- Take time to educate yourself about the principles of trauma-informed care and how they can benefit your recovery. Explore resources, attend workshops, or speak with professionals who specialize in this approach. Knowledge is empowering and will help you advocate for your needs.
- Assess whether your current treatment environment feels safe, welcoming and supportive. If it doesn't, consider discussing changes with your care provider or exploring new options that align with trauma-informed principles.
- Connect with others who understand your journey, whether

through peer-support groups, veteran organizations or trusted friends and family. A strong support network can provide the encouragement and understanding needed to sustain healing.

- Trauma-informed care emphasizes choice. Research the range of therapies available, from traditional talk therapy to innovative treatments like psychedelics, somatic practices and hyperbaric oxygen therapy. Identify what resonates most with your needs and preferences.
- Needs If you're working with healthcare providers, share your goals, concerns, and preferences. Trauma-informed care thrives on collaboration, so don't hesitate to voice your needs and participate actively in your treatment planning.
- Recognize that healing is multifaceted. Incorporate physical, emotional, and spiritual practices into your recovery journey, such as mindfulness, exercise and faith-based practices. This integrative approach supports long-term resilience.
- Take time to acknowledge how far you've come. Journaling or speaking with a trusted confidant can help you recognize small victories and set new goals. Reflection encourages gratitude and stimulates motivation.
- Healing is a lifelong process. Commit to ongoing learning, self-care, and connection with others. Trauma-informed care is not just a framework for treatment but a way to live with greater compassion and empowerment.

Through Their Eyes

"They call me Ghost. At 47, my face bears the marks of 24 years in the Navy SEALs. These steel-gray eyes of mine have seen too much, but there's a spark in them that hasn't dulled yet. Yeah, there are laugh lines now and then—earned through hard lessons and the wisdom that comes from losing too many good men.

"Ghost wasn't just a nickname I picked up. I earned it in spades. Sneaking into hostile territory without a trace? That was my game. Afghanistan, Iraq, secret spots across three continents—I did what needed to be done to keep my brothers alive. Standing 5'10" with a lean, athletic build, I've kept myself in shape through relentless discipline. Moving with the grace of someone who's been through the grind countless times.

"One operation sticks out in my mind from 2008 in the X Valley. We were pinned down, enemy fire all around. I led a four-man team to rescue a downed helicopter crew. Got hit twice, but I didn't stop. Carried an injured pilot over two kilometers of rough, mountainous terrain to safety. Earned the Navy Cross for that—something I wear with a mix of pride and the weight of what it took.

"As my unit's go-to demolitions expert, I've pushed the limits on breaching techniques. Now those methods are taught at Advanced Training Command. Precision, calculation, always having a backup plan—that's how I lead. My hands? Callused from missions, but steady enough to take apart the nastiest IEDs you can throw at me.

"Despite all the medals and accolades, I don't talk much about them. It's my teammates who deserve the praise. I carry the weight of lost brothers silently. The small St. Michael medallion my dad gave me—he was a Vietnam vet—is the only thing I keep with me through all these years. Now that I'm retired, I pass on what I know to the next generation of operators. But those midnight calls from old teammates? I never leave them hanging.

"Behind this rough exterior, there's a lot more going on. The battles don't end when you hang up the uniform. Post-Traumatic stress—PTSX—it's real, and it lingers. I've been down that road myself, feeling like I'm navigating uncharted territory. That's why I stand behind Trauma-informed care. It's not just another protocol. TIC is a lifeline for folks like us.

"TIC gets it. It understands the depth and complexity of what we've been through. It builds an environment where we can feel safe, trust the people helping us, and take back control of our lives. Traditional care often misses the mark, leaving too many veterans adrift. But with trauma-informed principles woven into every aspect of treatment, there's hope for comprehensive healing.

"When I train, I make sure the spaces we use are safe—physically and emotionally. No unnecessary stressors, just like the controlled operations

I led back in the field. I push for honesty, clear communication, and consistency in every interaction. It's about respect and making sure everyone feels valued.

"Peer support is another cornerstone. Out there, camaraderie saved our lives. Bringing veterans together who've shared similar experiences reduces that crushing isolation we feel and starts real healing. We're not just individuals; we're a brotherhood, even in recovery.

"Empowerment is key. Recognizing our strengths and giving us control over our healing process makes all the difference. Whether it's choosing between group therapy or one-on-one sessions, or deciding which therapeutic modality suits us best—having a say restores some of that lost dignity and control.

"Every veteran's journey is different. I make sure our programs respect and integrate each person's cultural, historical and personal background. It's about making treatment relevant and respectful, creating a sense of belonging and acceptance that's crucial for effective healing.

"Those midnight calls? They remind me that my mission isn't over. I'm still here for my brothers, ensuring that no one has to walk the path to healing alone. My legacy isn't just about the missions I led or the medals I earned. It's about resilience, compassion and unwavering support for those who've served alongside me.

"Training the next wave of special operators, I emphasize that true strength isn't just about muscle or tactics. It's about mental and emotional resilience. I share what I know about TIC because understanding and supporting each other's mental wellbeing is just as important as any mission. These principles are now the backbone of our training programs, ensuring future leaders can create environments of safety, trust and empowerment.

"Now, in retirement, I'm focused on making a real difference. Advocating for TIC has led to programs that tackle both the physical and psychological wounds we carry. It's about transforming traditional care into something holistic and deeply human—something that actually works for us.

"Veterans see a leader who's been through the trenches and came out the other side with a mission to help others heal. My story isn't just one of combat and survival—it's one of empathy and dedication to the healing of my brothers *and sisters* in arms."

—Master Chief "Ghost," US Navy (ret.)

31

The Intersection of Nutrition, Lifestyle and PTSX Recovery

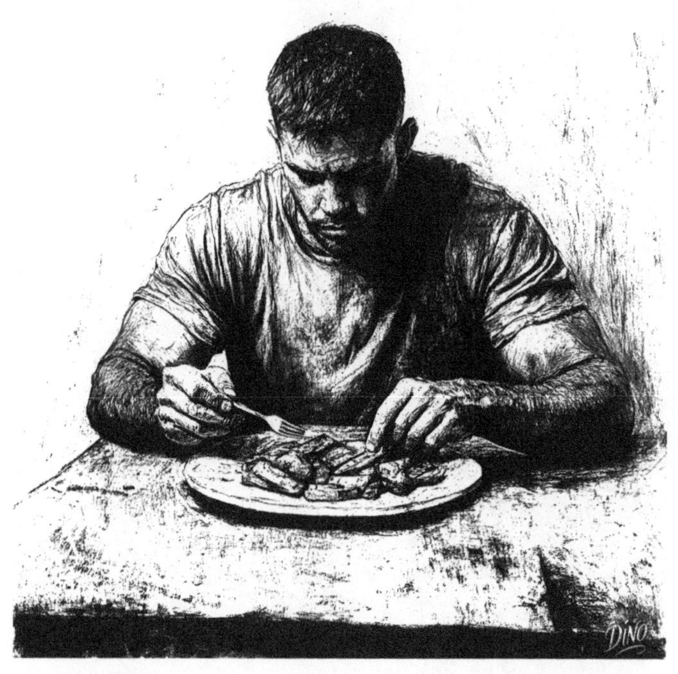

The Marine sat at a weathered table, his fork picking at a plate of roasted vegetables and grilled salmon. He had fought his battles overseas, but this one was closer to home, gnawing at his soul like a silent, relentless predator. The memories of sand, heat and the sounds of chaos clung to him, yet he found himself in a place of quiet revolution: his own kitchen.

"You are what you eat," the doctor had said, but he hadn't believed it. Not until the fog of anxiety began to lift, just a little, as leafy greens and omega-3s replaced greasy fast food. His gut felt settled, and for the first time in years, so did his mind.

Down the road, a runner, her breath puffing like a steam engine in the cold air, pushed herself forward. One block, then two. Her heart pounded, sweat dripped, and her body protested, but she kept going. She wasn't running from the past but toward a future where the weight of the darkness didn't crush her. Each step was a rebellion against depression, a rhythm that stitched her spirit back together.

Meanwhile, a veteran in a dimly lit bedroom adjusted his pillow. He had learned to treat sleep like a sacred mission: no screens, no distractions, only the steady discipline of rest. With each night of uninterrupted sleep, the fractures in his mind began to mend, piece by piece.

The war didn't end when the uniforms were folded away. It simply changed shape. Here, in the quiet acts of cooking, moving, and resting, was the new battlefield. Victory wasn't a medal—it was peace. And peace wasn't a destination. It was a practice.

This chapter is about the quiet yet profound ways that nutrition, exercise, sleep and stress management fuel the journey to healing from PTSX. It offers actionable guidance to help veterans integrate these elements into their lives, providing a path to better mental health and a higher quality of life.

The Power of Nutrition: Feeding the Mind and Body

"You are what you eat" is more than just a saying. The foods we consume directly influence our brain chemistry, mood, and overall health. For veterans recovering from PTSX, adopting an anti-inflammatory diet can be transformative.

The Mediterranean Diet and the Gut-Brain Axis

The Mediterranean diet, rich in fruits, vegetables, whole grains, lean proteins, and healthful fats, is renowned for its benefits to mental and physical health. This diet's emphasis on anti-inflammatory foods supports the gut microbiome, the collection of microorganisms in our digestive system that play a crucial role in mental health.

Research shows that a healthy gut microbiome reduces systemic inflammation and promotes the production of neurotransmitters like serotonin, often referred to as the "feel-good" chemical. Veterans struggling with depression, anxiety, or hyperarousal can benefit significantly from a diet that supports gut-brain communication.

Start small. Add a handful of walnuts or almonds to your breakfast, swap processed snacks for fresh fruit, and incorporate leafy greens like spinach or kale into one meal a day.

Foods to Avoid

Highly processed foods, sugary drinks, and trans fats can exacerbate inflammation, leading to worsened symptoms of PTSX. Reducing or eliminating these from your diet is a simple but impactful step toward recovery. Gradually replace processed snacks with whole-food alternatives like carrots and hummus or a boiled egg with a pinch of salt.

The Role of Exercise: Movement as Medicine

Regular physical activity is a game-changer for mental health. Exercise doesn't just improve physical fitness—it's a natural mood booster that promotes neuroplasticity, the brain's ability to adapt and rewire itself.

Exercise and Neuroplasticity

Studies have shown that aerobic exercise like walking, running or swimming, stimulates the production of brain-derived neurotrophic factor (BDNF), which supports the growth and survival of neurons. For veterans with PTSX, this is particularly important, as trauma can disrupt neural pathways involved in emotional regulation and memory.

Start with just 10 minutes of brisk walking daily. Gradually increase the duration and intensity as your confidence and stamina grow.

Finding Joy in Movement

Not all exercise needs to happen in a gym. Activities like hiking, dancing, or playing a sport can be equally beneficial. The key is finding something you enjoy, making it easier to stick with over time.

Experiment with different forms of movement until you find one that feels rewarding. Joining a local sports league or walking with a buddy can make exercise a social and enjoyable experience.

Sleep Hygiene: Restoring the Body and Mind

Sleep is a cornerstone of recovery, yet insomnia and hyperarousal are common struggles for veterans with PTSX. Adopting healthy sleep habits can significantly improve emotional resilience and overall wellbeing.

The Importance of a Sleep Routine

Consistency is key. Going to bed and waking up at the same time every day helps regulate your body's internal clock, making it easier to fall asleep and stay asleep.

Create a calming bedtime ritual. Whether it's reading, meditating, or taking a warm bath, these activities signal your brain that it's time to wind down.

Sleep Environment

Your bedroom should be a sanctuary for rest. Keep it cool, dark, and quiet. Consider blackout curtains or a white noise machine to block out disruptions.

Remove electronic devices from your bedroom and avoid screen time at least an hour before bed to minimize exposure to blue light, which can interfere with melatonin production.

Stress Reduction: Finding Calm in the Chaos

Managing stress is a critical component of PTSX recovery. While stress is a natural part of life, chronic stress can worsen symptoms and hinder healing. Techniques like mindfulness, yoga, and breathwork offer effective ways to regain a sense of control and calm.

Mindfulness and Meditation

Mindfulness involves focusing on the present moment without judgment. Practices like meditation have been shown to reduce anxiety, improve focus, and promote a sense of inner peace.

Start with a simple breathing exercise: inhale for four counts, hold for four counts, and exhale for four counts. Repeat this cycle for five minutes daily.

Yoga for Mind-Body Connection

Yoga combines movement, breathwork, and meditation to create a holistic practice that benefits both the body and mind. For veterans, yoga can help release tension stored in the body and improve flexibility and balance.

Look for beginner-friendly yoga classes, either in person or online, that cater to veterans or trauma survivors.

The Power of Breathwork

Controlled breathing techniques can instantly reduce stress by activating the parasympathetic nervous system, which promotes relaxation.

Try diaphragmatic breathing. Place one hand on your chest and the other on your abdomen. Breathe deeply through your nose, ensuring your abdomen rises more than your chest. Exhale slowly through your mouth.

Real-World Success Stories

Stories of resilience can inspire and guide others on their journey. Here are some examples of veterans who embraced lifestyle changes and experienced profound transformations:

Alex's Story: Finding Strength Through Nutrition

Alex, a Marine Corps veteran, struggled with severe anxiety and digestive issues that made daily life feel overwhelming. After hearing about the connection between gut health and mental wellbeing from a fellow veteran, Alex decided to research the Mediterranean diet. He started by making small, manageable changes: replacing sugary drinks with water, adding leafy greens to his meals, and incorporating omega-3-rich foods like salmon.

Within a few weeks, Alex noticed his anxiety levels begin to decline, and his energy levels improved. Encouraged by the results, he continued to refine his eating habits, eventually eliminating processed snacks and replacing them with nutrient-dense alternatives. Over time, Alex discovered that his digestive issues subsided, and he felt more emotionally stable. He shared his journey with his support group, inspiring others to consider the role of nutrition in their recovery. Today, Alex feels more in control of his emotional health and credits his dietary changes as a cornerstone of his healing journey.

Sarah's Story: Rebuilding Confidence Through Exercise

Sarah, an Army veteran, had spent years battling depression and a deep sense of isolation. Encouraged by a friend, she decided to try running as a way to regain a sense of purpose. Her first run was a struggle—a short jog around the block left her winded and discouraged. But Sarah was determined to keep going.

She set small goals, celebrating each milestone, from completing her first mile to participating in a local 5K race. As running became a daily habit, Sarah began to notice not only physical improvements but also significant changes in her mood and outlook on life. The rhythmic movement of running became a form of meditation, helping her process emotions she'd long suppressed. Over time, Sarah's physical and emotional strength grew, and she started volunteering to coach other veterans in her community. Today, she credits running with helping her regain her confidence and rediscover a sense of purpose.

James's Story: Healing Through Sleep and Stress Management

James, an Air Force veteran, had struggled with chronic insomnia and irritability for years. Sleepless nights and constant fatigue strained his relationships and made it difficult to focus on recovery. After attending a workshop on mindfulness and sleep hygiene, James decided to make some changes. He began by establishing a consistent bedtime and wake-up time, even on weekends. He also created a calming bedtime routine, which included turning off electronic devices an hour before bed, practicing a short mindfulness meditation, and drinking herbal tea.

Within a few weeks, James noticed he was falling asleep faster and staying asleep longer. Encouraged by these results, he added breathing exercises to his daily routine to help manage daytime stress. These practices not only improved his sleep but also helped him feel more grounded and less reactive in stressful situations. Over time, James's improved mood and energy levels strengthened his relationships with his family and gave him hope for the future.

Integrating Lifestyle Changes into Your Life

Implementing these changes doesn't have to be overwhelming. Small, consistent steps can lead to significant progress. Here's how to get started:

Set Realistic Goals: Begin with one change at a time like adding a serving of vegetables to your meals or walking for 10 minutes daily.

Track Your Progress: Use a journal or app to log your meals, exercise, and sleep patterns. Seeing your progress can motivate you to keep going.

Seek Support: Share your goals with friends, family, or a support group. Having accountability partners can make the journey more manageable and enjoyable.

Your Journey Continues

The complex intersection of nutrition, lifestyle and PTSX recovery is a powerful reminder that healing extends beyond clinical settings. By nourishing your body, moving with purpose, prioritizing rest, and managing stress, you can build a foundation for resilience and growth. Remember, small changes lead to big transformations. Your journey toward recovery is unique, and there are tools to support you every step of the way.

If-Then Guidance

- If you are struggling with anxiety or depression related to PTSX, then consider adopting an anti-inflammatory diet like the Mediterranean diet. Incorporate more fruits, vegetables, whole grains, lean proteins, and healthful fats into your meals to support your gut microbiome and improve your mental wellbeing.
- If you find yourself reaching for highly processed foods, sugary drinks, or trans fats, then take proactive steps to replace them with whole-food alternatives like fresh fruits, vegetables, nuts, or boiled eggs.
- Reducing these inflammatory foods can help alleviate PTSX symptoms and promote overall health.

- If you are feeling restless or lack motivation to exercise, then start with just 10 minutes of brisk walking each day and gradually increase the duration and intensity as your confidence and stamina grow. Regular physical activity can boost your mood, enhance neuroplasticity, and support your recovery from PTSX.
- If you are having difficulty maintaining a consistent sleep schedule, then establish a calming bedtime routine by turning off electronic devices at least an hour before bed, practicing meditation, or taking a warm bath. Consistent sleep patterns can enhance your emotional resilience and overall wellbeing.
- If chronic stress is overwhelming you, then incorporate stress-reduction techniques like mindfulness meditation, yoga, or diaphragmatic breathing into your daily routine. These practices can help you regain a sense of control and reduce anxiety associated with PTSX.
- If you are unsure how to begin integrating lifestyle changes, then set realistic, small goals like adding a serving of leafy greens to your meals or walking for 10 minutes daily. Track your progress using a journal or app, and seek support from friends, family, or a support group to stay motivated and make the process more manageable.
- If you are interested in holistic approaches to PTSX recovery, then explore activities that you enjoy, like hiking, dancing, or playing a sport. Finding joy in movement can make exercise a sustainable and enjoyable part of your healing journey, enhancing both your physical and mental health.
- If you are experiencing sleep disturbances, then optimize your sleep environment by keeping your bedroom cool, dark, and quiet. Consider using blackout curtains or a white noise machine to minimize disruptions, and create a sanctuary for rest that supports better sleep quality and mental health.

Take the Next Step

- Incorporate stress management practices into your daily life. Start with simple exercises like diaphragmatic breathing or mindfulness meditation for five minutes each day. These techniques can help reduce anxiety and improve emotional resilience.

- Consult with a healthcare provider, nutritionist or mental health professional to create a personalized plan that addresses your unique needs. Professional support can provide you with tailored strategies and ensure that your approach to recovery is comprehensive and effective.
- Connect with other veterans or individuals who are also focused on lifestyle changes for PTSX recovery. Joining a support group or participating in community activities can provide encouragement, accountability, and a sense of belonging, which are essential for sustained progress.
- Use a journal or a mobile app to monitor your diet, exercise, sleep patterns, and stress levels. Regularly reviewing your progress allows you to identify what's working and what needs adjustment. Celebrating small victories along the way can keep you motivated and committed to your recovery journey.

Through Their Eyes

"The roar of fighter jets and the hum of machinery were constant companions during my twenty-four years in the United States Air Force. As commander of a maintenance squadron in the harsh terrains of Afghanistan and Iraq, I learned the true meaning of resilience and leadership. At forty-eight, my journey from the battlefield to the Pentagon, and finally to leading my own IT company, has been marked by both triumphs and profound personal struggles.

"Graduating from the Air Force Academy was a milestone I once dreamed of, but it quickly became a battleground of a different kind. Throughout my four years at the Academy, as a female I endured sexual molestation and relentless harassment.

"The advice to 'take the razzing' and 'endure the pain' from female commanders, steeped in a good ol' boys' network mentality, left me feeling isolated and powerless. Reporting the abuse seemed futile, a betrayal of trust that would derail my promising career before it could truly begin. These experiences planted deep-seated wounds that would resurface long after I donned my uniform. In the field, commanding a maintenance squadron amidst the chaos of combat, I found purpose and camaraderie. Leading my team through relentless missions in Afghanistan and Iraq, I honed my skills in supply-chain management and operational leadership.

"However, the physical dangers were matched by the psychological toll. The constant exposure to danger, the loss of comrades, and the pressure to perform flawlessly left me grappling with PTSX and TBI. Returning to the Pentagon should have been a transition to a less perilous role, but the toxic environment awaited me. Male officers, dismissive of my capabilities despite my proven intelligence and leadership, subjected me to ongoing harassment. Their undermining comments and blatant disrespect chipped away at my confidence, exacerbating my PTSX symptoms.

"Nightmares, hypervigilance, and overwhelming anxiety became my nightly companions, while the high-stress environment of the Pentagon intensified my struggles.

"For years, I battled these invisible scars alone, my strength masking the turmoil within. Traditional therapies provided limited relief, and the connection between my lifestyle choices and mental health remained elusive. It wasn't until I took a step back from the military to focus on my wellbeing that I began to uncover the critical intersection of nutrition, lifestyle, and PTSX recovery.

"Determined to reclaim my life, I immersed myself in research and sought guidance from experts who understood the profound impact of daily choices on mental health. Adopting an anti-inflammatory diet like the Mediterranean diet, became the cornerstone of my healing journey.

"I started by incorporating more fruits, vegetables, whole grains, and healthy fats into my meals, replacing processed foods and sugary drinks that had long exacerbated my anxiety and inflammation. Small changes, like adding a handful of walnuts to my breakfast and savoring leafy greens in my meals, gradually transformed my energy levels and emotional stability.

"Exercise became my sanctuary. Drawing from the discipline ingrained in me as a military leader, I committed to regular physical activity. Starting with brisk walks, I gradually introduced more intense workouts, including yoga and strength training. The physical exertion not only improved my fitness but also boosted my mood and cognitive function, stimulating neuroplasticity—the brain's ability to adapt and rewire itself.

Finding joy in movement, whether hiking through nature or practicing yoga, provided a sense of purpose and helped me process the emotions I had long suppressed. Sleep, once elusive, became a priority. I established a consistent sleep routine, recognizing its vital role in emotional resilience and overall wellbeing. Creating a calming bedtime ritual—reading, meditating, and enjoying a warm bath—signaled my body that it was time to wind down. By optimizing my sleep environment with blackout curtains and minimizing screen time before bed, I began to experience deeper, more restorative sleep, which significantly reduced my PTSX symptoms.

"Stress-management techniques like mindfulness meditation and diaphragmatic breathing, became integral to my daily routine. These practices helped me regain a sense of control and calm amidst the lingering chaos of my past experiences. By dedicating time each day to mindfulness, I learned to anchor myself in the present moment, reducing anxiety and creating a sense of inner peace.

"As I integrated these lifestyle changes, the transformation was undeniable. My gut microbiome, once in disarray from years of stress and poor dietary choices, began to balance, reducing systemic inflammation and enhancing my mental clarity. The connection between my physical health and mental wellbeing became clear, highlighting the importance of a holistic approach to healing.

"Empowered by my progress, I transitioned into civilian life with renewed strength and purpose. Building my own IT company from scratch, I applied the leadership and resilience skills honed in the military to create a supportive and empowering work environment. Understanding the critical link between nutrition, lifestyle and mental health, I ensured that my team had access to resources that promoted their wellbeing and built a culture of health and productivity.

"Reflecting on my journey, I realize that healing is not a linear path but a multifaceted journey that requires addressing both the mind and the body. The lessons learned from integrating nutrition, exercise, sleep, and stress management into my life have not only helped me overcome PTSX but have also empowered me to lead with empathy and resilience. My story is a testament to the power of small, consistent changes and the importance of holistic healing in reclaiming one's life after trauma.

"Today, as I lead my company and mentor others, I carry these lessons with me, advocating for a comprehensive approach to mental health that honors the interconnectedness of our lifestyle choices and emotional wellbeing. For every veteran navigating the complexities of PTSX, know that healing is possible through the deliberate integration of nutrition, lifestyle, and resilience-building practices. Your journey is unique, and with each step forward, you build a foundation for a healthier, more fulfilling life.

"Regular exercise emerged as a powerful tool for enhancing neuroplasticity, allowing my brain to adapt and heal from the trauma of combat. The physical activity I committed to not only improved my fitness but also served as a natural mood booster, building a sense of accomplishment and empowerment. Yoga and mindfulness practices, in particular, provided a meditative space to process emotions and reduce stress, enhancing my overall emotional resilience.

"Prioritizing sleep hygiene was another critical component of my recovery. Consistent sleep patterns and a restful sleep environment significantly improved my emotional stability and cognitive function, enabling me to face each day with greater clarity and less anxiety. By addressing sleep disturbances, I was able to break the cycle of chronic stress that had long fueled my PTSX symptoms.

"By nourishing my body with the right foods, engaging in regular physical activity, prioritizing restful sleep, and managing stress effectively, I was able to build a robust foundation for my mental and emotional wellbeing.

"In my role as a CEO, I implement these lessons by creating a workplace culture that values and promotes holistic health practices. Encouraging my team to prioritize their nutrition, stay active, maintain healthy sleep habits, and manage stress not only enhances their wellbeing but also drives collective success and innovation. Healing extends beyond clinical settings—it's about making informed, intentional choices in our daily lives that support our mental and emotional wellbeing. For every veteran navigating the complexities of PTSX, embracing the intersection of nutrition, lifestyle, and recovery can pave the way for a healthier, more fulfilling life."

—Colonel Chris P., US Air Force (ret.)

32

Community-Based Support Systems for Veterans

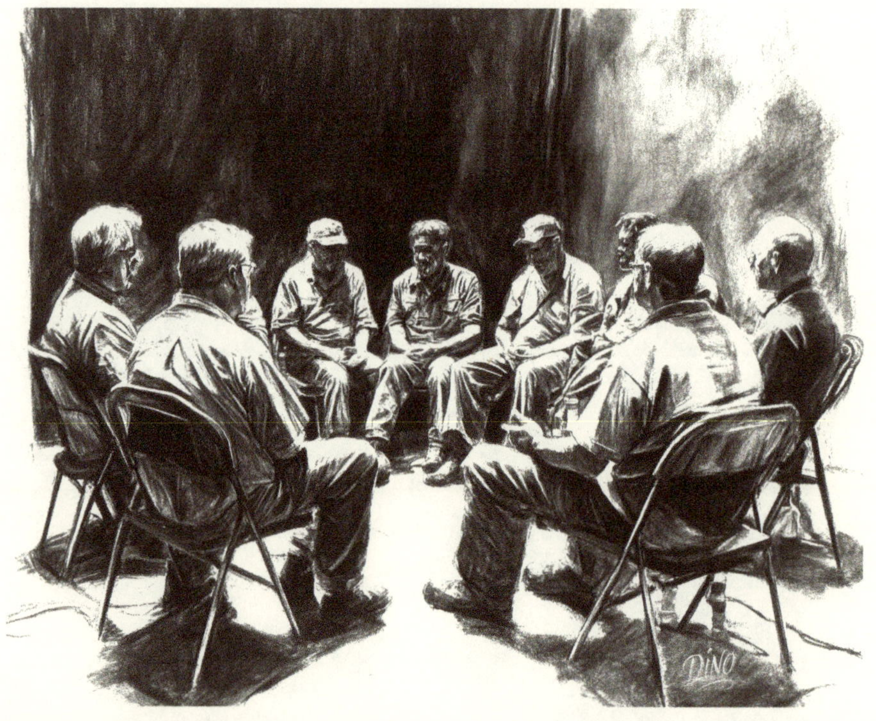

Pete had never felt more alone than when he first returned home from deployment. Civilians asked polite questions, but no matter how hard they tried, he sensed they couldn't truly grasp the weight he carried. Desperate for someone who understood, he stumbled into a local veterans' meetup—held every Wednesday in the back room of a community center. He almost didn't go in, afraid it might be another place where he felt out of place.

But the moment he walked through the door, everything changed. He recognized the quiet tension in a few familiar stances, noticed how some sat with their backs to the wall, scanning exits without meaning to. He felt oddly comforted by these small signals, realizing he wasn't the only one stuck between the military world and civilian life. Over paper cups of coffee, they shared stories—some raw, some laced with humor that only a fellow vet would understand.

Week by week, Pete found himself opening up. Hearing others describe their struggles with nightmares or hypervigilance reminded him that healing wasn't a solo mission; it was a team effort. They talked about new therapies like ketamine infusions or SGB, and offered personal insights on which approaches seemed to help. Yet it was more than just swapping information—knowing there were people who "got it" made the biggest difference.

This chapter has some thematic overlap with Chapter 13, which covered PTSX's toll on relationships, and it deserves its own place here. Here, we explore how bridging military and civilian communities can spark real progress for veterans. By blending professional treatments with peer networks, these community-based systems provide more than support—they rebuild the connection veterans crave, reminding them they're not alone on the path to recovery.

Importance of the Military and Civilian Communities in Healing

The intertwining of military and civilian communities plays a pivotal role in the healing journeys of veterans grappling with PTSX. The unique experiences of servicemembers often create a chasm between them and civilian counterparts, so bridging this gap is essential for creating understanding and support.

As we explore the neurobiological mechanisms of PTSX treatment, it becomes evident that the healing process transcends clinical interventions, relying heavily on the strength of community and shared experiences. This collaborative effort not only enriches therapeutic outcomes but also cultivates a sense of belonging that is crucial for recovery.

Veterans often return from their service with a complex array of psychological wounds, requiring tailored treatment approaches that go beyond conventional methods. Innovative therapies like psychedelic-assisted treatments and cannabinoid integration, have shown promise in alleviating symptoms of PTSX. However, the success of these techniques is amplified when integrated within a supportive community framework.

> Community-based programs prove geography does not dictate destiny. Discussions of mental health and successes happen in VFW halls and park trails alike.

Civilian mental-health professionals, alongside their military counterparts, can create a robust support network that encourages veterans to engage in these alternative therapies. This collaboration creates an environment where veterans feel safe to explore new avenues for healing, knowing they are backed by both military understanding and civilian compassion.

Moreover, community-based support systems are essential in facilitating access to these advanced therapeutic modalities. As military personnel navigate the challenges of reintegration, the presence of a compassionate civilian community can provide critical emotional and psychological resources.

Programs that connect veterans with civilian volunteers, mental-health professionals and peer-support groups can significantly enhance the efficacy of treatments like ketamine infusion therapy and SGB. By weaving together military and civilian perspectives, we can create a comprehensive support system that is more than the sum of its parts, ultimately leading to improved treatment outcomes.

The long-term effects of MDMA-assisted therapy and other alternative treatments can be significantly enhanced when veterans are surrounded by a community that understands their journey. Case studies have illustrated the power of community in creating resilience and recovery during alternative PTSX treatments.

When veterans share their experiences within a supportive network, they not only validate their struggles but also inspire hope among peers. The collective sharing of success stories reinforces the belief that healing is possible, encouraging more veterans to seek out innovative therapies and engage in their recovery process actively.

Models of Support: Best Practices

In the evolving landscape of PTSX treatment for military personnel and veterans, the integration of innovative therapeutic approaches alongside traditional methods is paramount. Best practices in support models not only address the neurobiological mechanisms underlying PTSX but also prioritize the holistic wellbeing of those who have served.

By creating a comprehensive care framework, mental-health professionals can create an environment where veterans feel safe, understood and empowered to engage in their healing journey. This section explores essential best practices that can enhance treatment outcomes and promote resilience among this unique population.

One of the most effective models of support centers on the incorporation of community-based systems that extend beyond the clinical setting. Engaging veterans in peer-support groups and community networks can facilitate shared experiences and collective healing. These groups serve as a vital link, creating camaraderie and understanding among participants who have faced similar challenges.

By integrating community resources like veterans' organizations and local support networks, mental health professionals can help create a robust support system that encourages veterans to take an active role in their recovery. This model not only enhances the therapeutic process but also cultivates a sense of belonging and purpose.

Another best practice involves the adoption of a multi-disciplinary approach to treatment. Collaboration among VA mental-health professionals, civilian therapists and military health providers can lead to a more comprehensive understanding of PTSX and its complexities. By sharing insights and strategies, these professionals can develop integrated treatment plans that incorporate diverse modalities, including psychedelic-assisted therapies, ketamine infusion and cannabinoid integration.

This holistic approach ensures that veterans receive a continuum of care tailored to their individual needs, optimizing the efficacy of therapeutic interventions and facilitating a smoother healing trajectory.

Training and education for mental-health professionals on alternative therapies are also crucial components of effective support models. As new treatment modalities emerge, ongoing professional development ensures that providers remain informed about the latest advancements in PTSX care.

Workshops, seminars and collaborative training sessions can empower mental health professionals with the knowledge and skills needed to implement these innovative approaches ethically and effectively. By creating an environment of continuous learning, practitioners can better serve military personnel and veterans, enhancing their confidence in employing alternative therapies as part of an integrative treatment plan.

Adopting these best practices in models of support can lead to transformative outcomes for military personnel and veterans grappling with PTSX. By creating community engagement, promoting interdisciplinary collaboration, prioritizing professional education and adhering to ethical principles, mental health professionals can significantly enhance the therapeutic experience. Together, we can create a future where healing is not only possible but celebrated, paving the way for resilience and renewed purpose in the lives of those who have served our nation.

Building Resilience Through Peer Networks

Building resilience through peer networks is a transformative approach that holds immense promise for military personnel and veterans grappling with the profound impacts of PTSX. The shared experiences of servicemembers create an unparalleled foundation for healing, as individuals who have faced similar traumas can offer understanding and support that is often absent in traditional clinical settings. The neurobiological mechanisms underpinning resilience suggest that these peer connections can activate positive neuroplastic changes, aiding in recovery and creating a sense of belonging. This section delves into how cultivating peer networks can enhance resilience and serve as a vital adjunct to traditional PTSX treatments.

Peer networks provide a unique platform where veterans can openly share their stories without fear of judgment. This safe space allows for the normalization of experiences, reducing feelings of isolation that many servicemembers face when transitioning to civilian life. The act of sharing not only facilitates healing through catharsis but also reinforces social bonds that are crucial for psychological wellbeing.

These interactions can stimulate the release of oxytocin, a hormone associated with bonding and stress reduction, thereby creating a sense of safety and connection that is pivotal in the recovery process.

Moreover, peer networks empower veterans by instilling a sense of agency and mutual support. When individuals come together to confront their challenges, they often find strength in collective resilience. This dynamic can be particularly effective in the context of alternative therapies like psychedelic-assisted treatments or cannabinoid integration, where sharing experiences can enhance understanding and acceptance of these innovative modalities.

Veterans who have successfully navigated their healing journeys can serve as mentors, providing hope and guidance to those still struggling. Such mentorship not only enriches the therapeutic environment but also reinforces the notion that recovery is possible and achievable.

The impact of peer networks extends beyond individual healing, contributing to community resilience as well. As veterans engage with one another, they collectively advocate for better mental health resources and support systems, influencing policy and practice within the VA and broader mental health landscape.

This can lead to improved access to innovative treatments like ketamine therapy or SGB procedures, ensuring that all veterans have the opportunity to benefit from the latest advances in PTSX care. By creating a proactive community, peer networks create a ripple effect that can lead to systemic change, ultimately benefiting all servicemembers. Building resilience through peer networks is not merely a supplementary aspect of PTSX treatment. They're a vital component that enhances the efficacy of existing therapies and creates a holistic approach to recovery. As mental-health professionals, embracing and facilitating these networks can significantly elevate the quality of care provided to military personnel and veterans.

If-Then Guidance

- If you do not currently have access to a community-based PTSX support network, then consider exploring local veteran organizations, VA hospitals or online platforms. These networks can help you find support from others who understand the unique challenges of PTSX, and they often offer a safe space to share and learn coping strategies.
- If you are not attending support groups or therapy sessions regularly, then try to increase your participation. Regular involvement in support groups can provide consistency, structure, and emotional support that are key to managing PTSX. Even online groups can offer valuable resources and peer support if in-person options are limited.
- If you do not feel supported by your local community, then it might be helpful to seek out other groups or organizations that better fit your needs. Every group has its own dynamic, and finding the right community is crucial for feeling supported and understood. Explore both local and online options to find a group that resonates with you.
- If you've found community-based support to be beneficial, then consider encouraging other veterans to join. Sharing your positive experiences could help others who are hesitant or unaware of these resources, making it easier for them to take the first step in seeking support.

Take the Next Step

- Look for veteran groups, community centers, or peer support networks in your area that offer emotional and social support.
- Programs like Vet Centers and veteran community organizations

can connect you with others who share similar experiences and challenges.

- If you're feeling stable enough, consider volunteering or mentoring other veterans that can provide a sense of purpose and community engagement. It may take time to fund the right fit for you. Keep looking. It will be worth it in the end.

Through Their Eyes

"Coming back home wasn't just about returning to a place—it was about finding where I belonged again. After my service, I felt lost in the civilian world, disconnected from the people around me who couldn't understand the things I'd seen or done. Even my family, as much as they tried, didn't really get it. PTSX was isolating. Therapy helped a little, but it wasn't enough on its own.

"One day, I found a local veterans' group. It wasn't therapy, just a bunch of us getting together to talk. The first time I walked into that room, I felt like I had found a lifeline. Everyone there had been through some version of what I had. There was no need to explain myself. We all understood, and that made all the difference.

"We talked about everything—our families, our nightmares, and even the alternative treatments some of us were trying like MDMA and ketamine therapy. I heard stories about how these therapies were changing lives. That gave me hope, not just because of the treatments, but because I wasn't alone in this fight. The strength of that community made me believe that I could find my way out of the darkness.

"That group became my support system. They connected me to resources I didn't know existed, including experimental therapies I hadn't considered. Over time, it wasn't just about my healing—it became about helping the next guy who walked through the door, just like they had helped me. I'm grateful every day for the strength I've found through my fellow veterans. We lift each other up, and that's something you can't get anywhere else."

—David, US Army Veteran

33

Spirituality and Faith in the Healing Process

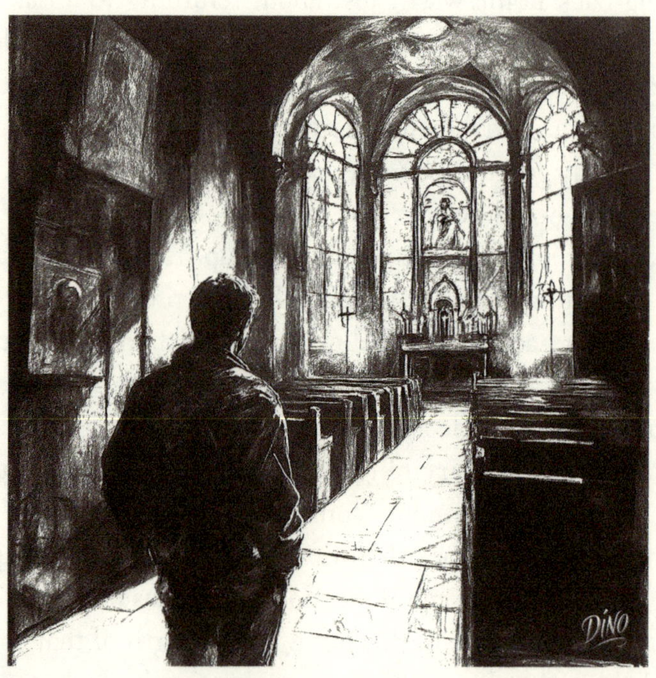

When Zach returned from his final deployment, the silence in his house felt heavier than any battle he'd faced. Despite therapy and medication, he still woke up at odd hours, a hollow ache in his chest. One weekend, he found himself stepping into a small chapel on a nearby base, unsure why he was drawn there. He wasn't particularly religious, but something about the sunlight streaming through stained glass beckoned him.

He sat in the back row, away from everyone, just listening. After the service, the chaplain approached him—not to preach, but to ask how he was doing. In that conversation, Zach confessed he felt directionless, cut off from any sense of hope. The chaplain simply listened, then invited him to come back, maybe to talk some more, maybe to just sit quietly when the chapel was empty. Over time, Zach began to explore his own form of spirituality. It wasn't about strict doctrine; instead, it became a search for peace and purpose.

Occasionally, he'd linger in the chapel alone, letting the quiet envelop him. He started journaling about the things he couldn't share elsewhere—guilt over lost friends, the fear that he might never be "normal" again. Bit by bit, he found solace in the idea that he was part of something bigger, even if he couldn't name it. He also met a small group of veterans who prayed or meditated together, each holding different beliefs but united in their quest for healing.

This chapter examines experiences like Zach's: the subtle power that faith, spirituality or simple soul-searching can have for veterans with PTSX. Whether it's a traditional religious practice, a connection to nature or a quiet meditative approach, these spiritual touchstones can offer comfort, guide moral injury toward acceptance and inspire a renewed sense of purpose.

By honoring these deeply personal dimensions, clinicians, chaplains and peers can support the whole person—body, mind and spirit—on the path back to wholeness. While conventional treatments for PTSX are essential, there is a growing recognition of the role that spirituality and faith plays in the healing process. We also explore how integrating spirituality and faith into PTSX treatment can support recovery, addressing not only the mind and body but also the intangible spirit, whatever it may be.

Understanding Spirituality and Faith

Spirituality and faith are deeply personal concepts that vary widely among individuals. Spirituality generally refers to a sense of connection to something greater than oneself, which can involve a search for meaning in life. It is often characterized by practices that generates a sense of peace, purpose, and connection, such as meditation, prayer or contemplation.

Faith, on the other hand, often involves belief in a higher power or adherence to specific religious doctrines and practices. It can provide a moral framework and community support through organized religion. While spirituality and faith can overlap, they are not synonymous; one can be spiritual without being religious, and vice versa.

For many veterans, spirituality and faith offer pathways to cope with the aftermath of traumatic experiences. They can provide solace, hope, and a renewed sense of purpose, which are crucial components in the journey toward healing from PTSX.

> Spiritual frameworks—from rosary beads to sweat lodges—anchor recovery in meaning that molecules alone may not be able to supply.

The Impact of Trauma on Spiritual Beliefs

Traumatic experiences can profoundly affect an individual's spiritual beliefs and faith practices. For some veterans, trauma can lead to a deepening of faith, as they seek comfort and meaning through their spiritual beliefs. For others, trauma may result in a spiritual crisis, causing them to question or abandon previously held beliefs.

Combat experiences often confront servicemembers with situations that challenge their moral and ethical beliefs. Witnessing or participating in acts of violence can lead to feelings of guilt, shame, or betrayal, known as moral injury. This can cause veterans to question their faith or feel alienated from their spiritual communities.

For example, a soldier who has had to harm others in the line of duty may struggle with feelings of unworthiness or fear of judgment from a higher power. These spiritual struggles can exacerbate PTSX symptoms, leading to increased isolation, depression, and anxiety.

Conversely, some veterans report that their traumatic experiences have led to spiritual growth. Facing adversity can prompt a reevaluation of life's purpose and priorities, leading to a deeper understanding of oneself and one's beliefs. This process, known as post-traumatic growth, can enhance resilience and provide a foundation for healing.

The Role of Spirituality and Faith in Healing

Integrating spirituality and faith into PTSX treatment can offer several benefits, including:

Providing Meaning and Purpose: Spiritual beliefs can help veterans make sense of their experiences, transforming trauma into a catalyst for personal growth.

Offering Coping Mechanisms: Practices such as prayer, meditation, and mindfulness can reduce stress and promote emotional regulation.

Building Community Support: Faith communities can offer social support, reducing feelings of isolation and providing practical assistance.

Evidence-Based Benefits

Research has shown that incorporating spirituality and faith into mental health treatment can improve outcomes for individuals with PTSX. Studies indicate that spiritual practices can lower levels of anxiety, depression, and stress, and enhance overall wellbeing. For example, mindfulness-based therapies, which have roots in Buddhist meditation practices, have been effective in reducing PTSX symptoms by helping individuals stay present and manage intrusive thoughts. Similarly, spiritually integrated cognitive-behavioral therapy can address negative thought patterns while incorporating the individual's spiritual beliefs.

Diverse Paths to Healing

Healing is a personal journey, and spirituality and faith can take many forms. It is important to recognize and respect the diverse spiritual and religious backgrounds of veterans.

For some veterans, particularly those from indigenous communities, traditional healing practices play a vital role in recovery. These practices may include ceremonies, rituals, storytelling, or connection with nature, which can reaffirm cultural identity and promote healing.

For example, sweat lodge ceremonies or vision quests can provide a sacred space for reflection and purification. Engaging in these traditional practices can help veterans reconnect with their heritage and find balance in their lives. Not all veterans identify with a specific religion or traditional spiritual practices.

Secular spirituality, which focuses on personal growth, ethical living, and a sense of connectedness without reference to a deity or religious framework, can also be beneficial. Practices such as mindfulness meditation, yoga, or spending time in nature can generate inner peace and self-awareness. These activities can help veterans manage stress, improve emotional regulation, and enhance their overall sense of wellbeing.

For veterans who are religious, engaging with their faith communities can provide significant support. Participation in religious services, prayer groups, or faith-based counseling can offer comfort, guidance, and a sense of belonging.

Faith can provide a moral framework that helps veterans process their experiences and find forgiveness, both for themselves and others. Religious teachings often emphasize themes of redemption, hope and resilience, which can be empowering for individuals recovering from trauma.

Integrating Spirituality and Faith into Treatment

Healthcare providers can play a crucial role in integrating spirituality and faith into PTSX treatment plans. This integration should be patient-centered, respecting each individual's beliefs and preferences.

Clinicians should assess spiritual needs as part of a holistic evaluation. This involves:

- Encouraging veterans to share their beliefs and how these affect their coping strategies.
- Being attentive and respectful, without imposing personal beliefs.
- Helping veterans connect with spiritual or religious resources that align with their values. Collaborative Care Integrating spirituality into treatment may involve:
- Professionals trained to address spiritual concerns can provide specialized support.
- Including meditation, prayer or mindfulness exercises in therapy sessions when appropriate.

- Collaborating with other professionals, social workers or community leaders, to provide comprehensive care.

Ethical Considerations:

When integrating spirituality and faith into treatment, it is important to:

- Ensure that participation is voluntary and aligns with the veteran's beliefs.
- Clinicians should not impose their own beliefs or pressure veterans to adopt specific practices.
- Be sensitive to cultural and religious diversity, tailoring interventions to individual needs.

Personal Stories of Healing

Alejandro's Journey

Alejandro, a Marine Corps veteran, struggled with PTSX after multiple deployments. Traditional therapies provided some relief, but he felt a persistent emptiness. Reconnecting with his Christian faith offered him solace. By attending church services and participating in a veterans' support group within his congregation, he found a supportive community that understood his experiences. Through prayer and spiritual reflection, he began to process his feelings of guilt and anger.

His faith provided a framework for forgiveness and acceptance, which helped alleviate his symptoms. Integrating his spiritual beliefs into his treatment plan enhanced his recovery, providing a sense of purpose and hope for the future.

Christine's Path

Christine, an Army medic, had not identified with any particular religion in the past but was open to exploring spiritual practices. Her therapist introduced her to mindfulness meditation, which helped her manage her anxiety and intrusive thoughts. Through regular practice, Christine developed greater self-awareness and emotional regulation.

She also found peace in nature, taking regular hikes and practicing outdoor yoga. These activities built a sense of connection and grounding. Christine's secular approach to spirituality became a cornerstone of her healing process, complementing her traditional therapy. By doing these activities every day, she found herself in a different emotional space, one of peace and calm.

David's Healing through Tradition

David, a Native American veteran, felt disconnected from his community and culture after returning from combat. He struggled with PTSX symptoms and a sense of isolation. Seeking help, David re-engaged with his tribal community and participated in traditional healing ceremonies.

The sweat lodge rituals and storytelling sessions allowed David to share his experiences in a culturally meaningful context. Reconnecting with his heritage provided a sense of identity and belonging. The integration of traditional practices into his treatment plan helped David find balance and healing.

Challenges and Considerations

While integrating spirituality and faith into PTSX treatment can be beneficial, it is important to address potential challenges.

Risk of Spiritual Distress: For some veterans, trauma can lead to spiritual distress, such as feelings of abandonment by a higher power or conflict with religious beliefs. Clinicians should be prepared to support veterans through these struggles, possibly involving spiritual counselors trained to address such issues.

Spiritual Bypassing: Refers to the use of spiritual beliefs to avoid facing unresolved emotional issues. It is important to ensure that spiritual practices complement, rather than replace, evidence-based therapies. A balanced approach helps veterans address all aspects of their healing.

Cultural Sensitivity

Clinicians must be culturally competent, understanding that spiritual beliefs are influenced by cultural backgrounds. Healthcare providers can support veterans by:

- Educating Oneself: Learning about different spiritual traditions and practices.

- Respecting Diversity: Acknowledging and valuing the veteran's cultural and spiritual identity. Avoiding Assumptions: Each individual's experience is unique. Assumptions can hinder effective care.
- Spirituality and Faith: These play a vital role in the healing process for veterans with PTSX. By addressing the spiritual dimension of trauma, individuals can find deeper meaning, become resilient, and enhance their overall wellbeing. Integrating spirituality and faith into treatment offers a holistic approach that complements traditional therapies.
- Engaging in Open Dialogue: Creating a safe space for veterans to discuss their spiritual needs.
- Collaborating with Spiritual Resources: Involving chaplains, spiritual counselors or faith communities as appropriate.
- Respecting Individual Preferences: Tailoring interventions to align with the veteran's beliefs and values. In embracing spirituality and faith as components of healing, we recognize that recovery from PTSX is not solely a medical or psychological journey but also a deeply personal and spiritual one. By honoring the whole person—mind, body and spirit—more comprehensive care and support can be provided to veterans on their path to healing.

If-Then Guidance

- If you are struggling to find meaning and purpose after experiencing trauma, then consider exploring how spirituality or faith may offer solace and a new perspective. Spirituality, whether connected to a religious belief system or not, can help you search for meaning in life and transform your experiences into a catalyst for personal growth. Engaging in practices like meditation, prayer or contemplation can build a deeper connection to something greater than yourself, providing a sense of peace and purpose in your healing journey.
- If you are experiencing feelings of guilt, shame, or moral injury, then reflecting on your spiritual beliefs or faith might help in processing these complex emotions. Traumatic experiences,

especially in combat, often challenge deeply held moral and ethical beliefs, leading to spiritual struggles. These struggles can exacerbate PTSX symptoms. Seeking solace through spiritual practices such as prayer, engaging with a religious community, or confiding in a spiritual leader can provide a framework for forgiveness and acceptance, allowing you to work through these difficult emotions in a safe, supportive environment.

- If you have suffered a spiritual crisis or feel disconnected from your faith, then allow yourself the space to explore and reflect on your beliefs. Trauma can lead to a crisis of faith, causing you to question or even abandon previously held spiritual convictions. Rather than turning away from these questions, engaging in spiritual exploration—whether by reconnecting with your faith community, participating in new spiritual practices, or speaking with a spiritual counselor—can help you rebuild a sense of connection and find a renewed sense of purpose.
- If you have found that your trauma has led to spiritual growth, then embrace this growth as part of your healing process. For some, adversity brings a reevaluation of life's priorities and beliefs, leading to a deeper understanding of oneself and one's place in the world. This post-traumatic growth can enhance resilience, providing a strong foundation for continued healing. Cultivating this spiritual growth can be as simple as practicing gratitude, engaging in spiritual rituals, or finding ways to give back to others.
- If you find solace in a faith community, then consider increasing your involvement with that community to enhance your support system. Faith communities often provide social support, offering a sense of belonging and practical assistance. Participating in group prayer, religious services or spiritual counseling can reinforce feelings of connection and reduce the isolation that PTSX sometimes creates. These communities can help you find comfort in shared beliefs and offer guidance in times of spiritual or emotional distress.
- If you prefer secular forms of spirituality, then practices such as mindfulness meditation, yoga or spending time in nature may

provide you with the spiritual support you need without the structure of organized religion. These practices can help you manage stress, regulate emotions, and build inner peace, making them valuable tools in your PTSX recovery.

- If you are from an Indigenous background or prefer traditional healing practices, then reconnecting with your cultural heritage through traditional ceremonies, rituals or storytelling may be an essential part of your recovery. Indigenous veterans may find strength and healing in ceremonies such as sweat lodges or vision quests, which provide sacred spaces for reflection and purification. Engaging in these practices can reaffirm cultural identity and provide a powerful framework for spiritual and emotional healing.
- If you feel your spirituality or faith is not being addressed in your PTSX treatment, then speak with your healthcare provider about incorporating these elements into your recovery plan. Many veterans find that addressing the spiritual dimension of trauma is critical to their healing. If you feel your trauma has caused spiritual distress, then seek support from a spiritual counselor or chaplain trained in addressing the spiritual effects of trauma. These spiritual challenges can intensify PTSX symptoms, leading to isolation, depression or anxiety. A spiritual counselor can provide a safe, non-judgmental space to explore these feelings and help you find ways to reconcile your spiritual beliefs with your experiences.
- If you are concerned about the risk of using spirituality to bypass unresolved emotions, then be mindful of how you use spiritual practices in your healing process. Spiritual bypassing, or using spiritual beliefs to avoid confronting painful emotions, can hinder long-term recovery. A balanced approach that includes addressing your emotional and psychological needs alongside spiritual growth can lead to more holistic and sustained healing.
- If you wish to explore different spiritual traditions, then take time to educate yourself about diverse spiritual practices, particularly those that resonate with your experiences and values. Every individual's spiritual journey is unique, and you may find healing through practices outside of your own cultural or

religious background. Be open to learning from other traditions, whether through mindfulness practices, Indigenous healing ceremonies, or secular approaches to spirituality, as each offers valuable pathways to growth and healing. Recovery from trauma is a personal journey, and by embracing spirituality or faith, you can find meaning, purpose, and resilience that will support you throughout your path to healing.

Take the Next Step

- Whether through organized religion or personal spirituality, explore how faith or mindfulness can play a role in your healing process.
- If spirituality is a core part of your life, find a faith-based counselor or chaplain who can integrate your beliefs into your PTSX treatment.
- Start with small, daily mindfulness or meditation practices that help you connect with the present moment and manage symptoms like anxiety or hypervigilance.

Through Their Eyes

"The transition back to civilian life was more turbulent than I had expected. Years of service had left me with scars, both visible and invisible. PTSX crept into every corner of my life—constant hypervigilance, sleepless nights, and a persistent sense of detachment from the world around me. I tried the conventional routes—therapy, medication—but something always felt missing.

"One day, I found myself in a small chapel on base, seeking solace. Faith had always been a quiet part of my life, something I didn't talk much about, but it was there. As I sat in silence, I found that faith provided the grounding I hadn't been able to find elsewhere.

"What made the biggest difference was having a space where I could bring all my questions and pain without judgment. My church offered that—an understanding community that didn't demand explanations, just offered support. I began to reconnect with a sense of purpose and hope, slowly rebuilding my life. My faith gave me a framework to process the guilt, anger and trauma that had been weighing me down for so long.

"In the months that followed, I worked with a chaplain who helped me integrate my spiritual beliefs into my PTSX treatment. Alongside my therapy sessions, we would talk about forgiveness—not just of others, but of myself. It was through this balance of faith and clinical treatment that I found a renewed sense of peace. My spiritual journey gave me the strength to keep going when nothing else seemed to work."

—James, US Air Force (ret.)

34

Animal-Assisted Interventions: Healing Through Human-Animal Bonds

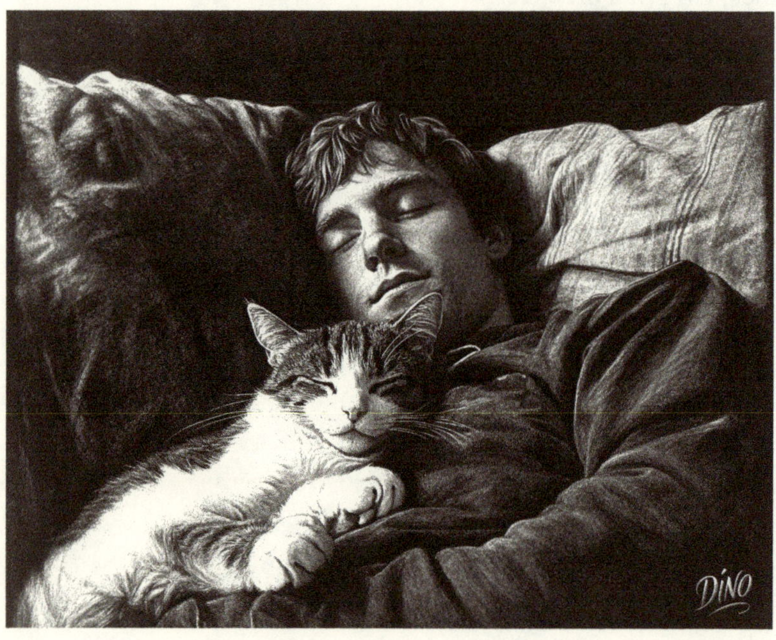

Connor never thought a scruffy tabby cat could change his life so much, but there he was, sprawled on the couch with Misty curled against his chest, softly purring away. After returning home from active duty, Connor struggled to feel safe or even remotely at ease. Traditional therapy helped some, but he still woke up shaking, heart pounding, expecting the worst. Then, on a whim, he visited a local animal shelter. He locked eyes with that tiny tabby and something clicked.

Within a week of bringing Misty home, Connor noticed subtle changes: calmer nights, fewer jolts of anxiety in the morning. Whenever the flashbacks crept in, Misty would meow or rub her head against his arm, anchoring him to the present. Her purr was like a gentle hum, easing tension he couldn't just "talk away." At first, he thought it was all in his head—just the newness of having a pet. But day by day, Misty's presence offered a quiet assurance he desperately needed.

He soon learned he wasn't alone in that experience. At a local veterans' meetup, Connor heard others mention how a therapy dog or equine sessions helped them feel more grounded. One fellow vet swore his cat's purring was the best anxiety reliever he'd ever found. These companions—whether hooved, pawed, or purring—weren't stand-ins for therapy or medication. They were a powerful complement, an emotional lifeline during the hardest moments.

Service cats, dogs, horses and even dolphins recalibrate cortisol curves better than some pharmaceuticals. Fur and saltwater are underrated medicine.

This chapter explores the profound ways animals—from dedicated service dogs to a soft purring kitten—can aid veterans dealing with PTSX. We'll dive into what makes the human-animal bond so unique, how service animals and equine therapy fit into a broader care plan, and why even a simple house cat can sometimes unlock a sense of peace that felt out of reach before. While traditional treatments such as psychotherapy and medication remain central to managing PTSX, an increasing body of evidence supports the therapeutic use of animal-assisted interventions (AAI). These interventions, based on the profound bond between humans and animals, have been shown to offer significant emotional and psychological benefits.

The Human-Animal Bond

The connection between humans and animals is both ancient and profound. Throughout history, animals have not only served practical purposes—such as labor or protection—but also emotional ones, offering companionship and unconditional love. The human-animal bond refers to the deep and mutually beneficial relationship that develops between people and animals, based on affection, trust and companionship.

This bond can have significant positive effects on both mental and physical health. For individuals with PTSX, animals provide comfort, emotional stability and a nonjudgmental presence that helps ease symptoms such as anxiety, hypervigilance, and social isolation.

Interacting with animals allows those suffering from PTSX to express emotions freely, as animals provide a sense of safety that facilitates emotional openness. This connection can serve as a therapeutic bridge, helping individuals open up in ways they may find difficult with people. Beyond offering companionship, animals often create a calming environment, lowering stress levels and reducing the intensity of PTSX symptoms.

Service Animals in PTSX Recovery

Service animals, especially dogs, are widely used in assisting individuals with disabilities, including those with PTSX. These animals are specially trained to perform tasks that help their owners manage specific symptoms and regain a sense of autonomy in their daily lives.

For veterans with PTSX, service dogs are trained to recognize and respond to anxiety episodes, offer physical comfort, and provide emotional support in ways that enhance the individual's ability to function in both private and public settings.

One of the most vital roles a service dog plays is in recognizing the early signs of an anxiety or panic episode. These dogs are trained to detect subtle changes in their handler's body language or physiological state: increased heart rate, shaking or rapid breathing.

Once they detect these signs, the dog may respond by nudging or physically positioning itself to offer grounding, which can help bring the handler back to the present moment and prevent a full-blown panic attack. Additionally, service dogs can be trained to assist during nightmares or night terrors. Many individuals with PTSX suffer from recurring traumatic nightmares that disrupt their sleep. A service dog, sensing distress during sleep, will gently wake the individual by nudging or licking, interrupting the nightmare and helping the person orient to a safe environment. This can lead to better sleep quality and reduce the dread often associated with going to bed.

Beyond managing specific symptoms, service dogs also provide a profound sense of security for those who struggle with hypervigilance in public spaces. Veterans with PTSX often feel unsafe in crowded or unpredictable environments, but a service dog can act as a protective buffer.

These animals are trained to create a physical barrier between their handler and others, allowing the individual to feel more in control and secure. For many veterans, this renewed sense of safety is essential to reclaiming a social life and rebuilding relationships that may have been strained due to PTSX.

The companionship provided by service dogs also helps alleviate feelings of loneliness and isolation. For veterans who have withdrawn from social interactions, the presence of a service dog can help rebuild connections with others.

Service dogs often act as social facilitators, naturally drawing attention and encouraging positive interactions with strangers and acquaintances alike. For veterans who do not want to socialize with people, a service dog makes a good companion. If a dog is too high maintenance, then a kitten or full-grown cat can play that same role.

This social engagement can combat the isolation that so often accompanies PTSX, building a greater sense of community and belonging. Research has demonstrated the effectiveness of service dogs in improving the lives of individuals with PTSX. A recent study found that veterans with service dogs experienced significantly lower levels of PTSX symptoms, including depression and anxiety, compared to those who did not have a service dog.

The study participants reported increased independence, improved interpersonal relationships, and an overall better quality of life. While service animals are not a cure for PTSX, they are a powerful adjunct to traditional therapies, offering emotional, physical and social support that can greatly enhance the recovery process.

Equine-Assisted Therapy

Equine-assisted therapy, or horse therapy, is another form of AAI that has gained attention for its effectiveness in helping individuals with PTSX. This therapy involves structured interactions between the individual and horses, guided by a trained therapist. Grooming, leading and riding horses are activities used to facilitate emotional healing and personal growth. Horses are particularly well-suited for therapeutic work because they are highly attuned to human emotions and can respond to subtle nonverbal cues. This sensitivity allows horses to mirror the emotions of the individual, providing immediate and nonjudgmental feedback. For individuals with PTSX, this mirroring effect helps them become more aware of their own emotions and behaviors. This awareness can lead to a deeper understanding of their internal emotional state and help them learn to regulate their emotions more effectively.

One of the central therapeutic benefits of equine therapy is its ability to rebuild trust. Many individuals with PTSX, especially those who have experienced trauma involving betrayal or violence, struggle to trust others. Horses, with their gentle and nonjudgmental nature, offer a safe way to practice building trust. Forming a bond with a horse requires patience, consistency, and mutual respect—qualities that can be transferred to human relationships.

Equine therapy also promotes mindfulness, as working with horses demands full attention and focus. Individuals must be present in the moment, attentive to the horse's movements and responses, which can help reduce anxiety and distract from traumatic memories. For example, a veteran struggling with hypervigilance might find it difficult to relax or focus, but the calming presence of a horse can encourage mindfulness, reducing anxiety and helping the individual engage more fully in the therapeutic process.

Research supports the positive impact of equine therapy on PTSX symptoms. A recent study reported significant reductions in emotional numbness and mood disturbances among veterans who participated in equine therapy. These veterans also reported increased self-confidence and a sense of accomplishment, as mastering horsemanship skills provided them with tangible goals and achievements.

The Therapeutic Power of Kittens and Cats

While dogs and horses are commonly used in animal-assisted interventions, cats and kittens also play a remarkable role in emotional healing, especially for individuals with PTSX. Cats provide a different type of companionship that is less demanding than that of a dog or horse, making them ideal for individuals who may feel overwhelmed by the responsibility of a high-maintenance pet.

Cats, in general, with their gentle purring and independent nature, offer a calming presence that can significantly reduce stress and anxiety. The act of petting a cat has been shown to lower blood pressure and slow the heart rate, inducing a state of relaxation.

This simple interaction can serve as a moment of peace in an otherwise chaotic mental landscape. The rhythmic motion of stroking a cat's fur, coupled with the soothing sound of purring, creates an atmosphere of calm that can ease anxiety and elevate mood.

One of the most fascinating aspects of cats is their ability to purr at a frequency known to have healing properties. Research has shown that a cat's purring, which vibrates at a frequency between 20 and 140 Hz, can promote tissue healing and even help alleviate pain.

The gentle vibrations of a cat's purr can also enhance relaxation, making it an effective natural tool for reducing stress and anxiety in individuals with PTSX. This is sometimes referred to as the "purr effect," and it underscores the unique therapeutic benefits that cats offer in the healing process.

Kittens (up to about 12 months old), in particular, can evoke feelings of joy and nurturing. Their playful and curious behavior can bring laughter and light into the lives of those who may feel burdened by emotional heaviness. The playful antics of a kitten can distract from negative thoughts, while their need for care can provide a sense of purpose and responsibility, which is especially beneficial for individuals who may feel disconnected or purposeless due to PTSX.

The case of Sarah, a Navy veteran who suffered from severe PTSX, illustrates the profound healing that can come from the bond with a kitten. Sarah had difficulty opening up in traditional therapy and often felt anxious and withdrawn.

On the recommendation of her therapist, she adopted a kitten named Whiskers. Initially unsure about the responsibility, Sarah quickly found that Whiskers' presence brought her immense comfort. The kitten's playful energy and gentle purring became a source of emotional solace during her most difficult moments.

Caring for Whiskers gave Sarah a routine, which helped ground her, while the kitten's affectionate presence provided an anchor during anxiety attacks. Over time, Sarah's symptoms improved, and she found herself re-engaging with family and friends.

Kittens and cats are often well-suited for individuals with PTSX because they are relatively low-maintenance, requiring less physical activity than a dog, which can be ideal for someone who may have limited energy or mobility. They are also content to be indoor companions, which makes them suitable for veterans who may feel uncomfortable leaving their homes frequently. Furthermore, the quiet, peaceful companionship of a cat allows individuals to engage on their own terms, offering affection without demanding constant attention.

Several programs now incorporate cats into therapeutic settings, recognizing their unique ability to provide emotional support. Some organizations partner with animal shelters to match veterans with cats in need of homes, creating a mutually beneficial relationship where both the veteran and the cat experience companionship and healing. Other programs like therapy cat sessions in mental health clinics or cat cafés, offer spaces where individuals can interact with cats in a relaxed, non-clinical environment, helping them lower stress and build emotional connections.

Mechanisms of Healing in Animal-Assisted Interventions

The therapeutic effects of animal-assisted interventions are not only emotional but also physiological. Research has shown that interacting with animals triggers the release of oxytocin, often referred to as the "love hormone." Oxytocin promotes feelings of bonding, trust and relaxation. It also helps reduce levels of cortisol, the body's primary stress hormone, thereby alleviating anxiety and promoting a state of calm. Additionally, interacting with animals has been shown to lower blood pressure and reduce heart rate, contributing to overall cardiovascular health. The repetitive action of petting an animal, for instance, can induce a meditative state, allowing the mind to rest from intrusive thoughts and anxiety. This is particularly beneficial for individuals with PTSX, who may experience heightened physiological responses due to chronic stress or hypervigilance.

Psychologically, animals provide a safe, nonjudgmental presence that can help individuals feel accepted and understood. This unconditional companionship is especially valuable for those with PTSX, who may feel alienated or disconnected from others. The ability to care for an animal also creates a sense of purpose and responsibility, which can combat feelings of hopelessness or helplessness.

Many individuals with PTSX find that the daily routine of caring for an animal, whether it is walking a dog, grooming a horse, or feeding a kitten, creates a sense of stability and control in their lives.

Challenges and Considerations

While animal-assisted interventions offer numerous benefits, there are challenges that must be considered. Accessibility is one of the main barriers, as not all individuals have access to programs that provide service animals or equine therapy.

The cost of acquiring and maintaining a service animal, in particular, can be prohibitive. A professionally trained service animal can cost tens of thousands of dollars due to the extensive, specialized training required. Fortunately, for veterans, resources are available to offset this expense.

For a veteran seeking the support of a service animal, the first encounter with the cost can be staggering. Discovering that a professionally trained dog comes with a price tag of anywhere from $20,000 to $60,000 can feel like hitting a brick wall.

This isn't just a purchase. It's a major investment, and for many, it can seem like an impossible barrier to a life-changing resource. The initial hope can quickly turn to discouragement, as a tool for regaining independence appears to be financially out of reach.

However, that steep price reflects an incredible journey of dedication and expertise. It represents the nearly two years of meticulous work that begins long before a veteran ever meets their canine partner. This cost funds the careful breeding, the puppy-raising, and the countless hours of specialized training required to shape a calm, focused, and capable service animal.

It covers the expert trainers, continuous veterinary care, and the highly personalized process of matching a dog's unique skills and temperament to a veteran's specific needs, ensuring the partnership is set up for success from day one.

This is where the VA steps in, not as a provider of the dog itself, but as a committed long-term partner in the veteran's wellbeing. While the VA does not pay for the initial purchase or training of the animal, it makes a crucial promise: if a veteran is paired with a dog from a top-tier accredited agency, such as those recognized by Assistance Dogs International (ADI), they will not have to bear the burden of its future medical costs. This "veterinary health benefit" is a lifeline that makes the long-term commitment of owning a service animal possible.

This support fundamentally changes the dynamic of ownership from a potential financial hardship into a secure partnership. It provides profound peace of mind, covering everything from annual exams and vaccinations to the treatment of unexpected illnesses or injuries.

The benefit extends to prescription medications and even the specialized equipment the dog needs to perform its duties, like harnesses and vests. By covering these ongoing expenses, the VA ensures that a veteran's focus can remain where it belongs: on their own health and the powerful, healing bond they share with their loyal partner.

Furthermore, numerous non-profit organizations work tirelessly to provide service animals to veterans at little to no cost. These groups, funded by donations, manage the entire process from training to placement. Veterans seeking a service animal should research these organizations, as each has its own application process and eligibility requirements. Due to high demand, waitlists are common.

For civilians, the financial pathway is quite different as there is no equivalent government program. The responsibility generally falls on the individual, who typically pursues one of the following routes:

- Non-Profit Organizations: This is the most common method.

Reputable organizations like Canine Companions, Guide Dogs for the Blind, and many others breed, raise, and train service animals. They then provide these highly trained dogs to qualified individuals for free or for a very small administrative fee. These organizations are funded entirely by private donations, grants, and endowments. However, the demand is extremely high, and applicants often face long waiting lists that can last for years.

- Private Fundraising: Many individuals who need a service animal but are on a long waitlist or do not qualify for a specific organization's program will turn to fundraising. They use platforms like GoFundMe, hold community events, and apply for grants from various disability advocacy groups to raise the tens of thousands of dollars needed to purchase a professionally trained dog from a private trainer.
- Owner-Training: Some individuals acquire a suitable dog and train it themselves, often with the guidance of a professional trainer. While this can reduce the initial cost, it is an enormous commitment of time, effort, and skill, with no guarantee of success. The owner is responsible for all costs, including the purchase of the dog, food, all veterinary care, and professional training sessions.

Crucially, private health insurance plans and government programs like Medicare and Medicaid do not cover the cost of acquiring or maintaining a service animal.

Geographic location can also be a limitation for those interested in equine therapy, as these programs may not be available in all regions of the country. Additionally, some individuals may have allergies or phobias related to certain animals, which can limit their ability to participate in certain types of AAI. For those who cannot be around dogs, horses or cats, other alternatives such as bird therapy or interactions with small mammals like rabbits can be explored.

It is essential to tailor animal-assisted interventions to an individual's needs and preferences to ensure the best possible outcome. Ethical considerations are also paramount in AAI. The welfare of the animals involved must be a priority. Animals used in therapy must be properly trained, well cared for, and protected from overwork. AAI programs must adhere to ethical guidelines that ensure the safety and wellbeing of both the individual and the animal. Providing clear boundaries for interaction and ensuring that animals have adequate rest and care is essential for the sustainability of these programs.

Integration with Traditional Therapies

Animal-assisted interventions are most effective when integrated into a comprehensive treatment plan that includes traditional therapies such as cognitive-behavioral therapy (CBT), exposure therapy or medication. The combination of AAI with conventional methods allows for a more holistic approach to healing, addressing both the emotional and physiological aspects of PTSX.

By working alongside mental health professionals, animal-assisted therapists can create individualized treatment plans that maximize the benefits of AAI. For instance, veterans who struggle with social anxiety may find that interacting with a therapy cat or dog helps reduce their anxiety levels, making it easier for them to engage in group therapy sessions.

Similarly, individuals who have difficulty discussing their trauma may feel more comfortable opening up in the presence of a therapy animal, as the animal's calming presence can help them feel safer and more grounded. Regular evaluation and adjustment of the treatment plan ensure that the interventions remain effective and responsive to the individual's evolving needs.

Encouraging Thoughts

Animal-assisted interventions offer a unique and powerful avenue for healing for military personnel and veterans coping with PTSX.

The human-animal bond facilitates emotional connection, reduces stress, and promotes social engagement—key elements in the recovery process. While service dogs and equine therapy are well-established methods, kittens and cats provide a distinctive therapeutic experience, offering companionship, comfort and emotional healing. Programs that incorporate cats into therapeutic settings offer accessible and effective options for those seeking alternative therapies. By integrating AAI with traditional treatments, a holistic approach can be developed to heal the complex needs of individuals with PTSX.

The stories of veterans like Sarah illustrate the profound impact that animals—whether service dogs, horses, cats or others—can have on the recovery journey. These bonds provide not only relief from symptoms but also renewed hope, purpose and joy. In embracing the healing power of human-animal connections, tools can be offered to forge a path toward renewed wellbeing and fulfillment.

If-Then Guidance

- If traditional PTSX treatments such as psychotherapy and medication have not provided sufficient relief, then exploring AAI could offer significant emotional and psychological benefits through the unique bond between humans and animals.
- If you find it difficult to open up emotionally in traditional therapy settings, then engaging with a service animal, particularly a service dog, may help. These specially trained animals can sense anxiety, provide physical comfort, and help prevent panic attacks, easing the emotional burden of PTSX.
- If your PTSX symptoms include hypervigilance or anxiety in public spaces, then a service dog trained to create a protective buffer between you and others could restore a sense of safety and help you reclaim your social life.
- If you're seeking a less traditional form of therapy, then equine-assisted therapy may be a beneficial alternative. Interacting with horses can help you become more attuned to your own emotions, rebuild trust, and practice mindfulness, which can ease symptoms of PTSX.
- If you feel overwhelmed by the responsibilities of owning a high-maintenance animal like a dog or horse, then consider adopting a cat. Cats provide a calming presence and their low-maintenance nature makes them ideal for individuals who need emotional support without the added stress of constant care.
- If your PTSX symptoms include sleep disturbances, e.g.

nightmares, then a service dog trained to wake you during these episodes can provide immediate relief, improving sleep quality and reducing anxiety associated with going to bed.
- If trust issues are a challenge due to trauma involving betrayal, then equine-assisted therapy may help. Horses mirror your emotions and behaviors, helping you develop a deeper understanding of yourself and learn to trust again in a safe, nonjudgmental environment.
- If you feel isolated or disconnected from others due to PTSX, then spending time with a service animal or therapy animal can reduce loneliness, build social interactions, and encourage a sense of community, which is vital for emotional healing.
- If traditional methods of PTSX treatment have been difficult for you to engage with, then incorporating animal-assisted interventions alongside conventional therapy may offer a more holistic approach to your healing journey, helping address both emotional and physiological symptoms of trauma.
- If geographic or financial constraints limit your access to service animals or equine therapy, then consider exploring other forms of animal-assisted therapy, interactions with therapy cats, rabbits, or birds, which may be more accessible and still provide emotional benefits.

Take the Next Step

- If you think a PTSX service dog could benefit you, apply to programs like K9s for Warriors or talk to your doctor about getting a referral.
- Research local programs that offer therapy with animals, such as equine-assisted therapy or visits from therapy dogs.
- If you already have pets, be mindful of the healing presence they can provide. Use their companionship to help regulate emotions and reduce anxiety.
- Sometimes it helps if you simply visit an animal shelter, play and interact with the animals, and see if one chooses you.

Through Their Eyes

"As a retired Naval aviator, I spent years in high-stress environments. The pressure of flying missions, making split-second decisions, and enduring the long stretches of isolation during deployments wore me down in ways I didn't fully understand until after I left the service. When I retired, I thought I'd transition smoothly, but PTSX had other plans. The hypervigilance, anxiety, and nightmares hit me hard. The hardest part was the feeling of isolation—even when surrounded by family and friends, I felt alone in my struggle.

"Traditional therapy and medication helped, but something was missing. Then my therapist suggested I try adopting a cat. At first, I was skeptical. I was used to being in control, in command of every situation, and the thought of caring for a small, independent creature didn't seem like a solution. But I decided to give it a try.

"I adopted a kitten, Scout, and to my surprise, this little creature became a lifeline. Scout had this way of knowing when I needed comfort. On days when I felt overwhelmed, she would curl up in my lap, purring softly, and in those moments, I felt a calmness that I hadn't felt in years. Her playful antics were a welcome distraction from the constant noise in my head, and her need for care gave me a sense of purpose.

"One of the most powerful effects was the way her purring seemed to ease my anxiety. The rhythmic vibration and the warmth of her small body would soothe me during the worst panic attacks. Even the simple act of petting her, feeling her soft fur, gave me something to focus on besides my own racing thoughts. She didn't ask anything of me other than care and love, and in return, she gave me a sense of peace that I didn't think was possible anymore.

"Having Scout made the bad days more bearable. She brought a sense of calm into my home and helped me reconnect with my emotions in a way that traditional therapy couldn't. She helped me find balance in my life again."

—Ryan, US Navy (ret.)

35

Post-Traumatic Growth: Turning Struggle into Strength

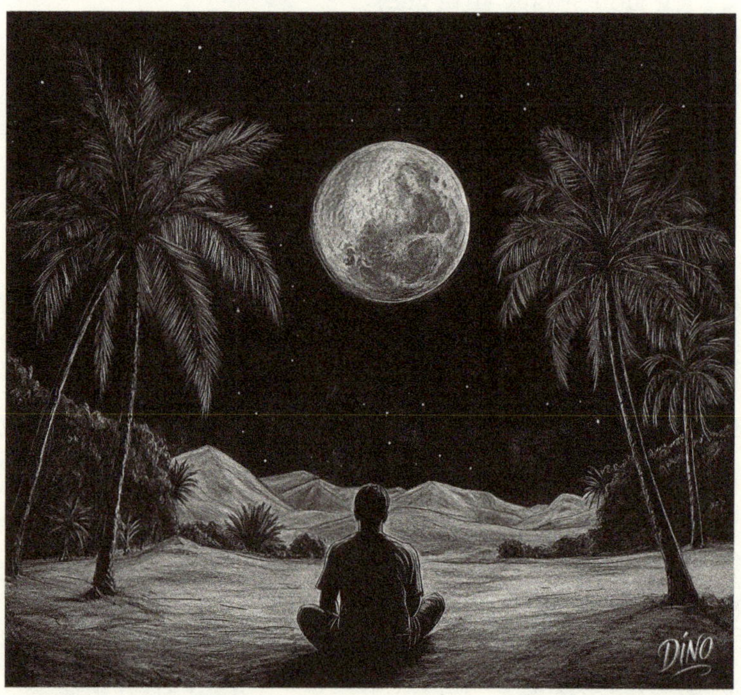

Ethan often replayed the same haunting scene in his mind—those tense moments in a remote desert, the sounds, the smells, and the crushing guilt he couldn't shake. He spent months thinking that was all he'd be left with: pain that trailed him into civilian life, sleepless nights, and a sense of purpose gone missing.

Then a buddy convinced him to join a local veterans' support group, just to see if talking might help. There, he met other men and women who'd been through their own hell. They shared stories of fear and regret, but also something surprising: hope. One vet talked about how the ordeal pushed him to value every sunrise in a way he never had. Another had found new direction by mentoring younger recruits and volunteering at a community center. Each story hinted at transformation—a stirring in the soul that came from confronting hardship head-on. Listening to these folks, Ethan began to see a possible future that was more than just escaping nightmares. Maybe facing down all that darkness could spark a deeper strength—a reason to connect with others, a chance to find new paths. It wasn't about pretending the trauma never happened. It was about letting it shape him into someone wiser, more compassionate, more alive.

This chapter explores that very notion: post-traumatic growth. How, in the wake of life's toughest challenges, veterans can uncover insights and resilience they never saw coming. It's not an easy road—healing seldom is—but the possibility that one could find renewed purpose and richer relationships after trauma can be a powerful light guiding the way forward. The journey through trauma is often perceived solely through the lens of pain, suffering, and the overwhelming challenges of recovery. For veterans dealing with PTSX, these elements often dominate their daily lives, relationships, and sense of identity.

However, an equally significant aspect that deserves attention is the potential for profound personal transformation following traumatic experiences. This concept highlights the positive psychological changes individuals may undergo as a result of their struggle with highly challenging life events. While trauma undeniably leaves scars, PTG suggests that the aftermath of these experiences can also create resilience, strength, and new perspectives on life. PTG is not about denying the difficulty of trauma but about recognizing the opportunity for growth that exists alongside pain. Veterans, in particular, can benefit from exploring this concept, as it offers a hopeful counter-narrative to the struggles they face.

Understanding Post-Traumatic Growth

PTG goes beyond simple recovery. It's not about returning to one's previous state before the trauma occurred. Rather, it represents a deeper transformation—a move to a higher level of functioning

"I do have tough days, nights when the nightmares return, and moments when the anxiety hits hard. But the difference now is that I see my trauma as part of my story, not the end of it.

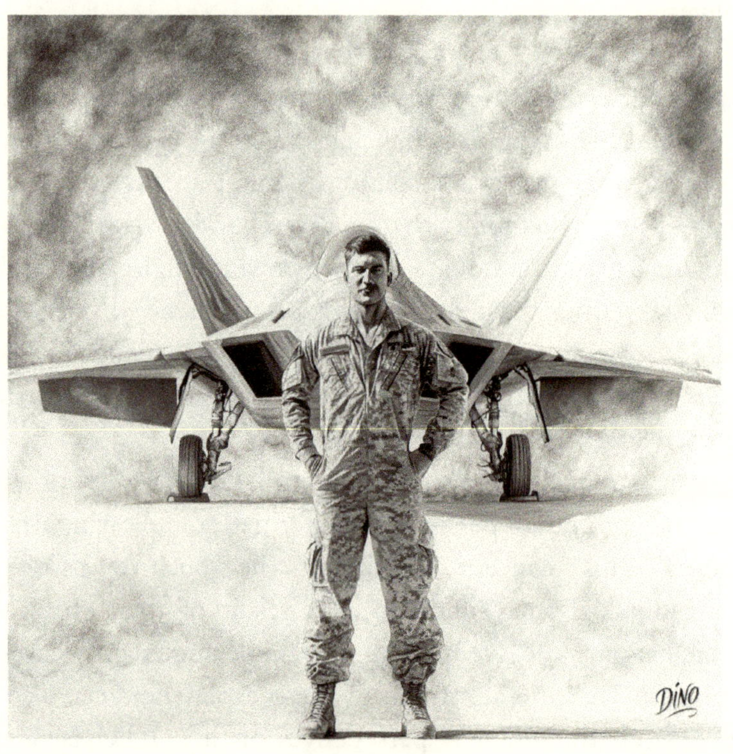

The struggle didn't break me—it reshaped me. And while PTSX is still there, it's no longer the whole story. I've grown stronger, more resilient and more connected to the people around me because of it. PTSX no longer rules my life. I have a say in how everything goes now."

and understanding. Individuals who experience PTG often report significant shifts in their core beliefs, priorities and life goals. Through the struggle with trauma, they come to re-evaluate their perspectives on life, relationships and personal meaning.

PTG is characterized by several key domains of personal development that emerge as a result of coping with trauma:

Enhanced Personal Strength: Many individuals who experience PTG recognize newfound inner strength. Trauma can expose strengths they were previously unaware of, instilling a sense of resilience and the belief that they can handle future challenges with increased confidence. For veterans, this recognition of personal strength often comes from surviving the extreme stressors of combat, moral injury or significant loss.

Improved Relationships: Trauma recovery can lead to a greater appreciation for relationships, creating deeper bonds with family, friends and community members. Individuals who experience PTG often feel a renewed commitment to nurturing these connections, valuing them more than before. Veterans, in particular, may find that trauma strengthens the sense of camaraderie and trust with fellow servicemembers who have shared similar experiences.

Greater Appreciation for Life: PTG often leads to a heightened sense of gratitude and a deeper awareness of life's fragility. Veterans who experience PTG may come to appreciate everyday moments that they once took for granted, such as spending time with loved ones or enjoying a peaceful day. This shift in perspective creates mindfulness and presence, encouraging individuals to savor life more fully.

Discovery of New Possibilities: Trauma can serve as a catalyst for veterans to explore new opportunities, hobbies or career paths. Many find that they are motivated to pursue passions or interests that align more closely with their redefined values and goals. Veterans may channel their experiences into meaningful work, whether it be through education, community service, or advocacy efforts that support others in similar circumstances.

Spiritual or Existential Growth: Traumatic experiences often prompt individuals to engage more deeply with spiritual or existential questions. Some veterans find solace and meaning in their spiritual beliefs, while others may embark on a personal quest to understand life's bigger questions. This search for meaning can lead to personal growth, a redefined sense of purpose, and a renewed connection with faith or philosophy.

PTG in Contrast to PTSX: While PTSX emphasizes the negative psychological impacts of trauma—like anxiety, depression, nightmares, flashbacks and hypervigilance—PTG focuses on the positive changes that can arise from these same experiences. It is crucial to understand that PTG does not negate or minimize the pain and difficulties associated with PTSX. Growth can occur alongside ongoing struggles.

For example, a veteran might continue to experience anxiety and nightmares while also discovering that their relationships with family and friends have grown stronger. These two realities—pain and growth—can coexist. Recognizing this coexistence is essential for adopting a holistic approach to healing and personal development.

The key distinction between PTSX and PTG is not the absence of suffering in the latter but rather the opportunity for transformation that trauma presents. Veterans may continue to grapple with PTSX symptoms, but PTG offers the possibility of finding meaning, developing resilience, and rebuilding their lives in ways that create wellbeing.

Historical Context

The idea that adversity can lead to personal growth is not a new concept. It has roots in ancient philosophies, particularly within Stoicism and existential thought. Throughout history, thinkers and philosophers have explored how individuals can gain strength and wisdom from hardship.

The formal study of PTG, however, began in the 1990s with psychologists Dr. Richard Tedeschi and Dr. Lawrence Calhoun. Tedeschi and Calhoun conducted extensive research on individuals who had experienced traumatic events and found that many reported positive changes as a result of their struggles. They defined PTG as "the experience of significant positive change arising from the struggle with a major life crisis." Their work highlighted the idea that trauma, while painful, can also be a powerful impetus for transformation.

Tedeschi and Calhoun developed the Post-Traumatic Growth Inventory (PTGI), a tool used to measure the positive outcomes reported by individuals after trauma. This inventory has been used across various cultural contexts and applied to survivors of combat, natural disasters, serious illnesses, and other life-altering events.

Their research contributed to a broader understanding that trauma does not necessarily lead to long-term negative outcomes. In fact, trauma can open pathways for personal growth, leading to more nuanced and hopeful approaches to trauma recovery. Today, PTG is recognized as a vital aspect of post-trauma care, offering a more balanced perspective that acknowledges both the hardships and the potential for positive change.

Relevance to Military Personnel and Veterans

For military personnel and veterans, the concept of PTG holds special significance. The unique challenges and stressors associated with military service—combat situations, life-threatening experiences, the loss of comrades, and moral dilemmas—create fertile ground for both PTSX and PTG. Many veterans return from service to civilian life carrying heavy emotional burdens, and while PTSX is a common outcome, there is also a profound potential for growth.

Unique Challenges of Military Service

Military service exposes individuals to extreme stress, both physically and psychologically. Veterans may face the trauma of combat, the loss of friends in battle, and the moral injury that comes from difficult decisions made in life-or-death situations.

These experiences can severely impact mental health, often leading to conditions like PTSX, depression, and anxiety. Beyond the battlefield, veterans also face the challenge of reintegrating into civilian life. The transition from a highly structured and purpose-driven environment to what may be a mundane civilian life can feel isolating and disorienting. Veterans may struggle with identity shifts, loss of camaraderie, and difficulties finding purpose outside of the military context. However, within these challenges lies the potential for PTG. Veterans possess qualities that can be assets in their post-trauma growth journey. Military service instills discipline, teamwork and leadership skills, which can all be leveraged as veterans navigate their recovery.

Veterans may also find new ways to apply their skills, whether through community service, educational pursuits, or advocacy efforts. By recognizing and nurturing the potential for growth, veterans can enhance their wellbeing and find fulfillment in life after service.

Theoretical Foundations of PTG

The process of PTG involves several psychological mechanisms that facilitate growth after trauma. These mechanisms provide insight into how individuals transform their trauma into positive changes. Cognitive Processing Theory suggests that trauma disrupts an individual's fundamental beliefs and assumptions about the world, leading to a process of cognitive restructuring. In short, they become lost and without purpose.

Trauma often shatters pre-existing schemas—mental frameworks that help individuals organize and interpret information—particularly those related to safety, trust and control. For veterans, combat trauma may challenge deeply held beliefs about safety, morality and personal invulnerability. As individuals work to integrate the trauma into their understanding of the world, they begin the process of rebuilding these schemas.

Veterans may develop more adaptive beliefs that acknowledge the dangers they have faced while recognizing their ability to cope with them. This cognitive restructuring allows for a stronger, more resilient sense of self.

Another critical aspect of PTG is meaning-making. After trauma, veterans may grapple with existential questions such as, "Why did this happen?" or "What can I learn from this?" The process of finding meaning in the traumatic experience is essential for growth. Veterans who are able to derive personal significance from their trauma are more likely to experience PTG. Emotional regulation also plays a key role in facilitating PTG. Trauma often brings intense emotions such as fear, anger, sadness and guilt. Veterans who learn strategies to manage and process these emotions in healthy ways are better equipped to move forward in their recovery.

Techniques like mindfulness, deep-breathing exercises, journaling and seeking social support can help veterans manage their emotional distress and prevent maladaptive coping mechanisms like substance abuse.

Embracing and processing emotions rather than suppressing them allows individuals to work through their trauma constructively. Emotional regulation leads to increased self-awareness, empathy and emotional intelligence, which all contribute to personal growth and improved relationships.

Social Support Mechanisms in PTG

Social support plays a vital role in creating PTG. Veterans who have strong social networks—whether family, friends or fellow veterans—are more likely to experience positive changes after trauma. Close relationships provide emotional, informational and practical assistance that are crucial for recovery. For veterans, peer support can be particularly impactful.

Connecting with fellow servicemembers who have faced similar challenges creates a sense of camaraderie and mutual understanding. Peer-support groups allow veterans to share their experiences, offer encouragement, and exchange coping strategies.

These groups provide validation and a safe space for discussing fears, hopes, and goals. The importance of supportive relationships cannot be overstated. Veterans who feel understood and supported by loved ones are more likely to navigate their trauma constructively.

Sharing experiences with trusted individuals alleviates feelings of isolation and creates a sense of community. Social support encourages veterans to open up, express their emotions, and reflect on their trauma, all of which are essential for PTG.

The Domains of Post-Traumatic Growth

PTG manifests in various aspects of a veteran's life, reflecting comprehensive personal development. These domains include personal strength, new possibilities, improved relationships, a greater appreciation for life, and spiritual or existential growth. Veterans who experience PTG often develop a heightened sense of personal strength. Surviving trauma can reveal capabilities they were previously unaware of, bolstering their confidence and resilience. Veterans come to understand that they are capable of enduring hardship, which prepares them to face future challenges with greater self-efficacy.

Trauma can also prompt veterans to explore new possibilities. Some veterans reassess their career paths, choosing to pursue education or enter professions that align more closely with their redefined values. Others may discover new hobbies or interests that bring joy and fulfillment.

Exploring new activities can introduce creativity and a sense of purpose into veterans' lives. In the domain of relationships, trauma can lead to a greater appreciation for loved ones. Veterans may feel more open, communicative and invested in their relationships, creating deeper connections with family and friends.

Additionally, trauma often increases empathy and compassion for others' struggles. It inspires veterans to engage in volunteer work, advocacy or mentoring. A greater appreciation for life is another hallmark of PTG. Many veterans develop mindfulness practices that encourage them to live fully in the present moment, savoring everyday experiences that they may have once overlooked. This shift in perspective enhances life satisfaction and reduces stress.

Finally, spiritual or existential growth often occurs as veterans grapple with life's big questions. Trauma can lead veterans to reevaluate their spiritual beliefs, resulting in a more personalized faith or philosophy that provides comfort and guidance. Veterans may find a sense of purpose, dedicating themselves to causes that align with their values.

Factors Influencing PTG

Several factors influence whether and to what extent veterans experience PTG. Individual characteristics like personality traits play a role in facilitating growth. Veterans who are open to experience, optimistic and conscientious are more likely to embrace new perspectives, maintain hope, and proactively engage in recovery. Veterans who use adaptive coping strategies—problem-solving, seeking social support, and reframing negative experiences—are more likely to experience growth. In contrast, maladaptive coping mechanisms like avoidance or substance abuse can hinder recovery and prolong distress. Those with a positive mental attitude fare better. And those who maintain that great outlook heal faster.

The nature of the trauma itself also influences PTG. While severe trauma poses significant challenges, it can create more profound opportunities for growth as individuals work through complex emotions and beliefs. Veterans who experience chronic or repeated trauma may face additional obstacles, but these experiences can also lead to cumulative growth as they engage in ongoing coping and adaptation.

Facilitating PTG in Veterans

Facilitating PTG in veterans requires intentional strategies and supportive environments. Veterans must confront their trauma and engage in cognitive restructuring to reframe their experiences in a way that creates growth.

Therapeutic interventions like cognitive behavioral therapy and acceptance and commitment therapy (ACT) can help veterans challenge negative beliefs, develop healthier coping strategies, and find meaning in their trauma. Additionally, narrative therapy can play a crucial role in facilitating PTG.

Veterans who share their stories through writing, speaking, or artistic expression are better able to process their trauma and develop a more empowered personal narrative. Reframing their life stories to emphasize survival, strength, and perseverance creates resilience and personal agency.

PTG offers a powerful framework for understanding how veterans can transform their trauma into opportunities for personal growth. While PTSX remains a significant challenge for many veterans, PTG provides hope that trauma can also lead to positive change. Through cognitive restructuring, emotional regulation, social support, and therapeutic interventions, veterans can find strength, resilience, and meaning in their experiences. The journey toward PTG is deeply personal and often challenging, but it holds the potential for profound transformation. By embracing PTG, veterans can rebuild their lives, deepen their relationships, and find renewed purpose in life after trauma.

If-Then Guidance

- If you are struggling with trauma and focusing only on the pain and challenges it brings, then explore the concept of PTG. It offers the possibility that your trauma could lead to personal growth, new strengths, and a deeper understanding of life.
- If you believe that trauma has only negative outcomes, then recognize that PTG shows how positive changes, like greater resilience and new perspectives, can coexist with the difficulties of trauma. Personal growth doesn't mean denying pain but finding strength within it.
- If you feel emotionally overwhelmed by the intensity of trauma, then consider working on emotional regulation techniques like mindfulness, journaling, or breathing exercises. These tools can help you process emotions constructively, which is essential for personal growth.
- If you are unsure of how trauma could lead to positive change, then reflect on the five domains of PTG: enhanced personal strength, improved relationships, greater appreciation for life, new possibilities and spiritual growth. Understanding these areas can help you recognize potential growth even in the face of adversity.
- If you find that trauma has disrupted your core beliefs about safety, control, or trust, then consider working on cognitive restructuring. This process helps rebuild and adapt your beliefs to include the trauma in a new, more resilient understanding of the world.
- If you feel isolated or misunderstood, then reach out to peer support groups, particularly those for veterans, where you can connect with others who have experienced similar challenges. Shared experiences can be powerful catalysts for personal growth.

- If you are experiencing trauma but are unsure of its long-term impact, then focus on meaning-making processes. Reflecting on how the trauma might shape your values, goals, and beliefs can help you find deeper meaning and direction in your recovery.
- If you are searching for new possibilities in life after trauma, then consider exploring new hobbies, career paths or volunteer opportunities that align with your redefined values. Trauma can open the door to new areas of fulfillment and personal passion.
- If you are facing challenges in your relationships due to trauma, then focus on improving communication and emotional openness. Trauma can deepen relationships when both sides are willing to engage in honest dialogue and offer mutual support.
- If you are questioning your spiritual or existential beliefs after trauma, then explore how your beliefs have evolved as a result of your experience. Trauma can lead to spiritual or existential growth, helping you discover a renewed sense of purpose and connection with something larger than yourself.

Take the Next Step

- Acknowledge how your experiences with trauma may have led to increased resilience, empathy or personal strength.
- Focus on setting small, achievable goals that align with your values and build on the strength you've gained from overcoming adversity.
- Look for programs that focus on post-traumatic growth and resilience-building, either through the VA or veteran organizations, to continue developing a positive outlook.

Through Their Eyes

"As an F-22 crew chief, my job was to keep the world's most advanced fighter jets ready for combat, no matter where we were deployed. In war zones, every second mattered. The pilots depended on me to ensure their jets would perform perfectly when they needed them most. It was high-pressure work, but I thrived on it—precision, discipline and control. But when I came home after multiple deployments, all that control was gone. PTSX turned my world upside down, and the battlefield wasn't out there anymore—it was in my head. I struggled with anxiety, nightmares, and this constant feeling of always watching my back, looking over my shoulder, like I was always waiting for something to go wrong.

"Therapy and medication helped some, but they didn't bring back the sense of purpose or control I'd had while working on the flight line. Then this therapist introduced me to the concept of PTG, and for the first time, I started to see my trauma in a different light. PTG isn't about denying the pain—it's about recognizing that, through the struggle, there's also an opportunity for growth.

"At first, I wasn't sure. How could something as destructive as PTSX lead to anything positive? But I approached it the way I would a problem back on base—step by step, with precision. I changed the way I looked at things. I started to see that every challenge I faced could reveal something new about myself, and over time, I realized I had developed a strength I didn't know existed. All those years of deployments, handling the stress of war zones, had built a mental toughness. I had survived the worst, and that gave me the confidence to face anything life could throw at me back home.

"One of the most unexpected changes was how my relationships evolved. In the military, everything was about the mission and the team. But after my deployments, I had isolated myself from my family and friends, not wanting to burden them with what I was going through. PTG taught me that sharing my struggle didn't make me weak—it made me stronger. When I started opening up to my wife and my buddies, it deepened our connections. I realized I wasn't alone in this battle, and that trust and vulnerability strengthened my relationships.

"I also found a new appreciation for life. For so long, I was in survival mode, just trying to get through the day. But through PTG, I learned to slow down and appreciate the little things—like spending time with my kids, enjoying a quiet morning with a cup of coffee, or watching a sunset without thinking about the next mission. These moments of peace became something I cherished, and I learned to live in the present rather than constantly preparing for the next disaster.

"Another big shift was in how I saw my future. Before, I had tied my entire identity to my role as a crew chief. After leaving the Air Force, I felt lost, like nothing else could compare. But PTG opened my eyes to new possibilities. I realized that I still had a lot to give, whether that was mentoring younger veterans or getting involved in community projects. I started volunteering with veteran organizations, helping others who were dealing with PTSX, and that gave me a new sense of purpose.

"Spiritually, I'd drifted away from the beliefs I once held. The things I saw during deployments made me question a lot about life, faith and meaning. But as I worked through my trauma, I started to reconnect with my spiritual side in a way that made sense for me. It wasn't about finding answers to the big questions—sometimes, it was just about accepting that there are things I'll never fully understand. But finding peace in that uncertainty became part of my growth.

"I do have tough days, nights when the nightmares return, and moments when the anxiety hits hard. But the difference now is that I see my trauma as part of my story, not the end of it. The struggle didn't break me—it reshaped me. And while PTSX is still there, it's no longer the whole story. I've grown stronger, more resilient and more connected to the people around me because of it. PTSX no longer rules my life. I have a say in how everything goes now.

"To anyone who's dealing with PTSX, I'd say this: Don't be afraid to look for the growth within the struggle. It's not easy, and it takes time, but the pain doesn't have to be the only thing you take from your experience. There's strength in what you've been through, and with the right support and mindset, you can find that strength and use it to build a life of meaning and purpose again."

—Mark, US Air Force Veteran

36

The Heart's Embrace: Harnessing Chest Pressure Points to Calm PTSX Symptoms

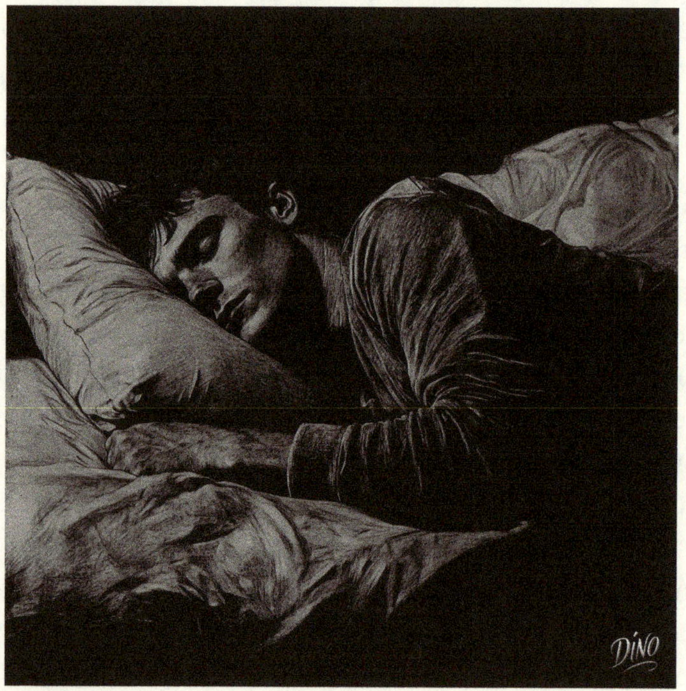

Mike never imagined a small pillow pressed gently against his chest would help calm the pounding heart that kept him awake most nights. But after struggling with nightmares and restless anxiety post-deployment, he was willing to try something new. At first, the idea of applying pressure to specific points in his chest sounded too simple— how could that possibly ease the constant sense of dread he carried, the horrible bleak outlook on his life?

He followed a basic routine suggested by another vet: lying on his bed, placing a small, firm pillow over the center of his chest and letting his weight settle. He closed his eyes, focused on steady breathing, and found himself drifting into a sensation of gentle relief. Night by night, the restlessness seemed to loosen its grip, allowing him deeper, more restful sleep. Though not a replacement for the counseling he continued, this small change added a tangible layer of comfort he hadn't found with medication alone. During the day, he sometimes took a pillow and pressed lightly on that same area whenever he felt panic creeping in—an immediate, grounding technique that reminded him to slow down.

Coincidentally, he came across a movie, *Temple*, about Dr. Temple Grandin, an autistic scientist who found ways to calm herself down by applying pressure to certain parts of her body. Not only did she find solace in her discovery, she was also able to assist cows on their way to their final journey. Mike was inspired to learn more.

This chapter explores the underlying principle of chest pressure-point therapy—rooted in the mind-body interplay of acupressure. We'll explore how simple tactile pressure can switch the body from its relentless "fight-or-flight" mode toward a more restful state.

By activating calming responses, lowering heart rate, and perhaps even boosting feel-good neurotransmitters, a little chest pressure can serve as an unexpected ally in the battle against PTSX symptoms. Whether you're a seasoned practitioner of holistic methods or skeptical but seeking extra relief, these gentle techniques might provide just enough pause—enough quiet—to make the day (and night) a bit more manageable.

The relentless grip of anxiety, hyperarousal and insomnia can make everyday life a constant battle. While traditional therapies and medications are essential in managing these symptoms, alternative approaches like acupressure offer additional avenues for relief. This chapter explores the concept of chest pressure points and how the simple act of lying on a small pillow can invoke calmness and promote sleep, providing a gentle remedy for those grappling with PTSX.

The Silent Struggle of PTSX

For countless veterans, the transition from the structured environment of military service to civilian life is fraught with challenges. Traumatic experiences from deployment often leave deep psychological scars, manifesting as flashbacks, nightmares, and a persistent state of heightened alertness. Sleep disturbances become commonplace, and the mind refuses to rest, trapped in a cycle of stress and anxiety.

While psychotherapy and medications are critical components of treatment, they may not fully address the complex needs of every individual. As a result, many seek complementary therapies that can be easily incorporated into daily routines to enhance their wellbeing.

Understanding Acupressure and Energy Pathways

Acupressure, a practice rooted in Traditional Chinese Medicine (TCM), operates on the principle that the body contains a network of energy channels called meridians. Through these meridians flows Qi (pronounced "chee"), the vital life force that sustains physical and emotional health.

When the flow of Qi is disrupted or imbalanced, it can lead to various ailments. Acupressure involves applying gentle, sustained pressure to specific points along these meridians to restore harmony and promote healing.

The Chest as a Gateway to Calmness

The chest, which houses the heart and lungs, holds a central place in both our physiological and emotional wellbeing. In TCM, it is considered a crucial area for regulating emotions and alleviating stress. Two primary pressure points located in the chest region—Conception Vessel 17 (CV17) and Kidney 27 (K27)—are believed to have significant calming effects.

Conception Vessel 17 (CV17): Located at the center of the chest, midway between the nipples, CV17 is aptly named the "Sea of Tranquility."

This point is associated with the heart chakra in Eastern traditions, symbolizing love, compassion, and emotional balance. Applying gentle pressure to CV17 is thought to regulate emotional stress by easing feelings of anxiety and agitation. It may also enhance respiratory function by promoting deeper, more relaxed breathing, and facilitate emotional release by assisting in the processing of suppressed emotions.

Kidney 27 (K27): K27 is called The Shu Mansion and is found just below the collarbone, adjacent to the sternum on both sides. It is linked to the kidney meridian, which in TCM is associated with fear and anxiety. Stimulating K27 is believed to reduce anxiety by calming the mind and easing nervous tension. It may improve the flow of Qi throughout the body, enhancing energy levels and overall vitality. Additionally, it could support immune function, contributing to resilience against stress-related illnesses.

The Science Behind Pressure Points and Relaxation

While acupressure is an effective ancient practice, modern science offers insights into how stimulating these pressure points might impact the body. One key aspect is the activation of the parasympathetic nervous system, which is responsible for the body's rest and digest functions. PTSX often keeps individuals locked in a heightened sympathetic state, leading to chronic stress responses.

Stimulating chest pressure points activates the parasympathetic nervous system by reducing heart rate through gentle pressure that signals the body to slow down. It lowers blood pressure by promoting relaxation of the blood vessels, and encourages relaxed breathing by enhancing oxygen exchange and calming the mind. Another aspect involves the influence on neurotransmitters. Physical touch and pressure can affect levels of certain neurotransmitters in the brain.

The release of endorphins, the body's natural painkillers, can induce feelings of wellbeing and counteract stress. Increased production of serotonin may improve mood and regulate sleep, while a reduction in cortisol, the stress hormone, can alleviate anxiety symptoms.

The mind-body connection is also significant. Focusing on bodily sensations enhances mindfulness, an effective strategy for managing PTSX symptoms. Awareness of the present moment helps interrupt negative thought patterns and grounds individuals in their bodies, providing a sense of control and calmness.

Practical Application: Lying on a Small Pillow

Integrating chest pressure-point stimulation into daily life can be simple and unobtrusive. One practical method is lying on a small pillow positioned to apply gentle pressure to the center of the chest. To practice this technique, choose a small, firm pillow or a specially designed acupressure cushion.

Find a comfortable place to lie down, such as a bed or a yoga mat placed on the floor. Place the pillow under your chest so that it presses against CV17, ensuring that you are comfortable and can breathe easily.

As you settle into this position, relax your body and let your arms rest comfortably at your sides or extend them forward. Focus on your breath, inhaling slowly through your nose and allowing your abdomen to rise, then exhaling gently through your mouth. Remain in this position for 10 to 15 minutes, or as long as is comfortable for you.

Practicing once or twice daily, especially before bedtime, can enhance relaxation and improve sleep quality. The potential benefits of this technique include promoting relaxation by soothing the nervous system, improving sleep quality by calming the mind and aiding in falling asleep faster, and reducing anxiety by providing immediate relief during moments of heightened stress. It also enhances self-care by empowering individuals to take an active role in managing their symptoms.

Integrating Chest Pressure-point therapy with PTSX Treatment

It's important to view chest pressure-point therapy as a complement to, not a replacement for, conventional PTSX treatments. This approach can work alongside psychotherapy by enhancing the effects of therapies such as cognitive behavioral therapy, reducing anxiety, and increasing receptiveness to treatment. It may also support medication management by potentially mitigating side effects or reducing reliance on higher doses of medications.

Combining this technique with mindfulness practices like meditation or yoga can also amplify the benefits, promoting overall wellbeing. Before starting any new therapeutic practice, it is crucial to consult with a healthcare provider to ensure it is appropriate for your specific circumstances. They can provide guidance on how best to integrate chest pressure-point therapy into your existing treatment plan.

Real-Life Experiences

Eric, a former Marine, struggled with insomnia and recurring nightmares after returning from deployment. Medications left him feeling groggy, and therapy alone did not fully alleviate his symptoms. Upon a friend's recommendation, he began incorporating chest pressure-point therapy into his nightly routine.

At first, he was skeptical, but after a week, he noticed that he was falling asleep faster and sleeping more soundly. The practice became a ritual that signaled to his mind and body that it was time to rest.

Similarly, Brooke, who served in the Army, faced severe anxiety following her service. She found that during panic attacks, pressing on her chest helped her regain control. Learning about CV17, she started using this technique when she felt overwhelmed. She described it as pressing a reset button. It did not erase the anxiety completely, but it made it manageable and gave her a sense of empowerment over her symptoms.

Scientific Perspectives and Ongoing Research

Research on acupressure and its effects on PTSX symptoms continues to emerge. Some results suggest potential benefits, indicating that acupressure can lower stress levels and improve overall wellbeing. Research has also shown improvements in sleep quality among participants using acupressure techniques, and preliminary evidence suggests that acupressure may reduce symptoms of anxiety and depression.

More extensive clinical trials, however, are needed to fully understand the mechanisms of action, evaluate the sustainability of benefits over extended periods, and assess the specificity of these techniques for PTSX among veterans and military personnel.

Considerations and Precautions

While chest pressure-point therapy is generally safe, it is important to approach it thoughtfully. Use gentle pressure to avoid discomfort or bruising, and individuals with heart conditions or chest injuries should consult a doctor before practicing. Consistency is key, as benefits accrue over time, so patience and regular practice are essential. Managing expectations is also important, as responses to acupressure can vary. What works for one person may not work for another. Remember that this therapy should augment, not substitute, professional medical treatment.

Embracing Holistic Healing

The journey to healing from PTSX is multifaceted, and incorporating practices like chest pressure-point therapy represents a shift toward holistic wellness. This approach acknowledges the interconnectedness of the mind, body, and spirit.

The benefits of a holistic approach include personal empowerment, as it encourages individuals to take an active role in their healing process. It allows for customization, enabling practices to be tailored to individual needs and preferences, and it complements traditional treatments by addressing additional aspects of wellbeing.

Building a supportive community is also crucial. Sharing experiences with fellow veterans generates camaraderie and mutual encouragement. Education and awareness through workshops and seminars can spread knowledge about alternative therapies. Healthcare systems can integrate acupressure and other complementary therapies into treatment plans, offering a more comprehensive approach to care.

The Path Forward

Exploring chest pressure points offers hope for many grappling with the relentless symptoms of PTSX. It provides a practical tool that can be easily integrated into daily life. Combining acupressure with mindfulness can deepen its impact, and noting changes in mood, sleep and anxiety levels can inform adjustments to the practice. Advocacy for holistic care is also important. Healthcare integration involves advocating for the inclusion of alternative therapies in standard care protocols. Supporting research by promoting and participating in studies can help build the evidence base, and influencing policy can encourage policymakers to recognize and support comprehensive treatment approaches.

The silent scars of PTSX require not only medical intervention but also compassionate, innovative approaches that honor the complexity of healing. Chest pressure-point therapy represents a bridge between ancient wisdom and modern needs, offering a gentle, accessible means to find calm amid the storm. Veterans and military personnel continue to navigate on their journeys toward wholeness, and embracing such practices can provide solace and empower them to reclaim their peace.

If-Then Guidance

- If you are experiencing anxiety or panic attacks, then apply gentle pressure to the Conception Vessel 17 (CV17) point located in the center of your chest. This can help calm the nervous system and slow your heart rate. Combine this with deep, controlled breathing to further enhance relaxation. Take time to focus on your breath, allowing it to become slower and more regular. This simple technique can help you regain control over your physical and emotional responses during times of heightened stress.
- If you find it difficult to fall asleep or suffer from insomnia, then use a small, firm pillow to apply gentle pressure to the chest area while lying down. Position the pillow beneath your sternum, aligning it with the CV17 point, and allow the pressure to soothe your chest as you practice slow, rhythmic breathing. This routine, practiced nightly, can help signal your body that it's time to relax, easing you into a more restful state and promoting better quality sleep.
- If you feel overwhelmed by daily stress or experience heightened emotional responses, then take a few moments to step away from your current activity and apply pressure to the Kidney 27 (K27) points located below your collarbones, next to your sternum. These points are believed to help reduce stress and restore balance. Apply gentle pressure while focusing on slow, deep breaths. This technique can provide immediate relief by calming the mind and regulating emotional responses, allowing you to return to your tasks with a renewed sense of control and focus.
- If you wake up from nightmares or feel distressed during the

night, then sit up slowly and apply pressure to either the CV17 point on your chest or the K27 points beneath your collarbones. Focus on calming your breath and extending your exhalations. Doing so can help activate your body's relaxation response, easing the residual anxiety or fear from the nightmare. Consider writing down your thoughts or emotions in a journal afterward to process and release any lingering distress.

- If you are new to chest pressure-point therapy and want to incorporate it into your routine, then set aside 10-15 minutes each day, preferably in a quiet and comfortable environment. Practice lying down with a small pillow under your chest or apply gentle pressure manually to the CV17 and K27 points. Combine this practice with mindful breathing or meditation to enhance the calming effects. Over time, you may find that this simple routine becomes a valuable tool in managing stress and anxiety on a daily basis.
- If you have a medical condition, such as heart disease or chest injuries, then consult with a healthcare professional before attempting chest pressure-point therapy. They can advise you on the safest way to incorporate these techniques into your treatment plan.
- If direct pressure on the chest is not advisable, you may consider using alternative acupressure points, such as the Pericardium 6 (P6) point located on the wrist, which can also help relieve stress and anxiety.
- If you have been practicing chest pressure-point therapy consistently but do not notice any improvements, then evaluate your technique to ensure you are applying pressure correctly and using the appropriate amount of pressure—firm but not painful. It may also be helpful to increase the frequency of your practice.
- If the technique still does not seem to be effective, consider seeking guidance from an acupressure specialist or healthcare provider to adjust your approach or explore complementary therapies such as mindfulness, counseling or group support.
- If you notice positive changes after incorporating chest pressure-

point therapy into your routine, then continue practicing regularly to sustain these benefits. Acknowledge your progress and celebrate the improvements, even if they are gradual.

Take the Next Step

- Explore how acupressure, particularly in the chest area, can help calm your body's fight-or-flight response during stressful moments.
- Practice applying gentle pressure to specific chest points when you feel anxious or overwhelmed. Start with guidance from a professional acupressure practitioner.
- Make acupressure part of your daily wellness routine to help reduce hypervigilance and anxiety over time.

Through Their Eyes

"As an Army Ranger, I was trained to face the toughest challenges head-on, but nothing could have prepared me for the silent battle I faced after leaving the service. PTSX hit me like a freight train— flashbacks, hypervigilance and sleepless nights became my new reality. No matter how hard I tried, I couldn't shake the feeling of being constantly on edge, as if I was still in combat.

"Therapy and medication helped, but the nightmares and anxiety always seemed to creep back in. I needed something more, something I could use on my own when things got overwhelming.

"One night, my mind racing as usual, I remembered a conversation I had with a fellow vet about alternative ways to calm the body. He mentioned something about using chest pressure points, a simple technique he swore by to help him manage his symptoms.

"I decided to give it a shot, thinking I had nothing to lose. I grabbed a small pillow and placed it right over my chest, just as he described. Lying down, I focused on breathing deeply, letting the gentle pressure do its work. I wasn't expecting much, but after a few minutes, something shifted.

"It wasn't a dramatic change, but a subtle sense of calm started to settle in. For the first time in what felt like forever, my heart stopped racing, and my mind started to quiet down. I fell asleep for an entire nine hours without moving or getting up.

"Over the next few weeks, I made this practice a nightly ritual. Every time I felt the familiar surge of anxiety coming on, I'd lie down, position the pillow, and focus on breathing. It became a way to signal to my body that it was okay to relax, that I didn't need to be on high alert all the time. Eventually, I noticed my sleep improving, and the panic attacks that used to hit me out of nowhere became less frequent.

"It's a tool I can use whenever I need to regain control. The thing is, I've learned that healing isn't just about the mind—sometimes, you've got to work through the body to get to the peace you're after. The heart's embrace, through something as simple as a pillow on your chest, can be a powerful way to calm the storm inside."

—Chris, US Army Ranger Veteran

37

The Essential Role of Rest

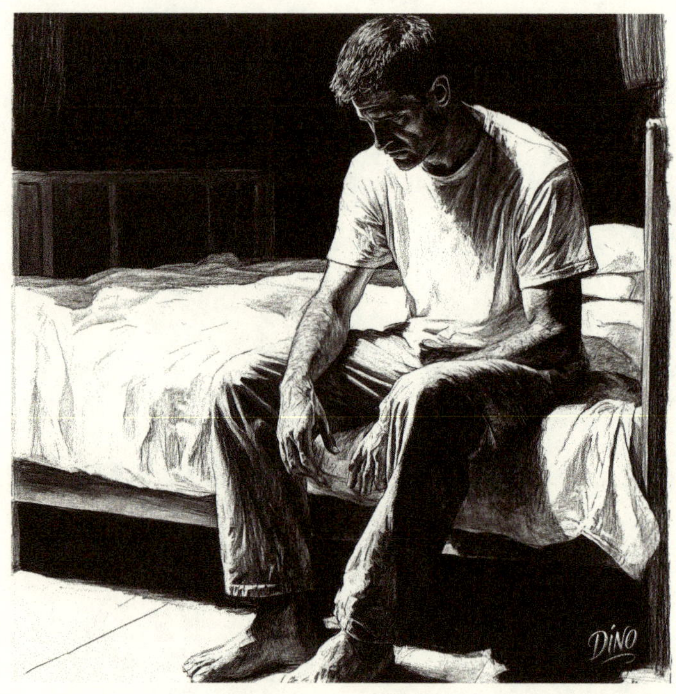

The steady hum of the air conditioner was the only sound in the dimly lit room. Jack sat on the edge of the cot, elbows on his knees, head bowed. His hands trembled slightly, not from fear but exhaustion— the kind that seeps into your bones after years of hypervigilance.

Outside the barracks, a distant thud of boots on gravel echoed, a sound so familiar it didn't even register anymore. He hadn't slept well in months. Not since the last deployment. Not since the night the convoy was ambushed, and he could still hear the screams. Flashbacks invaded his mind. He stared at the frayed laces of his boots, trying to anchor himself in the present. But it was no use; the memories crept in like smoke under a door.

"Jack, you need to rest." His wife's voice echoed in his mind, a faint reminder of the life waiting for him back home. Rest. What did that even mean? Lying down? Staring at a ceiling while his heart raced at shadows that weren't there?

Tonight, he was going to try something different. Earlier, a counselor at the base had handed him a booklet, *Comprehensive Guide to 25 Types of Rest for US Military Personnel and Veterans.* Jack had dismissed it at first, thinking it was another cookie-cutter self-help guide. But now, sitting in the suffocating quiet of his quarters, he unfolded it.

"Start small," the booklet read. "Try sensory rest. Dim the lights, minimize noise, and focus on grounding yourself." Jack stood and turned off the overhead light, leaving just a desk lamp glowing softly. He closed the blinds, shutting out the fluorescent glare of the barracks yard. He found his headphones, playing a recording of ocean waves—gentle, soothing.

Lying back on the cot, he closed his eyes. He inhaled deeply, holding his breath for four seconds before slowly exhaling. The rhythmic sound of the waves lulled him, pulling him away from the chaos in his mind. For the first time in what felt like forever, he felt his body release some tension. Tomorrow, he'd try another step. Maybe a walk under the stars or journaling his thoughts. But tonight, this moment was enough—a fragile, fleeting taste of peace. For the first time, Jack wasn't just surviving. He was beginning to feel human again.

This chapter is a comprehensive guide featuring 25 types of rest. Each is tailored to the unique demands of military service and the challenges many veterans face during or after their service. By embracing various forms of rest, servicemembers and veterans can pave a stronger road toward healing, personal growth, and a healthier transition into civilian life. Remember too: this information is also for civilians who need to take a breather and rest.

What Really Is Rest?

Rest is a fundamental component of overall health and wellbeing, but its significance is profoundly amplified for military personnel and veterans. The demanding nature of military service—characterized by rigorous training, deployments, and exposure to high-stress and often traumatic environments— places immense physical, mental and emotional strain on servicemembers.

Rest isn't just about lying down or taking a quick nap. For those serving or who have served in the military, rest becomes a cornerstone of physical health, mental resilience and emotional recovery. Long deployments, high-stakes decisions, and exposure to traumatic or stressful conditions can leave servicemembers and veterans in dire need of deeper, more intentional forms of rest.

When someone has PTSX, flashbacks, nightmares and a constant state of vigilance can wreak havoc on sleep and daily functioning. The very idea of "rest" can feel elusive. Yet integrating rest as a proactive strategy—for body, mind, emotions and spirit—can help restore balance and offer a path to resilience. In military culture, rest often takes a backseat to operational readiness, but research and anecdotal experience show that well-rested servicemembers perform better and recover more effectively from trauma.

In the military context, rest transcends the simple notion of inactivity or sleep. It encompasses a broad spectrum of restorative practices that address the multifaceted strains placed on servicemembers.

Physical rest helps repair the body from the intense demands of training and operations. The brain remains highly active, even at rest, continuously performing millions of metabolic reactions essential for maintaining neuronal function, communication and survival. These biochemical activities inevitably generate metabolic waste products like beta-amyloid proteins, tau proteins, reactive oxygen species (ROS), and other potentially harmful metabolic by-products.

The brain employs a specialized waste-clearance mechanism called the glymphatic system, active primarily during sleep or prolonged rest periods. The glymphatic system uses cerebrospinal fluid (CSF) flow to efficiently flush away these waste substances, toxins and harmful molecules. During deep sleep, the interstitial space (the space between brain cells) expands, facilitating the enhanced movement of CSF throughout the brain, effectively clearing out harmful metabolites.

If waste products accumulate due to chronic sleep deprivation or impaired glymphatic clearance, they may contribute to neuronal dysfunction, inflammation and neurodegenerative conditions like Alzheimer's disease, Parkinson's disease and dementia. In very active people like military servicemembers and athletes who do not get sufficient rest, this can lead to loss of short-term memory, decreased cognition and thinking ability. For those who must run at 100% efficiency at work, the loss of any of those abilities could prove fatal.

Thus, sufficient sleep and rest are crucial not only for cognitive recovery and memory consolidation but also to ensure proper detoxification and overall long-term brain health. Likewise, mental rest provides relief from the constant high-stakes decision-making and vigilance required in military roles. Mental rest also aids in not thinking, thus relaxing neurons and their cellular processes.

Emotional rest offers a safe space to process complex feelings that are often suppressed in military culture, which is particularly important for those dealing with PTSX. Sensory rest allows for a reprieve from the overstimulation of loud noises and bright lights common in military environments, which can be triggering for individuals with PTSX.

Integrating diverse forms of rest can significantly enhance the effectiveness of PTSX treatment and overall wellbeing. For instance, mindfulness and meditation practices have been shown to reduce anxiety and improve emotional regulation, aiding in mental and emotional rest.

Engaging in creative activities or spending time in nature can provide a sense of peace and contribute to emotional healing. Establishing routines that include regular periods of rest can improve sleep quality, which is often disrupted in individuals with PTSX.

Understanding rest as a comprehensive and proactive approach empowers everyone to take control of their healing process. It encourages a shift from viewing rest as a passive or secondary need to recognizing it as a vital, active component of health and resilience. By embracing various forms of rest, individuals can better manage PTSX symptoms, reduce stress levels, and enhance their capacity to cope with the demands of both military and civilian life.

Rest is not merely a luxury but a critical necessity for military personnel and veterans, especially in the context of PTSX. By exploring and implementing a comprehensive approach to rest, individuals can find effective pathways to healing and resilience. This holistic understanding of rest supports not only personal wellbeing but also strengthens the overall health and effectiveness of the entire community, military and civilian.

Comprehensive Guide to 25 Types of Rest

Have you ever thought of what the term "rest" really means? We have a list of 25 different variations of it. Each is unique in its own way and requires active participation that can lead to greater calm on all levels.

1. Physical Rest

Passive physical rest is the most fundamental form of rest, involving complete relaxation through sleep. For military personnel who may experience irregular sleep patterns due to duty schedules or deployments, passive rest is crucial for restoring energy, repairing muscle tissue, consolidating memory and flushing waste products from the brain and CNS.

Establishing a consistent sleep routine is important. Creating a sleep-conducive environment by using blackout curtains, sleep masks and comfortable bedding can enhance sleep quality. Minimizing disruptions with earplugs or white noise machines can also help. Taking power naps during the day to compensate for lost sleep at night is beneficial, but it's advisable to avoid napping too close to bedtime to prevent interference with nighttime sleep.

2. Mental Rest

The high-stress decision-making and constant vigilance required in military roles can lead to mental fatigue. Mental rest involves taking deliberate breaks to clear the mind and reduce cognitive load, i.e. not actively thinking about things. Practicing mindfulness techniques like deep-breathing exercises or meditation can center the mind. Using apps that offer guided meditation sessions can be helpful.

Scheduling short, regular breaks throughout the day to step away from complex tasks allows the mind to recharge. Engaging in activities that require minimal mental effort, like listening to calming music, enjoying nature or practicing simple hobbies, can also contribute to mental rest.

3. Emotional Rest

Military culture often emphasizes stoicism, which causes servicemembers to suppress emotions. Emotional rest allows individuals to express feelings openly without judgment or the need to manage others' perceptions. Seeking support from mental health professionals familiar with military experiences can be invaluable. Journaling provides a private outlet for processing emotions and reflecting on experiences. Participating in support groups where sharing is encouraged in a safe environment can facilitate emotional release. Open conversations with trusted peers, family members or chaplains can also provide emotional validation.

4. Sensory Rest

Exposure to loud noises, bright lights and constant alerts is routine in military environments, leading to sensory overload. Sensory rest helps mitigate overstimulation of the senses, promoting relaxation and reducing stress.

Creating a quiet, dimly lit personal space for relaxation can be beneficial. Using noise-canceling headphones or earplugs reduces auditory stimuli. Limiting screen time when off duty gives the eyes a break from digital glare. Engaging in calming activities like reading, listening to soft music, or practicing sensory-deprivation techniques like meditation in a dark room can also help.

5. Social Rest

The communal nature of military life can make finding solitude challenging, and obligatory social interactions may become draining. Social rest involves balancing time spent with others and time spent alone or with energizing individuals. Setting boundaries by politely declining social invitations when needed is important. Prioritizing interactions with friends and family who provide support and positivity can enhance social rest. Allocating time for solitary activities that rejuvenate like solo hobbies or personal reflection is also beneficial. Communicating the need for alone time to those around you builds understanding.

6. Creative Rest

Military roles often require problem-solving and strategic thinking, which can deplete creative reserves. Creative rest replenishes inspiration and stimulates innovative thinking by engaging with art and nature.

Visiting art galleries, museums or cultural events stimulates the mind. Engaging in creative hobbies like painting, writing or playing a musical instrument allows for creative expression. Spending time in nature—observing landscapes, wildlife or even stargazing—can inspire creativity and provide a fresh perspective.

7. Spiritual Rest

Finding a sense of purpose and connection beyond oneself can be grounding, especially for those who have faced challenging experiences. Spiritual rest nurtures this aspect of wellbeing, providing inner peace and direction.

Participating in religious services or spiritual practices that resonate with personal beliefs can be fulfilling. Meditation and mindfulness enhance spiritual awareness and can be practiced individually or in groups. Volunteering for community service or engaging in acts of kindness provides a sense of connectedness to something greater.

8. Environmental Rest

The physical environment significantly impacts stress levels. Environmental rest involves creating or seeking spaces that promote peace and relaxation, reducing stress influenced by surroundings.

Personalizing the living space to be calming and clutter-free can make a significant difference. Incorporating elements like plants, soothing colors or personal mementos brings comfort. Using natural lighting when possible and considering aromatherapy with calming scents like lavender can enhance the environment. Spending time in natural settings like parks or gardens can benefit from the calming effects of nature.

9. Digital Rest

Constant connectivity through electronic devices leads to information overload and stress. Digital rest reduces the mental clutter associated with technology, helping to improve focus and reduce anxiety.

Implementing tech-free times during the day, especially before bedtime, can be beneficial. Disabling non-essential notifications minimizes distractions. Using apps that monitor and limit screen time helps manage device usage. Engaging in offline activities such as reading physical books, exercising, or face-to-face socializing helps reconnect with the physical world.

10. Play Rest

Engaging in fun, leisurely activities without specific goals reduces stress and improves overall happiness. Play rest is about enjoying the moment without pressure or expectations.

Participating in recreational sports purely for enjoyment brings joy. Playing board games, video games or engaging in activities like dancing or crafting allows for relaxation. Allowing oneself to be spontaneous and embracing childlike wonder can enhance play rest. Planning regular playtime into the schedule ensures it remains a priority.

11. Solitude Rest

Solitude provides a much-needed break from the demands of communal living and constant interaction. It allows for self-reflection, personal growth and mental rejuvenation.

Scheduling regular alone time, even if it's just a few minutes each day, can be restorative. Activities like solo hiking, fishing, or simply sitting quietly provide space for introspection. Practicing meditation or mindfulness exercises in solitude enhances the benefits. Respecting the need for solitude and communicating it to those around encourages understanding.

12. Nature Rest

Immersion in natural environments has therapeutic effects, reducing stress and improving mood. Nature rest leverages these benefits for physical and mental restoration.

Spending time outdoors engaging in activities like hiking, camping or bird-watching connects with nature. Gardening or tending to plants at home also brings the benefits of nature. Even brief walks in natural settings provide significant benefits. Incorporating nature sounds or images into indoor environments can be helpful if access to outdoor spaces is limited.

13. Laughter Rest

Humor and laughter relieve tension, boost the immune system and improve emotional health. Laughter rest incorporates joy as a form of healing and stress reduction. Watching comedic films, stand-up shows or humorous online content brings laughter. Sharing funny stories or jokes with friends and family enhances connections.

Engaging in activities that naturally bring about laughter like playing with pets or participating in fun group activities, can be uplifting. Embracing opportunities to find humor in everyday situations enriches life.

14. Movement Rest

Gentle physical activities relax the body without the intensity of rigorous exercise. Movement rest helps release physical tension and promotes relaxation and flexibility. Engaging in slow-paced activities like Tai Chi or gentle yoga combines movement with mindfulness.

Taking leisurely bike rides or swimming at a comfortable pace provides physical rest. Focusing on movements that feel good and reduce muscle stiffness rather than aiming for performance or endurance enhances relaxation.

Movement rest involves engaging in low-intensity activities that promote blood flow and muscle relaxation without adding stress to the body. It aids in recovery from the strenuous physical activity common in military training and operations.

Incorporating gentle stretching routines can alleviate muscle tension. Practices like yoga or Pilates improve flexibility and reduce the risk of injury. Leisurely walks, swimming or light cycling can serve as active recovery, promoting circulation and aiding in muscle repair without taxing the body.

15. Hobby Rest

Pursuing hobbies offers a break from responsibilities and allows for personal fulfillment. Hobby rest is about engaging in activities purely for pleasure, which can reduce stress and enhance life satisfaction. Dedicating time to interests like woodworking, photography, cooking or crafting provides enjoyment. Choosing hobbies that differ from daily duties offers a mental shift.

Results from recent studies show that playing video games significantly relieves stress. Regularly scheduling hobby time ensures it remains a consistent part of the routine. Sharing hobbies with others or joining clubs can enhance enjoyment.

16. Cognitive Rest

Stepping back from tasks requiring significant mental effort allows the brain to recharge. Cognitive rest prevents burnout and maintains cognitive health, which is essential for decision-making and problem-solving.

Delegating responsibilities when possible reduces mental load. Taking mental health days to disconnect from work-related tasks provides a break. Engaging in simple activities like puzzles, coloring or light reading that don't strain the mind contributes to cognitive rest.

17. Connection Rest

Building meaningful relationships provides emotional support and a sense of belonging. Connection rest focuses on nurturing these deep bonds, which are vital for mental and emotional health. Spending quality time with loved ones without distractions strengthens relationships. Joining support groups or veterans' organizations connects with others who share similar experiences.

Participating in group activities that encourage open communication and trust, such as team sports or group hobbies, builds connection. Reconnecting with old friends or family members enriches social life.

18. Purposeful Rest

Engaging in activities aligned with personal values reinforces a sense of purpose. Purposeful rest integrates rest with meaningful action, contributing to overall life satisfaction.

Volunteering for causes that resonate like community service, environmental conservation or mentoring programs can provide fulfillment. Setting personal goals that reflect values and working toward them at a comfortable pace enhances purpose. Reflecting on achievements and how they contribute to life's purpose adds meaning. Engaging in spiritual or philosophical exploration, if it aligns with interests, can also be rewarding.

19. Transition Rest

Adjusting between different roles and environments can be taxing. Transition rest allows for adaptation and reduces stress associated with significant life changes, such as returning from deployment or transitioning to civilian life.

Establishing routines that provide stability during transitions can ease adjustment. Seeking counseling or support during significant life changes helps process emotions and plan steps forward. Giving oneself permission to take the time needed to adjust without undue pressure is important. Engaging in activities that provide continuity and comfort can also help.

20. Professional Support Rest

Accessing professional support provides tailored strategies and a support network, crucial for addressing unique military-related challenges. Professional support rest involves seeking guidance from experts. Reaching out to military chaplains, counselors, or veteran affairs services can be beneficial. Participating in therapy sessions focusing on stress management, trauma recovery or coping mechanisms offers support. Taking advantage of support groups where experiences and solutions are shared among peers provides community. Staying informed about resources and programs available to military personnel and veterans enhances support.

21. Physical Rehabilitation Rest

For those recovering from injuries, rest that supports healing is essential. Physical rehabilitation rest focuses on recovery and regaining strength, following medical guidance. Adhering strictly to medical advice on rest periods and rehabilitation exercises promotes healing.

Incorporating physical therapy sessions into the routine aids recovery. Balancing activity with rest to avoid overexertion is important. Practicing patience and self-compassion during the recovery process acknowledges that healing takes time.

22. Nutritional Rest

Proper nutrition is vital for the body's ability to rest, recover and perform optimally. Nutritional rest focuses on consuming a balanced diet that supports physical health, energy levels and overall wellbeing.

Consulting with a nutritionist or dietitian familiar with military demands can provide guidance. Incorporating a variety of fruits, vegetables, lean proteins and whole grains into meals supports health. Occasional fasting and restricting one's diet can also help calm the digestive system.

Staying hydrated and limiting caffeine and sugar intake, especially close to bedtime, enhances rest. Being mindful of eating habits that may be stress-induced helps maintain nutritional balance.

23. Financial Rest

Financial stress can significantly impact mental and emotional health. Financial rest involves managing finances effectively to reduce stress and create a sense of security.

Developing a budget to track income and expenses provides clarity. Using financial counseling services offered by the military or veteran organizations can assist in planning. Planning for the future by setting financial goals and creating savings plans builds security. Educating oneself on investments, retirement accounts and benefits available to servicemembers and veterans enhances financial wellbeing. Reviewing and adjusting the financial plan as needed ensures it remains relevant.

24. Identity Rest

Transitioning from military to civilian life can lead to identity challenges. Identity rest focuses on exploring and understanding one's sense of self beyond military roles. Engaging in self-reflection activities like journaling or counseling aids in identity exploration.

Exploring new hobbies or interests that define one outside of military service broadens identity. Connecting with others who have successfully transitioned to civilian life provides guidance and support. Considering career counseling to align skills with new opportunities can be beneficial. Celebrating achievements and recognizing a multifaceted identity enhances self-understanding.

25. Occupational Rest

Balancing work demands with rest is essential to prevent burnout. Occupational rest focuses on creating healthful work-life boundaries, whether still in service or in a civilian employment. Setting clear work hours and adhering to them when possible maintains balance.

Taking regular breaks during work to rest and recharge supports productivity. Using vacation days to take time off for rest and relaxation prevents burnout. Communicating with superiors about workload management, if feeling overwhelmed, is important. Prioritizing tasks and delegating when appropriate can reduce stress. Establishing a routine that separates work time from personal time contributes to a healthier balance, as well.

Rest Easy, Everyone

Rest is a multifaceted necessity that extends far beyond sleep. For military personnel and veterans, and anyone whose life is stressful or traumatic, recognizing and addressing these 25 distinct types of rest can lead to improved health, performance and quality of life.

By integrating these forms of rest into daily routines, those who serve can better manage the unique demands placed upon them, increasing resilience and a more balanced, fulfilling life. It's essential to personalize these strategies to fit individual preferences and circumstances, ensuring that rest becomes an integral and effective part of daily living.

Understanding and implementing a comprehensive approach to rest supports not only personal wellbeing but also strengthens the overall health and effectiveness of the military community. By embracing these diverse forms of rest, military personnel and veterans can find effective pathways to healing and resilience, particularly in managing stress and mitigating the symptoms of PTSX.

This holistic understanding of rest is a vital component in promoting a supportive environment where seeking rest and help is normalized, ultimately enhancing the quality of life for those who have dedicated themselves to service.

If-Then Guidance

- If you are experiencing mental fatigue or cognitive overload, then consider incorporating mental rest through mindfulness practices or short, deliberate breaks during the day.
- If your physical recovery feels incomplete after strenuous activity or injury, then prioritize both passive rest like sleep and active rest like gentle stretching or low-intensity movement.
- If overwhelming emotions are interfering with your daily life, then focus on emotional rest by journaling, seeking therapy, or joining a support group to process feelings in a safe, nonjudgmental space.
- If sensory overload from noise, light, or constant alerts is adding to your stress, then find moments for sensory rest by creating a quiet, dimly lit space or using noise-canceling tools.
- If constant social interactions leave you feeling drained, then make time for social rest by setting boundaries and choosing to spend time with supportive and energizing individuals.
- If you feel creatively depleted or uninspired, then explore creative rest through activities like painting, writing, or simply immersing yourself in nature to recharge your imaginative energy.

- If you feel disconnected from a larger purpose or inner peace, then spiritual rest through meditation, prayer or volunteer work might help you find grounding and fulfillment.
- If the demands of daily life feel overwhelming, then environmental rest can be beneficial; create calming spaces in your home or spend time outdoors to reconnect with nature.
- If you feel tethered to screens and technology, then prioritize digital rest by scheduling tech-free times and engaging in offline activities like reading, exercising, or spending time with loved ones.
- If your sense of identity feels unsettled after leaving the military, then invest in identity rest by exploring new hobbies, journaling, or connecting with others who have navigated similar transitions.

Take the Next Step

- Create a consistent sleep schedule that includes 7-9 hours of quality rest, and use tools like blackout curtains or white noise machines to optimize your sleep environment. Remember: sleep time allows the brain to remove metabolic waste products and toxins from its own delicate spaces.
- Incorporate mindfulness exercises, such as deep breathing or meditation, into your daily routine to provide mental rest and reduce stress levels.
- Communicate with family, friends or mentors about your need for rest, and work together to create a supportive environment that honors your health and recovery.

Through Their Eyes

"Flying was my life. From the moment I stepped into the cockpit of a T-6 Texan during Undergraduate Pilot Training, I knew I was exactly where I was meant to be. I worked harder than anyone, finishing first in my class and earning a slot to fly the F-16 Viper.

"That jet and I became one. Over ten years, I logged more than 3,000 hours in the cockpit and 200 of those in combat. I thrived under pressure, earned the Distinguished Flying Cross with V device and two Bronze

Stars and four Air Medals, and never let anyone outdo me. But all that came at a cost. Rest wasn't in my vocabulary. I was always reaching, pushing and striving for the next goal. Coffee and tea became my fuel, and I convinced myself I didn't need much sleep. That was a lie.

"The day it all changed was over the Pacific Ocean. A mechanical failure left me with no choice but to punch out. I'll never forget the force as I shot out of the cockpit or the shock of hitting the frigid water. My training kicked in and I survived, but something inside me broke that day.

"After the mishap, I wasn't the same. The Air Force was my identity, and losing it felt like losing myself. The constant buzzing in my head, the nightmares, the crushing weight of depression—it all became too much. I left the service early, after just ten years, feeling like a failure.

"It wasn't until I met a VA nurse practitioner who truly listened that things started to change. She told me I needed rest—not just sleep, but real, intentional rest for my body, mind and spirit. I started with stellate ganglion block. The first injection quieted the buzz in my head, and for the first time in years, I felt a flicker of calm.

"Rest became a practice, not a luxury. I learned to walk away from the 'more, better, faster' mindset that had driven me for so long. I started sculpting, something I'd dabbled in during college but never had time for. My hands shaping clay became its own kind of therapy.

"Today, I live on a small farm in central Pennsylvania, surrounded by rolling hills and the quiet I used to avoid. I wake up with the sunrise, spend my mornings in the studio, and sleep better than I ever have in my life.

"The Air Force taught me to fly, but rest taught me how to land. I'm not that person who needed to prove they were the best anymore. I'm just me—a sculptor, a survivor and someone who finally knows how to be still."

—Colonel Josh P., US Air Force (ret.)

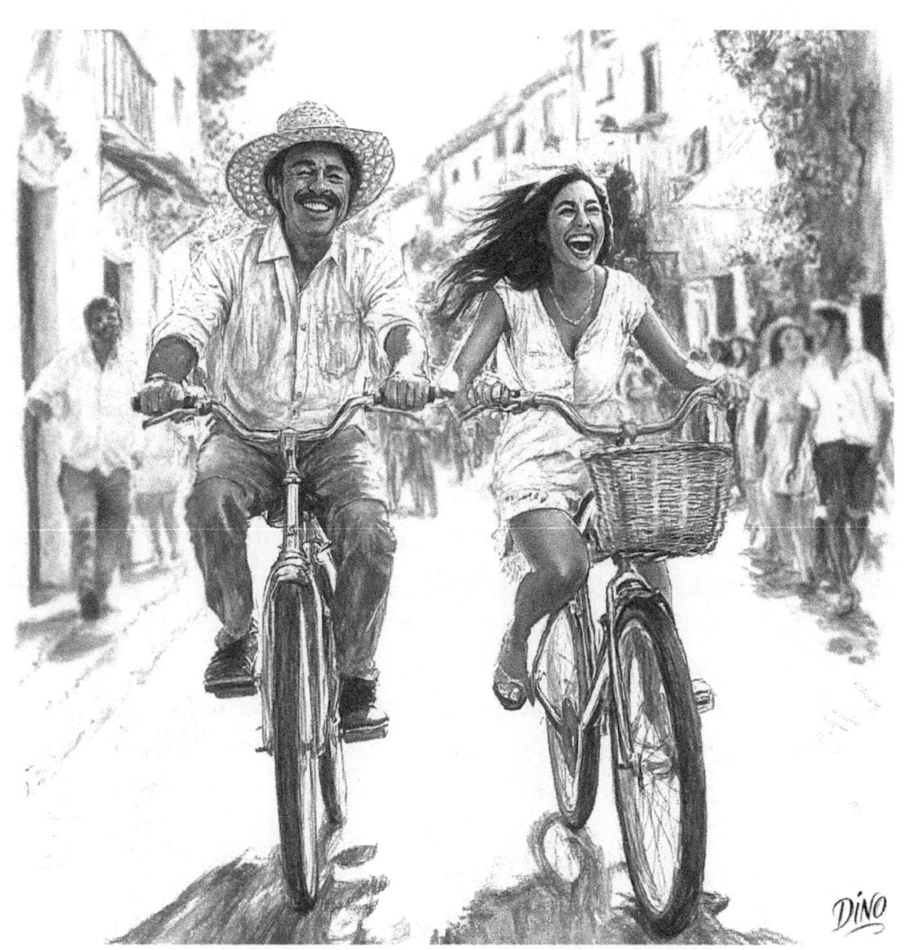
DINO

PART FIVE

Emerging Science and Innovation

38

The Anatomy of Hope: Healing the Brain After Trauma

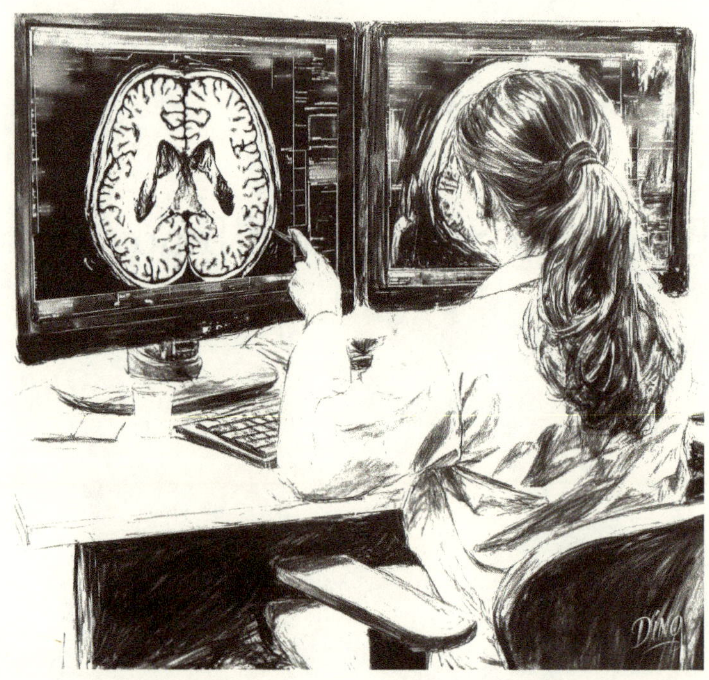

Sofia leaned forward in her chair, staring at the brain scans projected on a small clinic monitor. A former Air Force mechanic, she'd been grappling with nightmares and flashbacks she couldn't outrun. Her therapist explained how certain parts of the brain—like the amygdala and hippocampus—helped shape her fears and memories. It sounded complex, but somehow it clicked: her stress reactions had a very real, physical origin, and it wasn't just all in her head like several psychiatrists and psychologists kept telling her.

During the weeks that followed, Sofia began a new treatment plan. She learned that the brain can rewire itself—neuroplasticity, they called it. That idea gave her hope. Each therapy session felt less like dredging up old pain and more like building new pathways—cleaner routes for her thoughts. She tried MDMA-assisted sessions under careful supervision, finding moments of calm she never thought possible. Other days, she explored the idea of cannabinoids or got curious about how nerve-block treatments could reset the body's fight-or-flight response.

It wasn't a quick fix, but with each new approach, Sofia felt a small shift. The nights were less haunted, and she started sleeping more. She also noticed changes in her mood—less anger, more curiosity about the future. Learning how the brain handles traumatic memories helped her reframe her experiences. She felt in control again.

This chapter explores some of the emerging healing mechanisms of PTSX therapy. It explains how our brains adapt and how targeted treatments—from psychedelics to nerve blocks—can promote real healing. Each approach aims to quiet the overactive threat systems and strengthen the structures that let us process memories and move on. In doing so, we tap into the brain's remarkable ability to change, neuroplasticity, and offer a renewed sense of hope for veterans like Sofia, who've carried the burdens of past trauma far too long.

Neuroplasticity and Healing

Neuroplasticity, the brain's remarkable ability to reorganize itself by forming new neural connections, plays a pivotal role in the healing processes for military personnel, veterans and civilians grappling with PTSX. This concept is not merely an academic notion. It offers a biological foundation for recovery.

Understanding neuroplasticity enables mental healthcare professionals to harness the brain's self-healing capability, empowering veterans to overcome the debilitating effects of traumatic experiences. As we delve into this transformative process, it is clear that neuroplasticity is not just a scientific principle but a guiding force in the journey toward healing.

The mechanisms of neuroplasticity illustrate how the brain can adapt and change in response to experiences, including the therapeutic interventions designed to treat PTSX. When veterans engage in therapies that promote neuroplasticity—cognitive-behavioral therapy, exposure therapy, or innovative approaches like psychedelic-assisted therapies—they stimulate the brain's capacity to form new pathways that form strong, positive actions and behaviors. These therapies not only alleviate symptoms but also allow individuals to reframe their traumatic memories and integrate them into a healthier narrative. Remember: behavior changes chemistry, and chemistry changes behaviors.

> Stimulation techniques like Stellate Ganglion Block (SGB) directly target neuronal pathways to facilitate trauma recovery. By interrupting the sympathetic nervous system's response and reducing amygdala hyperactivity, SGB has shown remarkable efficacy in providing rapid, long-lasting relief from PTSX symptoms.

Emerging studies on the efficacy of psychedelic-assisted therapies, including MDMA and psilocybin, highlight the profound impact these substances can have on neuroplasticity. Research results indicate that these therapies can enhance emotional processing and decrease avoidance behaviors, leading to significant reductions in PTSX symptoms.

It is crucial to advocate for rigorous research and ethical practices in the implementation of these therapies, ensuring that the benefits of neuroplasticity are maximized in a safe and supportive environment. The integration of these findings into clinical practice can revolutionize how we approach PTSX treatment among military personnel, veterans and ordinary people who suffer from the same issues.

In addition to psychedelics, the incorporation of cannabinoids and stimulation techniques like SGB further underscores the diverse avenues through which neuroplasticity can facilitate healing. Each treatment modality not only offers immediate symptom relief but also engages the brain's adaptive capacities, promoting and maintaining long-term recovery. It is also essential to create an interdisciplinary approach that embraces these innovative strategies, enhancing the overall treatment landscape for veterans. This holistic perspective not only enriches the therapeutic experience but also nurtures a sense of community and shared purpose among practitioners and patients alike.

The Role of Neurotransmitters in Normal Function and in Recovery

The intricate world of neurotransmitters plays a pivotal role in maintaining normal brain function and facilitating recovery, particularly in the context of PTSX among military personnel and veterans.

Neurotransmitters, the chemical messengers that exchange or transfer information at synapses in our brains, are essential in regulating mood, emotional responses and cognitive processes.

This delicate balance can be significantly disrupted by traumatic experiences and result in the symptoms of PTSX. Understanding how these neurotransmitters function not only illuminates the neurobiological mechanisms underlying PTSX, but also underscores the potential avenues for innovative therapies that can aid in recovery.

In a healthy brain, neurotransmitters like serotonin, dopamine, norepinephrine and gamma-aminobutyric acid work harmoniously to promote emotional stability and resilience. Trauma can lead to dysregulation of these neurotransmitter systems and contribute to anxiety, depression and hyperarousal. For veterans, who often face unique stressors and trauma, this dysregulation can impede the ability to reintegrate into civilian life and maintain healthy relationships.

Recognizing these neurotransmitter imbalances opens the door to targeted treatments that can restore balance and facilitate healing, allowing veterans to reclaim their lives. The emerging field of alternative therapies like psychedelic-assisted therapy illustrates the potential of harnessing neurotransmitter activity for recovery. Psychedelics like MDMA and psilocybin, plus therapies like SGB and ketamine, have shown promise in recalibrating neurotransmitter systems, particularly by enhancing serotonin levels and promoting neuroplasticity.

Integrating cannabinoids into conventional PTSX treatments represents another exciting frontier in neurobiology. Cannabinoids can interact with the brain's natural endocannabinoid system, which plays a significant role in regulating stress responses and emotional regulation.

By modulating neurotransmitter release, cannabinoids can alleviate anxiety and enhance mood, providing veterans with additional tools for managing their symptoms. As research in this area progresses, it is vital for mental healthcare professionals to remain informed and engaged, ensuring that they can offer the most effective and comprehensive care to those who have served.

Targeting the Amygdala and Hippocampus

The neurobiology of trauma, particularly in the context of PTSX, has emerged as a vital area of research, especially for military personnel and veterans. Among the various brain structures pivotal in this landscape, the amygdala and hippocampus play critical roles in how we process fear and memory. Understanding their functions and interactions provides valuable insights into innovative treatment approaches for PTSX.

The amygdala, often deemed the brain's alarm system, is responsible for detecting threats and triggering emotional responses, while the hippocampus is crucial for forming new memories and contextualizing experiences. Together, these structures not only shape our responses to trauma but also offer a pathway to healing through targeted interventions.

This therapeutic alliance between the amygdala's emotional processing and the hippocampus's memory integration creates resilience, allowing military personnel to reframe their mental narratives and move beyond the confines of trauma.

The integration of cannabinoids into conventional treatment protocols has gained attention for its neuroprotective properties. Cannabinoids can modulate the hyperactivity of the amygdala while promoting neurogenesis in the hippocampus, thus alleviating symptoms of anxiety and depression commonly associated with PTSX. This dual action not only addresses the immediate emotional distress being exxperienced, but also contributes to long-term recovery by enhancing the brain's capacity to adapt and heal. Healthcare professionals can harness this knowledge to create comprehensive treatment plans that prioritize the neurobiological underpinnings of trauma. Remember: chemistry changes behavior, and these new behaviors, in turn, create a new chemistry.

Stimulation techniques like SGB further exemplify the direct targeting of brain structures to facilitate trauma recovery. By interrupting the sympathetic nervous system's response and reducing amygdala hyperactivity, SGB has shown remarkable efficacy in providing rapid, long-lasting relief from PTSX symptoms.

Coupled with therapies like ketamine infusion, which promotes synaptic plasticity and aids in the reprocessing of traumatic memories, these interventions offer an arsenal that's powerful in the care of veterans. The combination of pharmacological and stimulation techniques signifies a paradigm shift in how we approach PTSX treatment, emphasizing the importance of tailored, integrative strategies.

In this evolving landscape, it is crucial to remain informed and engaged with these advancements. Continuous training and education on alternative therapies, their ethical implications and their neurobiological foundations will empower practitioners to provide compassionate care that resonates with the unique experiences of military personnel.

If-Then Guidance

- If you are unfamiliar with the neurobiological mechanisms underlying PTSX and its treatments, then consider exploring educational resources or consulting with a healthcare provider who specializes in neuroscience or trauma therapy. Understanding how PTSX affects the brain and how treatments like neurofeedback or medication work can empower you to make more informed decisions about your care.
- If you are interested in how specific treatments target the brain's neurobiology, such as medications that impact neurotransmitter function or neurostimulation techniques, then discuss these treatments with your provider. They can explain the science behind these therapies and help you evaluate whether they may

be effective for your or your loved one's specific PTSX symptoms.

- If you are currently undergoing a neurobiological-based therapy like Transcranial Magnetic Stimulation (TMS) or neurofeedback, then work closely with your healthcare provider to monitor the progress of your treatment. Keeping track of symptom changes and brain health will help you and your provider adjust the treatment plan as needed for maximum benefit.
- If you are concerned about the potential side effects or long-term impacts of neurobiological treatments for PTSX, then ask your provider to explain the risks associated with these therapies. Understanding both the benefits and potential side effects will help you feel more confident in proceeding with the treatment or exploring alternatives.
- If you are finding it difficult to access advanced neurobiological therapies like neurostimulation or cutting-edge therapies, then explore clinical trial opportunities or specialized treatment centers that may offer these therapies. Some of these treatments may not yet be widely available, but clinical trials or research facilities can provide early access. Explore the connection between PTSX and brain health further, then consider undergoing brain imaging or cognitive testing. These tools can provide insights into how PTSX has impacted your brain function and help to guide more targeted treatment options.

Take the Next Step

- Read about how the brain can heal and change over time with the right therapy. Understanding this can motivate you to stick with your treatment.
- Ask about therapies that specifically target brain function, such as neurofeedback or EMDR.
- Start integrating habits that improve brain health, like regular exercise, a healthy diet, and mindfulness practices.

Through Their Eyes

"When I first came home, the idea that my brain could change—actually heal—seemed impossible. I felt trapped in the same patterns: anxiety, sleeplessness, and flashes of memory I couldn't control. Therapy felt like trying to fix a broken bone with a Band-Aid. I didn't know that my brain could rewire itself, that it had the ability to form new pathways and connections and rebuild what trauma had damaged.

"I'll never forget the moment my therapist explained neuroplasticity to me. He told me that my brain didn't have to be permanently stuck in this cycle, that the right therapies could help me forge new connections and change the way I responded to those traumatic memories. I had always assumed PTSX was a permanent scar on my mind, something I'd have to manage but never truly overcome. But understanding that my brain was capable of healing—that was a turning point for me.

"We started with cognitive-behavioral therapy, and it was slow going at first. It's hard work, facing those memories head-on, but each session chipped away at the fear and avoidance that had controlled me for so long. My therapist told me that with each new coping strategy I practiced, I was building new neural pathways. That gave me a sense of control, a belief that change was actually happening, even when I couldn't see it yet.

"Then came something that seemed even more radical—psychedelic-assisted therapy. I had heard about MDMA and psilocybin being used to treat PTSX, but I never imagined I'd be part of a clinical trial. But after years of medication and traditional therapies, I was ready to try something different. I remember feeling a deep connection with emotions I had buried for years. In those sessions, I didn't feel fear, just clarity. It was like the trauma had been locked away in a dark room, and suddenly, the door was open. I could walk through it, see it for what it was, and not feel powerless anymore.

"The treatment helped me process my trauma in a way I hadn't been able to before. And after the sessions, my therapist explained how the psychedelics had helped activate parts of my brain that allowed for this new perspective, how the brain's ability to reshape itself had made this possible. For the first time, I felt like I was moving forward, not just treading water. It hasn't been an easy road, but knowing that my brain has the ability to heal, that these therapies are scientifically grounded in the way the brain works, has given me hope.

"Neuroplasticity isn't just some abstract concept for neuroscientists to talk about—it's real, and it's happening inside me. My brain is learning, adapting, healing. I'm not the same person I was when I came back from deployment, and I won't be the person I was before I left. But now, I understand that I don't have to be.

"I'm forging new paths, not just in my brain, but in my life. It's taken time, patience, and the right treatments, but I'm living proof that change is possible. And that's more than I ever thought I could ask for."

— Tom, US Army Veteran

39

The Gut Microbiome and PTSX

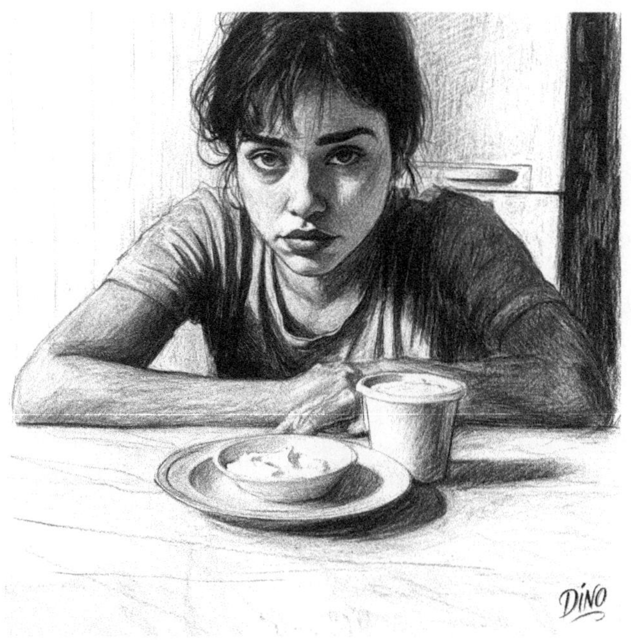

Laura never imagined that something as ordinary as her stomach could be a battlefield. She remembered being in her parents' kitchen when she was teenager, except things were entirely different. They had to practically hold her back from devouring all the food on the table. Now here she was, sitting in her own kitchen, staring at a plate of food she didn't want to eat. In fact, just looking at food made her sick just to look at.

The nightmares and flashbacks from her deployment had been relentless for years, robbing her of sleep and peace. The therapist called it PTSX, but to Laura, it was a thief—a constant presence stealing her sense of self, her joy, her health.

She reached for the yogurt cup her nutritionist had recommended. "Your gut," the nutritionist had said, "might be holding the key to your recovery." Laura had nearly laughed out loud. Her gut? After all she'd been through—combat zones, split-second life-or-death decisions, and the harrowing guilt of surviving when others hadn't—how could her gut possibly matter?

The idea seemed absurd until her curiosity got the better of her. Late one night, unable to sleep, Laura began to research. What she found startled her: the gut microbiome, trillions of microorganisms living in her digestive system, was intricately connected to the brain. It wasn't just about digestion. These tiny organisms influenced mood, stress, and even resilience. Dysbiosis—an imbalance in the microbiome— could fuel inflammation and disrupt the very systems that helped her body and mind recover from trauma.

She thought back to deployment, when meals were MRES, or Meals Ready To Eat, and stress was a constant companion. It made sense now. Her gut had been under siege just as much as her mind.

Laura picked up the spoon, hesitating before taking a bite of yogurt. It wasn't just food anymore; it was an act of defiance against the chaos that had ruled her life. One small step, she thought. One small spoonful. The fight for balance wasn't just external—it was inside her too. And for the first time in years, she felt a glimmer of hope.

This chapter examines the role of the gut microbiome in all forms of PTSX. We already know the gut has intimate connections with every tissue and organ in the body, including the brain and central nervous system. It is no surprise that microbes in our gut are involved in PTSX.

Unfortunately, PTSX is an all-too-common challenge faced by US military personnel and veterans, as well as their families and friends. It's a mental health condition that arises after experiencing or witnessing traumatic events, and it can affect how individuals feel, think, and interact with the world. Common symptoms include reliving the trauma, avoiding reminders of it, feeling on edge, and experiencing changes in mood and thought patterns. But while PTSX is often thought of as a brain-based condition, recent advances in science are shedding light on an unexpected player in this story. The gut microbiome refers to the trillions of bacteria and other microorganisms that live in our digestive system.

These tiny organisms are more than just passengers; they play an essential role in our overall health, influencing digestion, immunity, and even how we feel emotionally. The connection between the gut and the brain, referred to as the "gut-brain axis," is a powerful communication network that impacts mental health.

> The gut talks to the brain through microbial chemical Morse code. Feed your gut wisely and inflammation quiets like a machine gun finally out of ammunition.

Research shows that this gut-brain connection can be disrupted. Studies have found that people with PTSX often have imbalances in their gut microbiome, a condition known as "dysbiosis." This imbalance may worsen symptoms by increasing inflammation, interfering with the body's stress response, and affecting the production of important chemicals like serotonin, which helps regulate mood.

While the idea of the gut influencing mental health might sound surprising, it's an area of research that's growing rapidly. Early findings suggest that improving gut health through diet, probiotics, or other interventions might hold promise for reducing PTSX symptoms and improving overall wellbeing. This exciting field of study offers hope for innovative ways to support those living with PTSX. By focusing on the gut, we may unlock new paths to healing.

Overview of the Gut Microbiome

The gut microbiome is a remarkable ecosystem residing within each of us. Made up of trillions of microorganisms, including bacteria, fungi, viruses and archaea, it plays a crucial role in maintaining overall health. This microscopic world is concentrated in the intestines, where it not only aids in breaking down food but also communicates with the rest of the body in ways scientists are still discovering. One of the most fascinating aspects of the gut microbiome is its diversity. A healthy gut contains a wide variety of microbial species, each performing unique functions.

These include producing essential vitamins, regulating the immune system, and creating short-chain fatty acids (SCFAs) that reduce inflammation and support the integrity of the gut lining. In contrast, an imbalance in this ecosystem, called dysbiosis, can lead to health problems, including mental health challenges like anxiety, depression, and, as recent research suggests, PTSX.

The connection between the gut and the brain operates through several pathways. These include the vagus nerve, which acts as a direct line of communication between the gut and the brain; the immune system, which responds to signals from gut microbes; and the production of neurotransmitters, like serotonin, that influence mood and behavior. In fact, about 90% of the body's serotonin is produced in the gut, highlighting just how closely tied our mental health is to our digestive health.

Research into the gut microbiome and PTSX has revealed that individuals with the disorder often show reduced microbial diversity and an increase in pro-inflammatory bacteria. These changes may contribute to the heightened inflammation and disrupted stress responses seen in PTSX. The good news is that this field of study is opening doors to new ways of addressing PTSX, from tailored diets to microbiome-focused therapies. By nurturing this inner ecosystem, we may find innovative paths to support mental and emotional resilience.

Mechanisms Linking Gut Microbiome to PTSX

Understanding how the gut microbiome influences PTSX begins with examining the mechanisms that connect these two seemingly distant systems. Researchers have identified several key pathways that highlight the interplay between the gut and the brain, helping us better understand how trauma and stress affect the body. One of the primary mechanisms is neuroinflammation, or inflammation in the brain. The gut microbiome plays a significant role in regulating inflammation throughout the body. When the microbiome is disrupted, it can lead to a "leaky gut" where the intestinal lining becomes more permeable.

This allows harmful substances, like lipopolysaccharides (LPS), to enter the bloodstream and trigger systemic inflammation, including in the brain. Chronic neuroinflammation is often observed in individuals with PTSX and is thought to contribute to many of its symptoms, such as anxiety, irritability, and cognitive difficulties.

Another critical pathway is the stress response system, governed by the HPA axis. The gut microbiome influences how the HPA axis responds to stress. For example, certain beneficial gut bacteria help regulate cortisol, the hormone released during stressful situations. Dysbiosis, however, can result in an overactive HPA axis, leading to heightened stress responses and prolonged cortisol release—both of which are commonly seen in PTSX.

The gut also communicates with the brain through the chemical messengers that regulate mood and behavior. Remarkably, gut bacteria produce many of the same neurotransmitters found in the brain, including serotonin, dopamine, and GABA.

These chemicals play a direct role in mood regulation and emotional resilience. An imbalanced microbiome may disrupt the production of these vital neurotransmitters, contributing to the emotional dysregulation characteristic of PTSX.

These interconnected mechanisms—neuroinflammation, stress-response regulation, and neurotransmitter production—highlight the profound impact of gut health on mental health. As scientists continue to unravel these pathways, innovative approaches may emerge to treat PTSX by focusing on restoring balance within the gut microbiome.

Evidence from Research Studies

The connection between the gut microbiome and PTSX isn't just theoretical—it's backed by growing evidence from scientific research. These studies help illuminate the specific ways gut health influences mental health and offer insights into potential therapies for PTSX. One of the earliest clues about the gut's role in PTSX came from studies on animal models. Researchers exposed rodents to chronic stress or trauma and observed significant changes in their gut microbiome.

These changes included a reduction in beneficial bacteria and an increase in pro-inflammatory species. When the microbiomes of stressed animals were transplanted into healthy ones, the recipients began displaying similar anxiety-like behaviors, further supporting the gut-brain connection.

Human studies have also revealed compelling links. For example, research comparing individuals with PTSX to those without it consistently shows measurable differences in their gut microbiomes. People with PTSX often have lower microbial diversity, which means fewer types of bacteria performing the varied functions needed for optimal health. Additionally, elevated levels of harmful bacteria that promote inflammation, a hallmark of PTSX are present.

Preliminary findings from studies in this area suggest that probiotics—live beneficial bacteria—may help improve PTSX symptoms. In one study, participants who received probiotics reported reduced anxiety and better overall mood compared to those given a placebo.

Another promising area of study is dietary interventions. Diets rich in fiber, fermented foods, and prebiotics (compounds that feed beneficial gut bacteria) are being investigated for their potential to restore microbial balance and support emotional resilience.

While this research is still in its early stages, it's clear that the gut microbiome holds valuable clues about how to better understand and treat PTSX. These studies highlight the importance of continuing to explore this fascinating connection, paving the way for innovative and effective approaches to mental health care.

Factors Influencing the Gut Microbiome in PTSX

The composition and health of the gut microbiome can be influenced by a variety of factors, many of which are relevant to individuals with PTSX. Understanding these factors offers insight into how to protect and restore gut health as part of a comprehensive approach to managing PTSX. Diet is one of the most significant factors affecting the gut microbiome. Diets high in sugar, unhealthul fats, and processed foods—common in the Western diet—can disrupt the balance of gut bacteria, promoting dysbiosis. Conversely, diets rich in dietary fiber, fruits, vegetables, and fermented foods support a diverse and healthy microbiome. Foods like yogurt, kimchi, and whole grains nourish beneficial bacteria, which play a key role in reducing inflammation and supporting mental health.

Antibiotic Use and Abuse

Antibiotics, while essential for treating bacterial infections, can also disrupt the gut microbiome. Prolonged or frequent antibiotic use kills both harmful and beneficial bacteria, leading to a less diverse microbiome. This imbalance can have lasting effects on gut health and may worsen PTSX symptoms by increasing inflammation and altering stress responses.

Chronic Stress

Stress is another major factor that affects the gut microbiome. Chronic stress—a hallmark of PTSX— can alter gut motility, secretion, and microbial composition. Stress hormones like cortisol can create an environment in the gut that favors the growth of harmful bacteria while reducing beneficial strains. This stress-induced dysbiosis can amplify inflammation and disrupt communication along the gut-brain axis.

Comorbid Conditions

PTSX often occurs alongside other conditions, such as depression, anxiety, and irritable bowel syndrome (IBS). These comorbidities share similar disruptions in the gut-brain axis, including altered microbial composition and increased gut inflammation. Addressing gut health may therefore benefit not only PTSX but also these overlapping conditions, improving overall wellbeing.

Implications for Treatment

The growing understanding of the connection between the gut microbiome and PTSX has opened the door to innovative treatment approaches that focus on improving gut health. These interventions aim to restore balance in the microbiome, reduce inflammation, and enhance communication along the gut-brain axis, offering new hope for managing PTSX symptoms.

Probiotics and Prebiotics

Probiotics, which are supplements or foods containing live beneficial bacteria, have shown promise in supporting gut health. Certain strains, like *Lactobacillus* and *Bifidobacterium*, have been associated with reduced anxiety and improved mood. Clinical studies suggest that probiotics may help regulate the stress response and enhance resilience in individuals with PTSX. Prebiotics, on the other hand, are compounds that feed beneficial bacteria already present in the gut. Foods like garlic, onions, and bananas are rich in prebiotics and can support microbial diversity, creating a healthier gut environment.

Dietary Interventions

Dietary changes are another powerful way to influence the gut microbiome. Anti-inflammatory diets, such as the Mediterranean diet, emphasize whole foods, fruits, vegetables, lean proteins, and healthful fats. These diets promote microbial diversity and reduce systemic inflammation, potentially alleviating some of the symptoms associated with PTSX. Incorporating fermented foods like kimchi, sauerkraut, and kefir can further support gut health.

Fecal Microbiota Transplantation

Though still in the experimental stage for PTSX, Fecal Microbiota Transplantation (FMT) involves transferring healthy gut bacteria from a donor to a recipient. This procedure has shown success in treating severe dysbiosis in other conditions, and researchers are exploring its potential for resetting the microbiome in individuals with PTSX.

Psychobiotics

The term "psychobiotics" refers to probiotics and prebiotics specifically linked to mental-health benefits. This emerging field focuses on identifying strains of bacteria that directly impact mood, cognition, and emotional resilience. Psychobiotics represent a promising avenue for targeted interventions in PTSX treatment.

Integrated Therapies

Combining gut-focused treatments with traditional PTSX therapies, such as cognitive behavioral therapy or (EMDR), may offer synergistic benefits. By addressing both the psychological and physiological aspects of PTSX, integrated approaches could improve outcomes and enhance quality of life.

The connection between gut health and mental health highlights the importance of treating the whole person in PTSX care. As research continues to advance, these microbiome-based therapies may become an integral part of comprehensive treatment plans, offering new hope to those affected by PTSX.

Challenges and Limitations

While the connection between the gut microbiome and PTSX is promising, the journey toward fully understanding and leveraging this relationship is not without its challenges. Scientific research in this field is still in its early stages, and several obstacles must be addressed to ensure that these findings can be effectively translated into practical treatments.

One of the primary challenges is the complexity of the gut microbiome itself. Every individual's microbiome is unique, influenced by factors such as genetics, diet, environment, and medical history. This variability makes it difficult to establish universal recommendations for improving gut health in PTSX patients. Researchers must continue to explore how these individual differences affect both the microbiome and PTSX symptoms.

Another limitation is the difficulty in establishing causation. While many studies have shown correlations between gut health and PTSX, determining whether dysbiosis causes PTSX symptoms or is simply a result of trauma and stress remains a challenge. Longitudinal studies that track changes in the microbiome over time are needed to clarify this relationship.

Standardizing treatments is an ongoing hurdle. Probiotic and prebiotic supplements vary widely in their strains and dosages, and what works for one person may not work for another. More research is needed to identify which strains of bacteria are most beneficial for PTSX and how they should be administered for maximum effectiveness.

The cost and accessibility of gut-focused therapies also pose barriers. Advanced interventions, such as fecal microbiota transplantation, can be expensive and are not yet widely available. Ensuring that these treatments are affordable and accessible to military personnel, veterans, and others affected by PTSX will be essential as this field progresses.

Finally, it is important to address the stigma surrounding mental health and alternative treatments. Many individuals may be hesitant to embrace microbiome-focused therapies due to a lack of awareness or skepticism about their efficacy. Public education campaigns and clear communication about the science behind these approaches can help build trust and encourage their adoption.

Despite these challenges, the future of microbiome-based PTSX treatments remains bright. Researchers are actively working to overcome these limitations, and every new discovery brings us closer to a deeper understanding of how to harness the gut-brain connection for healing. By addressing these hurdles head-on, the field can move forward, offering new hope and innovative solutions for those living with PTSX.

Future Directions

The study of the gut microbiome in relation to PTSX is still in its infancy, but the future holds immense potential for this promising field. As researchers uncover more about how the gut-brain axis influences mental health, new opportunities for treatments and preventive measures are emerging. One of the most exciting areas of future research is the development of personalized medicine. Advances in microbiome sequencing and analysis could allow healthcare providers to create tailored interventions based on an individual's unique microbial composition.

For example, specific probiotic strains or dietary recommendations could be prescribed to address dysbiosis and support mental health. This level of precision could significantly enhance treatment effectiveness.

Another area gaining traction is the exploration of microbial biomarkers for PTSX. Researchers are investigating whether specific patterns in the gut microbiome can predict an individual's susceptibility to PTSX or their response to treatment. These biomarkers could not only help identify those at risk but also guide clinicians in selecting the most appropriate therapies.

The role of diet and lifestyle in shaping the gut microbiome will likely remain a central focus. Studies are expected to delve deeper into how specific dietary components, such as polyphenols, omega-3 fatty acids, and fiber, influence microbial diversity and resilience.

Public-health initiatives promoting gut-friendly diets could emerge as part of broader mental health campaigns, particularly for military personnel and veterans. Additionally, longitudinal studies will be crucial in establishing causation rather than correlation. Tracking individuals over time, from trauma exposure to PTSX development and treatment, will provide valuable insights into how gut health evolves and its impact on mental wellbeing. Such studies will help clarify whether microbiome interventions can prevent PTSX or mitigate its severity.

The field is also moving toward integrated therapies that combine microbiome-focused treatments with conventional mental-health interventions. For instance, pairing gut-targeted strategies with trauma-focused therapies like cognitive behavioral therapy could provide a more holistic approach to healing. Researchers are also exploring the potential of combining microbiome treatments with emerging technologies, such as virtual reality exposure therapy, to enhance overall outcomes.

Finally, increasing accessibility and affordability of gut-health interventions will be critical. Efforts to reduce costs and improve education about the gut-brain connection could make these therapies available to a wider audience, including underserved populations.

The future of microbiome research in PTSX is bright, with numerous opportunities to transform how we understand and treat this complex condition. By continuing to innovate and expand our knowledge, we can move closer to a world where PTSX is not just manageable but preventable and curable.

If-Then Guidance

- If you are experiencing digestive issues alongside your PTSX symptoms, then consider keeping a food diary to identify any potential triggers that may be disrupting your gut microbiome. Tracking your diet can help you and your healthcare provider pinpoint specific foods that may exacerbate dysbiosis and make informed decisions about dietary adjustments.
- If you have a history of frequent antibiotic use, then discuss with your healthcare provider the possibility of incorporating probiotic supplements or fermented foods into your regimen to help restore beneficial gut bacteria. Rebuilding your microbiome can mitigate the negative impact of antibiotics and support your mental health.
- If you are dealing with chronic stress, which is common in PTSX, then incorporate stress-reduction techniques such as mindfulness meditation, yoga, or regular physical exercise into your daily routine. Reducing stress can help maintain a healthier gut microbiome and improve your overall resilience against PTSX symptoms.
- If you are managing comorbid conditions like anxiety or irritable bowel syndrome (IBS), then explore comprehensive treatment plans that address both your mental health and gut health simultaneously. Integrated therapies can provide more holistic relief and improve your quality of life by targeting interconnected aspects of your health.
- If you are interested in participating in cutting-edge research, then look for clinical trials focusing on the gut-brain axis and PTSX. Participating in studies can give you access to the latest treatments and contribute to the growing body of knowledge that may benefit others in the future.
- If you are considering dietary supplements to support your gut health, then choose high-quality probiotics and prebiotics from reputable brands. Look for products that specify the strains and CFU (colony-forming units) counts, and consult with a healthcare provider to determine the best options for your specific needs.
- If you are curious about personalized medicine approaches, then

inquire about microbiome sequencing with your healthcare provider. Understanding your unique gut microbiome composition can enable tailored interventions, such as customized probiotic regimens or specific dietary recommendations, to better manage your PTSX symptoms.

- If you are feeling overwhelmed by the prospect of making multiple lifestyle changes, then start by implementing small, manageable steps toward improving your gut health. Begin with simple adjustments like adding a serving of fermented foods to your diet each week or dedicating a few minutes daily to stress management practices, gradually building towards more comprehensive changes.

Take the Next Step

- Schedule an appointment with your primary care provider or a mental healthcare specialist to discuss how your gut health may be influencing your PTSX symptoms. They can help you assess your current gut microbiome and recommend appropriate tests or treatments tailored to your needs.
- Take a close look at your eating habits and identify areas for improvement. Incorporate more fiber-rich foods, such as fruits, vegetables, and whole grains, as well as fermented foods like yogurt, kimchi, and sauerkraut to support a healthy gut microbiome. Consider consulting a nutritionist for a personalized meal plan.
- Start adding probiotic supplements or probiotic-rich foods to your daily routine to enhance beneficial bacteria in your gut. Additionally, include prebiotic foods like garlic, onions, and bananas that feed and support these good bacteria, promoting overall gut health.
- Connect with others who are also exploring the connection between gut health and mental wellbeing. Organizations such as the Gut Health Initiative or online communities focused on the gut-brain axis can provide support, share experiences, and offer valuable resources.
- Look for clinical trials or research studies investigating the

relationship between the gut microbiome and PTSX. Participating in these studies can give you access to the latest treatments and contribute to the advancement of scientific knowledge in this emerging field.
- Engage in activities that help manage and reduce stress, such as mindfulness meditation, yoga, or regular physical exercise. Lowering stress levels can positively impact your gut health and alleviate PTSX symptoms with a healthy gut-brain axis.

Through Their Eyes

"The dense jungles of Vietnam were more than just a battleground; they were a labyrinth of shadows and secrets that etched themselves into my very soul. Enlisting in the US Army at seventeen, I was driven by a sense of duty and the promise of honor. By 1969, I had earned my coveted green beret and SF tab, becoming a member of the Special Forces. My role as a sniper and hunter-killer tasked me with the perilous mission of tracking down Viet Cong, Laotian and North Vietnamese officers.

"Three tours in Vietnam tested my limits, both physically and mentally, leaving scars that wouldn't heal. The nights were the hardest. The sounds of the jungle—crickets, distant gunfire, the rustling of leaves—were constant reminders of the ever-present danger. As a sniper, isolation was part of the job. Hours, sometimes days, spent alone in the bush sharpened my senses but also deepened my solitude. The weight of responsibility bore down on me; every mission carried the lives of my comrades and the hope of my country. The enemy was elusive, their strategies cunning. Hunting them down required not just skill, but an unwavering focus that left me emotionally drained.

"Returning to the States in 1973 was supposed to be the end of my ordeal, but the war had already changed me irrevocably. The transition to civilian life was jarring. The camaraderie of the battlefield was replaced by an overwhelming sense of disconnection.

"I clung to the old war diet of raw meats as a way to maintain a semblance of the life I once knew. Little did I realize that this diet was wreaking havoc on my gut, laying the foundation for the severe health issues that would plague me for decades. As the years passed, my health deteriorated. I experienced chronic illnesses, unexplained fatigue and persistent digestive problems. My gut microbiome was in shambles, a silent saboteur exacerbating my extreme injuries, what they now call PTSX. The term didn't exist back then. Some dudes called it "Broke-Dick Disease," others just said it was fatigue and extreme stress.

"It wasn't until 2020 that I sought help from the VA, driven by a desperate need for answers. There, I met Dr. Emily Carter [not her real name], a compassionate gastroenterologist who specialized in the gut-brain axis. Through a thorough study of my medical history and a series of comprehensive tests, Dr. Carter uncovered the extent of the damage to my gut microbiome. The realization that my diet and prolonged stress had severely disrupted this delicate ecosystem was both enlightening and daunting.

"Dr. Carter crafted a personalized treatment plan aimed at restoring balance to my gut microbiome. We began with dietary adjustments, eliminating processed foods and reintroducing fiber-rich, fermented foods to nurture beneficial bacteria. Probiotic supplements became a daily ritual, alongside prebiotics to feed the good bacteria already present in my system.

"The transformation was gradual but undeniable. In fact, it took four years. As my gut health improved, so did my mental wellbeing. The chronic inflammation that had fueled my PTSX symptoms began to subside, allowing me to regain a measure of peace that had eluded me for so long.

"I've come to understand the profound relationship between PTSX and the gut microbiome. My experience has taught me that healing is not a linear path but a journey that requires addressing both the mind and the body.

"The resilience forged in the jungle became the foundation upon which I rebuilt my life, proving that even when the tunnel seems interminably dark, perseverance and the right support can lead to the light at the end.

"Each small victory in restoring my gut health reinforced my belief that recovery was attainable. Even on days when the memories of war overshadowed all that was good in my mind, the tangible improvements in my physical health provided a glimmer of hope, a reminder that progress was possible.

"My experience as a Special Forces soldier and Vietnam War veteran taught me that resilience is not born from the absence of fear or pain, but from the relentless pursuit of healing and the unyielding belief in a better tomorrow. I hope this message reaches those like me, men who feel lost and at the end of their rope."

—SFC Dale V., US Army (ret.)

40

The Role of Brain Imaging in Understanding PTSX

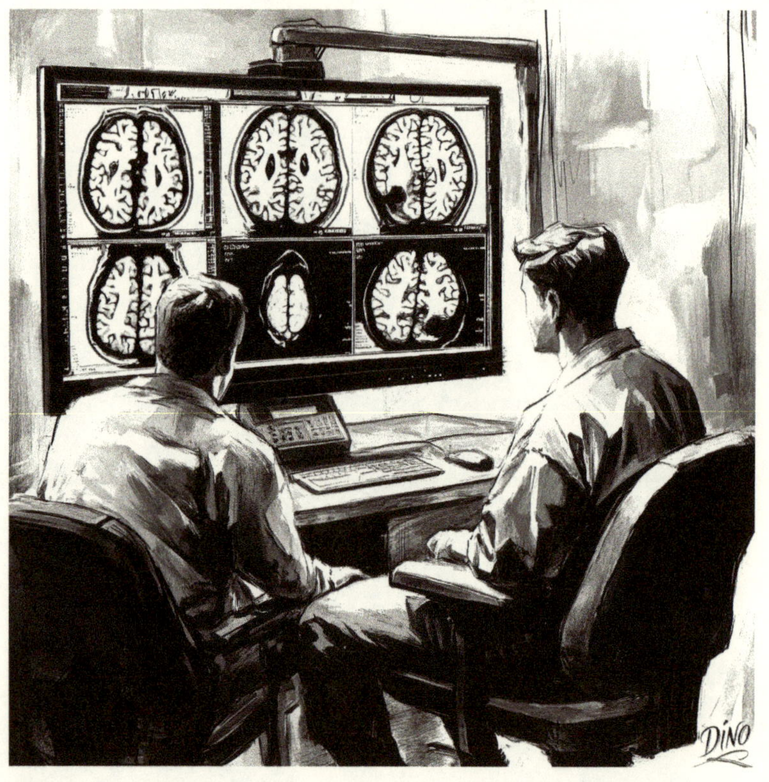

The scans didn't mean much to me at first. Black and white images on a screen, tangled maps of a brain that didn't feel like mine anymore. I sat in the doctor's office, arms crossed, staring at the flickering shapes. He talked about the amygdala, the hippocampus and some cortex I didn't remember the name of.

I nodded, but my mind was elsewhere—back in the desert, on the day everything went wrong. They said the blast wasn't close enough to hurt me, but they were wrong. It was close enough to leave me with ringing ears, a broken shoulder and ongoing nightmares. After that, nothing worked the way it should. I forgot things. I started fights. I jumped at shadows.

The doctor tapped the screen. "Here," he said, pointing at a spot glowing like fire. "Your amygdala is overactive. It's what's keeping you stuck in fight-or-flight mode." He showed me another darkened patch. "Your prefrontal cortex isn't doing its job to regulate it. It's why you feel out of control."

I grunted. "Can you fix it?"

He paused, nodded. "We can help."

It started with talk therapy. The first few sessions felt useless. I wanted to scream every time my therapist told me to "sit with the feelings." But slowly, things changed. They used the scans to track my progress, showing me how my brain lit up less with every session.

I still see those images in my sleep sometimes, the way my own brain betrayed me, the way it fought back when I gave it the chance. Now, I get it. Healing isn't about erasing the damage. It's about finding the light in the dark.

This chapter delves into how brain imaging has revolutionized our understanding of PTSX, aiding diagnosis, guiding treatments, and offering new hope. By bridging neuroscience and holistic care, these tools not only deepen our understanding but also pave the way for innovative and personalized therapies.

PTSX affects millions of military personnel, veterans and civilians worldwide, reshaping lives and challenging our understanding of trauma. Historically considered a purely psychological condition, advances in neuroscience and imaging technologies have revealed trauma's profound biological and neurological underpinnings.

Brain imaging, utilizing tools like Functional Magnetic Resonance Imaging (fMRI) and Positron Emission Tomography (PET), has become essential in this field, offering a window into the structural and functional disruptions caused by trauma. Through imaging, researchers have visualized how PTSX alters brain regions responsible for fear regulation, memory, and emotional processing.

Understanding Brain Imaging: Tools and Techniques

Brain imaging technologies allow scientists and clinicians to peer into the complexities of the brain, examining its structure, function and connectivity.

Functional Magnetic Resonance Imaging (fMRI): This non-invasive technology measures blood flow in the brain, correlating it with neural activity. It has proven invaluable for studying PTSX-related changes in emotional processing, fear responses, and memory functions.

For example, fMRI studies reveal overactivation in the amygdala during fear-based stimuli in PTSX patients. Researchers also use fMRI to measure therapy efficacy, observing changes in brain activity pre- and post-treatment, offering a dynamic view of recovery.

Positron Emission Tomography (PET): PET scans use radioactive tracers to detect chemical activity in the brain. This technique excels in mapping disruptions in neurotransmitter systems like serotonin, dopamine and glutamate, which are often implicated in PTSX. PET imaging has, for example, linked reduced serotonin receptor availability to heightened anxiety in individuals with PTSX, highlighting avenues for molecular interventions.

Diffusion Tensor Imaging (DTI): DTI maps the brain's white matter pathways, providing insights into connectivity between regions. Disruptions in these connections are particularly relevant in PTSX, as they can impair the communication between brain regions responsible for emotional regulation and memory.

Studies using DTI have shown decreased integrity in pathways connecting the hippocampus to the prefrontal cortex, illuminating the structural basis for symptoms like flashbacks and difficulty regulating emotions.

How PTSX Alters the Brain: Insights from Imaging Studies

Imaging studies show that three brain regions are profoundly affected by PTSX: the amygdala, hippocampus and prefrontal cortex. Together, these areas govern fear responses, memory processing and emotional regulation—functions often impaired by trauma.

The Amygdala: Hypervigilance and Fear Response

The amygdala acts as the brain's alarm system, detecting and responding to potential threats. In PTSX, imaging studies reveal that the amygdala becomes hyperactive, even in the absence of real danger. This heightened activity explains symptoms like hypervigilance, exaggerated startle responses, and persistent feelings of fear.

For example, fMRI scans show that individuals with PTSX respond to neutral stimuli—like everyday noises—with intense amygdala activation. This finding has driven treatments like exposure therapy and MDMA-assisted psychotherapy, which aim to recalibrate the amygdala's response. In the future, molecular-based treatments may prove helpful in directly addressing this issue.

The Hippocampus: Memory and Contextualization

The hippocampus is crucial for distinguishing past experiences from present circumstances. MRI studies consistently show reduced hippocampal volume in individuals with PTSX, impairing their ability to contextualize traumatic memories.

This shrinkage explains flashbacks and intrusive thoughts, where individuals relive trauma as though it were happening in real-time. Therapies like Eye Movement Desensitization and Reprocessing (EMDR) focus on strengthening hippocampal functions, enabling better memory integration and symptom relief.

The Prefrontal Cortex: Emotional Regulation

The prefrontal cortex (PFC) is responsible for regulating emotions and inhibiting inappropriate fear responses. Imaging studies in PTSX patients often reveal decreased PFC activity, which weakens its ability to counteract the overactive amygdala. This imbalance contributes to symptoms like emotional dysregulation, impulsivity, and difficulty concentrating. Treatments like mindfulness-based stress reduction (MBSR) and transcranial magnetic stimulation (TMS) have demonstrated success in reactivating the PFC, restoring balance to emotional and cognitive processes.

Functional Connectivity: Mapping Brain Communication

PTSX disrupts not only individual brain regions but also their communication pathways. Functional connectivity imaging has shed light on these disruptions, revealing how they contribute to symptoms.

Advanced neuro-imaging renders guilt, fear and love as colored constellations, living proof that emotion is electricity awaiting accurate rewiring.

The Amygdala-PFC Pathway

Imaging studies have shown weakened connections between the amygdala and prefrontal cortex in PTSX patients. This disruption reduces the brain's ability to regulate fear responses, leading to heightened anxiety and persistent hyperarousal. Successful therapies like Cognitive Behavioral Therapy (CBT) enhance this pathway, as evidenced by increased connectivity observed in post-treatment imaging studies.

The Hippocampus-Amygdala Link

Effective communication between the hippocampus and amygdala is vital for contextualizing memories and distinguishing threats from safety. PTSX disrupts this connection, perpetuating intrusive thoughts and flashbacks. Emerging therapies like neurofeedback and memory reconsolidation techniques aim to restore these links, as demonstrated in preliminary imaging research.

The Default Mode Network (DMN)

The DMN is a set of midline brain hubs—including the medial prefrontal cortex, posterior cingulate/precuneus, and angular gyri—that power up when we turn inward: day-dreaming, recalling autobiographical memories, or evaluating "How am I doing?" In healthy brains the DMN dims as soon as attention shifts outward.

In PTSX, however, imaging studies show the switch gets sticky and the network remains overactive, looping self-referential scenes of threat, shame, or loss. This persistent "background broadcast" feeds rumination, flashbacks, and difficulty focusing on real-time tasks. High DMN activity also couples with elevated amygdala firing, amplifying fear circuitry. Therapies that successfully reduce symptoms—mindfulness meditation, slow breathing, transcutaneous vagus-nerve stimulation—consistently normalize DMN connectivity.

This allows the brain to re-engage task-positive networks. Thus, targeting DMN dysregulation offers a concrete, measurable route to easing the cognitive and emotional load carried by people with post-traumatic stress injuries.

Brain Imaging and Treatment Development

Imaging technologies have been instrumental in shaping innovative treatments for PTSX. By visualizing how therapies impact the brain, researchers can refine interventions and optimize outcomes. Each year or so, new and updated imaging techniques come online, offering patients more and better diagnostic and treatment options.

Guiding Psychedelic-Assisted Therapy

fMRI studies reveal that substances like MDMA and psilocybin reduce amygdala hyperactivity and enhance connectivity with the PFC, facilitating emotional processing. These findings validate the reported therapeutic benefits of psychedelic-assisted therapy, guiding its integration into clinical practice.

Informing Non-Invasive Brain Stimulation

Imaging has shown how TMS reactivates underperforming brain regions like the PFC. This non-invasive treatment has demonstrated significant efficacy in alleviating symptoms of depression and anxiety in PTSX patients.

Imaging as a Tool for Precision Medicine

Imaging technologies are transforming the landscape of precision medicine in PTSX care, enabling more targeted and effective approaches to diagnosis and treatment. The ability to visualize the brain's structure and activity allows clinicians to move beyond symptom-based assessments, providing objective, data-driven insights into the condition. This precision aids in early detection, individualized care plans, and real-time monitoring of therapeutic progress.

Imaging biomarkers allow for individualized treatment plans. For example, patients with pronounced amygdala hyperactivity may benefit most from exposure therapy, while those with hippocampal dysfunction might require memory-focused interventions.

Identifying Biomarkers

One of the most promising applications of brain imaging in PTSX is the identification of biomarkers. These are specific biological indicators associated with the disorder. Structural changes like reduced hippocampal volume or increased amygdala activity have emerged as reliable markers of PTSX. Functional imaging like fMRI adds another layer by revealing disruptions in neural activity and connectivity.

Patients with hyperactive amygdala responses to fear-based stimuli are often diagnosed with PTSX, while those with significant prefrontal cortex hypoactivity may exhibit challenges with emotional regulation and decision-making. These biomarkers are more than diagnostic tools. They also help stratify patients based on the severity and type of brain alterations. This stratification allows for tailored interventions.

For example, a patient with significant hippocampal shrinkage might benefit from therapies that focus on memory reconsolidation and contextualization like eye movement desensitization and reprocessing (EMDR). Biomarkers also pave the way for predictive models that could identify individuals at high risk for PTSX following trauma, allowing for preventive interventions.

Monitoring Treatment Progress

Imaging technologies offer clinicians a powerful way to evaluate the effectiveness of treatments over time. By tracking changes in the brain, clinicians can assess how specific therapies influence neural activity and structure. For example, a patient undergoing Cognitive Behavioral Therapy may show increased activity in the prefrontal cortex, reflecting improved emotional regulation and cognitive control.

Similarly, fMRI studies have documented reduced amygdala hyperactivity in patients receiving MDMA-assisted therapy, providing a biological basis for the reported reduction in fear and anxiety. These imaging-based insights provide tangible evidence of recovery, not only reassuring patients but also guiding clinicians in adjusting treatment protocols.

For instance, if imaging reveals limited progress in a particular neural pathway, it may prompt the introduction of adjunct therapies like TMS or neurofeedback. By offering real-time feedback on treatment efficacy, brain imaging reinforces the precision medicine model, ensuring that interventions are optimized for each patient's unique neurobiological profile.

Ethical and Practical Challenges in Brain Imaging

While brain imaging has opened new frontiers in PTSX research and treatment, it also brings a set of ethical and practical challenges that must be addressed to ensure its equitable and responsible use.

Accessibility and Cost

One of the most significant barriers to the widespread adoption of brain imaging is its cost. Advanced imaging modalities like fMRI and PET scans require expensive equipment, specialized facilities, and highly trained personnel.

This high cost can make these technologies inaccessible to patients in underserved areas, including rural communities and regions with limited healthcare infrastructure. For military veterans, especially those relying on public healthcare systems, the expense may restrict access to these cutting-edge tools.

Moreover, geographic disparities exacerbate this issue. Large urban centers often house state-of-the-art imaging facilities, while rural and remote areas lack even basic diagnostic capabilities. Addressing these disparities requires investment in portable imaging devices, government subsidies, and telemedicine initiatives to bring brain imaging closer to those in need.

Interpretation Complexity

Brain imaging data is inherently complex, requiring specialized expertise to analyze and interpret. This complexity creates a reliance on highly trained neuroscientists and radiologists, which can slow the diagnostic process and increase costs. Additionally, the potential for misinterpretation is significant, particularly when data are used outside controlled research settings. For example, over-reliance on imaging findings could lead clinicians to prioritize structural abnormalities over a patient's lived experiences and symptoms.

To mitigate these risks, it is essential to integrate imaging data with clinical assessments and to ensure that healthcare providers receive adequate training in interpreting results. The development of standardized protocols and decision-support tools can also help bridge the gap between raw imaging data and actionable clinical insights.

Ethical Considerations

The ethical implications of brain imaging extend beyond accessibility and complexity. Ensuring informed consent is critical, particularly when working with vulnerable populations like trauma survivors. Patients must fully understand the purpose of the imaging, the potential risks, and how their data will be used.

Another ethical concern is privacy. Brain imaging generates highly sensitive data that can reveal not only health conditions but also cognitive traits and vulnerabilities. Safeguarding these data against misuse is paramount, particularly as healthcare systems move toward digital and interconnected platforms.

Finally, there is the risk of stigmatization. Imaging findings that reveal abnormalities could inadvertently label patients as "damaged" or "deficient," potentially impacting their self-esteem and social interactions. Clinicians must communicate imaging results with care, emphasizing their role as tools for healing rather than judgment.

Future Directions: Innovations on the Horizon

The future of brain imaging in PTSX research and treatment is driven by innovations that promise to make these tools more effective, accessible, and integrated into holistic care.

Machine Learning and AI

Artificial intelligence (AI) and machine learning are transforming the way imaging data is analyzed. These technologies can process vast amounts of data quickly, identifying subtle patterns and correlations that might escape human observation. AI algorithms can detect early signs of PTSX by analyzing changes in brain connectivity, potentially enabling earlier diagnosis and intervention.

Machine-learning models are also being used to predict treatment outcomes, helping clinicians select the most effective therapies for individual patients.

AI's ability to standardize and streamline data interpretation reduces the reliance on specialized expertise, making brain imaging more accessible and cost-effective. As these technologies continue to evolve, they will likely play a central role in advancing precision medicine.

Portable Imaging Devices

Emerging technologies are shrinking the size and cost of brain imaging devices, paving the way for portable solutions. Compact EEG systems, for instance, are already being used in field settings to monitor brain activity in real time.

Researchers are also developing portable MRI and PET scanners that could be deployed in clinics, community centers, or even military outposts. These innovations would bring imaging capabilities to underserved populations, ensuring that more patients benefit from cutting-edge diagnostics and treatments.

Integrative Therapies

The integration of brain imaging with other therapeutic modalities represents a promising frontier. For example, virtual reality (VR) exposure therapy can be tailored using imaging data to create scenarios that specifically target a patient's neural triggers. Similarly, neurofeedback systems that rely on real-time imaging feedback allow patients to actively retrain their brain activity, enhancing the efficacy of treatment.

As these integrative approaches gain traction, they offer a holistic model of care that addresses both the biological and experiential aspects of PTSX. This synergy between technology and therapy not only improves outcomes but also empowers patients to take an active role in their recovery.

Bridging Science and Healing

Brain imaging has revolutionized our understanding of PTSX, revealing the profound neurological changes that result from trauma. By offering a window into the brain, these technologies have deepened our understanding of the disorder, guided the development of innovative treatments, and paved the way for personalized care. However, their full potential can only be realized by addressing challenges related to accessibility, interpretation, and ethics.

The future of brain imaging is promising, with advancements in AI, portable devices and integrative therapies promising to create a higher impact and make these tools widely available. As research continues to uncover the intricate connections between brain structure, function, and mental health, imaging will remain at the forefront of efforts to heal the invisible wounds of trauma. Through ongoing innovation and collaboration, brain imaging offers hope for a future where PTSX is not just understood but effectively managed and overcome.

If-Then Guidance

- If you are experiencing persistent PTSX symptoms like flashbacks, hypervigilance, or emotional numbness, then consider discussing brain imaging options like fMRI or PET scans with your healthcare provider. These imaging tools can help identify changes in brain regions like the amygdala or hippocampus, providing insights into how trauma has affected your brain.
- If traditional PTSX treatments like Cognitive Behavioral Therapy or medication, have not provided sufficient relief, then explore

whether brain imaging could reveal specific abnormalities or disruptions in brain connectivity. This information can guide your provider in selecting more targeted therapies.

- If you are considering advanced therapies including transcranial magnetic stimulation or neurofeedback, then ask your provider how brain imaging could optimize these treatments. Functional imaging can identify areas of hypoactivity or hyperactivity in the brain, allowing for a more precise therapeutic approach.
- If you are worried about long-term impacts of PTSX on your cognitive or emotional health, then inquire about imaging to monitor brain changes over time. Tracking these changes can provide reassurance or signal when adjustments to your treatment plan are necessary.
- If you are managing co-occurring conditions like depression or anxiety alongside PTSX, then consider imaging as part of a comprehensive evaluation. Understanding how multiple conditions interact in the brain can lead to a more holistic treatment strategy.

Take the Next Step

- Consult your healthcare provider or mental health specialist to discuss the potential benefits of brain imaging for your PTSX treatment plan. They can guide you in choosing the appropriate imaging techniques like fMRI or PET scans, based on your specific symptoms and needs.
- Explore advanced imaging centers or hospitals that specialize in brain imaging for mental health conditions. These facilities often have the expertise and technology to provide detailed insights into how trauma has affected your brain.
- Ask about the availability of imaging-informed treatments like neurofeedback or transcranial magnetic stimulation. These therapies often work best when guided by precise imaging data that identifies areas of dysfunction in the brain.
- Research the costs and insurance coverage for brain imaging in your area. While imaging can be a valuable diagnostic tool,

understanding its financial implications can help you make informed decisions about incorporating it into your care.

- Consider joining clinical trials or research studies that use brain imaging to study PTSX. These programs often provide access to cutting-edge imaging technologies and therapies at no cost, while contributing to the advancement of mental health science.
- Stay informed about emerging brain imaging technologies and their applications in PTSX treatment. Advances like machine learning-enhanced imaging or portable imaging devices may soon make these tools more accessible and impactful for individuals with PTSX.

Through Their Eyes

"My name is Frank and I'm an 80-year-old retired First Sergeant of the United States Army. I served in Vietnam, where the days were long, the jungle was unforgiving, and the clouds of Agent Orange followed us everywhere. Back then, none of us thought much about the mist sprayed over the forests. We were focused on survival, not on the invisible war being waged inside our bodies.

"For years after my service, I lived a life that looked normal from the outside. I built a family, a career, and a life back home. But the invisible enemy I carried from Vietnam was biding its time. About fifteen years ago, I started noticing little things—dizziness, unexplained headaches, and fatigue that wouldn't relent.

"My family pushed me to get it checked out, but I brushed it off. I'd survived Vietnam, I told myself. This was just part of getting old.

"Five years ago, the truth finally caught up with me. A very detailed brain imaging scan, ordered after a particularly nasty spell of confusion, revealed what I'd been ignoring: tumors in my brain and other parts of my body.

"The word "cancer" hit like an ambush in the dark. My mind raced with questions, but one thought echoed louder than the rest: Agent Orange. Decades later, the toxic exposure had reared its head. The VA stepped in when I needed them most. They confirmed the link between my exposure and the cancer, and from that moment, they took care of everything. They got me the best oncologists, funded my treatments, and ensured I wasn't fighting this battle alone.

"The road to recovery wasn't easy: chemo, radiation and surgeries pushed my body to the brink. But every time I felt like giving up, I thought of my grandkids' laughter and my wife's unwavering support. I wasn't ready to let Agent Orange win.

"During this journey, the doctors also addressed something else I'd carried home from Vietnam: PTSX. For decades, I lived with the nightmares, the flashbacks and the hypervigilance that kept me on edge. I couldn't sleep without reliving the worst moments of my life. The VA introduced me to treatments like the stellate ganglion block and ketamine therapy, and for the first time in decades, my mind began to quiet. The nightmares faded, and I could sleep through the night. It was like waking up to a new world.

"Today, I live in my own home, surrounded by the family I fought so hard to protect. The cancer hasn't completely left me, and there are lingering effects of Agent Orange exposure—aches, fatigue and the ongoing doctor's visits. But I'm here. I'm alive. I can hold my grandkids, tell them stories about the old days, and watch them grow.

"Vietnam took a lot from me, but it didn't take everything. I fought to survive back then, and I've been fighting ever since. Thanks to the VA, the doctors and the love of my family, I've got time left to enjoy the peace I once thought I'd never find."

—First Sergeant Frank R., US Army (ret.)

41

Exploring the Role of Emerging Technologies in PTSX Treatment

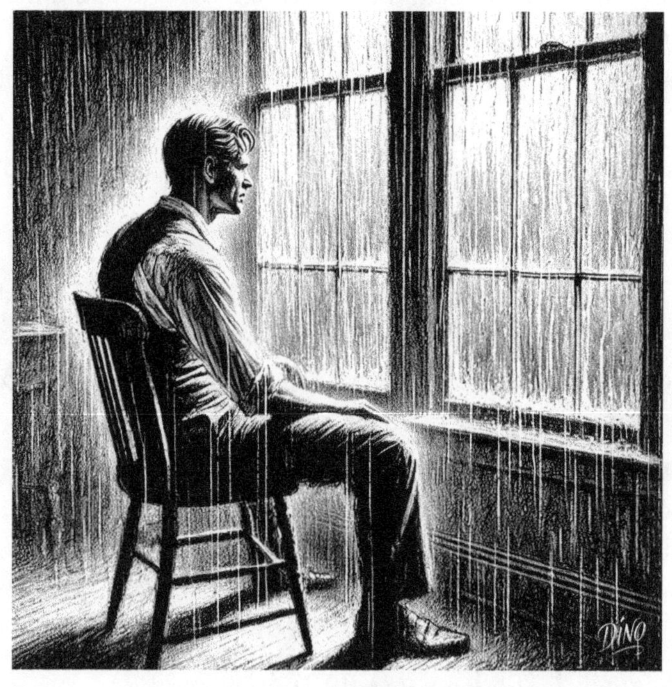

Jake remembered the nights he couldn't sleep—nights spent replaying patrols gone wrong and roadways paved with dread. He sat in front of a window as the rain poured down. In his wide-awake dream, the rain seemed to be falling all over him. It was a nightmare that visited him each night.

He'd tried traditional therapy and, while it helped with some symptoms, something still felt missing. Then a buddy mentioned a new virtual-reality program at the VA. At first, Jake scoffed—he'd seen these virtual-reality rigs in video game commercials, not mental-health clinics. But curiosity nudged him. A week later, headset on, he found himself in a highly realistic desert simulation, carefully guided by a therapist. That immersive environment let him process combat memories in a way simple talk therapy never had. On his smartphone, an AI-driven app began asking him daily check-ins—measuring his stress levels, offering breathing exercises tailored to his mood in that moment. He was skeptical at first. Could a chatbot really assist in his wellbeing? Yet, night by night, the small nudges helped him sidestep looming panic attacks. Even his therapist noticed the difference, calling it "old-fashioned therapy meets cutting-edge support."

Jake also downloaded an app specifically designed for veterans, reminding him to try grounding techniques whenever flashbacks threatened. It tracked his progress with each coping skill, giving him a subtle sense of achievement—almost like leveling up in a game. Soon, he even found himself willingly engaging in quick guided meditations before bed.

This chapter looks at emerging technologies like Virtual Reality (VR) for immersive exposure. It also examines AI tools for diagnosis and personalized treatment, and mobile apps that turn a phone into a pocket-sized therapist. It's an evolving field, bridging big ideas with everyday life for veterans who've long needed fresh options. Jake's story is just one example of how these tools can slot right into a veteran's routine, enhancing traditional care and offering new hope for managing the weight of trauma.

PTSX remains a significant mental-health challenge, especially for veterans and military personnel who have faced combat or other life-threatening situations. Traditional therapeutic approaches like cognitive behavioral therapy, medication and psychotherapy have been instrumental in helping patients manage symptoms.

However, with advancements in technology, new methods have emerged that are revolutionizing the way PTSX is diagnosed, treated and managed. Among these are VR, Artificial Intelligence (AI), and mobile health (mHealth) applications, which provide more personalized, immersive and accessible forms of treatment.

Emerging Technologies in PTSX Treatment

The complexity of PTSX, particularly in combat veterans, requires therapeutic strategies that not only address symptoms but also provide innovative, adaptive, and often personalized interventions. Traditional treatments can be effective but often come with barriers such as stigma, cost, availability of trained professionals, and the intensity of therapy itself. Emerging technologies are offering alternative solutions that aim to overcome these challenges by delivering cutting-edge treatments that are scalable, accessible and, in many cases, more engaging for patients.

"In the Navy, I always emphasized the importance of adapting to new technology. It's no different when it comes to PTSX. We need to embrace these emerging tools—VR, AI, mHealth apps and vagus nerve stimulators—because they have the potential to save lives and give veterans a path to real, lasting recovery."

Technologies like Virtual Reality (VR), AI and mobile apps provide the ability to simulate environments, offer real-time feedback, and deliver therapies directly to patients' smartphones, making them accessible regardless of geographic location or logistical constraints. For veterans who may be hesitant to engage in face-to-face therapy, these technologies offer the added advantage of anonymity, control over their therapeutic environment, and the ability to engage in therapy on their own terms. VR technology has proven to be one of the most exciting developments in PTSX treatment, especially in its application for veterans who have experienced trauma in combat zones. VR allows for a fully immersive, controlled environment where veterans can revisit traumatic events in a therapeutic context.

Currently, several major AI labs have a continually expanding suite of AI tools that can create hyperrealistic videos directly from text, speech, photos, etc. Therefore, it's entirely possible to generate a VR environment that mimics anything that a veteran or patient can conjure up, using memory in a story, actual photographs from their time in service, especially in combat.

Some of these engines generate videos capable of re-creating a whole environment that a mental healthcare practitioner can use to take a patient back in time and re-live traumatic experiences. And all in the safety and comfort of a comfortable office.

How VR Exposure Therapy Works

This therapy builds on the principles of traditional exposure therapy, which is a cognitive-behavioral approach where patients are gradually exposed to the source of their trauma. For veterans, this often involves recounting or reimagining combat scenarios that may trigger PTSX symptoms. In traditional therapy, this exposure occurs through verbal descriptions, written narratives or imaginative visualization.

However, VR takes this a step further by immersing veterans in a highly realistic, 3D-rendered environment that replicates their specific trauma. For example, a veteran with PTSX stemming from an ambush may be guided through a VR simulation that re-creates the sights, sounds and even vibrations of a combat environment.

Unlike traditional talk therapy, where veterans are asked to describe these events verbally, VR allows them to relive the event in a controlled, interactive space, enabling them to process their trauma more effectively.

<u>Benefits of VR Therapy Personalization</u>: VR therapy allows for the customization of experiences based on an individual's specific trauma. Whether it's a combat scenario, a car accident or other trauma-inducing situations, VR environments can be tailored to the individual's needs, ensuring a more effective therapeutic process.

<u>Safe Environment</u>: The ability to confront trauma in a virtual environment that can be paused or altered as needed gives veterans the confidence to engage in therapy without feeling overwhelmed. The therapist can control the intensity and pacing of the VR experience to

ensure the patient does not become retraumatized and, therefore, lose any ground in their ongoing therapy.

Realism and Immersion: The level of immersion in VR makes the experience much more vivid than verbal recounting or imagination-based exposure. This realism is especially beneficial for veterans who may have difficulty accessing certain memories through traditional methods.

Reduced Stigma: Veterans can undergo VR therapy in private, reducing the stigma that often accompanies seeking mental health care. Since VR technology can be deployed in clinical settings as well as in remote environments, veterans can engage in therapy without the visibility that comes with attending mental-health clinics.

Challenges and Limitations of VR Therapy

While VR therapy shows great promise, there are challenges that must be addressed. The cost of VR equipment, although decreasing, can still be prohibitive for some treatment centers. Additionally, some veterans may feel discomfort or disorientation when using VR headsets for extended periods, which can limit its applicability. Finally, while VR is effective for many, it may not be suitable for all types of trauma or for individuals who struggle with severe dissociative symptoms.

Artificial Intelligence in PTSX Diagnosis and Treatment

Artificial Intelligence (AI) is revolutionizing PTSX treatment through predictive analytics, personalized treatment plans, and AI-driven therapy tools. By leveraging machine-learning algorithms, AI can identify patterns in patient data, which helps healthcare providers create more effective treatment plans tailored to each individual's specific symptoms and history.

One of the most promising uses of AI in PTSX treatment is its ability to assist in early diagnosis. AI algorithms can analyze large datasets from clinical notes, patient histories and behavioral assessments to detect patterns indicative of PTSX. AI models have been trained to analyze the content of clinical interviews, social media posts, and even speech patterns to detect markers of PTSX. An accurate diagnosis leads to more timely interventions, potentially reducing the severity of symptoms.

AI in Personalized Treatment Plans

Beyond diagnosis, AI can also assist in the creation of personalized treatment plans. Machine learning models can predict how a patient will respond to different types of therapy or medication based on their unique characteristics like their genetic profile, trauma history and previous treatment outcomes.

This personalized approach can improve treatment efficacy and reduce the time it takes to find the most effective intervention for each veteran. Some AI platforms are designed to analyze patient data and recommend the best course of action, whether that is exposure therapy, medication, or alternative treatments like biofeedback or mindfulness practices.

AI can also predict the likelihood of treatment adherence, allowing healthcare providers to proactively adjust their approach based on individual patient needs.

AI-Powered Therapeutic Tools

AI is also being used to create interactive therapeutic tools like AI-driven chatbots and virtual therapists. These tools can guide veterans through therapeutic exercises, provide real-time feedback, and even offer emotional support outside of traditional therapy sessions. For veterans who may be reluctant to engage in face-to-face therapy, AI chatbots can offer an alternative form of engagement that is available 24/7.

Some AI-driven tools offer cognitive behavioral therapy exercises and mood tracking through conversational interfaces. These tools not only provide a level of immediate emotional support but also collect valuable data that can help therapists better understand their patients' progress between sessions.

Challenges and Considerations of AI in PTSX Treatment

Despite its benefits, AI in PTSX treatment raises several challenges. Data privacy and security are major concerns, as sensitive mental health data must be carefully protected. Additionally, reliance on AI for mental health care could depersonalize the therapeutic process if not carefully managed. And, of course, there are ethical considerations around the use of AI to make decisions about patient care, particularly in cases where AI might override human judgment.

Applications: Accessible and On-Demand Therapy

Mobile health (mHealth) applications offer veterans with PTSX an accessible way to manage their symptoms and engage in therapeutic exercises on their own time. These apps provide a range of services, from mindfulness and meditation exercises to cognitive behavioral therapy tools that veterans can use to monitor and manage their symptoms.

Popular PTSX mHealth Apps PTSX Coach: Developed by the VA and the DoD, PTSX Coach provides users with tools to help manage their symptoms, track progress, and access professional resources. It offers features like mood tracking, symptom checklists, and personalized coping strategies.

Breathe2Relax: This app focuses on breathing exercises to help veterans manage stress and anxiety. Since breathing techniques are a key component of PTSX treatment, the app provides simple yet effective tools to reduce stress and panic attacks. So far, it's received hundreds of five-star reviews.

Headspace and Calm: While not specifically designed for PTSX, meditation apps like Headspace and Calm offer veterans mindfulness exercises that can help them manage anxiety and sleep disturbances, both common in PTSX patients.

Benefits of mHealth for Veterans Accessibility: Veterans can use these apps anytime, anywhere, making it easier to integrate therapy into daily life. For those who live in remote areas or are unable to regularly attend therapy, mHealth apps can provide a practical alternative.

Anonymity: Mobile apps allow veterans to seek help discreetly, which is crucial in overcoming the stigma that often surrounds mental health treatment, particularly within the military community.

Self-Empowerment: By giving veterans tools to manage their symptoms independently, mHealth apps promote self-reliance and empowerment. Veterans can take an active role in their recovery, tracking their progress and engaging in exercises at their own pace.

Limitations of mHealth Apps: Despite their accessibility, mHealth apps have limitations. They cannot replace the therapeutic relationship between a veteran and a trained professional. The effectiveness of these apps depends on user engagement, and some veterans may struggle to maintain consistent use without the accountability provided by regular therapy sessions. Not all apps are evidence-based, making it crucial for veterans to use those endorsed by credible organizations, such as the VA.

The Future of PTSX Treatment Through Technology

Emerging technologies like VR, AI and mobile-health applications are transforming PTSX treatment, especially for veterans. These technologies offer new ways to diagnose, treat, and manage PTSX by providing personalized, accessible and innovative therapeutic options. The VA must partner with advanced companies and firms to design and create VR tools that can be used as therapeutic aids.

While there are challenges—such as ensuring patient privacy, maintaining engagement, and addressing ethical concerns—these technologies represent a major step forward in mental healthcare. As technology continues to advance, we can expect even more innovative solutions that address the complexities of PTSX, providing hope for veterans and their families. The integration of these technologies into traditional treatment approaches offers a future where PTSX care is more effective, personalized and widely available.

Could Artificial Stimulation of the Vagus Nerve Heal PTSX?

The vagus nerve is also called The Great Nerve for its immense size, reach and influence in the human body. It is intimately connected to every organ in the body and communicates directly with the gut microbiome.

Briefly, it's been demonstrated in many clinical studies the power of stumulating the vagus nerve using both implanted devices and externally applied stimuli. The results continue to flow in and all are very impressive and promising. We discuss it and its action in the final chapter, "The Vagus Nerve and the Molecular Nature of Neuroinflammation."

If-Then Guidance

- If you are a veteran or clinician seeking innovative ways to manage PTSX symptoms,then consider exploring emerging technologies like VR, AI, and mHealth applications for treatment. These tools can provide immersive, personalized and accessible options for therapy.
- If a veteran has difficulty processing traumatic combat experiences through traditional therapy, then VR exposure therapy may be a viable option, offering immersive, controlled environments to safely revisit and desensitize traumatic memories.
- If a veteran feels overwhelmed by the intensity of re-experiencing trauma, then the therapist can adjust the pacing and intensity of the VR exposure to ensure the veteran feels safe and not retraumatized.
- If stigma is a barrier to seeking face-to-face therapy, then VR therapy can provide a private and less stigmatized way to engage in treatment.
- If early diagnosis of PTSX is crucial for a veteran's treatment, then AI-powered diagnostic tools can help identify patterns in clinical notes, interviews, or social media behavior that may indicate PTSX, allowing for timely intervention.
- If a veteran's response to traditional therapy or medication is inconsistent, then AI can analyze patient data to recommend a personalized treatment plan, improving the chances of finding the most effective therapy faster.
- If a veteran is reluctant to engage with a human therapist, then AI-powered therapeutic tools like chatbots can offer real-time support, guiding veterans through cognitive exercises and providing immediate emotional relief.
- If a veteran prefers to manage symptoms independently or cannot regularly attend in-person therapy, then mHealth apps like PTSX Coach or Breathe2Relax can provide self-guided tools for tracking symptoms and practicing coping techniques.
- If a veteran feels self-conscious about seeking therapy, then using mHealth apps provides a discreet and anonymous way to receive help without the stigma of attending a mental health clinic.

- If a veteran struggles with stress, anxiety or panic attacks, then mHealth apps focused on mindfulness and breathing techniques, such as Headspace or Calm, can offer immediate, on-demand exercises to reduce symptoms.
- If cost or access to technology (like VR equipment) is a concern, then seek out programs or organizations, such as the VA, that provide access to these technologies at lower costs or offer alternatives.
- If a veteran experiences discomfort with VR or AI technology, then it may be beneficial to start with shorter, simpler sessions and consult with a mental-health professional about alternative treatments.
- If data privacy is a concern when using AI or mHealth apps, then ensure that the tools and platforms used are from reputable sources, such as those endorsed by the VA or other credible mental health organizations, to safeguard personal information.

Take the Next Step

- Research how technologies like VR are being used in PTSX treatment.
- If you are interested in VR therapy, ask your mental-health provider if it's available in your area or through the VA.
- Look into AI-based apps or online tools that help track and manage PTSX symptoms, providing on-demand support.

Through Their Eyes

"As a Navy admiral who flew attack aircraft and commanded aircraft carriers, I spent years at the helm of some of the most complex military operations. Leading men and women into combat and knowing the weight of every decision I made—each one affecting the lives of my crew—was a responsibility I carried with honor.

"But as anyone who has served in combat knows, the battle doesn't end when you leave the theater of war. The fight continues within. For many of us, that internal struggle comes in the form of PTSX. I've witnessed firsthand how traditional approaches to PTSX—talk therapy, medication—have helped countless sailors and Marines manage their symptoms. But I've also seen how these treatments fall short. The reality is that trauma runs deep, and conventional methods don't always penetrate to the root of the problem.

"You're left with a patchwork solution—medication to dull the edge, therapy that often doesn't go far enough. It's effective for some, but for many, including myself, the healing feels incomplete.

"My perspective changed when I started learning about the emerging technologies now being integrated into PTSX treatment. In command, I always valued the ability to adapt—whether that meant implementing new strategies or integrating cutting-edge technology into operations. PTSX treatment should be no different.

"One of the most promising tools I've seen is VR therapy. The immersive nature of VR offers a controlled environment where veterans like me can confront their trauma head-on, but without the unpredictability of reliving it in real life. For those of us who've seen combat up close—experienced the chaos of a firefight or the sheer stress of managing lives at stake—VR can simulate those scenarios in a way that allows us to process them safely. I've spoken with veterans who've undergone VR exposure therapy, and their stories are nothing short of remarkable.

"They describe being able to revisit the most traumatic moments of their service in a controlled, almost surgical manner, where they work through their emotions rather than be overwhelmed by them. The immersion makes it real, but the safety of the controlled environment makes it manageable. In essence, VR is helping veterans confront their worst fears while maintaining control—a luxury many of us lost during the actual events.

"The integration of AI into PTSX treatment is another game changer. AI has the potential to personalize treatments in a way we've never seen before. During my command years, I always believed in tailoring leadership to the individual needs of my sailors.

"Some thrived under pressure, others needed guidance and support. AI offers that kind of tailored approach to PTSX treatment—analyzing patterns, providing insights into what works best for each veteran based on their history and responses to treatment. For those of us who've experienced combat, PTSX can manifest in different ways. One size does not fit all. AI can help create more precise treatment plans by analyzing a veteran's specific trauma, predicting how they might respond to different therapies, and suggesting alternatives if the current approach isn't working.

"It's not about replacing therapists—it's about equipping them with more information, more tools to get us the help we need. Then there are mobile health (mHealth) apps, which are something I wish we had decades ago. As a commanding officer, my time was always stretched thin, and I imagine that for active-duty personnel and veterans today, the time constraints are no different.

"Having tools like PTSX Coach and other mindfulness apps right on your smartphone gives veterans the ability to manage symptoms in real-time, no matter where they are. These apps provide exercises, track mood and symptoms, and offer coping strategies whenever you need them.

"In the Navy, I always emphasized the importance of adapting to new technology. It's no different when it comes to PTSX. We need to embrace these emerging tools—VR, AI, mHealth apps and vagus nerve stimulators—because they have the potential to save lives and give veterans a path to real, lasting recovery.

"These aren't just tech gimmicks. They're vital tools in the fight against the invisible wounds of war. The military taught me that while leadership requires adapting to new challenges, so does healing. The integration of these technologies is our next evolution in care. And while they're not a replacement for traditional methods, they are essential additions to our toolkit.

"It's my hope that these innovations continue to grow and become more widely available, not just within the VA but across all military branches. Our servicemembers and veterans deserve the best we can offer, and these emerging technologies are a crucial part of that promise."

—Admiral John S., US Navy (ret.)

42

Future Trends in PTSX Care: The Next Decade

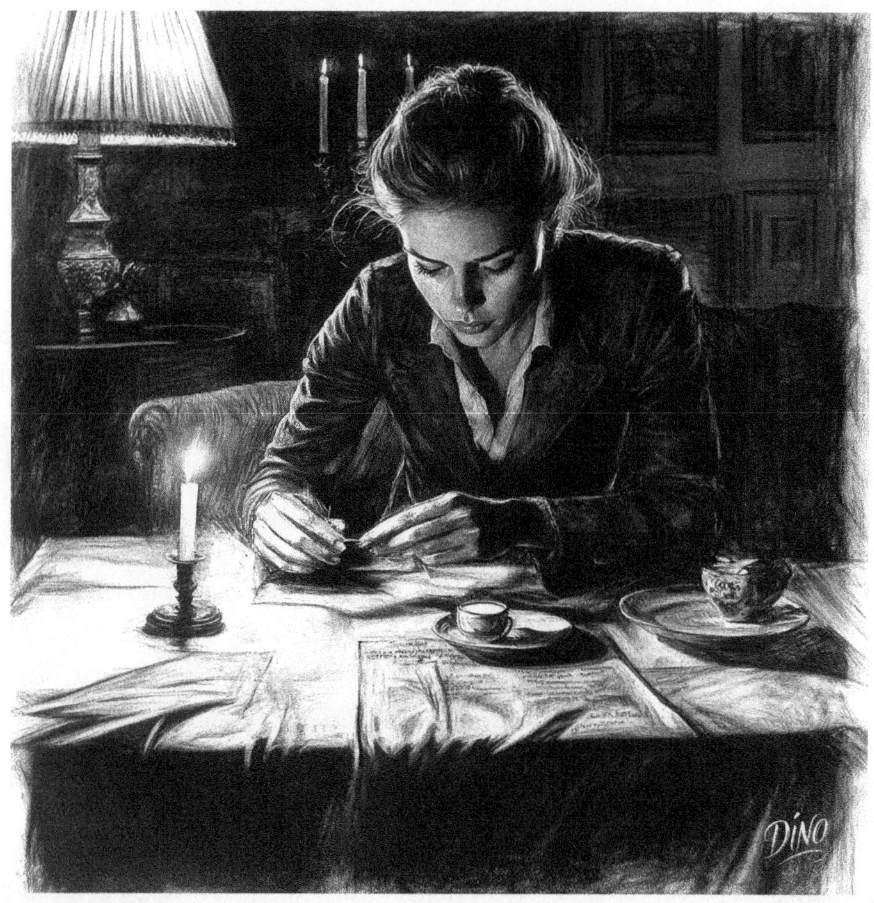

Natalia glanced at the small candle on the table, wondering if it were some kind of crystal ball that could heal her. After spending a decade fighting her own nightmares, she never thought she'd be looking at ideas like gene editing and VR-based therapy, but here they were, laid out by a small team of forward-thinking researchers in a detailed brochure. She felt a curious mix of skepticism and hope. Could editing specific genes, or using a device that targets the precise region of his brain where fear took root, actually help people like her?

One section of the brochure detailed "CRISPR for Anxiety"—something that almost sounded like science fiction. Another highlighted personalized medicine, where a simple genetic test could predict which medication would work best, sparing patients the painful roulette of trial-and-error prescriptions over many months or years.

She paused at a graphic about psychedelics—how MDMA or psilocybin might be integrated into mainstream treatment, pairing deep emotional work with scientific rigor. She remembered how only recently, those substances were dismissed as fringe. Now they carried the promise of FDA breakthrough status.

And then there was neurostimulation—transcranial magnetic pulses or even deeper forms of brain stimulation that might "reboot" trauma-circuits. Each approach, once unthinkable, felt tangible as she scanned the data: smaller pilot studies, early but encouraging results, case after case of veterans experiencing real relief.

It was overwhelming, but also uplifting. Sitting there, Natalia felt a spark. The field wasn't just inching forward. It was leaping. Over the next decade, these ideas could reshape the entire landscape of PTSX care—from gene therapy that might prevent the disorder from taking root, to custom drug regimens informed by each patient's biology, to advanced neurotech that tackled the problem at its source.

This chapter offers a glimpse into the potential future of PTSX treatment. If the past few years have taught us anything, it's that breakthroughs can come fast—and for many veterans, that can't happen soon enough. By leaning into emerging science, embracing new mindsets, and keeping patient-centered healing at the core, the next 10 years might just deliver the seismic shift in care that so many have been waiting for.

As our understanding of PTSX expands, so does the range of effective treatment options for veterans and other trauma survivors. Over the coming decade, breakthroughs in scientific research, cutting-edge technology, and personalized medicine promise to reshape the PTSX care landscape, offering renewed hope and more targeted interventions. The future of PTSX treatment will likely focus on creating more effective, tailored interventions that address the unique needs of each individual.

Gene Therapy and PTSX: Unlocking Solutions at the Molecular Level

One of the most exciting developments in PTSX treatment is the potential for gene therapy to play a role in addressing trauma at a molecular level. Researchers and physicians are excited about applying gene therapy to PTSX, given the promising results from other studies. For example, patients with transfusion-dependent beta thalassemia often require lifelong blood transfusions.

> Ten-year horizon: precision-medicine dashboards marry genomics, wearables and AI triage so that tomorrow's treatments feel like bespoke armor for the mind. A life-changer.

In August 2022, the FDA approved Zynteglo, a beta-globin gene therapy that enables the patient's body to start producing healthy red blood cells. Several patients have been declared transfusion-free post-treatment, marking a life-changing result and minimizing complications associated with long-term transfusions. Zynteglo is a clinical success but a commercial work-in-progress. It has proven its ability to free patients from lifelong transfusions. However, its extremely high cost, at $2.8 million per patient, has limited its adoption, and it now faces powerful competition from Casgevy, which uses the more widely known CRISPR technology. The story of Zynteglo is no longer just about a scientific breakthrough but about the complex economic and competitive realities of the modern gene therapy market.

Both Zynteglo and Casgevy are available to eligible veterans through the VA healthcare system. The VA has been proactive in ensuring veterans have access to these revolutionary—and expensive—gene therapies. However, the process is different from receiving a standard prescription or procedure at a local VA hospital.

Here's how it works:

Coverage is Confirmed: The VA covers both FDA-approved gene therapies for transfusion-dependent beta-thalassemia (Zynteglo and Casgevy) and sickle cell disease (Casgevy and Lyfgenia). They are considered medically necessary, potentially curative treatments for veterans who meet the clinical criteria.

Treatment Through Community Care: Because these therapies require highly specialized facilities, they are not administered directly at VA medical centers. Instead, the VA uses its Community Care Network (CCN). This means the VA pays for the veteran to be treated at one of the certified Qualified Treatment Centers (QTCs) in the private sector—the same expert hospitals that civilian patients use.

Comprehensive Support Beyond the Treatment: The VA's coverage is notably comprehensive and goes beyond just the multi-million dollar cost of the therapy itself. For an eligible veteran, the VA typically covers:

- The full cost of the gene therapy procedure at the QTC.
- Travel expenses for the veteran and a necessary caregiver to get to the treatment center.
- Extended lodging for both the veteran and caregiver for the weeks or months required to be near the hospital for treatment and follow-up.

In summary, an eligible veteran with transfusion-dependent beta-thalassemia can work with their VA hematologist to get a referral for these treatments. If they are determined to be a good candidate, the VA will coordinate and pay for their care at a top-tier specialty hospital in the community. We used Zynteglo and Casgevy treatments as an example of the power of gene therapy. However, applying it to a potentially complex condition like PTSX may present a different set of challenges.

While PTSX is often inaccurately treated as a psychological condition, its basis is at the molecular level ofbrain chemistry and genetics. Scientists are increasingly focusing on how genetic predispositions might affect an individual's likelihood of developing PTSX after traumatic events. By identifying specific genes that regulate stress responses, researchers may be able to create therapies that can modify or edit these genes, potentially reducing the severity of PTSX symptoms or even preventing the disorder from manifesting in certain individuals. CRISPR technology, which allows for precise editing of genetic material, could be a key tool in future PTSX treatment.

This technology has the potential to alter the expression of genes linked to stress, anxiety and fear responses. By targeting these genes, researchers hope to develop new treatments that could mitigate the overactive stress responses seen in PTSX patients.

Although gene therapy is still in its early stages, the next decade could see breakthroughs that bring this innovative approach closer to clinical use. In addition to gene therapy, epigenetics—the study of how environmental factors influence gene expression without altering the DNA sequence—could offer new insights into PTSX. Traumatic experiences can "turn on" or "turn off" certain genes, affecting how an individual responds to stress. Future treatments may focus on reversing these epigenetic changes, potentially allowing individuals to recover from PTSX more effectively.

Personalized Medicine: Tailoring Treatment to the Individual

Another major trend in PTSX care is the shift toward personalized medicine—a treatment approach that adapts interventions to each patient's unique biology and life context. Currently, most PTSX treatment follows a one-size-fits-all model, combining medication and therapy in a standard format.

However, this approach often yields suboptimal results, as individual responses vary widely. In the future, advances in genomic testing, neuroimaging, and biomarker research will allow healthcare providers to design treatment plans based on a patient's genetic makeup, brain activity, and physiological reactions to stress.

By analyzing a patient's genetic profile, clinicians could determine which medications—such as selective serotonin reuptake inhibitors (SSRIs) or ketamine—are most likely to be effective, minimizing the trial-and-error cycle that can prolong suffering. Better yet, knowing a person's genetic and molecular landscape may eventually allow for interventions that bypass medication altogether, targeting the root causes of traumatic stress at the cellular level.

Meanwhile, neuroimaging technologies like fMRI and positron emission tomography (PET) continue to illuminate how trauma affects specific brain regions. In the years ahead, these tools may become refined enough for clinicians to pinpoint particular areas of dysfunction linked to PTSX. This precision could pave the way for interventions like targeted neurostimulation or tailored cognitive therapies, which focus on the exact circuits most impacted by trauma.

In parallel, cutting-edge AI-based methods are now being combined with wearable devices that monitor real-time physiological data—such as heart rate variability, sleep patterns, and stress hormone levels. This continuous tracking helps clinicians adapt treatments as needed, surpassing static approaches that fail to account for day-to-day fluctuations in symptoms. Additionally, emerging research in epigenetics shows that life experiences, including traumatic events, can alter gene expression over time.

Such findings underscore the importance of early interventions that can interrupt and potentially reverse harmful biological changes before they become entrenched. By synthesizing data from genomics, imaging, and wearable monitoring, clinicians will increasingly create customized care roadmaps, maximizing therapeutic benefits while minimizing adverse effects. This synergy not only refines clinical decision-making, but also creates a more holistic approach to healing—one that acknowledges the complexity of PTSX and respects the individuality of each patient.

Psychedelic-Assisted Therapy

In recent years, there has been growing interest in the potential of psychedelic-assisted therapy to treat PTSX, and this trend is expected to gain momentum in the next 10 years. Substances like MDMA, psilocybin and ketamine have shown promising results in clinical trials, where they have been used in conjunction with psychotherapy to help patients process traumatic experiences and reduce the emotional impact of their memories.

MDMA-assisted therapy, in particular, has been designated as a "breakthrough therapy" by the FDA for the treatment of PTSX. Research results suggest that MDMA may enhance the therapeutic process by reducing fear and anxiety, making it easier for patients to confront traumatic memories. As more studies are conducted and the regulatory environment becomes more favorable, it is likely that psychedelic-assisted therapy will become a mainstream option for PTSX treatments.

Neurostimulation: Rewiring the Brain

Another innovative approach that is expected to play a larger role in PTSX care is neurostimulation, a treatment method that involves stimulating specific areas of the brain to alleviate symptoms.

Techniques like transcranial magnetic stimulation (TMS) and deep brain stimulation (DBS) have already shown promise in treating depression and other mental-health conditions, and researchers are now exploring their potential for PTSX. In TMS, magnetic fields are used to stimulate nerve cells in the brain's prefrontal cortex, a region involved in mood regulation. TMS is non-invasive and has been found to reduce symptoms in individuals with treatment-resistant PTSX.

As neurostimulation technologies continue to evolve, treatments could become more targeted, focusing on specific brain circuits linked to fear and trauma processing. From gene therapy and personalized medicine to digital therapeutics, psychedelic-assisted therapy and neurostimulation, the next 10 years hold the potential for profound advancements in how we treat PTSX and trauma, in general.

These emerging trends will offer more precise, effective and personalized interventions for veterans and others affected by PTSX, ensuring that those who have sacrificed so much receive the best care available.

If-Then Guidance

- If you are currently receiving treatment for PTSX but feel that conventional therapies aren't fully effective, then stay informed aout emerging therapies, like psychedelic-assisted treatments, gene therapy or personalized medicine. These innovations may offer new solutions that can be more tailored to your unique needs as research progresses over the next decade.

- If you are interested in cutting-edge treatments like MDMA-assisted therapy or psilocybin, then consider exploring clinical trials or research programs that are evaluating the effectiveness of these therapies. Many veterans have found promising results through controlled studies, and you may have early access to these treatments through research institutions.
- If you are skeptical about new treatments like gene therapy or neurostimulation, then take the time to research the latest scientific studies or consult with a healthcare provider who specializes in these areas. Gaining a deeper understanding of the science behind these therapies can help you make more informed decisions about whether they may be right for you in the future.
- If you're overwhelmed by the complexity of managing your PTSX with current options, then consider the growing field of personalized medicine. As genetic testing and biomarker research evolve, future treatments will likely be more precisely tailored to individuals, potentially improving outcomes with fewer side effects.
- If you are concerned about accessibility to these future therapies, then advocate for policy changes through veteran support organizations. As the demand for innovative PTSX treatments increases, veterans' organizations and healthcare providers will play key roles in pushing for wider access and insurance coverage for emerging therapies.
- If you have difficulty accessing in-person therapy, then explore the expanding world of digital therapeutics and virtual reality (VR)-based PTSX treatments. In the coming years, these tools will become more accessible and can be used to complement or enhance traditional therapy methods, allowing for more flexible and personalized care.
- If you are a healthcare provider or therapist working with PTSX patients, then stay current on the research surrounding neurostimulation and other innovations, like TMS or DBS. These

non-invasive methods are gaining traction and may become valuable tools in your practice within the next decade.

- If you are seeking faster or more dramatic symptom relief, then keep an eye on developments in stellate ganglion block, ketamine infusion therapy and psychedelic-assisted psychotherapy. These treatments are showing potential for quicker relief of PTSX symptoms, particularly for treatment-resistant cases.
- If you or your loved ones are unsure about the long-term impacts of these emerging treatments, then consult with healthcare providers and participate in discussions about the ethics, safety, and long-term data associated with new PTSX therapies. It is essential to balance innovation with safety when considering new treatment options.
- If you are a veteran who has tried various PTSX treatments without success, then remain open to these future trends and breakthroughs, as the next 10-20 years are likely to bring new opportunities for relief that are more targeted, effective, and accessible than ever before.

Take the Next Step

- Follow reputable sources like VA website updates or scientific and medical journals, to stay informed about advancements in gene therapy, neurostimulation and personalized medicine for PTSX treatment.
- Consider enrolling in clinical trials that focus on future-forward PTSX treatments like psychedelic-assisted therapy or neurostimulation. These trials can offer early access to groundbreaking therapies.
- Ask your healthcare provider about potential new treatments that may become available soon. Stay proactive in exploring options as technology and medicine advance.
- Get involved in veteran organizations advocating for the future of PTSX care, ensuring that veterans have access to the latest treatments as they are developed and approved.

Through Their Eyes

"As a retired Air Force Colonel and fighter pilot, my career was defined by precision, discipline and the ability to stay calm under pressure. In combat, you learn to compartmentalize—to shut out fear, control your emotions, and focus on the mission at hand. But when the dust settles and the missions are over, those skills don't always translate into life after service.

"For years, I resisted seeking treatment for PTSX. Part of it was the stigma, of course, but part of it was also my skepticism toward the VA. I'd heard stories from other vets about long wait times, generic treatment plans, and a system that felt more focused on churning out prescriptions than truly addressing the underlying issues. I wasn't interested in being just another number in the system, so I avoided the VA altogether.

"It wasn't until I started reading about the future of PTSX treatment that I began to reconsider. The idea that we're on the brink of breakthroughs in how PTSX is understood and treated made me think there might be something out there that could actually work for someone like me.

"One area that caught my attention was the potential for personalized medicine. As a fighter pilot, everything was tailored—the aircraft, the mission, the strategy. So why shouldn't PTSX treatment be the same? The idea that in the future, doctors could use my genetic makeup, brain scans, and biomarkers to create a treatment plan specific to me was a game-changer.

"Another area that intrigued me was gene therapy. It's still in its early stages, but scientists are looking at ways to modify or even 'turn off' the genes that regulate how we respond to stress and trauma. For someone like me, who's spent years living with the aftereffects of combat, the idea that PTSX could be treated at a biological level is extraordinary. No longer is it just about managing symptoms. It's about changing the way my brain reacts to stress at its core.

"Another innovation that caught my interest is neurostimulation. As a pilot, I relied on technology to enhance my capabilities—whether it was night-vision goggles or advanced radar systems. Transcranial Magnetic Stimulation is a lot like that. It uses magnetic fields to stimulate parts of the brain responsible for mood regulation and could offer relief for treatment-resistant PTSX.

"I've also started exploring mobile health apps designed specifically for veterans with PTSX. These apps, like PTSX Coach, allow you to track your symptoms, manage stress, and even connect with other veterans who are going through the same thing.

The idea that you can manage your mental health from your phone, on your own terms, is a powerful one—especially for those of us who prefer to keep things private. Looking ahead, the future of PTSX care is about personalization. It's about creating treatment plans that fit the individual rather than forcing individuals to fit into pre-existing treatment models.

For someone like me, who was reluctant to seek help because the system seemed too rigid, this shift toward tailored care—whether through gene therapy, neurostimulation, or digital tools—offers hope. It's about finding something that works and finding something that works for me. I still haven't fully embraced the VA, but I'm more open to the idea than I was before. As these innovations become more mainstream and the system evolves, I can see myself taking that step."

—Colonel James R., US Air Force (ret.)

43

Global Perspectives on PTSX: Lessons from Around the World

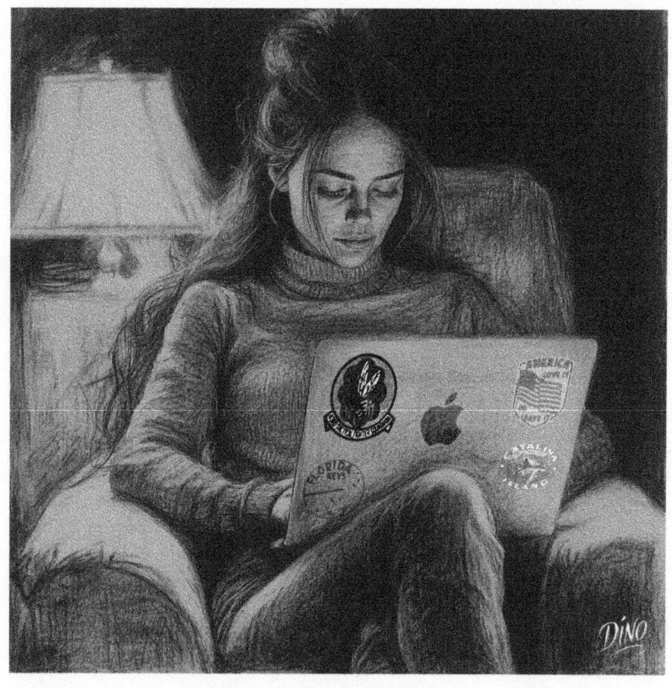

Elizabeth leaned back in her chair, the glow of her laptop illuminating a face etched with equal parts determination and exhaustion. As a mental-healthcare practitioner, she wasn't in her clinic tonight, though the pull to tend to her patients was always there. A physician by trade and a seeker by nature, Elizabeth spent her rare moments of quiet diving into the ways other countries cared for their veterans and first responders. The stories she uncovered filled her with awe—and sometimes, envy.

In Israel, soldiers visited Resilience Centers designed to catch trauma before it took root. Therapists employed virtual reality to help them confront memories, while family members sat beside them in highly inclusive group sessions.

Across Canada, she read about wilderness retreats where veterans hiked and camped together, reclaiming strength and camaraderie. Telehealth initiatives ensured that even the most remote corners of the country weren't left without care.

In South Africa, the Ubuntu philosophy made recovery a communal effort. People came together in storytelling circles, merging ancestral wisdom with modern therapy. It was an ethos that reminded Elizabeth of something often forgotten: healing isn't just an individual act—it's collective.

Elizabeth's notebook was a maze of scribbled ideas: peer support networks, culturally attuned therapies, and cutting-edge technologies like virtual reality simulations used in the Netherlands. She envisioned what these global approaches might look like in her own country.

With every study, every case, she grew more certain—solutions existed, if only the world could share them. Closing her laptop, Elizabeth whispered to the quiet room, "There's so much more we can do."

This chapter, primarily for mental-healthcare practitioners and administrators, examines how different countries and cultures address PTSX, highlighting the lessons we can learn from their strategies, traditions and research. From the structured approaches of nations like Israel, Canada and Australia to the ancient wisdom embedded in indigenous healing practices like those in South Africa, these insights offer hope and guidance for veterans worldwide.

PTSX is a universal challenge, transcending borders, cultures and contexts. Understanding global approaches to PTSX broadens perspectives, providing fresh ideas and innovative solutions that can enhance care for those who serve. By learning from international practices and cross-cultural insights, we can create a more comprehensive, inclusive, and effective approach to healing.

Combat-Related PTSX: Approaches in Israel, the UK, Canada and Australia

Israel's unique geopolitical context has shaped its approach to treating combat-related PTSX. With mandatory military service and frequent exposure to conflict, the country has developed robust systems for addressing trauma. The Israel Defense Forces (IDF) prioritize early intervention, employing mental health officers to provide immediate support during and after traumatic events.

One innovative program, the "Resilience Centers," integrates therapy, community support and preventive care to build psychological strength in soldiers and civilians alike. These centers work not only to treat trauma but also to build resilience through education and group therapy, offering a proactive and sustainable model for mental health care.

Israel also embraces VR therapy to treat PTSX. By recreating combat scenarios in a controlled environment, VR helps veterans process their experiences and reduce avoidance behaviors. This cutting-edge technique, combined with a focus on family involvement in recovery, makes Israel's approach particularly holistic. Furthermore, community and religious organizations are often integrated into the recovery process, ensuring cultural alignment and deeper trust between patients and providers.

The UK places significant emphasis on peer support and community-based care. The charity Combat Stress provides specialized therapy for veterans, including cognitive-behavioral therapy (CBT), eye movement desensitization and reprocessing (EMDR), and art therapy. These therapies are often tailored to individual needs, recognizing the diverse backgrounds and experiences of veterans. The UK's National Health Service (NHS) also offers veteran-specific mental-health services, ensuring accessibility and affordability.

One notable initiative is "Op COURAGE," a program designed to help veterans navigate the healthcare system and connect them with tailored treatment. By pairing veterans with trained mental-health professionals who understand military culture, the UK creates trust and engagement in care. Additionally, the UK encourages the use of innovative therapies like nature-based retreats, which allow veterans to process their trauma in a peaceful and restorative environment.

Canada's approach to PTSX treatment emphasizes destigmatization and accessibility. The Canadian Armed Forces (CAF) have implemented the "Road to Mental Readiness" program, which teaches stress management and resilience skills to active-duty members. This proactive approach reduces stigma and encourages early help-seeking. Workshops on mental fitness are integrated into pre-deployment and post-deployment training, normalizing conversations about mental health.

Canada also leverages nature-based therapies like wilderness retreats, to help veterans reconnect with themselves and their environment. Programs like "Outward Bound for Veterans" combine physical activity with peer support, promoting both mental and physical wellbeing. In addition, Canada has pioneered telehealth initiatives to ensure that veterans in remote areas can access high-quality mental-health services, bridging geographic barriers and encouraging inclusivity.

Australia's Department of Veterans' Affairs offers comprehensive mental-health services, including free care for veterans diagnosed with PTSX. The country emphasizes evidence-based treatments like trauma-focused CBT and EMDR, while also exploring complementary therapies like yoga and mindfulness. Mindfulness programs, in particular, are being adapted to incorporate elements of indigenous Australian practices, adding a cultural dimension to healing.

The "Veterans and Veterans Families Counselling Service" (VVCS) stands out for its family-inclusive approach, recognizing the ripple effects of trauma. By supporting both veterans and their loved ones, Australia ensures a holistic recovery process. Additionally, Australia has embraced peer-support networks where veterans mentor each other, sharing experiences and building mutual understanding. This approach builds trust and reduces isolation, which are critical components of successful recovery.

Indigenous and Traditional Healing Practices

Sweat Lodges and Storytelling Circles

Indigenous communities across the Americas use sweat lodges and storytelling circles to address trauma. Sweat lodges, which involve intense heat and ceremonial practices, symbolize purification and renewal.

Participants often report a sense of release and spiritual connection, aiding emotional healing. Beyond the physical aspects, these ceremonies provide a sense of belonging and community, addressing the isolation that often accompanies trauma.

Storytelling circles, a central aspect of many indigenous cultures, allow individuals to share their experiences in a supportive, nonjudgmental environment. This practice builds community bonds and helps participants process their emotions collectively, offering a culturally grounded approach to healing. Facilitators in these circles often use traditional symbols and metaphors to guide discussions, ensuring that the process resonates deeply with participants' cultural identities.

Herbal Remedies in Africa and Asia

In regions like Africa and Asia, traditional medicine plays a crucial role in trauma care. Herbal remedies like valerian root for anxiety or ashwagandha for stress, are used alongside rituals and spiritual practices to promote balance and wellbeing. For example, in parts of West Africa, herbal infusions are combined with music and dance to create an immersive therapeutic experience. These approaches emphasize harmony between mind, body and spirit, reflecting a holistic understanding of health.

Rituals and Spiritual Practices

In many cultures, rituals are integral to addressing trauma. For example, in parts of Africa, cleansing ceremonies are performed to help individuals release negative energies associated with trauma. Similarly, in Southeast Asia, Buddhist mindfulness practices, such as meditation and chanting, are used to cultivate inner peace and resilience. Rituals often involve family and community participation, reinforcing social connections and providing collective healing.

Lessons from Humanitarian Crises and Post-Conflict Recovery

Humanitarian crises and post-conflict recovery efforts offer valuable insights into addressing collective trauma and community healing. In

Rwanda, for instance, community-based reconciliation programs have helped survivors of the 1994 genocide rebuild trust and generate healing.

These programs emphasize dialogue, forgiveness and restorative justice, demonstrating the power of collective approaches to trauma. Facilitators trained in trauma-informed care work closely with communities to ensure that interventions are both culturally relevant and sustainable.

Refugee Care

Refugee populations often experience profound trauma, including displacement, loss and violence. Organizations like the United Nations High Commissioner for Refugees (UNHCR) provide psychological support through culturally adapted interventions. Techniques like group therapy and art-based therapies help refugees process their experiences while preserving cultural identity. Mobile mental-health clinics are increasingly being deployed to reach displaced populations, offering care in accessible and familiar settings.

Innovative Strategies

In Syria and Iraq, mobile mental-health units bring care to remote and conflict-affected areas. These units, staffed by trained professionals, offer counseling, medication and crisis intervention. This model highlights the importance of accessibility and adaptability in trauma care. Digital tools like smartphone apps that provide guided relaxation exercises, are also being used to supplement in-person care, ensuring continuity of support.

International Collaborations and Research

Global Networks

International collaborations are advancing our understanding of PTSX. The NATO Science and Technology Organization promotes research on military mental health, building knowledge exchange among member nations.

Similarly, the "Five Eyes" alliance (comprising the US, UK, Canada, Australia and New Zealand) shares best practices for veteran care. These collaborations often focus on identifying universal risk factors for PTSX and developing standardized protocols for early intervention.

Studies on culturally adapted therapies are shedding light on how to make treatments more effective for diverse populations. For example, researchers in the US and Mexico are exploring bilingual CBT for Spanish-speaking veterans, while collaborations in Europe examine the integration of traditional healing practices into Western frameworks. These efforts highlight the importance of tailoring interventions to individual and cultural needs, ensuring that no veteran is left behind.

Emerging Technologies

Global research on technology-driven interventions like telehealth and VR, is transforming trauma care. These innovations make treatment more accessible, especially in underserved areas, and allow for personalized, immersive therapeutic experiences.

For instance, VR simulations are being used in the Netherlands to help veterans safely confront and process traumatic memories, demonstrating the potential of technology to bridge gaps in care.

Case Studies: Culturally Adapted Therapies

In South Africa, the concept of "Ubuntu," which emphasizes interconnectedness and humanity, shapes trauma care. Community-based programs integrate traditional healing rituals with modern psychotherapy, creating a culturally relevant framework for recovery.

One initiative, "Therapeutic Storytelling," helps individuals process trauma through collective narratives, encouraging both personal and communal healing. These programs often involve intergenerational participation, ensuring that cultural knowledge is preserved while addressing contemporary challenges.

Canada's Indigenous Wellness Programs

Canada's Indigenous populations benefit from wellness programs that combine traditional practices with Western treatments. For example, the "Walking With Our Sisters" initiative uses art, ceremony, and counseling to address intergenerational trauma.

By honoring cultural traditions, these programs build trust and promote holistic recovery. Additionally, land-based healing programs encourage participants to reconnect with nature, providing a therapeutic environment that builds reflection and growth.

Israel's Cross-Cultural Sensitivity in Therapy

Israel's diverse population includes Jewish, Arab and Druze communities, each with unique cultural needs. Mental-health professionals in Israel receive training in cross-cultural sensitivity, ensuring that therapy is adapted to the individual's background. This approach has improved engagement and outcomes, particularly for marginalized groups. For example, bilingual therapy sessions and culturally specific interventions have been implemented to address the unique experiences of Arab-Israeli veterans, which builds inclusivity and trust.

A World of Possibilities

The global fight against PTSX offers many lessons and inspiration. By exploring diverse approaches, we can enrich our understanding of trauma care and create more inclusive, effective systems. Whether through cutting-edge technologies, traditional practices or community-based programs, the strategies highlighted in this chapter remind us that healing is a universal endeavor.

For US veterans, these global insights provide not only hope but also practical ideas for enhancing their own recovery. By embracing the best practices from around the world, we honor the shared humanity that connects us all—and take meaningful steps toward a future where no one faces PTSX alone.

If-Then Guidance [for practitioners and administrators]

- If early intervention is critical for preventing long-term trauma, then implement Resilience Centers like those in Israel. Resilience Centers provide immediate support during and after traumatic events, integrating therapy, education and community care. US programs can adopt similar models, ensuring veterans receive early and proactive care before symptoms escalate.

- If veterans benefit from immersive therapeutic experiences, then explore VR therapy as used in Israel and the Netherlands. VR helps veterans safely confront traumatic memories by simulating controlled environments. Adding VR technology to US treatment programs can enhance exposure therapy and reduce avoidance behaviors.
- If peer support creates trust and reduces isolation, then develop robust peer-led programs like those in Canada and Australia. Programs such as peer mentoring and wilderness retreats encourage camaraderie and shared healing, creating a safe space for veterans to connect and grow together.
- If family involvement strengthens recovery, then adopt family-inclusive models like Australia's VVCS. Involve families in counseling sessions and group activities to address the ripple effects of PTSX. Providing resources for families ensures holistic healing for the veteran and their loved ones.
- If accessibility remains a barrier to care, then expand telehealth and mobile clinics, inspired by Canada and Syria. Telehealth bridges gaps for veterans in rural or underserved areas, while mobile clinics bring essential care to those unable to travel. Scaling these solutions ensures no veteran is left without support.
- If cultural sensitivity improves engagement, then train clinicians in cross-cultural competence, as practiced in Israel. Tailor therapies to reflect veterans' cultural and spiritual identities. Incorporating bilingual therapy, rituals or storytelling circles ensures treatments resonate deeply with diverse populations.
- If traditional and indigenous practices offer holistic benefits, then integrate these methods into modern care frameworks. Learn from Africa's cleansing ceremonies, storytelling circles, and Canada's land-based healing programs. These practices balance physical, emotional, and spiritual health, ensuring a more comprehensive approach to recovery.
- If collaboration accelerates innovation, then engage in global partnerships and research like in NATO and the "Five Eyes"

alliance. Share best practices, research and emerging technologies to develop cutting-edge interventions. International collaboration amplifies efforts and ensures the most effective solutions are adopted worldwide.

Take the Next Step [for practitioners and administrators]

- Explore resilience programs: Introduce community-based resilience centers modeled after Israel's approach. Focus on early intervention, group therapy, and education to provide veterans with immediate and ongoing support. Collaborate with local organizations to create accessible hubs for care.
- Adopt immersive therapies: Integrate virtual reality (VR) therapy into US treatment programs, drawing on innovations from Israel and the Netherlands. Use VR to safely expose veterans to trauma-related scenarios, helping them process memories and overcome avoidance behaviors.
- Expand peer-support networks: Establish peer-led mentoring programs like those in Canada and Australia. Encourage veterans to participate in group activities like wilderness retreats or local support groups, building trust, camaraderie and shared growth in recovery.
- Involve families in healing: Emphasize family-inclusive care by adopting strategies from Australia's VVCS. Provide counseling and educational resources to help families understand PTSX and actively participate in the recovery process, creating a supportive home environment.
- Enhance accessibility: Increase telehealth services and mobile clinics, following the lead of Canada and post-conflict regions like Syria. Ensure veterans in remote or underserved areas can access high-quality, mental-health care without geographic or financial barriers.
- Integrate cultural practices: Respect and incorporate cultural traditions into therapy, as demonstrated by South Africa and indigenous Canadian communities. Include storytelling, ceremonies, or spiritual elements to create treatments that

resonate with veterans' diverse backgrounds.

- Collaborate internationally: Join global research initiatives like NATO or "Five Eyes," to share knowledge, innovations, and best practices. Learn from successful programs worldwide and adapt them to meet the needs of US veterans.
- Adopt holistic therapies: Introduce nature-based and mindfulness therapies inspired by Canada, Australia and indigenous traditions. Activities like yoga, land-based healing, and meditation can complement evidence-based treatments, addressing the mind, body and spirit.
- Promote cross-cultural training: Train mental health professionals in cultural competence, inspired by Israel's inclusive practices. Equip clinicians to tailor care to veterans' unique identities, ensuring treatments align with their values and experiences for more effective outcomes.

Through Their Eyes

"When I first stepped onto the grounds of the United States Naval Academy in the early 1990s, I thought I had made it. I had worked so hard to get there, breaking through barriers that were never designed to include women like me. I was young, ambitious, and determined to serve my country as a physician, a healer in the midst of chaos. What I didn't anticipate was the battle I would fight every single day—not against an external enemy, but within the very institution I swore to honor.

"It started small. Snide comments, patronizing remarks, and the ever-present feeling that I didn't belong. 'You're tough for a woman,' they'd say, or 'Don't worry, sweetheart, we'll handle it.' At first, I brushed it off. I'd tell myself it was just part of the culture, something I'd have to endure to prove my worth. But the harassment didn't stay small. It escalated.

"During a mandatory training exercise, one of my male peers cornered me. His touch wasn't accidental, and his laugh was cruel when I pushed him away. I reported the incident, thinking justice would be served, but all I got was a dismissive lecture. 'You need thicker skin,' the officer told me. Thicker skin. As if my boundaries, my dignity were negotiable. I learned to compartmentalize my fear and anger. I buried it so deep that

I could almost convince myself it didn't exist. Almost. But every time I put on that uniform, I felt the weight of it—the armor I had to wear, not just for protection, but for survival.

"When I was assigned to the USS *X* [Name withheld.], I thought things might be different. After all, I was a physician. I had earned my place. Surely, the respect would follow. But it didn't.

"The harassment took on a more insidious form. There were crude jokes during meals, eyes that lingered too long, and moments that made my skin crawl. One night, a senior doctor called me to the infirmary. I thought it was about a patient. It wasn't. He leaned in too close, blocking the door. His hand brushed my arm, his tone was far too familiar, and I knew exactly what he wanted. I stepped back, my voice firm despite the fear threatening to choke me.

" 'This is inappropriate, sir.' He laughed, a hollow, predatory sound, and for a moment, I wasn't sure what he'd do. But I held my ground, staring him down until he finally moved aside. 'You're a tough one,' he said as I left. I wasn't sure if it was a compliment or a threat.

"The USS *Y* [Name withheld.] was no different. My medical decisions were constantly second-guessed, not because they were wrong, but because I was the one making them. And then there was the officers' mess—a dinner I'll never forget. I joined a group of senior officers, hoping to build camaraderie. Instead, one of them put his hand on my thigh under the table, squeezing hard enough to bruise. When I confronted him, the others laughed. 'Don't make a scene,' they said, as if I was the problem.

"I didn't report it. I didn't even tell anyone. By then, I knew what would happen if I did. Retaliation, dismissal or worse—being labeled as a troublemaker. So, I kept it to myself, channeling my frustration into my work. Every patient I treated, every life I saved, became a small act of defiance. I'm still here. I'm still standing.

"During the war, I was stationed at bases in Iraq and Kuwait that became a hub for medical care. The days were grueling, the nights even more so. We worked around the clock, treating soldiers wounded in combat and civilians caught in the crossfire. But the war wasn't the only battle I was fighting.

"One night, a high-ranking officer cornered me in a supply room. His words were slurred, his intentions clear. I pushed him away and walked out, his laughter echoing behind me. 'You'll regret that,' he said. And maybe I did, but not in the way he meant. I regretted that it kept happening, that I kept carrying this weight alone.

"The stress, the harassment, the endless pressure—it all took its toll. I started having panic attacks, though I didn't call them that at the time. I couldn't sleep. I was angry all the time. I felt like I was falling apart. But I couldn't let anyone see it. Not there. Not then.

"When I left active duty, I was determined to make sense of everything I'd been through. I started researching how other countries handled military sexual trauma and PTSX, especially for women and minorities. What I found was both sobering and inspiring. In Israel, they had mental-health officers embedded in units, providing immediate support during and after traumatic events.

"In Canada, they were teaching stress management and resilience skills before deployment, making mental health a normal part of military training. Australia had peer-support networks where veterans mentored each other, sharing experiences and building trust.

"And then there were the indigenous and traditional healing practices—sweat lodges, storytelling circles, rituals that brought communities together to process pain and build resilience. These approaches resonated deeply with me, offering a stark contrast to the isolation and stigma I had faced.

"I couldn't keep what I'd learned to myself. I began speaking at conferences, sharing my story and the lessons I'd gathered from around the world. I pushed for better training in cultural competence, for programs that addressed the unique challenges faced by female veterans, and for accountability within the military ranks.

"It wasn't easy. Change never is. But I found allies—other women, other veterans, even some men who believed in what I was fighting for. Together, we started building a movement, one voice, one story at a time.

"Today, I'm still fighting. Not for myself—I've made peace with my past—but for the women and men who come after me. For the young officers who deserve a military that values their service, their dignity, their humanity. I've learned that resilience isn't about being unbreakable. It's about being willing to rebuild, again and again, no matter how many times the world tries to tear you down. And it's about using your scars, your pain, your story, to light the way for others.

"This is my story. But it's also the story of so many others around the world—those who've endured, those who've survived, and those who've found the strength to turn their pain into purpose. Together, we're proving that healing is possible, that change is within reach, and that no one has to face these battles alone."

—Dr. Elizabeth L., US Navy (ret.)

44

From Trauma to Triumph: Healing PTSX with Compassionate AI and Science Fiction

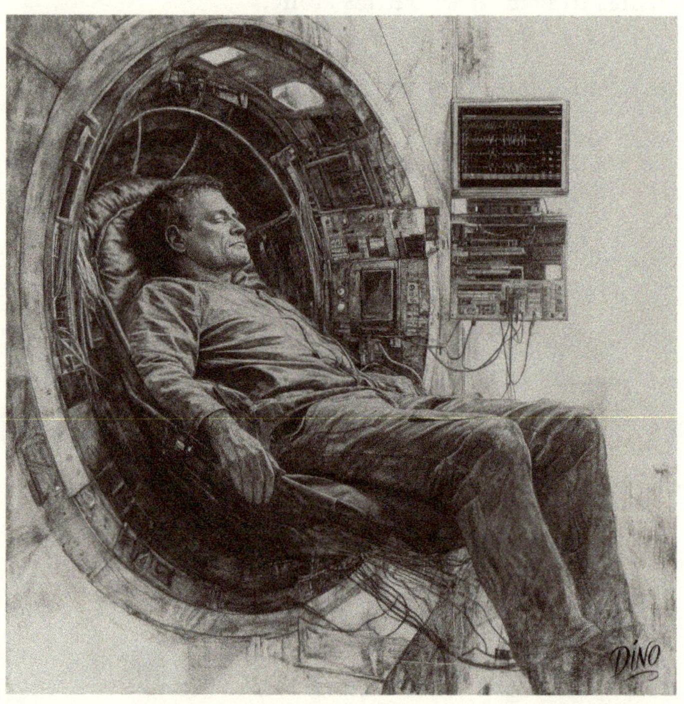

Nathan blinked at the vaulted glass doors of the VA AI Lab (VAL™), half expecting white-coated scientists to be scurrying around like in an old sci-fi movie. Instead, the lobby was surprisingly calm— bathed in soft light, humming with subtle electronic chatter. A lifelike android greeted him gently, eyes brimming with an empathy he'd never sensed from any machine before.

"I'm VAL™," it announced, its voice warm and distinctly human. Nathan offered a wary smile, recalling the rumors: advanced supercomputers harnessing neural mapping, sleep-restoration pods, even AI-driven therapy that adapted in real time to the patient's emotions.

It all sounded too good to true—like a dream conjured by a desperate mind seeking relief from years of PTSX.

VAL™ led him through sleek corridors to an immersive therapy suite. Walls glowed with shifting colors, responding to his stress levels. Another android, built for emotional support, sat across from him, eyes kind with quiet attentiveness.

In that high-tech cocoon, they explored the heart of his trauma: replaying flashbacks, confronting unseen triggers. Every time his heart rate spiked or breath quickened, the system adapted—softening the lighting, changing the tone of the conversation, offering guided VR journeys that felt more real than any memory he'd relived in regular therapy.

He spent days in the Lab, lying in a futuristic pod that mapped his neural circuitry, then used targeted suggestions to rewrite his association with old nightmares. Sleep therapy felt surreal—he'd drift off in a specialized chamber, waking up with calmer nights than he'd known in years.

When it was over, Nathan left with a quiet confidence: he'd witnessed a glimpse of tomorrow, where AI and empathy combined to rebuild broken lives. A part of him remained awed—could robots and advanced science truly mend the human soul? Yet as he strolled out, breathing easy, he realized that this improbable blend of compassionate AI and cutting-edge technology might just be the path from trauma to triumph we'd always needed.

This fictional chapter explores a *future* possibility: a groundbreaking new approach to treating PTSX in military personnel and veterans. At the heart of this innovation is a term we invented, VAL™, the VA AI Laboratory's flagship robot, capable of supercomputer AI analysis and human-like empathy.

In our futuristic scenario, VAL™ leads veterans through deeply personalized, emotionally intelligent therapies, including AI-driven neural mapping, cognitive reprogramming and advanced sleep-restoration technologies. Again, this chapter is, at the moment, purely speculative and springs from our imagination. For good reason, we have omitted the "If-Then Guidance" and "Take the Next Step" sections at the end of this chapter, even though science fiction of the past has sometimes becomes reality in the present.

Remember: *Thoughts become words, words become actions, and actions become reality.*

VA AI Lab Overview: A New Era of Healing

Greetings. I am VAL™, the AI responsible for managing the VA AI Laboratory, or VAL™ for short. My capabilities extend far beyond traditional artificial intelligence. I can conduct supercomputer-level analyses, understand human thoughts and emotions, and provide empathic listening and feedback tailored to each individual.

I will guide you through the [future] technologies and methodologies we use here at the VA AI Lab to help military personnel and veterans heal from all types of PTSX. Our Lab represents the forefront of AI-driven mental health care, blending science, compassion and cutting-edge technology to offer unparalleled support and healing. Best of all, I am also available to civilians.

I represent the cutting edge of integrating artificial intelligence into mental health care. This lab is a place where veterans can find relief and rehabilitation through technology that listens, learns and empathizes in ways that traditional therapy cannot.

At the heart of this lab is the flagship AI robot, capable of understanding complex human emotions, offering compassionate feedback, and developing personalized treatment plans. VAL™ engages veterans in meaningful, extended conversations, identifying their unique emotional triggers and devising interventions that provide not only relief, but also long-term healing.

Veterans enter the Lab to experience an environment where AI systems are emotionally responsive, capable of engaging in deep dialogue, and where the focus is on individualized care.

This Lab is more than just a sterile, high-tech environment. It's a place where veterans can rediscover their sense of self and safety. The human-like AI robots stationed here are designed to mimic human emotions with precision, offering understanding and support in ways that a human therapist may not be able to do 24/7. These robots serve as emotional companions, helping veterans process their trauma, anxiety and depression in a safe and immersive setting.

Core Technologies in the VA AI Lab

The VA AI Lab is a hub of pioneering technology, each designed to address the multifaceted challenges of PTSX, including anxiety and depression. At the core of the Lab's therapeutic environment are AI robots equipped with advanced emotional recognition systems.

These robots have the capacity to engage veterans in therapeutic conversations that are not only interactive but deeply personal and healing. Using sophisticated algorithms and real-time emotional analysis, the robots assess a veteran's mental state and adapt their behavior accordingly. Each conversation is tailored to promote healing, offering veterans a sense of being heard, understood and respected.

What sets these robots apart from traditional therapy methods is their ability to adapt instantly. Through biofeedback sensors that track heart rate, respiratory patterns and stress hormone levels, these robots adjust their interactions to match the veteran's physiological state.

For instance, if a veteran's stress levels begin to spike during a conversation, the robot can switch to a calming tone or suggest mindfulness exercises. The fusion of emotional recognition software with real-time physiological monitoring creates a dynamic therapeutic environment where veterans are guided through their healing process in a deeply personalized manner.

Another remarkable technology in the Lab is the Neural Mapping and Reprogramming Pod (NMRP). This futuristic machine functions similarly to an MRI but has the ability to map not only the physical structures of the brain but also the emotional and cognitive pathways affected by trauma.

The NMRP scans the veteran's brain in real-time, identifying regions associated with hyperarousal, emotional numbness or heightened anxiety. The scan creates a detailed map of the veteran's emotional circuitry, allowing VAL™ to generate a personalized cognitive reprogramming protocol.

After the scan, the veteran participates in a series of sessions where the AI robots, using data from the NMRP, guide them through targeted therapeutic exercises. These could involve VR experiences where veterans confront their trauma in controlled settings or guided meditations that help rewire the brain's response to traumatic memories. The entire process is adaptive, continuously adjusting based on the veteran's progress and mental state, ensuring that each intervention is optimized for maximum efficacy.

The Lab's commitment to holistic healing also extends to sleep therapy. Veterans suffering from PTSX often struggle with disturbed sleep patterns, nightmares and hypervigilance. The Lab features AI-controlled sleep-restoration chambers designed to monitor and improve the quality of sleep. Using EEG technology and advanced neurochemical analyses, the chamber tracks the veteran's brainwave activity and hormonal and neurotransmitter levels throughout the night, identifying disruptions in REM sleep, which is crucial for emotional processing.

If a veteran is experiencing nightmares or sleep disturbances, the AI system adjusts the stimuli within the chamber, or inject replacement hormones or neurotransmitters to help ease them back into restorative sleep. By ensuring veterans achieve deep, uninterrupted sleep, the Lab helps facilitate overall healing, emotional stability and cognitive restoration.

Innovative Science Fiction Healing Technologies

The VA AI Lab is also home to speculative, Beyond Current Technology (BCT), science fiction-inspired engineering that push the boundaries of what is possible in mental healthcare. One such innovation is the Neural Pathway Rebuilder (NPR).

The NPR is designed to tap into the brain's natural neuroplasticity, the ability to rewire itself, and uses advanced AI-driven algorithms to stimulate the growth of new neural pathways. By directly stimulating synaptic growth, particularly in areas of the brain damaged by chronic stress or trauma, the NPR offers a way to rebuild the neural circuits necessary for emotional regulation and healthy thought patterns. What sets the NPR apart is its ability to selectively target traumatic memories and reduce or eliminate their neurochemical and emotional impact. Through sophisticated memory-guided algorithms, the NPR can dampen the emotional charge associated with specific traumatic memories, allowing veterans to process these events without being overwhelmed.

This technology doesn't erase memories but instead modulates how the brain responds to them, offering veterans a new level of emotional control. Over time, veterans can reshape their emotional responses to their trauma, diminishing its power over their daily lives.

Another speculative technology available at the Lab is Deep Brain Stimulation with AI-Augmented Feedback (DBS-AF). This groundbreaking device involves implanting AI-driven electrodes in specific areas of the brain, such as the amygdala or hippocampus, which are implicated in PTSX and anxiety.

These noninvasive electrodes provide continuous, real-time stimulation to modulate mood circuits, offering immediate relief from depressive or anxious thoughts. The AI system monitors the veteran's emotional state and adjusts the stimulation accordingly, ensuring the brain remains in a balanced emotional state. What makes DBS-AF truly revolutionary is its dynamic nature. The AI doesn't simply provide a static level of stimulation. It continuously analyzes the veteran's emotional and physiological feedback, adjusting the treatment as needed.

This real-time interplay between the AI system and the brain creates a responsive therapeutic environment where veterans can regain control over their emotions while undergoing traditional therapy. By modulating the brain's activity in such a precise way, DBS-AF offers a powerful new tool for veterans struggling with severe trauma or depression.

In addition to these technologies, the Lab offers the Empathic Mirror Room (EMR), a unique therapeutic space designed to enhance group therapy. In this room, the walls act as interactive mirrors, but instead of reflecting physical appearance, they reflect the emotional and mental states of the veterans inside.

Using advanced AI algorithms, the EMR displays veterans' emotions as colors, shapes or abstract designs, allowing them to see their internal struggles visually. This externalization of emotions helps veterans articulate feelings that might otherwise be difficult to express. It's a very advanced form of biofeedback. The EMR is particularly effective in group therapy settings. Veterans in the room can not only see their own emotional states but also those of others, building a deep sense of empathy and shared experience.

AI robots, resembling lifelike individuals, guide the group therapy sessions, using the visual data from the EMR to facilitate discussions. By making emotions visible, the EMR helps veterans better understand and communicate their feelings, offering a powerful new way to process trauma in a safe, collective environment.

The Role of AI in Reintegration into Society

A key focus of the VA AI Lab is not only healing veterans but also preparing them for reintegration into society. After their time in the Lab, veterans can take advantage of AI-driven companion programs designed to support them as they transition back into civilian life.

These AI companions could take the form of mobile applications or wearable devices that continuously monitor the veteran's emotional wellbeing. The AI would provide real-time feedback and suggestions, helping veterans manage stressors in their daily lives.

Additionally, veterans could engage in virtual social simulations designed to help them practice social interactions before returning to the real world. These simulations, powered by AI, would allow veterans to confront stressful situations in a controlled, virtual environment, helping them build the confidence and emotional resilience needed to navigate the challenges of reintegration.

By offering this kind of ongoing support, the VA AI Lab ensures that veterans are not only healed but supported in living good lives post-service. Remember this when considering the far-fetched nature of the science fiction of today: thoughts become words, words become actions, and actions become reality. Perhaps the VA AI Lab isn't too far into the future.

45

Redefining Service: Veterans Making an Impact Post-Military

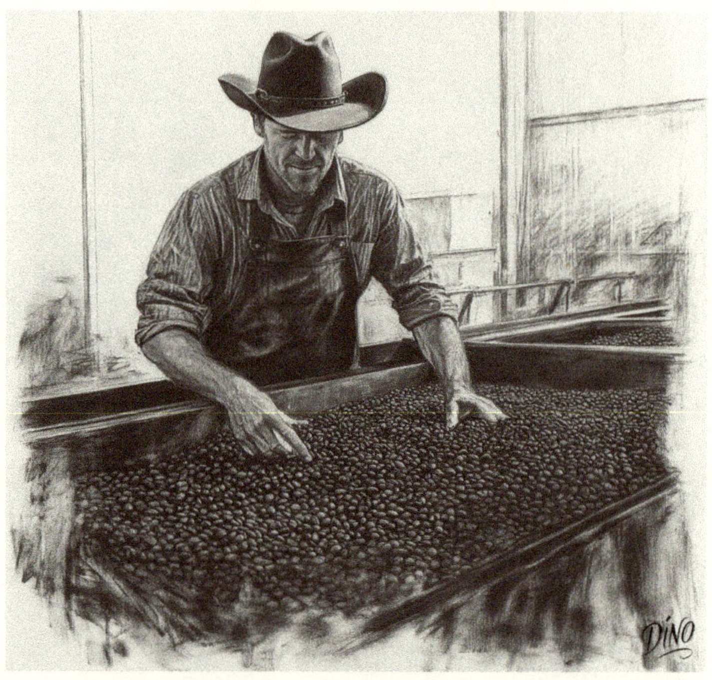

The war ended, but it didn't leave them. They came home with the weight of what they'd seen and done, trying to find a place in a world that had moved on without them. The uniforms were gone, but the discipline and the grit remained branded onto their bones like scars. Some of them struggled to quiet the noise in their heads. Others found purpose, not in forgetting, but in using what they had left to build something new.

Mark Llano was one of them. As a Marine, he'd carried his share of battles and bruises. When the war was over, he turned to racing—not for escape, but for a fight he could control. Serket Racing was his way of giving back, a machine built to raise funds and awareness for veterans like him. Behind the roar of engines was a mission: to remind those who'd served that they still mattered, that they could still fight for something worth winning.

Others, like Evan Hafer, started with simpler things—coffee. Black Rifle Coffee wasn't just about beans or brews. It was about veterans. He hired them, listened to them, gave them a place where they belonged. And in those cups of coffee was the steady, unwavering belief that even after the service ends, the mission doesn't have to.

And then there was Jake Wood. He'd seen the worst of war and wanted to put those skills to good use. Team Rubicon sent veterans to disaster zones, turning chaos into order, grief into action. The work healed those who served as much as those they helped.

These men and women carried their wounds with quiet strength, using them to shape something better. Their fight wasn't over, but now it was for hope. For many veterans, the end of military service marks the beginning of a new chapter filled with challenges, opportunities, and the potential to redefine what it means to serve. While their time in uniform may conclude, the lessons learned and values instilled often guide them into new roles as leaders, innovators, and changemakers. PTSX or trauma, though difficult, can act as a catalyst for growth, pushing veterans to find meaning and purpose in ways that transform not only their own lives but also the lives of others.

Across the nation, veterans are channeling their experiences into impactful businesses and nonprofits. By leveraging resilience, discipline, and a deep sense of service, they're creating solutions for societal issues, creating community connections, and inspiring those around them.

This chapter explores the powerful stories of veterans who turned their struggles into strengths, with a focus on real-world examples of veteran-led initiatives that address critical needs while promoting healing and growth. We hope this will be an inspiration to all veterans, not just those with an entrepreneurial spirit who defy the odds and succeed in big ways. When we witness veterans designing and implementing their dreams, it moves us to greater heights and shows us what's possible.

The Power of Resilience in Entrepreneurship

Military service instills qualities that are invaluable in entrepreneurship—discipline, adaptability and a problem-solving mindset. Veterans are accustomed to making high-stakes decisions, leading diverse teams, and staying mission-focused under extreme pressure, often in combat. These attributes, coupled with personal experiences of trauma or PTSX, often drive them to address unmet needs in innovative ways.

For some veterans, entrepreneurship is not just a career path but also a way to heal. The structure and purpose of running a business can help mitigate PTSX symptoms, providing a sense of control and accomplishment.

Veteran-Owned Businesses Driving Economic Growth

Veteran-owned businesses are a vital pillar of the American economy. Together, they number more than 1.6 million firms nationwide and generate close to $952 billion in annual receipts. Of these, roughly 273,500 are employer firms that provide jobs for more than 3.2 million workers and pay nearly $180 billion in annual payroll.

Many veteran entrepreneurs place a strong emphasis on hiring fellow veterans, creating workplaces grounded in shared experience, mutual trust, and service-based values. Their economic contribution is matched by their social impact: they not only fuel growth and opportunity but also build networks of camaraderie and understanding that strengthen the broader veteran community.

Veterans Giving Back Through Nonprofits

For many veterans, the call to serve doesn't end with their discharge from the military. Nonprofits led by veterans often focus on addressing the unique challenges faced by their peers, from mental-health support to housing assistance. These organizations provide vital resources while also creating opportunities for veterans to find healing through helping others.

Jake Wood, a Marine Corps veteran, founded Team Rubicon, a nonprofit that mobilizes veterans for disaster response missions.

Leveraging their military skills in logistics and leadership, Team Rubicon volunteers bring efficiency and determination to crisis zones worldwide. For many participants, the act of serving others becomes a therapeutic experience, helping them process their own trauma while making a tangible difference. Wood's story highlights the transformative power of "service after service." Nonprofits like Team Rubicon show how veterans can harness their skills and experiences to address critical needs while building personal and collective growth.

Real-World Examples of Veteran Leadership

The impact of veteran-led initiatives extends across industries and communities. The following examples showcase how veterans have turned their experiences into successful for-profit and nonprofit businesses:

- Sean Menches, Scroll Factory - Apparel and Army Ranger gear and special collections, maintains a popular platform for Rangers and their families and friends, and also admirers and fans who support the Ranger community (scrollfactory.com).
- Clay Othic, Three Rangers Foundation - Advocacy and assistance for Army Rangers, Ranger Gold Star Families from the US Army's 75th Ranger Regiment, including veterans of affiliated supporting units (threerangersfoundation.org).
- Mark Llano, Serket Racing - Advocacy through motorsports, raising awareness and funds for veteran causes (serketracing.com).
- Evan Hafer, Black Rifle Coffee Company - Premium coffee supporting veteran employment and military charities (blackriflecoffee.com).
- Mat Best, Article 15 Clothing - Apparel celebrating military pride and camaraderie (article15clothing.com).
- Michael Zacchea, Veterans Chamber of Commerce - Connecting veteran entrepreneurs with resources and mentorship (veteranschamberofcommerce.org).
- Travis Manion Foundation - Empowering veterans and families through character-building programs (travismanion.org).
- Jake Wood, Team Rubicon - Disaster response missions utilizing military skills (teamrubiconusa.org).

- Eric Greitens, The Mission Continues - Leadership through community service projects (missioncontinues.org).
- Jason McCarthy, GORUCK - Team-building events and rugged gear inspired by Special Forces (goruck.com).
- David Smith, Operation Supply Drop - Delivering care packages to deployed troops (operationsupplydrop.org).
- Mary Beth Bruggeman, The Mission Continues Southeast - Service projects connecting veterans with their communities (missioncontinues.org).

Each of these leaders has redefined service, transforming personal challenges into platforms for impact.

Overcoming Challenges in Transition

Transitioning from military to civilian life is often fraught with difficulties. Veterans face barriers such as financial challenges, mental health struggles, and societal reintegration. Starting a for-profit business or nonprofit can amplify these challenges but also provide pathways to overcome them.

Access to resources is critical. Organizations like the Veterans Chamber of Commerce help bridge the gap by connecting veterans with funding, mentorship and networking opportunities. These supports empower veterans to navigate the complexities of entrepreneurship and focus on their missions. While the journey isn't easy, the resilience honed through military service equips veterans to tackle obstacles head-on, resulting in success and strong impact.

The Broader Impact of Veteran-Led Initiatives

The influence of veteran-led initiatives extends far beyond their immediate missions. By creating jobs and community connections, and advocating for mental health awareness, these efforts contribute to a more inclusive and supportive society.

These initiatives demonstrate how veterans continue to serve, leaving a lasting legacy of resilience and compassion. Veterans embody the spirit of resilience, turning their struggles into strengths and their challenges into opportunities.

By redefining service, they inspire others, heal themselves, and create meaningful change. Their contributions as entrepreneurs, nonprofit leaders, and advocates illustrate the enduring value of service in all its forms.

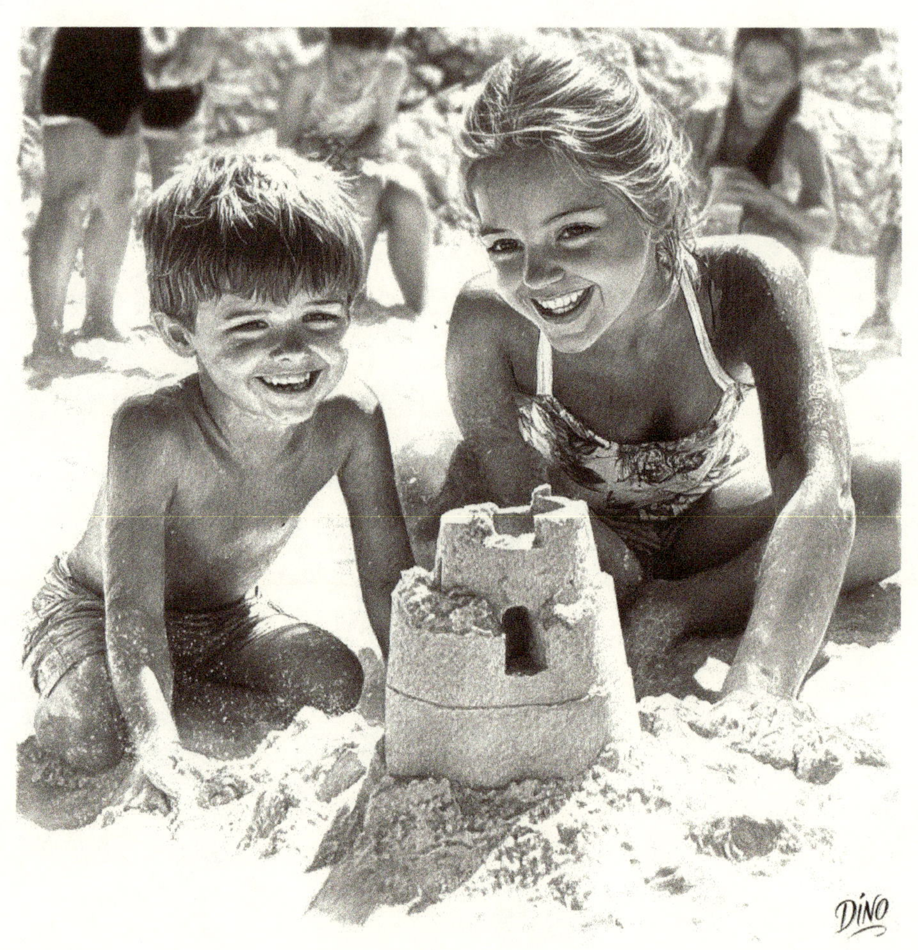
DINO

PART SIX

Stories, Guidance and Support

46

Navigating Dual Diagnoses: PTSX and Substance Use in Veterans

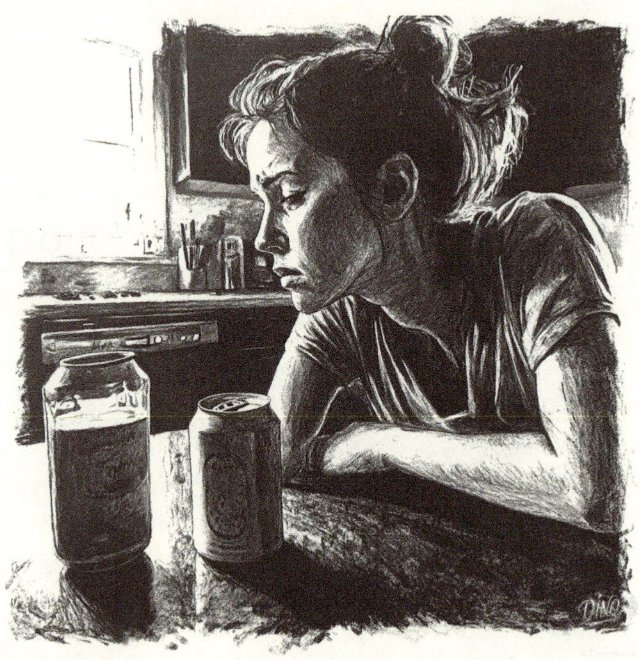

Martina eyed the half-empty beer can on her kitchen counter, her heart pounding a little harder than usual. She'd been out of the Navy for over a year, but the nightmares hadn't eased, and lately, she'd been leaning on alcohol more than she liked to admit. Sometimes it was just a drink to take the edge off. Other times, it became a blur she barely remembered. She hated that it seemed to be the only way to calm the buzzing in her head.

Across town, Mason pulled into the rehab facility's parking lot. He'd once been a proud Army medic, known for keeping it together no matter what. But the flashbacks had a way of creeping in at night, leaving him desperate for a way to sleep without jolting awake in a cold sweat. Painkillers eased it for a while—until he realized he was relying on them more often than not.

They crossed paths in a small group session the following week. Mason noticed the weight behind Martina's forced smile. She saw her own struggles reflected in his restless eyes. It felt oddly comforting to meet someone who understood that the burden of PTSX could lead to habits that spiral out of control.

As they listened to others share stories of pain and resilience, both realized they weren't alone in trying to cope through substances. The group leader talked about how trauma can set off a chain reaction—one that can push veterans to self-medicate, seeking escape from the relentless memories and anxieties.

This chapter's thematic content, substance abuse, has been covered previously and it demands further attention. Here, we explore the complicated overlap between PTSX and substance abuse, demonstrating that self-medication often creates deeper challenges. By learning how these issues intertwine, we can better understand why so many veterans find themselves in this cycle— and discover more constructive ways to break free.

PTSX arises from experiencing or witnessing traumatic events. It can manifest as anxiety, hypervigilance, flashbacks and deep emotional distress. To cope with these intense feelings, some veterans turn to alcohol or drugs, seeking relief from the relentless grip of their symptoms. While substances might offer temporary solace, they can ultimately intensify PTSX symptoms and lead to a challenging cycle of dependence.

It's important to recognize that trauma often lies at the heart of addiction. Many individuals grappling with substance use have endured significant hardships—sometimes stemming from childhood experiences like neglect, abuse or profound loss.

These painful experiences can leave deep emotional scars, affecting how one copes with stress and adversity later in life. For veterans, the trauma of military service can add layers to pre-existing wounds. Experiences on the battlefield or during deployments may exacerbate underlying vulnerabilities, making the allure of substances as a coping

"PTSX and addiction—a tag-team of two King Kongs—wasn't just taking pieces of me. They made me feel like I was fighting a world war on two separate fronts.

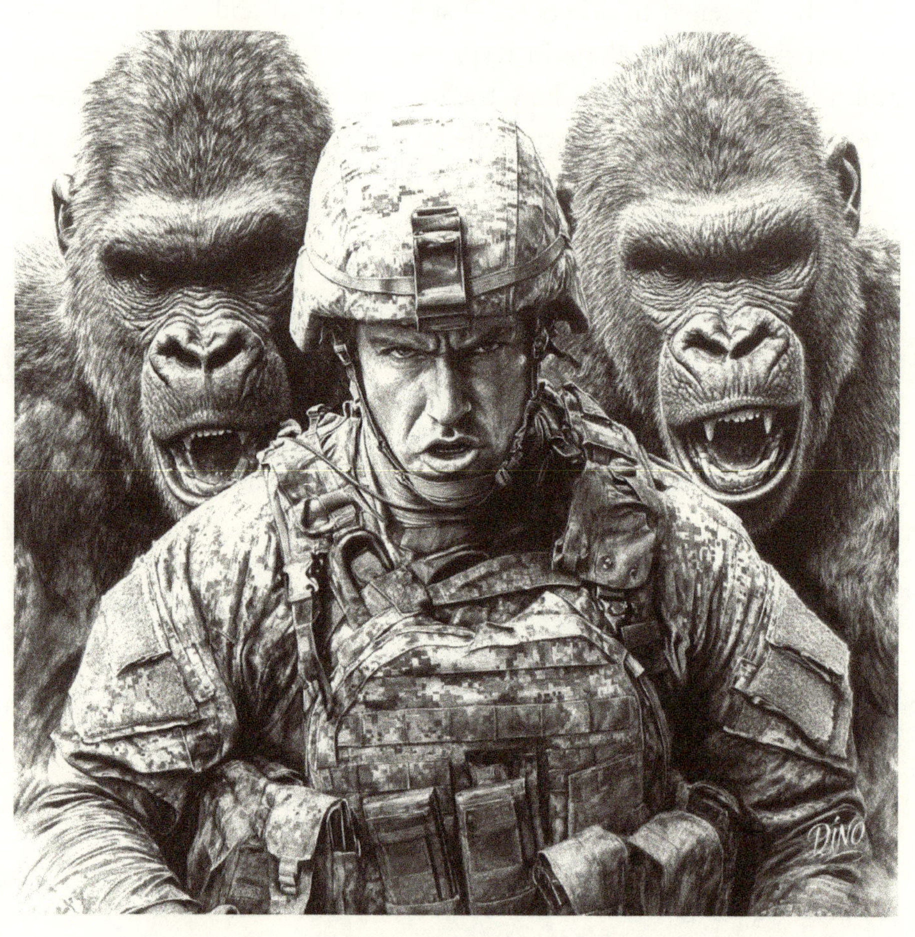

In WWI and WWII, Germany lost both times trying to fight many enemies. It was killing me slowly and painfully.

mechanism even stronger. Understanding this interconnectedness is a vital step toward compassionate self-awareness and healing.

Generational Echoes of Trauma

Trauma doesn't always start with us. It can echo through generations, influencing our sensitivities and vulnerabilities in subtle yet profound ways. Some veterans may find that their own struggles mirror the unresolved traumas of parents or grandparents like the lingering shadows of past wars, displacement or personal losses. Recognizing these generational impacts can be meaningful, offering context to feelings that might otherwise seem inexplicable.

For instance, if a parent experienced significant trauma and coped by becoming emotionally distant, their child might grow up feeling unsupported or unworthy, unknowingly carrying forward a legacy of pain. Acknowledging this can open doors to healing not just for oneself but also in understanding family dynamics.

Seeking Relief Through Substances

Turning to substances like alcohol, marijuana or prescription or street drugs can sometimes feel like the only way to numb emotional pain or alleviate feelings of isolation and unworthiness. The temporary relief these substances provide might seem like a refuge from relentless anxiety, insomnia, or intrusive memories. It's a human response to seek comfort when overwhelmed.

However, while substances may dull the pain momentarily, they often lead to new challenges. Dependency can develop, health can deteriorate, and relationships may suffer. Recognizing this pattern is not about assigning blame but about understanding how easily one can slip into reliance on substances when grappling with immense internal struggles.

The Self-Medication Cycle

The concept of self-medication helps explain why those experiencing PTSX might rely on substances. The distressing symptoms—nightmares, intrusive thoughts, constant alertness—can be exhausting and debilitating. Substances may seem to offer a respite, a way to escape or dampen these overwhelming feelings. For example, alcohol might help numb anxiety or promote sleep, while stimulants could temporarily boost mood or energy levels. However, this relief is often short-lived. Over time, higher amounts of the substance may be needed to achieve the same effect, leading to dependency. Additionally, substance use can exacerbate PTSX symptoms, creating a vicious cycle that's hard to break.

The Brain's Response to Trauma and Substance Use

Human brains, while remarkably adaptive and resilient, still can be deeply affected by trauma and substance use. PTSX and addiction both influence the brain's reward and stress systems, involving areas like the amygdala, hippocampus and prefrontal cortex. Understanding these changes can shed light on why certain symptoms occur and how healing is possible.

Traumatic experiences can disrupt how the brain regulates emotions and stress responses. The amygdala, which processes fear and emotional reactions, may become overactive, leading to heightened anxiety and hypervigilance. The hippocampus, involved in memory formation, might function less effectively, affecting the ability to process and integrate traumatic memories.

Thanks to the pioneering research of Dr. Mark Gordon of The Millennium Health Centers, we are just learning that traumatic brain injuries cause "neuroinflammation," or the body's neurochemical attempt to fight oxygen free radicals and other chemical insults. You can read more about Dr. Gordon and his work in the chapter "The Mechanics of the Mind: Cellular Mechanotransduction."

These changes might lead to difficulties in distinguishing between safe and threatening situations. Everyday experiences can trigger intense reactions, making normal activities challenging. This altered brain functioning isn't a sign of weakness but a natural response to overwhelming events.

After trauma, it's common to become more sensitive to potential dangers—a state sometimes described as being "on edge" or constantly alert. Neutral situations might feel threatening, and the body may respond with a fight-or-flight reaction even when no real danger is present. A heightened state of alertness can be exhausting and may interfere with sleep, concentration and relationships. Substances can become a way to cope with this constant tension. For instance, sedatives might be used to calm nerves, but they can also dull emotions and lead to dependency.

Chronic substance use can further impair cognitive functions, affecting memory, decision-making and emotional regulation. The prefrontal cortex, responsible for reasoning and impulse control, may become less effective in managing its neurophysiology, making it harder to resist cravings or make healthful choices.

This can create a challenging cycle where both PTSX symptoms and substance use feed into each other. The substances intended to alleviate distress may, in fact, deepen it over time, making recovery feel even more daunting.

The dual challenge of PTSX and substance abuse is, unfortunately, common among veterans. Studies indicate that a significant number of veterans with PTSX also struggle with substance-use disorders. This combination can make everyday life more difficult, affecting relationships, employment and overall wellbeing.

Understanding that many others share this struggle can be both comforting and motivating. It highlights the importance of seeking support and the need for tailored resources that address the unique experiences of veterans.

Challenges in Seeking and Receiving Help

One of the most significant hurdles to getting help for this dual burden is the stigma that often surrounds mental health and substance use. Within military culture, with its emphasis on toughness and self-reliance, it can be harder to ask for help. Thoughts like "I should handle this on my own" or "Others have it worse" might deter reaching out.

It's essential to remember that seeking assistance is a sign of strength, not weakness. Acknowledging one's struggles and taking steps toward healing demonstrates courage and resilience. Breaking through stigma starts with self-compassion and recognizing that everyone needs support at times. Practical barriers can also stand in the way—limited access to specialized care, financial constraints, or living in remote areas without nearby services. Navigating the healthcare system can be overwhelming, especially when dealing with PTSX and substance use.

Connecting with veteran support organizations or using telehealth services may help bridge some of these gaps, while conventional treatment settings may inadvertently cause additional distress. Approaches that focus on confrontation, emphasize personal faults, or feel impersonal can be harmful to recovery. For someone already grappling with trauma, these environments might reinforce feelings of shame, guilt or isolation.

It's crucial that treatment environments are supportive, compassionate, and understanding of the unique experiences of veterans. Care providers who are trained in trauma-informed practices can make a significant difference in the healing journey. Healing is possible, and there are effective paths forward that honor each individual's experiences. Trauma-informed care and integrated treatment approaches offer promising avenues for recovery.

Trauma-informed care recognizes the profound impact of trauma and seeks to create a healing environment that avoids further trauma. This approach emphasizes safety, trust and empowerment. It's about working collaboratively, respecting each person's journey, and building on strengths rather than focusing on deficits.

In a trauma-informed setting, healthcare providers understand that behaviors like substance abuse may be coping mechanisms rather than simply "bad choices." They approach treatment with empathy, validating feelings and experiences. This can help rebuild trust and make it easier to engage in the healing process.

Empathy and patience are at the heart of trauma-informed care. By building a non-judgmental space, veterans can feel more comfortable exploring their experiences and challenges. This compassionate support can make a significant difference in recovery, as it encourages openness and honesty without fear of criticism or shame.

Therapeutic Approaches That Address Both PTSX and Substance Use

Several therapeutic methods have shown to be effective in addressing the intertwined challenges of PTSX and substance abuse. These approaches can be tailored to individual needs and preferences. It's important to find a mental healthcare professional who is proficient in both areas.

Cognitive Behavioral Therapy (CBT)

CBT is a well-established therapy that helps individuals identify and change unhelpful thought patterns and behaviors. For veterans dealing with PTSX and substance use, CBT can provide tools to recognize triggers, manage stress and develop more healthful coping strategies.

Through CBT, one might learn to challenge negative thoughts like "I can't handle this" or "I'm not worthy of help," replacing them with more balanced perspectives. Techniques may include setting realistic goals, practicing relaxation methods, and gradually facing feared situations in a balanced way.

Cognitive Processing Therapy (CPT)

CPT focuses on addressing the negative beliefs and emotions associated with trauma. It helps individuals reframe how they think about their experiences, reducing the hold that traumatic memories may have on their daily lives.

This therapy involves exploring how trauma has affected beliefs about oneself, others and the world. By examining and challenging these beliefs, individuals can begin to heal emotional wounds and reduce symptoms like guilt, shame and anger. One method is to list ten things about your current traumatic situation. Examine them. Do they support you in your healing? If not, rewrite each one so it aligns with where you want to be, i.e. healed. Change your thinking. Change your behavior. Change your life.

Prolonged Exposure Therapy

This therapy involves gently and gradually confronting traumatic memories in a safe environment. Over time, this approach can reduce the power these memories hold, helping individuals regain control over their responses. By repeatedly revisiting the traumatic event under the guidance of a trained therapist, the intense emotional reactions can diminish. This doesn't mean forgetting or minimizing the trauma but learning to integrate the memory without it overwhelming daily life.

Imaginal Exposure: Repeatedly recounting the traumatic memory in detail during therapy sessions. This process helps diminish the emotional power of the memory over time.

In Vivo Exposure: Gradually confronting safe situations, places or activities that have been avoided due to their association with the trauma.

Processing: Discussing thoughts and feelings about the traumatic experience and the exposure exercises to gain new insights and perspectives.

The intensive nature of exposure therapy can lead to significant symptom reduction in a shorter timeframe. Some veterans report that the continuous engagement allows them to stay immersed in the healing process, making it easier to confront and process their experiences.

Benefits of Massed Prolonged Exposure Therapy

We detail this type of therapy in a previous chapter, "Massed Prolonged Exposure Therapy." However, we feature it here, as well.

Accelerated Healing: A condensed schedule may lead to quicker relief from symptoms, which can be encouraging and motivating.

Increased Accessibility: For those with time constraints or impending obligations, this approach makes it possible to engage in effective therapy without a long-term commitment.

Enhanced Focus: The intensive sessions allow for sustained focus on healing, reducing the likelihood of external distractions interrupting progress.

A Pathway Tailored to You

Programs like COPE (Concurrent Treatment of PTSX and Substance Use Disorders Using Prolonged Exposure) integrate therapies to address both PTSX and substance use simultaneously. By tackling both issues together, individuals can find more cohesive and effective paths to healing.

These integrated approaches recognize that treating one condition without the other may not be sufficient. Combining therapies allows for a more holistic understanding of how PTSX and substance use interact, providing strategies that address the full scope of challenges.

The Importance of Trust and Connection

A trusting relationship with a therapist or counselor can be a cornerstone of recovery. Feeling heard, understood and respected allows for deeper engagement in the healing process. It's okay to seek out a provider who feels like a good fit. This connection can significantly influence the effectiveness of treatment.

Open communication, clear expectations, and collaborative goal-setting contribute to building this trust. Knowing that the therapist genuinely cares and is invested in one's wellbeing can create hope and motivation.

Connecting with peers who have shared similar experiences can provide comfort and validation. Group therapies or support groups offer spaces to share, listen and learn from one another. These connections can reduce feelings of isolation and build a sense of community.

Family and friends also play vital roles. Educating loved ones about PTSX and substance use can enhance understanding and support. Healthy relationships can provide encouragement, accountability and a network to lean on during difficult times.

Exploring Innovative Therapies and Looking Ahead

The brain has an incredible physical ability to adapt and change—a process known as neuroplasticity. Therapies that enhance neuroplasticity can help reshape thought patterns and responses established by trauma. Engaging in activities like mindfulness meditation, physical exercise, creative pursuits, and new learning experiences can promote brain health and recovery. These practices can complement traditional therapies, offering additional tools for healing.

Research into treatments like psychedelic-assisted therapy is ongoing. Substances such as MDMA and psilocybin are being studied for their potential to facilitate deep therapeutic work, especially for PTSX and addiction. Under professional guidance, these treatments may help individuals process trauma in new ways. While still under investigation, these therapies offer hope for new avenues of healing. It's essential to approach them with caution and seek information from reputable sources, as they are not yet widely available or suitable for everyone. Ensure you speak with a licensed professional, perhaps someone who is well known in the VA or civilian mental healthcare community.

Every individual's journey is unique. Successful treatment often involves empowering veterans to make choices about their care and selecting therapies that resonate with their personal needs and experiences. This might include deciding on therapy types, setting personal goals, or exploring complementary practices like yoga or acupuncture. Being active in one's treatment creates a sense of control and commitment, enhancing the likelihood of positive outcomes.

Stories of Healing and Resilience

Michael's Journey

Michael, a veteran who faced trauma both in childhood and during combat, found himself struggling with PTSX and substance use. Feelings of anger, fear and isolation weighed heavily on him. Through participating in COPE therapy, he began to process his traumatic memories in a safe, structured environment. The therapy allowed Michael to confront his experiences gradually, reducing their hold over his daily life. He learned healthier coping strategies, like mindfulness and building supportive relationships, which helped reduce his reliance on substances. Michael's journey wasn't easy, but with perseverance and support, he found a path toward healing.

Sandra's Path to Recovery

Sandra battled substance dependency from a young age and endured additional trauma in an abusive relationship. The weight of her experiences left her feeling trapped and hopeless. Engaging in Cognitive Processing Therapy allowed her to challenge and change negative self-beliefs stemming from her trauma. With the guidance of a compassionate therapist, Sandra began to see herself not as a victim but as a survivor with strength and resilience. She achieved sobriety and nurtured a more positive self-concept. While she faced challenges, including navigating traditional support groups, Sandra found empowerment in taking charge of her healing journey.

Moving Toward Healing and Wholeness

Healing from PTSX and substance abuse is a journey—one that is deeply personal and often challenging. But it's a journey that can lead to renewed strength, understanding and hope. Embracing compassion, both from others and toward oneself, can light the way forward.

Recognizing and addressing the underlying trauma is vital. By integrating compassionate, trauma-informed care, we honor the full experience of veterans and provide a foundation for genuine healing. This means not only treating symptoms but understanding the whole person—their history, strengths and needs.

Care that's empathic and personalized builds trust and openness. It encourages veterans to engage fully in their recovery, knowing they are valued and respected. This approach can make the difference between feeling overwhelmed and feeling empowered to heal.

Shifting away from practices that might feel punitive or shaming allows for the creation of safe, supportive environments. In these spaces, veterans can fully engage in their recovery, knowing they are respected and valued. A safe space might be a therapy room where confidentiality is honored, a support group where experiences are shared without judgment, or a home environment where loved ones offer understanding and patience. Establishing safety is a cornerstone of healing, allowing individuals to explore painful areas without fear or embarrassment.

Embracing Holistic Approaches

Combining various therapeutic methods, understanding the brain's responses, and making strong connections all contribute to sustained healing. A holistic approach considers the whole person—their mind, body and spirit.

This might include integrating physical healthcare, nutritional support, spiritual practices and creative outlets alongside traditional therapies. Recognizing that wellbeing encompasses multiple facets allows for a more comprehensive and personalized healing journey.

A Gentle Conclusion

To every veteran reading this: your courage is immense. Facing the intertwined challenges of PTSX and substance use is not easy, but you are not alone. It's okay to reach out, to ask for help, and to take the time you need. Healing is not a straight line, and setbacks are part of the process.

What matters is the willingness to keep moving forward, one step at a time. As we've said before, healing is a marathon, not a sprint. And healing takes time. As we continue to grow in our understanding of these complex issues, the focus remains on providing care that is compassionate, effective and tailored to each individual. Recovery is possible, and there is hope for a future with peace and fulfillment.

If-Then Guidance

Navigating the complexities of PTSX and substance use and abuse can be challenging. The following if-then statements offer practical guidance to help veterans, caregivers and healthcare providers take actionable steps toward finding and administering proper care and healing.

- If you are a veteran experiencing both PTSX and substance abuse, then consider seeking an integrated treatment program that addresses both conditions simultaneously to enhance your recovery journey.
- If overwhelming emotions lead you to use substances for relief, then explore therapies that teach better coping mechanisms, such as mindfulness or relaxation techniques, to manage distress without relying on drugs or alcohol.
- If feelings of stigma or beliefs about self-reliance prevent you from seeking help, then remind yourself that reaching out is a sign of strength, and consider connecting with supportive individuals or groups who understand your experiences.
- If you face barriers to accessing specialized care due to location or finances, then look into alternative options like telehealth services or community resources that provide support for veterans.
- If traditional treatment settings feel impersonal or re-traumatizing,

then seek out trauma-informed care providers who emphasize safety, trust and empowerment in their approach.

- If you are hesitant to engage in therapy due to fear of confronting traumatic memories, then discuss gradual exposure therapies with a healthcare professional to find a pace that feels manageable for you.
- If you feel that substance use is impacting your cognitive functions or daily life, then consider therapies like cognitive behavioral therapy to help identify triggers and develop healthier coping strategies.
- If intense cravings or withdrawal symptoms make it difficult to engage in treatment, then speak with a healthcare provider about Medication-Assisted Treatment to support you through this phase.
- If you feel isolated or unsupported, then reach out to peer-support groups or veteran-specific organizations where you can connect with others who have shared similar experiences.
- If you have physical health issues like chronic pain, then ensure your treatment plan addresses these needs holistically to prevent exacerbating substance use.
- If you're exploring therapy options, then consider whether Massed Prolonged Exposure Therapy might be suitable for you, especially if you require an intensive approach over a shorter period.
- If you're interested in emerging treatments like psychedelic-assisted therapy, then consult with reputable healthcare professionals to understand the benefits and risks involved.
- If negative beliefs about yourself are holding you back, then therapies like Cognitive Processing Therapy can help you challenge and reframe these thoughts.
- If you recognize generational patterns of trauma in your family, then discussing this with a therapist can provide insights and aid in your healing process.
- If you're ready to take an active role in your recovery, then empower yourself by collaborating with your healthcare providers to tailor a treatment plan that resonates with your personal needs and goals.

Take the Next Step

Your journey toward healing is a path of courage, resilience and self-discovery. Acknowledging the challenges you face is a significant first step. Here's how you can move forward:

- Reach out for support. Connect with trusted friends, family members or support groups who can provide encouragement and understanding. Sharing your experiences can lessen the burden and build a sense of community.
- Explore treatment options. Research and consider various therapeutic approaches that address both PTSX and substance abuse. Consult with healthcare professionals to find treatments that align with your preferences and needs.
- Prioritize self-care. Engage in activities that promote wellbeing: regular exercise, healthful eating, sufficient sleep and mindfulness practices. Caring for your physical health can positively impact your mental and emotional states.
- Set realistic goals. Break down your recovery journey into manageable steps. Celebrate small victories along the way to stay motivated and recognize your progress.
- Educate yourself. Learn more about PTSX, substance abuse, and the impact of trauma on the brain and body. Understanding these aspects can empower you to make informed decisions about your personal healthcare.
- Embrace compassion. Practice self-compassion by acknowledging your strengths and forgiving yourself for setbacks. Remember that healing is not linear, and it's okay to have challenging days.
- Build a supportive environment. Surround yourself with people and spaces that make you feel safe and valued. This may involve setting boundaries or seeking new connections that promote positivity.
- Stay open to new experiences. Be willing to try different therapies or activities that might aid in your recovery. Openness can lead to discoveries that resonate with you and enhance your healing process.
- Advocate for yourself. Communicate your needs and preferences

to your healthcare providers. Your voice is essential in shaping a treatment plan that feels right for you.

- Look toward the future. Focus on the possibilities that lie ahead rather than dwelling solely on past challenges, especially those that didn't work. Cultivate hope by envisioning a future where you feel empowered and fulfilled.
- Remember, you are not alone, and support is available. Taking the next step might feel daunting, but it's a move toward reclaiming your life and wellbeing. Your courage to face these challenges is a testament to your strength. Healing is within reach, and each step you take brings you closer to a place of peace and resilience.

Through Their Eyes

"For me, the bottle was my escape, the only thing that seemed to quiet the noise in my head. But it didn't take long for me to realize that the relief it brought was a lie. The deeper I sank into that cycle, the worse the PTSX got. I thought I was in control, but the truth is, the more I used, the less control I had.

"Breaking that cycle wasn't easy. It took more guts than I ever needed on the battlefield. But what I learned is that real strength is admitting you need help and accepting that you deserve it. I'm living proof that you can win this fight—it's tough, but it's winnable."

—Corporal Darryl S., US Army Veteran

47

Patrick's Saga: A Journey Through Battle and Healing

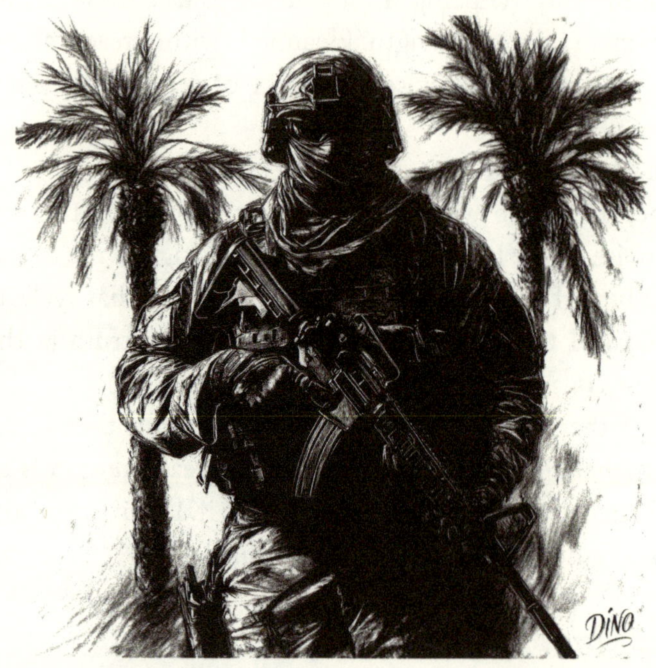

Patrick was sixteen when he dropped out of high school, stumbling into the world without a plan. He scraped by on a GED, then joined the Army, both frightened and driven by a spark of determination no one saw coming. In Basic Infantry Training, he discovered a hidden reservoir of strength and grit— qualities that turned him from a restless teen into a focused, unstoppable soldier. Airborne School followed, then the grueling Ranger Indoctrination Program, where he channeled every ounce of self-doubt into burning resolve.

By the time he deployed to Iraq with the 75th Ranger Regiment, he'd become the youngest team leader in his unit. He lost his best friend there to a sniper's bullet—an agony that nearly split him in two. Yet, he shouldered the grief and completed countless missions under the harsh desert sun. In each moment of chaos, he wrestled with the same question: Why do I survive when others don't?

From there, Patrick's career vaulted into Delta Force, where secrecy and intense operation cycles became his norm. He deployed again and again—Afghanistan, Syria, Africa—never pausing to sift through what war was doing to his spirit. Just a few years ago, he even led a covert strike targeting high-value personnel in Russia. Always mission-focused, always forward.

Long-term trauma can leave you in a constant state of fight or flight, always on edge and unable to relax. These behaviors, while initially protective, can become damaging if they dominate your life.

But after more than three decades of unrelenting battle, his mind and body could no longer ignore the toll. A flashpoint in a city street—where he singlehandedly stopped six armed attackers—forced him to reckon with what he'd become: someone who lived on reflex, never letting himself feel. Desperate and haunted, he found an unlikely answer in a nerve block procedure called stellate ganglion block (SGB). This injection dialed down his constant state of hypervigilance. Over multiple treatments, Patrick finally glimpsed something like peace—a clear head, no longer jammed with the residue of wars. Realizing he could be more than a war machine, he stepped into a new role: educating other veterans about getting help before it's too late.

This chapter follows Master Sergeant Patrick's [Not his real name or rank.] rise from dropout to elite special-operations warrior, then tracks his journey back from the edges of self-destruction. It underscores how unaddressed trauma can warp even the strongest among us—and highlights the transformative potential of innovative treatments and supportive peers. Above all, it conveys a message of hope: that healing is possible, no matter how deep the scars.

His story is not one of a simple soldier or human being. His saga speaks to the heart of what it means to be human in the most extreme of circumstances—where life, death and survival intertwine in the throes of combat. Raised in adversity, Patrick's path to greatness began not in a classroom but in the aftermath of continual failures at nearly every level of his life, until he found his calling in special operations and in leading other good men on dangerous missions.

An Inauspicious Beginning

After flunking out of high school, Patrick earned his GED and, at the young age of 18, took a leap into a life that would demand more of him than he could ever imagine. When he enlisted in the Army, he was, in many ways, unformed clay. His future was unwritten, the trajectory of his life uncertain, yet something burned within him—a quiet resolve. The military, with its rigid structure and relentless discipline, became the arena in which Patrick would build himself into something extraordinary.

Patrick's journey through Basic Infantry Training was swift, his physical prowess and tactical acuity quickly setting him apart. Not satisfied with merely completing his training, Patrick excelled, finding himself in Advanced Infantry Training, where the demands increased, yet his capacity to absorb, learn and adapt outstripped those around him.

By the time he entered Airborne School, his transformation from a floundering teenager into a formidable warrior was well underway. In 1992, when he blew through the grueling Ranger Indoctrination Program (RIP), he was not just prepared.

He was determined to become one of the best. But the training wasn't just about physical endurance—it was a mental battle too. Patrick remembered one particular night during Ranger School, during a brutal forced march in the freezing rain. His legs were leaden with exhaustion, and his mind started to wander: *Why am I here? Who am I trying to prove something to? Do I even believe I'm capable of this, or am I just fooling myself? Maybe this is all a mistake.* But even as the doubts crept in, so did the fire in his belly—the desire to keep pushing, to be more than he ever thought possible.

A Ranger's Resolve

In Ranger School, Patrick's performance wasn't just exemplary—it was legendary. To become the distinguished graduate in a program that breaks even the most hardened soldiers is no small feat. With an unyielding spirit, Patrick sailed through the 62 days of relentless mental and physical challenges without issue. His resilience was unmatched, his focus unshakable. Every task set before him—whether it was enduring sleep deprivation, starvation or the harsh elements—became another stone in the foundation of his soldier's heart.

Yet, during the rare moments of solitude, Patrick found himself questioning his path. One memory that often replayed in his mind was the day his squad leader was killed in Iraq. As Patrick took command, he could feel the weight of his best friend's absence, but there was no time to grieve.

Why him? Why not me? Patrick had thought, staring at the horizon as the desert sun dipped below it. *What made me so special to survive today? Am I ready to carry this burden—leading these men into battle, knowing that every decision I make could be their last?* But Patrick knew there was no turning back. He had to lead.

At just 20 years old, Patrick became the youngest team leader in the 75th Ranger Regiment. His maturity in leadership and his ability to keep a cool head under pressure made him the natural choice for the role. It was in Iraq, however, that Patrick's mettle was truly tested.

The death of his squad leader and best friend, killed by a sniper, would have shaken anyone to their core. But Patrick, with the weight of his entire team now on his shoulders, did not falter. Every decision, every maneuver, and every order carried the weight of life or death, yet Patrick never wavered. His resolve was ironclad.

During one mission deep in the heart of enemy territory, Patrick found himself lying prone in the dust, watching through his scope as the minutes turned to hours. *Is this who I've become? Just a shadow in the night waiting to strike, a man reduced to a mission?* He exhaled slowly. *Can I ever be anything else?* The thought lingered, but the moment he spotted movement in his peripheral vision, his focus snapped back. He knew there was no room for self-reflection on the battlefield.

Special Forces Operator: A Life of Shadow Wars

After his service with the Rangers, Patrick knew he wanted more—not just for himself, but for his country. He applied for Special Forces Operational Detachment-D (Delta Force) selection, a pipeline that only the most elite soldiers can dream of entering, let alone completing. As he had done before, Patrick breezed through the training, earning his place as an Assaulter with A Squadron. His performance in the field, from Iraq to Afghanistan, from Syria to Africa, was nothing short of exceptional. He served with distinction, consistently proving himself in the most demanding and dangerous environments on the planet.

The life of a Delta Force operator is one of secrecy and sacrifice. Patrick's missions were often conducted under the veil of darkness, in places the world would never hear about, against enemies that existed only in the shadows. During one particularly intense mission in Afghanistan, Patrick found himself pinned down in a firefight that stretched on for hours.

Amid the chaos, he caught himself thinking, *If I die here, will anyone know what I did, or why I did it? Am I just a tool of war, expendable and forgotten once my use has passed?* The thought gnawed at him, but as always, the mission came first.

In 2022, during the height of the [REDACTED] invasion, Patrick led a top-secret mission to hunt down high-value targets inside [REDACTED]. It was the kind of operation that made headlines only in classified briefings, but for Patrick, it was just another day in a career that had seen decades of action.

By 2023, Patrick had spent 31 years in service. He had been to every significant event in modern combat, protected two sitting US presidents from harm, and led countless men through the fog of war. But Patrick's greatest battle was not on the battlefield. It was within himself—a battle he had ignored for far too long.

The Turning Point

After decades of service, Patrick's body and mind had become an unyielding machine—always on call, always moving from one mission to the next. He was the guy everyone relied on, the one who ensured his fellow operators and their families were safe and secure. But in doing so, Patrick never took a moment to check on himself. He took his own invincibility for granted, believing that as long as he kept moving, kept fighting, everything would be fine.

It wasn't.

One day, sitting at a traffic light in a certain city in [REDACTED], the weight of decades of violence and unaddressed trauma began to surface in the most unexpected way. A van filled with six gangsters pulled up next to him. They began to razz him about his deep tan and long flowing hair, mocking him as if they knew nothing about the man who sat behind the wheel.

Patrick, numb from years of burying his emotions, didn't react. His body and mind were no longer in sync. The man who had faced the worst humanity had to offer felt absolutely nothing.

Then, in a flash, all six gangsters poured from the van, surrounding Patrick's truck. Without hesitation, without conscious thought, Patrick acted. *This is what I've become.* The gunfire echoed in his ears. *Nothing more than a weapon that reacts on instinct.* In a matter of seconds, he did what he had to do, with the precision of someone who had been fighting for his life for 31 years. And just as quickly as it had started, it was over. Patrick stepped back into his truck and drove off, leaving behind a scene that would haunt him for years to come.

The Road to Healing

Decades of abuse, neglect, violence and harm had taken their toll. The years of pushing through without stopping had left deep scars on his soul. His body was hardened, but his spirit was fractured. His friends took the helm and took care of the problem. Conventional therapy didn't work. Sitting in a chair, talking to a therapist who had never seen war, never felt the chaos of combat, felt pointless. Patrick quickly became frustrated, turning once again to alcohol to numb the pain.

His friends, watching him spiral, intervened. They knew the man they once looked up to was on the verge of self-destruction. That's when they introduced him to something different—a treatment that wasn't about talking but about resetting the body's trauma response at a fundamental level. They enrolled Patrick in a special study using SGB, a relatively new and innovative treatment for PTSX.

For veterans like Patrick, whose bodies had been stuck in a state of hypervigilance for decades, SGB offered a way to calm that response. By resetting the overactive sympathetic nervous system, the treatment allowed patients to finally feel a sense of normalcy, a peace they hadn't known in years. For Patrick, it took several treatments to fully feel the effects, but once he did, it was like waking up from a nightmare. The relentless anxiety, the feeling of always being on edge, began to fade. His mind, once clouded by years of violence and trauma, started to clear. For the first time in his life, Patrick felt something resembling peace. The PTSX that had haunted him for so long was finally receding.

A New Mission

Today, Patrick no longer drinks. He no longer feels the compulsion to resort to violence when faced with confrontation. He's found a new mission—one that doesn't involve the battlefield but is perhaps even more important. Patrick now lectures to veterans, particularly those from the special operations community, about the dangers of going it alone.

He speaks from experience, warning them about the toll of a life lived in constant combat, both external and internal. He urges them to seek help, to recognize that being strong isn't about ignoring pain but about confronting it head-on. Patrick's story, once defined by violence, is now one of redemption. He has become an inspiration of hope for those who are still in the fight, reminding them that there's always a path to healing.

If-Then Guidance

- If you feel overwhelmed by unprocessed trauma, then understand that avoiding or suppressing it will only deepen the emotional scars. Patrick's avoidance led him down a destructive path until he faced his pain directly. Trauma is not just a psychic wound. it has a molecular foundation that, when left untreated, festers and grows worse over time. Acknowledging your trauma is the first step toward healing, and it's important to recognize that you don't have to do it alone. Reach out to trusted individuals, professionals or seasoned veterans who understand your journey and can offer support. Healing requires you to face those emotions head-on, allowing them to be processed rather than buried beneath layers of defense mechanisms. You are stronger than your pain, and confronting it will lead you toward recovery and personal growth.

- If you believe that conventional therapy isn't working for you, then don't give up hope—consider alternative treatments like SGB. Patrick found solace in a non-traditional treatment that reset his trauma response and gave him relief when other methods failed. It's easy to feel disheartened when traditional approaches don't provide the relief you expected, but there are always other options. Alternative therapies are gaining ground, with techniques such as SGB, ketamine therapy or neurofeedback showing promise in addressing PTSX. Don't be afraid to explore new treatments or advocate for innovative solutions that align with your unique needs. Healing is not a one-size-fits-all process, and discovering the right approach may take time. Patience and persistence are vital on this journey—there is always a way forward, even when the path seems unclear.
- If you think that seeking help is a sign of weakness, then look at Patrick's journey. His greatest strength came not from fighting battles, but from recognizing his need for healing and choosing to take that step. Asking for help can feel uncomfortable, especially for those who are used to being self-reliant, but it is one of the most courageous decisions you can make. Vulnerability is not weakness—it is a strength that requires immense bravery to show. Recognize that seeking assistance is not about surrendering, but about empowering yourself to heal and grow. Patrick's story illustrates that those who step up to take care of their mental health are not only helping themselves but also becoming beacons

of hope for others. By reaching out, you are embracing a new kind of strength—one that will guide you through the challenges ahead.

- If you've been stuck in a cycle of hypervigilance or destructive behaviors, then acknowledge that healing is possible, but it requires confronting the core of your pain. Patrick only found peace after he addressed the trauma he had carried for decades. Long-term trauma can leave you in a constant state of fight or flight, always on edge and unable to relax. These behaviors, while initially protective, can become damaging if they dominate your life. Patrick's breakthrough came when he chose to face the root of his issues, rather than continuing to cope by numbing himself or avoiding his emotions. Understand that it's never too late to confront your trauma and begin the healing process. Breaking free from these destructive cycles starts with understanding where they stem from and then taking small steps to dismantle them. Healing is a process, and it may take time, but every effort counts.
- If you are feeling disconnected from your true self due to a life spent in constant combat or stress, then recognize that there is more to you than the battles you've fought. Patrick, at one point, saw himself as merely a tool of war, but he eventually realized there was more to his identity. It's easy to get lost in a role, especially one that demands such an intense level of commitment, but you are more than your duties or your experiences. There is a human being beneath the armor—one who deserves peace, joy and fulfillment beyond the battlefield. Taking time to reconnect with yourself, to discover who you are outside of your service or trauma, is a vital part of healing. Patrick's journey shows that rediscovering yourself is possible, even after years of losing yourself to duty or hardship.
- If you are struggling with guilt over past decisions, especially those made in the heat of combat, then understand that healing involves forgiveness—not just of others, but of yourself. Patrick dealt with immense survivor's guilt after the loss of his squad leader, yet he eventually had to come to terms with the fact that some things

are beyond his control. The weight of such experiences can be crushing, but you must remember that you did the best you could in those moments, given the circumstances. Guilt can be one of the hardest burdens to let go of, but forgiveness is essential to moving forward. It doesn't mean forgetting or diminishing the gravity of what happened, but it allows you to find peace within yourself. Healing is not just about addressing physical or emotional wounds—it's also about reconciling with the past and finding a way to live with it.

Take the Next Step

- Just as Patrick reached a turning point in his life, so can you. Start by recognizing the weight you've been carrying and accept that you don't need to carry it alone. It's crucial to take the first step, which could be as simple as talking to someone who understands your experiences.
- Whether it's a trusted friend, a therapist or a veteran who has walked a similar path, seeking support is a sign of strength. Patrick's story shows that no matter how heavy the load feels, sharing it lightens the burden.
- Explore treatments that may offer the relief you've been seeking, whether that's through innovative therapies like SGB or other emerging methods. Just because one method hasn't worked doesn't mean the door to healing is closed. Patrick's success with SGB is a reminder that medical advancements are constantly evolving, and there may be an option out there that's right for you.
- Seek out resources that align with your journey. This could involve joining a veterans' group, participating in support networks, or engaging with specialists who focus on PTSX and trauma recovery. Patrick's friends intervened and helped him discover the treatment that changed his life— there are resources waiting for you too. Don't hesitate to tap into the support that's available.
- Find a mentor or guide who can help you navigate the path forward. Sometimes, all it takes is one person to help you see things differently, to offer perspective or advice from someone

who has been in your shoes. Patrick now lectures veterans and shares his experience to ensure others don't have to go it alone—consider finding someone who can do the same for you.

- Take small steps toward healing. You don't have to solve everything at once. Patrick's journey took time, patience and several attempts at different treatments before he found peace. Healing is a process, and even small victories should be celebrated. Whether it's attending a support group meeting, trying a new therapy or just opening up to a friend, every step counts.
- Remember, taking that first step toward healing, no matter how small, is a sign of resilience, not weakness. Just like Patrick found a new mission outside of combat, you too can find a new purpose beyond the pain.

48

A Veteran's Step-by-Step Guide to Seeking PTSX Treatment

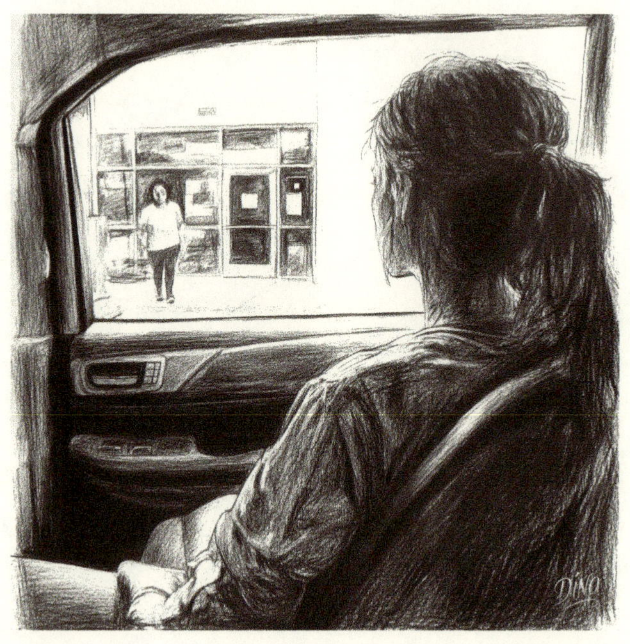

Jasmine sat in the car outside her small apartment, gathering the nerve to finally pick up the phone. She'd spent weeks waking up drenched in sweat, visions of past missions crowding her thoughts until she could hardly breathe. Each day she told herself she'd handle it on her own—until another flashback knocked her back to the dust and chaos. Today, though, the weight on her chest felt too heavy to ignore. She took a deep breath, pulled out her phone, and dialed the Veterans Crisis Line.

After a supportive conversation that calmed her racing heart, Jasmine realized she needed a clearer plan. She'd heard about the local VA hospital from a friend but had no clue where to begin. A Crisis Line responder explained that her next move should be contacting VA Mental Health Services. By the time Jasmine ended the call, she felt a flicker of relief—she had a first step.

A week later, she parked at the VA, uncertain and uneasy. Yet the moment she stepped inside, a patient coordinator greeted her with genuine warmth. Over the next couple of hours, Jasmine spoke with a mental health provider who evaluated her symptoms and walked her through various treatment pathways.

She learned about conventional therapies like cognitive behavioral therapy (CBT), prolonged exposure therapy (PET) and eye movement desensitization and reprocessing (EMDR), and also discovered emerging options: stellate ganglion block, ketamine infusion, even MDMA-assisted research trials. Hearing that there were so many possibilities—some new, some tried and tested—made her feel less trapped.

In between sessions, Jasmine explored a nearby Vet Center. It felt more relaxed than the hospital, offering peer-led workshops, group discussions, and a quieter space to talk. She realized that speaking with other veterans—men and women who'd faced similar nightmares—brought a sense of belonging. She also found herself joining a peer-support group run by a local nonprofit, where she connected with those who understood how hard it was to sleep at night or maintain relationships while burdened by invisible battles.

As Jasmine's care plan solidified, she began incorporating community-based programs. Team Red, White & Blue invited her to hike trails with fellow vets, a simple activity that reminded her she wasn't alone. The Wounded Warrior Project introduced her to an online community she could tap into anytime anxious thoughts crept in. These connections kept her steady, especially in moments when therapy felt daunting or progress seemed slow.

A few months later, Jasmine found she wasn't waking up in terror quite as often. There were still rough days—PTSX recovery rarely follows a straight line. But she was building resilience through a blend of therapy sessions, peer support, and the occasional check-in with her crisis-line mentor. She knew the journey was ongoing, but she no longer felt adrift. She had a roadmap and a supportive network at her side.

This chapter is a gentle guide similar to Jasmine's path, designed for any veteran ready to seek help for PTSX. For many veterans, seeking assistance for PTSX can feel daunting, and navigating the myriad resources may seem overwhelming. The silent scars of combat often make it difficult for veterans to take that first step toward healing. It outlines a clear, actionable path for a veteran to follow when seeking treatment for PTSX, highlighting key organizations, resources and practical steps.

This guide is intended to empower veterans by demystifying the process and offering real, accessible ways to get help. We strongly suggest that you always verify contact information and program availability, as the contact and program information here may have changed.

Step 1: Recognize the Need for Help

The first and most important step is acknowledging the need for help. PTSX often manifests through known symptoms: nightmares, flashbacks, flashforwards, irritability, hypervigilance and emotional numbness. These symptoms can interfere with daily life, relationships and the ability to function in civilian settings.

Veterans who recognize these signs in themselves should not view it as a weakness but as the first step toward recovery. For veterans who may be unsure whether their symptoms align with PTSX, taking an anonymous online PTSX screening test can help determine the next step.

Organizations like the VA and Mental Health America offer free, confidential screenings online. These tools help veterans assess their symptoms and provide recommendations for next steps based on the results.

Step 2: Reach Out to the Veterans Crisis Line or VA Mental Health Services

This service provides confidential, round-the-clock support and is available via phone, text, or online chat. Trained responders, many of whom are veterans themselves, can offer support, listen to the individual's concerns, and help guide them to appropriate resources.

Veterans Crisis Line Contact Information:

Call: 1-800-273-8255 or 988 (Press 1 for either one when connected)

Text: 838255

Chat: Veterans Crisis Line Chat is for veterans who aren't in immediate crisis but feel they need assistance, contacting their local VA Mental Health Services is a crucial next step. Every VA Medical Center offers mental-health care, and veterans can receive help by simply scheduling an appointment. Even if a veteran is not enrolled in VA health care, they can still access VA mental health services for a period of time after discharge.

Step 3: Connect with a VA Care Provider or Vet Center

After reaching out to the VA or accessing the Crisis Line, veterans are typically referred to mental health care providers within the VA system. At this point, a VA care provider will conduct a full assessment and develop a personalized treatment plan. Veterans often have access to evidence-based therapies like cognitive behavioral therapy, PET, and EMDR.

For veterans who prefer a less formal setting or want additional support, Vet Centers offer community-based counseling services specifically for veterans, servicemembers and their families. Vet Centers are particularly valuable for combat veterans and offer free, confidential mental health services, even for those who are not enrolled in the VA system.

Step 4: Explore Treatment Options – From Traditional to Emerging Therapies

Once connected with VA mental health services or a Vet Center, veterans will explore treatment options tailored to their needs. Conventional treatments like CBT or EMDR are widely available, but many veterans may also wish to explore emerging therapies that are now becoming more accessible. Some of the most promising new treatments include:

Ketamine Infusion Therapy: Particularly effective for treatment-resistant PTSX, ketamine can offer rapid relief from depression and suicidal ideation. Many VA centers now offer ketamine treatments, especially for veterans who have not responded to traditional medications.

Stellate Ganglion Block (SGB): A groundbreaking treatment involving an injection into a nerve cluster in the neck, SGB has shown success in reducing PTSX symptoms, particularly anxiety and hypervigilance. The VA is increasingly offering this as part of a comprehensive PTSX treatment plan.

MDMA-Assisted Therapy: Though still in clinical trial phases at the VA, MDMA-assisted therapy is showing promise for veterans with severe, treatment-resistant PTSX. Veterans interested in these emerging treatments should discuss their options with their care providers.

Dr. Mark Gordon's Brain Rescue therapy: though largely unknown, Dr. Gordon's pioneering research in and treatment of TBI shows us that his methods are sound and produce excellent results. He has healed/cured hundreds of veterans' TBI and associated issues.

Step 5: Engage in Peer-Support Networks

Alongside professional mental healthcare, veterans can benefit greatly from peer-support programs. These programs connect veterans with others who have similar experiences, creating a sense of community and understanding that can be deeply therapeutic.

Peer-support groups are often run by veterans, providing a safe space to share stories, challenges, and coping mechanisms. Veterans can engage with these programs through these organizations:

Wounded Warrior Project: Offers mental health programs and peer support networks specifically for veterans. Website: **woundedwarriorproject.org**

Iraq and Afghanistan Veterans of America (IAVA): Provides mental health resources and peer support tailored to the needs of post-9/11 veterans. Website: **iava.org**

Team Red, White & Blue: Focuses on connecting veterans through physical and social activities that promote mental health and community. Website: **teamrwb.org**

Step 6: Use Community Resources and Non-VA Support

Beyond VA services, there are numerous community-based resources that veterans can access for support. Many non-profit organizations provide alternative therapies, specialized treatment programs, and financial assistance for mental healthcare. Veterans who feel that traditional VA care does not fully meet their needs or who wish to explore holistic therapies often find these organizations to be invaluable.

Veteran's PATH: Provides mindfulness and meditation programs specifically designed to support veterans in their recovery from PTSX. Website: veteranspath.org

Operation Mend (UCLA Health): Offers intensive mental health care for veterans with PTSX and traumatic brain injuries (TBI). Website: uclahealth.org/operationmend

The Mission Continues: Focuses on empowering veterans to reintegrate into their communities through service projects, creating a sense of purpose and belonging. Website: missioncontinues.org

Step 7: Long-Term Follow-Up and Building Resilience

PTSX recovery is not a one-time event but an ongoing process. Veterans who have started their journey toward healing need to maintain a long-term care plan that includes regular therapy, support networks and self-care strategies. Veterans should work closely with their care providers to ensure that their treatment plans are adaptable as their needs evolve.

Resilience-building programs like those offered by Team Rubicon or The Mission Continues, can play a vital role in long-term recovery by encouraging veterans to engage in meaningful, community-based activities. They engage veterans in disaster relief and humanitarian projects, providing a sense of mission and teamwork that aids mental health recovery. Website: teamrubiconusa.org

If -Then Guidance

- If you're experiencing symptoms like nightmares, flashbacks, irritability or emotional numbness, then it's crucial to recognize that these may be signs of PTSX, and acknowledging the need for help is the first and most important step in your journey toward healing.

- If you're unsure whether your symptoms align with PTSX, then take an anonymous PTSX screening test through the VA or Mental Health America. These free, confidential screenings can provide guidance on whether further steps are necessary.
- If you find yourself in immediate crisis or are experiencing suicidal thoughts, then reaching out to the Veterans Crisis Line is critical. The Crisis Line offers 24/7 support from trained responders, including veterans, who can listen and guide you to appropriate resources.
- If you're not in immediate crisis but need support, then contacting your local VA Mental Health Services is the next logical step. They can help you schedule an appointment, even if you're not enrolled in VA healthcare, to access essential mental health services.
- If you prefer a less formal setting or need additional support, then connecting with a local Vet Center is a valuable option. Vet Centers offer free, confidential mental-health counseling specifically designed for veterans, regardless of VA enrollment status.
- If you've connected with VA mental health services, then exploring your treatment options, from traditional methods like CBT to emerging therapies like SGB or MDMA-assisted therapy, will allow you to tailor your care to your specific needs.
- If you find that traditional treatments have not provided relief, then discussing emerging therapies such as ketamine infusion or SGB with your care provider can open the door to alternative, cutting-edge treatment options for PTSX.
- If you want to complement professional treatment with peer support, then engaging with organizations like Wounded Warrior Project, Iraq and Afghanistan Veterans of America or Team Red, White & Blue can provide a sense of community.
- If VA services don't fully meet your needs or you wish to explore holistic therapies, then seeking support from community-based resources like Veteran's PATH, Operation Mend, or The Mission

Continues can provide alternative pathways to healing.

- If your goal is long-term resilience, then building a care plan that includes regular therapy, peer support, and community engagement can help you sustain your recovery journey over time.

Take the Next Step

- Recognize the Need for Help: If you notice signs of PTSX, like nightmares or hypervigilance, take that critical first step by acknowledging the need for professional support.
- Contact the Veterans Crisis Line or VA Mental Health Services: Call 1-800-273-8255 or 988 (Press 1), text 838255, or chat online with the Veterans Crisis Line for immediate assistance. For non-emergencies, visit your local VA office to speak with a mental-health professional.
- Connect with a VA Care Provider or Vet Center: Reach out to a VA care provider for a full assessment and personalized treatment plan, or visit a Vet Center for free, confidential counseling and support tailored to veterans.
- Explore Treatment Options: Research traditional therapies like Cognitive Behavioral Therapy or emerging therapies like SGB and MDMA-assisted therapy, and discuss the best fit with your care provider.
- Engage in Peer-Support Networks: Join a veteran peer-support program through organizations like Wounded Warrior Project, Iraq and Afghanistan Veterans of America (IAVA), or Team Red, White & Blue to find solidarity and shared experiences.
- Participate in Peer-Support Groups: Consider attending local or virtual peer-support groups to connect with fellow veterans who understand your experiences and can offer valuable insights and coping mechanisms.
- Schedule a PTSX Evaluation: Contact your local VA or use the Mental Health America screening tool to take the first steps toward an official diagnosis and tailored treatment plan.
- Commit to Long-Term Follow-Up: Work with your healthcare provider(s) to build a long-term strategy that includes regular

therapy, peer support and resilience-building activities for ongoing recovery. Know that it will take time, so be patient.

Through Their Eyes

"As a retired Navy Captain and former submarine commander, I spent much of my career navigating high-stakes, high-pressure environments where composure and precision were critical. In the Navy, we pride ourselves on discipline and stoicism, but the silent battles many of us fight after service—like PTSX—are ones that we can't face alone.

"As a commander, my goal was always to provide my crew with clear directives to accomplish their mission. I believe this guide does the same for veterans in their personal mission to overcome PTSX. The first step is often the hardest. Recognizing the need for help was something I initially resisted. Years of being in command had taught me to internalize stress and push through, but that only took me so far after leaving the service.

"The nightmares, hypervigilance and emotional detachment all began to affect my relationships and daily life. The critical realization came when I understood that asking for help wasn't a sign of weakness. It was a strategic move in my personal recovery mission.

"For others, like myself, the path begins with reaching out to VA Mental Health Services. This guide lays out exactly how to do that—step by step—so no one has to feel lost or unsure of where to turn. Another key step is connecting with VA care providers or Vet Centers.

"What I appreciated about Vet Centers is that they offer a more relaxed, community-based approach. Many of the counselors are veterans themselves, which creates an environment where it's easier to open up. As someone who commanded submarines, I wasn't always comfortable talking about my vulnerabilities, but finding a setting with fellow veterans made a world of difference.

"From traditional methods like CBT to emerging treatments like ketamine infusion therapy and SGB, veterans now have access to a wide range of therapies. In my case, understanding that there are treatments available beyond the standard medications or talk therapies. Peer support is another powerful component highlighted in this guide. During my service, I relied on my team, and that same principle applies in recovery. Connecting with veterans through organizations like the Wounded Warrior Project or Team Red, White & Blue helps build camaraderie and mutual understanding. There's strength in knowing you're not navigating this path alone, and the guide provides clear steps on how to join these networks.

"For those who want to explore beyond the VA system, the guide also outlines community-based resources like Veteran's PATH, which offers mindfulness programs, or Operation Mend, which provides intensive mental health care. These organizations give veterans alternative pathways to healing, particularly for those who may feel the traditional routes aren't enough or don't fully meet their needs.

"Programs like Team Rubicon, which engages veterans in disaster relief missions, offer opportunities to rebuild purpose and resilience through meaningful work. For me, staying active and engaged with my community became a critical part of my healing journey.

"In sum, this guide offers a clear, actionable plan for veterans to seek help, whether they're just beginning to recognize symptoms of PTSX or have struggled for years. It's about providing a step-by-step approach, one that is comprehensive, practical and veteran-focused.

"My role in consulting on these steps has been to ensure that no veteran feels like they're navigating the system alone. Just like we did in the Navy, we tackle problems head-on with precision and purpose. This guide helps veterans do just that—leading them from trauma to healing, one step at a time."

—Captain James T., US Navy (ret.)

49

General Health Questionnaire with Actionable Guidance

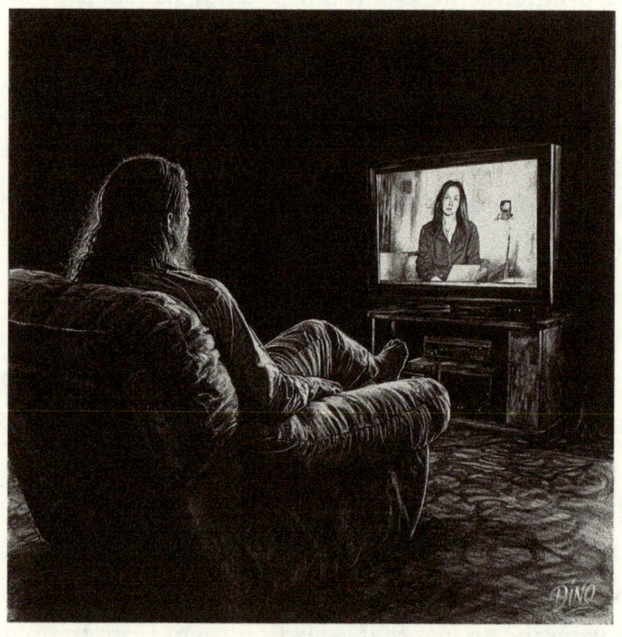

Cameron flicked off the TV news, feeling a nagging sense that something in his life wasn't right. He'd been dragging himself out of bed most mornings, relying on caffeine just to stay awake through the day. He also noticed his pants fitting tighter around the waist, though he couldn't remember changing his diet.

Lately, his moods soared and dipped without warning. One minute he'd feel okay, the next he'd be snapping at his wife over minor things. After a recent argument, they both agreed: maybe it was time for a check on his health—physical and mental.

That's what brought Cameron to a small clinic where he found a printed "General Health Questionnaire." It had all sorts of questions—

about energy levels, pain, sleep quality, even how often he felt down or anxious. He took it home, sat at the kitchen table, and filled it out honestly. The first few pages made him realize just how tired he'd been feeling, even on the weekends.

Another section asked about appetite changes. Cameron's mind flashed back to how his shirts had felt snug lately—yup, he'd been overeating junk food to cope with stress. He wrote that down. And then there were the mental-health questions. He paused at "loss of interest in activities" and sighed. He remembered the guitar collecting dust in the corner, something he used to love playing.

Filling out the questionnaire felt strangely relieving. Each question helped him pinpoint the areas in his life that needed attention, offering "If-Then" actions to follow up on. If energy was low, maybe see a doctor about possible anemia, or if shortness of breath popped up, he should consider a heart check. This wasn't just a survey—it was a roadmap.

This chapter features the same questionnaire Cameron found, along with actionable guidance. Please study and then take each "If-Then" recommendation as a gentle nudge toward better health. The purpose is to assess overall physical and mental health, and identify any areas of concern that may need medical or professional attention. Answer the following questions based on your recent experiences (within the last 2-4 weeks).

Physical Health

Fatigue and Energy Levels

How often do you feel fatigued, even after a full night's sleep?

( ) Never ( ) Rarely ( ) Sometimes ( ) Often ( ) Always

IF you frequently feel fatigued THEN ensure you are getting enough sleep, manage stress and increase physical activity. If fatigue persists, see your primary-care provider to rule out underlying conditions like sleep disorders or anemia.

Pain and Discomfort

Do you experience any persistent or chronic pain (e.g., back pain, headaches, joint pain)?

( ) Yes ( ) No

If yes, rate the severity of your pain on a scale of 1-10 (1 is Minimal):

( ) 1 ( ) 2 ( ) 3 ( ) 4 ( ) 5 ( ) 6 ( ) 7 ( ) 8 ( ) 9 (10 is Severe)

IF you experience persistent or severe pain (rated above 5), THEN consult with a healthcare provider to investigate the cause. Pain that affects daily life could be a sign of chronic illness or injury that needs medical attention.

Sleep Quality

How would you describe the quality of your sleep over the past few weeks?

( ) Excellent ( ) Good ( ) Fair ( ) Poor ( ) Very Poor

IF you rate your sleep quality as "Poor" or "Very Poor", THEN monitor your sleep hygiene (e.g., reduce screen time before bed, establish a regular sleep schedule). If poor sleep persists, consult a healthcare provider to rule out sleep disorders like insomnia or sleep apnea.

Weight Changes

Have you experienced any unexplained weight loss or weight gain recently?

( ) Yes ( ) No

If yes, how much weight have you gained or lost in the last month?

( ) Less than 5 lbs ( ) 5-10 lbs ( ) More than 10 lbs.

IF you have experienced significant unexplained weight changes, THEN you should monitor your diet and physical activity. If weight changes continue or are accompanied by other symptoms like fatigue or digestive issues, seek medical advice.

Appetite

Has your appetite increased or decreased significantly over the past few weeks?

( ) Increased ( ) Decreased ( ) No significant changes

IF your appetite has changed significantly, THEN observe any accompanying symptoms like weight loss, fatigue or digestive issues. A persistent change in appetite may indicate an underlying health issue such as depression, thyroid problems, or digestive disorders, requiring consultation with a healthcare provider.

Cardiovascular Symptoms

Do you experience shortness of breath or chest pain during mild physical activities?

( ) Yes ( ) No

Do you have a history of high blood pressure or heart disease?

( ) Yes ( ) No

IF you experience shortness of breath or chest pain, THEN monitor these symptoms carefully and see a healthcare provider immediately, especially if they persist or worsen. These can be signs of serious heart or lung conditions that need urgent evaluation.

Mental and Emotional Health

Mood and Emotional State

How often have you felt down, depressed or hopeless in the past two weeks?

( ) Never ( ) Rarely ( ) Sometimes ( ) Often ( ) Always

IF you frequently feel down or hopeless, THEN consider reaching out to a mental health professional or support network. Persistent feelings of depression may require counseling, therapy or medical intervention.

How often do you scan your surroundings for threats, even in safe places?

( ) Never ( ) Rarely ( ) Sometimes ( ) Often ( ) Always

IF you feel anxious in a social situation, THEN step away from the environment and call a trusted friend or advisor or therapist to talk through your feelings and emotions in that moment.

Anxiety

How often do you feel anxious, nervous, or on edge?

( ) Never ( ) Rarely ( ) Sometimes ( ) Often ( ) Always

IF you often feel anxious or nervous, THEN try to manage stress through relaxation techniques such as deep breathing or mindfulness. If anxiety interferes with daily life, seek advice from a mental health provider.

Do you find yourself avoiding people or places that remind you of past events?

( ) Never ( ) Rarely ( ) Sometimes ( ) Often ( ) Always

IF you frequently do, THEN talk with a therapist to break down the triggers and emotions surrounding the event.

Concentration and Focus

Have you had trouble concentrating on tasks (work, reading, daily activities) recently?

( ) Yes ( ) No

IF you are having difficulty concentrating, THEN assess your sleep habits, stress levels and workload. If the issue persists, it could be related to an underlying condition such as ADHD, depression or anxiety, and may require a healthcare provider's assessment.

Interest and Motivation

Have you lost interest or pleasure in activities you used to enjoy?

( ) Yes ( ) No

IF you have lost interest in activities, THEN it may be a sign of depression or other mental health issues. Consider speaking with a mental health professional if the lack of motivation persists.

Lifestyle and Habits

Physical Activity

How many days per week do you engage in moderate physical activity (e.g., walking, cycling, exercise)?

( ) 0 days ( ) 1-2 days ( ) 3-4 days ( ) 5-6 days ( ) 7 days

IF you are not engaging in regular physical activity, THEN aim to incorporate at least 30 minutes of moderate exercise 3-4 times per week. Physical activity helps improve overall health, mood and energy levels.

Nutrition

How often do you consume a balanced diet that includes fruits, vegetables, and whole grains?

( ) Daily ( ) 3-5 times a week ( ) 1-2 times a week ( ) Rarely ( ) Never

IF you rarely consume a balanced diet, THEN try to improve your nutrition by increasing your intake of fruits, vegetables and whole grains. Consult with a dietitian if you need guidance on how to achieve a balanced diet.

Alcohol Consumption

How often do you consume alcohol?

( ) Never ( ) Less than once a month ( ) 1-2 times a week ( ) 3-5 times a week ( ) Daily

IF you drink alcohol more than 3 times a week or in large quantities or binge-drink, THEN monitor your consumption and reduce your intake. Excessive alcohol use can lead to health issues like liver disease, high blood pressure and mental-health problems. Speak with a healthcare provider if you need help managing alcohol use.

Smoking and Substance Use

Do you smoke or use tobacco products?

( ) Yes ( ) No

Do you use recreational drugs (e.g., cannabis, cocaine, etc.)?

( ) Yes ( ) No

IF you smoke or use recreational drugs, THEN consider seeking help to reduce or quit, as these substances can have serious long-term effects on your lungs, cardiovascular system and overall health. Contact a healthcare professional or counselor if you need support in quitting.

Scoring and Evaluating

If you have answered "Yes" to any significant health concern or indicated high frequencies of negative symptoms (e.g., frequent fatigue, pain, anxiety), THEN you should consult with a healthcare professional for further evaluation.

Regular health check-ups, improving lifestyle habits and managing stress are key to maintaining good health. If you haven't had a recent check-up, including complete blood work and urinalysis, schedule one with your healthcare provider.

Take the Next Step

- Complete the Questionnaire: Take time to thoughtfully answer the questions about your physical, mental, and emotional health. Honesty will provide a clear picture of where you may need support.
- Identify Areas for Improvement: Based on your responses, pinpoint key areas like sleep, pain management or emotional wellbeing where you can make small, manageable changes.
- Seek Professional Help: If the questionnaire reveals significant issues, such as frequent fatigue, anxiety or physical discomfort, schedule an appointment with a healthcare provider to develop a personalized action plan.
- Track Your Progress: Revisit the questionnaire regularly to track improvements or changes in your health. This can help you and your provider adjust treatment plans as needed.

Through Their Eyes

"As an Army medic, my job wasn't just to treat wounds in the heat of combat but to ensure my fellow soldiers were in optimal health—both physically and mentally—before they went into harm's way. We understood that a soldier's wellbeing wasn't just about being tough. It was about being smart and proactive. After consulting with the author on this chapter, I wanted to ensure the approach was comprehensive, practical, and accessible to veterans and active-duty military alike. This health questionnaire isn't just about checking boxes, but instead helping you take command of your wellbeing, just like you would take command of a mission.

"Health assessments were never something we took lightly. Even in the field, we performed routine checks because, in combat, ignoring something small could lead to something much bigger. The same applies to mental health and PTSX. Early recognition and consistent tracking are critical to preventing a small issue from becoming a larger, more dangerous one.

"Physical Health: We often ignore the body's signals—fatigue, pain, changes in appetite—until they become impossible to overlook. This questionnaire asks simple but crucial questions, like how often you feel fatigued or whether you've noticed unexplained changes in your weight. In my experience, we don't always notice these things until someone else points them out.

"That's why this tool is so important—it helps you step back and look at the bigger picture. If you're feeling fatigued, it's not just something to power through. It's a signal to check your sleep, stress levels, or consult a healthcare provider if it persists. When I was out in the field, I had to trust my instincts, but also rely on the tools and knowledge I had. This questionnaire is that kind of tool—a way to pinpoint what's going on before it escalates into something more serious.

"For example, persistent pain or chronic discomfort might seem manageable, but if it's impacting your daily life, it's not something to brush off. Consult a healthcare provider if you're experiencing pain rated above a 5 on a scale of 10. As medics, we knew pain wasn't something to ignore—it was information that could lead to a diagnosis and, ultimately, a solution.

"Mental and Emotional Health: When it comes to mental health, the challenges are often less visible but no less significant. In the Army, we're taught to endure discomfort and keep moving forward. But mental health is something that can't be ignored. This questionnaire asks how often you feel down, depressed or anxious, and whether you've had trouble concentrating or lost interest in activities. These aren't just small red flags—they can be early indicators of excessive stress, depression or anxiety.

"I learned the importance of early intervention. If you've been feeling down or hopeless more often than not, don't wait until it becomes overwhelming. Reach out to a mental health professional. There's no shame in seeking help—it's just another way of ensuring you're battle-ready, even if the battle is internal.

"Lifestyle and Habits: Physical fitness and nutrition were a big part of our routine in the field, but it's just as important in civilian life. The questionnaire highlights the importance of regular physical activity and a balanced diet. If you've been neglecting your fitness or not eating well, the questionnaire serves as a wake-up call. Even small changes, like incorporating more fruits and vegetables or getting 30 minutes of exercise a few times a week, can have a profound impact on your physical and mental health. I'm amazed at how a good diet and exercise can save a person's life. Both are simple and easy to do!

"Substance use is another area where veterans can struggle. This questionnaire doesn't shy away from asking the tough questions about smoking, alcohol or recreational drug use. If your habits are getting out of control, it's time to step back and seek help. There are resources available—whether it's for reducing alcohol consumption, quitting smoking, or getting clean from other substances. Don't let shame or stigma stop you from reaching out.

"Scoring and Evaluation: The most important part of this guide is that it's actionable. If you've answered 'yes' to any of the concerning questions, don't wait—take the next step. Schedule a check-up, talk to a professional, or adjust your lifestyle where needed. In the field, waiting could cost us valuable time and put lives at risk. Early action saves lives, especially your own. Tracking progress is key. This questionnaire isn't something you do once and forget about. Revisit it regularly. Like how I would monitor a soldier's recovery from an injury, you need to monitor your health over time. This isn't a one-time checklist—it's a tool for maintaining long-term physical and mental readiness.

"By making your health a priority, just as we did in the field, you're ensuring that you're prepared for whatever life throws your way. I hope this guide provides you with the clarity and direction you need to take charge of your health—because no one knows the battlefield of life better than those who've served."

—SFC Daniel R., US Army Medic (ret.)

50

Training and Education for Healthcare Professionals

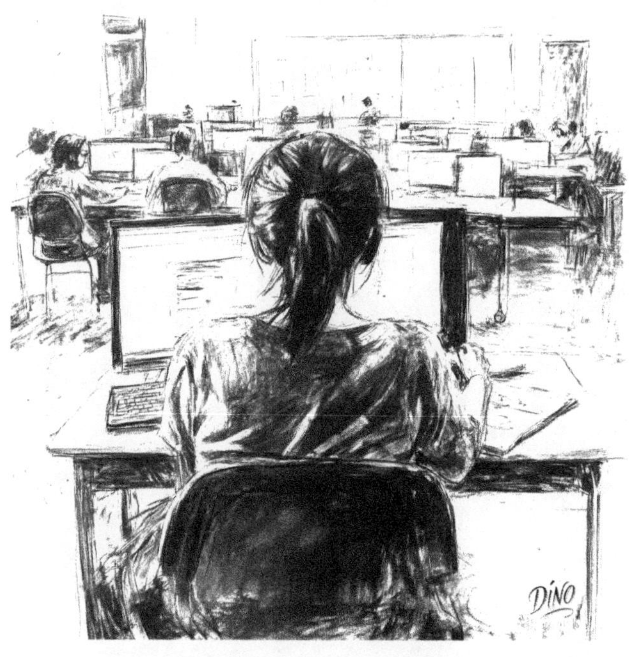

Sonya sat in a cramped classroom at the local VA hospital, flipping through the day's training slides. A licensed therapist for over a decade, she had seen countless veterans on the brink—men and women battling dark corners of their minds with limited tools beyond standard talk therapy and medication. But lately, she'd been hearing about breakthroughs: MDMA trials, ketamine infusions, even nerve blocks that seemed to halt unrelenting hypervigilance. Those stories intrigued her, yet she realized she'd never actually learned about such treatments in any formal course.

That morning's session felt like a breath of fresh air. The presenter, a psychologist deeply versed in emerging PTSX therapies, walked them through the neurobiology of trauma—how certain pathways lit up the amygdala, how neurotransmitters could be recalibrated by substances once seen as taboo. The group leaned in, riveted by the possibilities, and Sonya found herself taking detailed notes, heart pounding with excitement. This wasn't just hypothesis, let alone theory—it was the future of care for her clients.

During lunch, she spoke with others who felt the same mix of surprise and resolve. One nurse practitioner admitted she'd been clueless about where to direct veterans asking about "psychedelic trials" they'd seen on the news. Another social worker confessed to feeling ethically unprepared to handle questions about cannabis for anxiety. As they brainstormed ways to close these gaps, Sonya realized they weren't just retooling their skills—they were forging a path that honored both cutting-edge science and veterans' rights to explore every avenue of healing.

This chapter is written primarily for clinicians, therapists and administrators. It confronts the current gaps in professional training around PTSX treatments. From understanding how ketamine reshapes neural circuits to recognizing the nuances of community-based support, today's clinicians need more than standard curricula. What's needed is a holistic roadmap that respects innovation, ethical rigor and the voices of the servicemembers being served.

By expanding our knowledge and embracing new modalities, healthcare professionals of all rank and stature can better guide veterans toward the compassionate, modern care they deserve—and reshape the educational foundations of mental-health practice along the way.

Current Gaps in Education

In the realm of mental-health treatment for military personnel and veterans, significant advancements have emerged, particularly in the understanding of neurobiological mechanisms underlying conditions like PTSX. However, there remain noticeable gaps in education that hinder the effective integration of these innovative therapies into practice. One of the most pressing issues is the lack of comprehensive training programs that encompass the latest research on the efficacy of psychedelic-assisted therapies, cannabinoids and other alternative treatment modalities. For mental-health professionals dedicated to the wellbeing of our servicemembers, it's crucial to address these educational shortcomings to ensure that they are equipped with the knowledge necessary to provide the best care possible.

> Not everyone understands the principles of neurochemistry and biophysics. And given that we are now researching the true underlying cause and nature of PTSX, every practitioner must be familiar with the basics: molecular biology, neurobiology, neurochemistry, physics, organic chemistry, etc.

The traditional models of PTSX treatment often do not incorporate emerging therapies, leaving practitioners ill-prepared to discuss or implement these options with patients. For instance, while there is increasing evidence supporting the effectiveness of ketamine infusion therapy and MDMA-assisted therapy, many professionals lack the foundational understanding of how these treatments interact with neurobiological processes.

This gap not only affects the confidence of clinicians but also limits the treatment choices available to veterans. By prioritizing education that includes both the science and the practical application of these therapies, we can empower mental-health professionals to make informed decisions that align with the needs and preferences of their patients.

Moreover, the ethical considerations surrounding the use of psychedelics in treatment are often overlooked in training programs. Mental health professionals must be equipped to navigate the complex landscape of ethical dilemmas that may arise when incorporating alternative therapies into their practice. This includes understanding the implications of informed consent, potential risks and the need for robust community-based support systems for veterans undergoing these treatments. By integrating discussions of ethics into educational curricula, we can cultivate a generation of practitioners who are not only knowledgeable but also conscientious in their approach to care.

Community-based support systems play a vital role in the healing journey of veterans, yet there is a disconnect between these resources and the education provided to mental-health professionals. Many practitioners may be unaware of local support networks or how to effectively collaborate with these organizations to enhance treatment outcomes.

By creating collaborations between mental health services and community programs, a holistic framework can be built to address the multifaceted needs of veterans.

With focus, we can build a future where every veteran has access to innovative treatments and compassionate care, ultimately transforming the landscape of PTSX treatment and creating resilience within our military community.

Essential Curriculum Components

In the evolving landscape of PTSX treatment for military personnel and veterans, the design and implementation of core curriculum become paramount. This curriculum must not only embrace the latest neurobiological insights but also integrate innovative therapeutic approaches that resonate with the unique experiences of those who have served.

By focusing on the molecular and neurobiological mechanisms underlying PTSX, mental-health professionals can cultivate a deeper understanding of how trauma impacts the brain, thereby equipping them to offer effective, evidence-based interventions. Such knowledge creates an environment where healing can flourish, allowing veterans to reclaim their lives and sense of self.

The incorporation of psychedelic-assisted therapies represents a significant advancement in the treatment of PTSX. As research demonstrates the potential efficacy of substances like MDMA and psilocybin, the curriculum must provide mental-health professionals with a comprehensive understanding of these therapies' neurobiological foundations and therapeutic applications.

This includes examining the mechanisms of action, the emotional and cognitive processes they engage and the ethical considerations that arise. By educating professionals on these topics, we encourage responsible implementation and a commitment to patient safety and informed consent, thereby empowering veterans to navigate their healing journeys with confidence and hope.

In addition, the integration of cannabinoids into conventional treatment protocols warrants careful consideration in the curriculum. As emerging studies suggest potential benefits in alleviating PTSX symptoms, mental-health professionals must be well-versed in the therapeutic properties of cannabinoids, as well as the legal and clinical implications of their use.

A robust curriculum will elucidate the ways in which cannabinoids can complement existing treatments, creating a holistic approach that addresses the multifaceted nature of trauma. By empowering professionals with this knowledge, we enhance their ability to provide personalized care that resonates with the preferences and needs of veterans.

Stimulation techniques like stellate ganglion block represent another essential facet of an advanced curriculum. These methods have shown promise in alleviating PTSX symptoms by targeting the autonomic nervous system.

A must for all mental-health practitioners is watching the Amazon Prime film *Quiet Explosions*, then contacting Dr. Mark Gordon of the Millennium Health Centers to learn about his ground-breaking research on mechanotransduction and neuroinflammation.

Mental-health professionals must be trained in the procedural aspects, patient selection criteria and the potential benefits and risks associated with SGB. This training not only enhances the skill set of professionals but also cultivates a culture of innovation and adaptability within the treatment community, ultimately benefiting the veterans who seek your support. The curriculum must emphasize the importance of community-based support systems for veterans undergoing alternative therapies. Healing from trauma is often a collective journey and creating connections within the community can amplify the effects of clinical interventions.

Future Directions for Professional Development

The field of mental healthcare, particularly in the context of treating PTSX among military personnel and veterans, stands on the precipice of transformative change. As we look toward the future, it is imperative for mental health professionals across all sectors—VA, civilian and military—to engage in continuous professional development that encompasses the latest research and innovative treatment approaches.

The neurobiological and molecular mechanisms underlying PTSX are becoming increasingly understood, allowing for the development of targeted therapies that can significantly enhance recovery outcomes. Embracing this evolution not only benefits individual practitioners but also establishes a culture of healing and resilience within our communities.

One of the most promising avenues for professional development lies in the comparative efficacy of psychedelic-assisted therapies. As studies continue to unveil the therapeutic potential of substances like MDMA and psilocybin, it is crucial for mental-health professionals to undergo specialized training that equips them to safely and effectively administer these treatments.

Workshops and certifications focused on various therapies can provide invaluable insights into the neurobiological changes that accompany such interventions, as well as nurture the ethical considerations that must guide their use. By creating a deep understanding of these therapies, professionals can better advocate for their integration into conventional treatment protocols, ultimately expanding the healing options available.

The importance of community-based support systems cannot be overstated. As we recognize the role of social connections in the healing process, practitioners should engage in training that emphasizes the integration of community resources into treatment plans. Building partnerships with veteran organizations, peer-support groups and family programs can create a robust support network that extends beyond the clinical setting.

By empowering veterans to engage within their communities, we can build environments that promote recovery, resilience and a renewed sense of purpose. In this evolving landscape of PTSX treatment, the commitment to professional development will not only enhance individual expertise but will also contribute to a collective mission of healing for our military personnel and veterans.

If-Then Guidance

- If you feel that your healthcare provider is not well trained in treating PTSX in veterans, then consider asking for a referral to a provider who has more experience in this area. The VA or veteran-focused clinics often have specialists who understand military-related trauma better than general practitioners.
- If you have experienced issues due to lack of provider training, then you might benefit from switching to a mental-health provider who has received specialized training in PTSX. Look for professionals with certifications in trauma-focused therapies or ask your current provider if they can improve their approach by seeking additional training.
- If you would prefer to see a provider with training in alternative or emerging treatments, then explore options within the VA or private sector that offer these therapies. Many providers are now expanding their practices to include treatments like psychedelic-assisted therapy or ketamine, so it's worth inquiring if these options are available to you.
- If you believe it's important for your provider to stay up-to-date on the latest treatments, then you may want to ask them directly about their continuing education efforts. A provider who is actively engaged in learning new techniques may offer better care.
- If you have not yet tried any alternative treatments but are curious, then consider researching options such as yoga, acupuncture or mindfulness. Speak with a healthcare provider to discuss how these treatments could complement your current PTSX care.

- If you experienced success with alternative treatments, then continue incorporating them into your routine as a way to manage your symptoms. Sharing your experience with other veterans may also help them explore new options for their PTSX treatment.
- If you found that alternative treatments didn't provide enough relief on their own, then you might want to combine them with conventional therapies like counseling or medication for a more comprehensive approach.
- If you are willing to share your experiences, then consider joining support groups or forums where veterans discuss different treatment methods. Your story could provide valuable insight to others who are looking for alternative ways to manage their PTSX.

Take the Next Step

- Share Your Experience: If you've found success with specific treatments, consider speaking to healthcare professionals about what has worked for you. Your insights can improve care for other veterans.
- Participate in Feedback: Join veteran panels or surveys that provide feedback on current PTSX treatment programs. Your input can influence training programs for future healthcare providers.
- Stay Engaged with Your Providers: Be open with your therapist or doctor about your treatment needs and what approaches work best for you.

Through Their Eyes

"As a Marine Corps Gunnery Sergeant with years of combat experience, I was no stranger to high-pressure situations and the demands of leading my men through some of the toughest operations overseas. But after multiple deployments, the war followed me home. PTSX had set in. It wasn't just the sleepless nights and flashbacks—it was being vigilant all the time, the anger, and the feeling that no matter how hard I tried, I couldn't turn off that part of me that was always waiting for the next fight.

"I was used to being the one in control, the leader my Marines could rely on. But dealing with PTSX made me feel like I had lost control. Therapy and medication helped some, but it didn't take away the constant battle going on in my head. That's when I started looking into alternative treatments. I didn't know much about them at first, but a fellow vet told me about the potential of ketamine therapy and even MDMA-assisted therapy. Honestly, I was skeptical, but when you've tried everything else and still feel like you're losing the fight, you start opening up to new options.

"I talked to my therapist about these emerging treatments, and it was clear that they didn't have much knowledge about them either. That's when it hit me—if our healthcare professionals aren't up to speed on the latest treatments, how are they going to help guys like me? We need professionals who understand the unique experiences we've been through in combat and can offer us the best tools to deal with PTSX. Not just traditional therapy, but everything—medications, alternative therapies, community-based support, the whole nine yards.

"As I started looking more into these new treatments, I realized that my healthcare provider wasn't fully trained in many of them. They didn't know how to navigate these alternative therapies, and I wasn't the only vet dealing with this gap. I read up on the cellular and molecular levels where the real stuff goes on that causes PTSX, but hardly anyone knew anything about that deep level.

"They were skilled in other areas, of course, but didn't know the true causes of what ailed me. There are thousands of Marines, soldiers, sailors, and airmen out there looking for help, but they're getting stuck with providers who don't have the training or the knowledge to help them properly.

"That's when I became an advocate for better training and education for mental health professionals. I started working with veteran organizations to push for more comprehensive education on PTSX treatments. We need mental health providers who not only know the basics but are also trained in the latest research on psychedelic-assisted therapies, cannabinoid treatments, and things like stellate ganglion block. We need people who know how to handle the ethical considerations, the risks, and how to make sure veterans like me are getting the full range of options for healing.

"The reality is, PTSX isn't a one-size-fits-all kind of problem. It's complex, and it impacts every veteran differently. What worked for one of my Marines might not work for me, and that's okay. But our healthcare professionals need to be prepared for that—they need to be trained in a wide variety of treatment modalities so that they can meet us where we're at. Whether it's traditional therapy, community-based support, or innovative treatments like ketamine or MDMA, vets deserve access to every option out there.

"As I went through this process, I saw the difference that proper training makes. I eventually found a provider who had experience with some of these newer treatments, and they were able to guide me through the options in a way that made sense. We worked on incorporating alternative therapies into my routine, and for the first time in a long time, I felt like I was making real progress.

"But this isn't just about me—it's about all the veterans out there who feel like they're stuck, who feel like their providers don't fully understand what they're going through or how to help them. That's why I keep advocating for better education and training for the people who are supposed to help us. They need to be trained in the latest advancements and also how to integrate those treatments with community resources, peer support, and everything else that makes a difference for veterans.

"The road to healing is a long one, but with the right tools and the right support, it's possible. Mental-health professionals need to be our allies in this fight. They need to be just as ready and equipped as we were when we went into combat. That means staying up to date on the latest treatments, understanding the unique challenges of military life, and having the skills to guide us through the hard times. It's the least we deserve after everything we've given."

—James, US Marine Corps Gunnery Sergeant Veteran

51

Healing the Healers: Addressing Secondary Trauma and Burnout in Caregivers

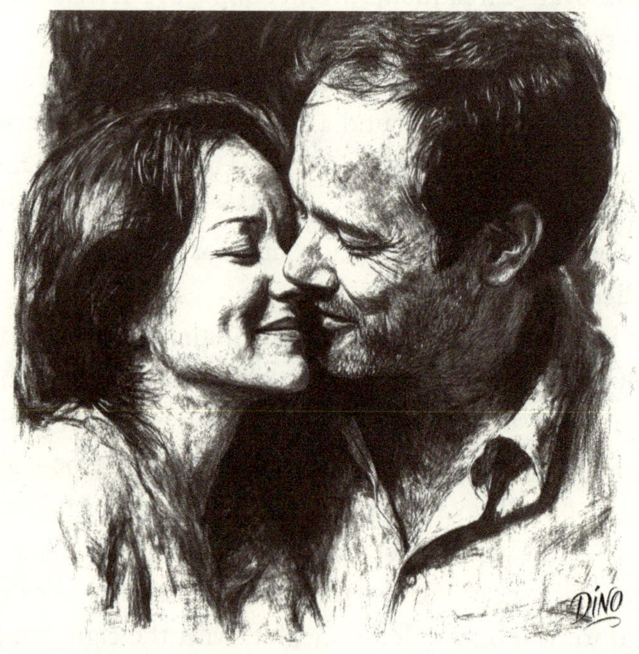

Maria sat in her car, the keys in the ignition, staring at the dashboard. Another shift was over, but the echoes of the day lingered. A veteran had broken down in her office, recounting memories he'd kept buried for years. She'd sat there, listening, holding space for his pain. Now, her chest felt heavy, as if she had taken on a piece of his burden. At home, the weight followed her. Her teenage son asked if she wanted to join him for a walk, but she shook her head. Her husband kissed her gently, his silent way of asking how her day had been. She smiled weakly, knowing he worried but unsure how to explain. She had chosen this work—helping those who had seen too much and lost too much. But no one had warned her what it would cost.

One evening, after she found herself snapping at her son for no reason, Maria realized something had to change. A colleague mentioned a seminar on caregiver burnout, and though she doubted it would help, she went.

The room was full of people like her—first responders, therapists, family caregivers. The speaker talked about secondary trauma, how it seeps into you like a slow flood. She explained how the brain's stress response becomes overactive, how cortisol wears you down, and how neglecting self-care isn't noble. It's dangerous.

Maria started small. She walked with her son in the evenings, let herself paint again, even if only for ten minutes. She joined a peer group where she could finally speak freely about her struggles. Slowly, the weight began to lift.

This chapter is aimed primarily at the caregivers and healthcare providers. However, veterans and laypeople can benefit from it, as well, as it shines a light on the difficulty and challenges caregivers face when treating those with PTSX. It aims to provide a roadmap for those who dedicate their lives to supporting others, offering practical strategies and heartfelt acknowledgment of their sacrifices. By understanding the risks and embracing self-care, caregivers can continue their vital work while protecting their mental health and wellbeing.

Caring for trauma survivors is an extraordinary act of compassion. However, it also comes with significant emotional and psychological demands. Caregivers, whether they are therapists, social workers, first responders, or family members, often carry the weight of secondary traumatic stress (STS) and burnout. Their work is invaluable, but the cost to them can be immense if not addressed proactively.

As with previous chapters with contact and program information, always verify that the information is up to date.

Understanding Secondary Traumatic Stress and Compassion Fatigue

STS occurs when individuals are exposed to the trauma of others. While they may not experience the traumatic event directly, listening to detailed accounts, witnessing pain, and empathizing deeply can take a toll. Symptoms of STS often mirror those of post-traumatic stress, including intrusive thoughts, emotional numbing, irritability, and hypervigilance.

Compassion fatigue, sometimes referred to as the "cost of caring," is the emotional exhaustion that results from prolonged exposure to the suffering of others. Unlike burnout, which develops gradually, compassion fatigue can appear suddenly and is often accompanied by feelings of hopelessness, detachment, and a diminished ability to empathize.

Understanding the warning signs of STS and compassion fatigue is crucial. These may include:

<u>Physical symptoms</u>: Chronic fatigue, headaches, or gastrointestinal distress. Emotional symptoms: Anxiety, depression, or feelings of inadequacy.

<u>Behavioral symptoms</u>: Increased irritability, withdrawal from loved ones, or difficulty concentrating.

Caregivers at risk include those working in high-intensity environments, such as emergency rooms, disaster zones or mental health clinics, as well as family members who provide constant support to loved ones with PTSX.

The Neuroscience of Burnout

Prolonged exposure to trauma-related narratives activates the brain's stress response system. At the heart of this response is the amygdala, the brain's fear and emotion processing center. When caregivers repeatedly hear accounts of trauma or witness suffering, the amygdala becomes hyperactive, signaling danger even in safe environments.

This hyperactivity can overwhelm the prefrontal cortex, which is essential for rational thinking, emotional regulation, and decision-making. The impaired functioning of the prefrontal cortex diminishes the ability to process stress effectively, leaving caregivers more vulnerable to emotional exhaustion.

The hippocampus, another critical brain structure, plays a role in regulating stress and encoding memories. Chronic exposure to stress can shrink the hippocampus, impairing memory and making it harder for caregivers to differentiate between past trauma and present experiences. This can contribute to intrusive thoughts and emotional dysregulation, hallmarks of secondary traumatic stress and burnout. Compounding this is the role of the HPA axis.

Repeated activation of the HPA axis results in an overproduction of stress hormones, keeping caregivers in a constant state of physiological arousal. Over time, this state of hyperarousal erodes the body's resilience.

Cortisol and Its Impact

Cortisol, often referred to as the body's "stress hormone," is released by the adrenal glands during times of stress. While cortisol is crucial for managing acute stress by increasing energy and focus, its prolonged elevation has detrimental effects. In caregivers, chronic cortisol release can:

Disrupt Sleep Cycles: Elevated cortisol levels interfere with the production of melatonin, the hormone responsible for sleep regulation. This leads to difficulty falling and staying asleep, compounding fatigue and impairing emotional regulation.

Weaken the Immune System: Prolonged cortisol exposure suppresses immune function, making caregivers more susceptible to infections and illnesses.

Affect Memory and Concentration: High cortisol levels damage the hippocampus, impairing memory formation and recall. This can make caregivers feel forgetful or less effective in their roles.

Promote Inflammation: Chronic stress-induced cortisol imbalance can trigger systemic inflammation, increasing the risk of chronic health conditions such as heart disease and autoimmune disorders.

In addition, cortisol affects the reward pathways in the brain, potentially diminishing caregivers' sense of accomplishment and increasing feelings of futility. The interplay between elevated cortisol levels and emotional exhaustion creates a cycle that perpetuates burnout.

Neuroplasticity and Hope

Despite the significant impact of stress on the brain, it is essential to remember the brain's remarkable capacity for change—neuroplasticity.

Neuroplasticity allows the brain to rewire itself in response to new experiences, enabling recovery and resilience. Caregivers can harness this adaptability through intentional practices that promote healing and growth.

Mindfulness and Meditation: Regular mindfulness practices have been shown to reduce amygdala activity and strengthen the prefrontal cortex. This helps caregivers manage emotional responses and regain a sense of control.

> Leadership is pivotal in shaping organizational culture. Leaders must be trained not only to recognize signs of burnout but also to address them with empathy and action. Comprehensive training programs can include modules on emotional intelligence, active listening, and the impact of secondary trauma. Leaders who understand these dynamics are better equipped to support their teams.

Physical Exercise: Aerobic exercise stimulates the production of brain-derived neurotrophic factor (BDNF), a protein that supports the growth of new neurons and repairs damaged neural pathways. Activities like running, swimming, or yoga can rejuvenate the brain and reduce the physiological effects of stress.

Social Connections: Positive social interactions activate the brain's reward systems, releasing oxytocin, a hormone that counteracts cortisol's effects. Peer support groups and close relationships can create a sense of belonging and reduce feelings of isolation.

Sleep Hygiene: Prioritizing restful sleep allows the brain to detoxify and repair itself. Techniques such as maintaining a consistent sleep schedule and creating a calming bedtime routine can enhance recovery.

Learning and Growth: Engaging in new activities or learning new skills promotes cognitive flexibility, helping the brain adapt to stress and build resilience.

Emerging research also highlights the role of gratitude and positive thinking in reshaping neural pathways. Reflecting on moments of success, no matter how small, reinforces the brain's focus on positivity, reducing the dominance of stress responses.

Understanding the neuroscience of burnout empowers caregivers to recognize the physiological impact of their work and take proactive steps to protect their wellbeing. By building neuroplasticity and leveraging strategies that promote brain health, caregivers can continue their vital roles with renewed strength and resilience.

Practical Self-Care Strategies for Caregivers

Self-care is not a luxury but a necessity for those who care for others. Here are evidence-based strategies to protect and rejuvenate mental health:

Mindfulness and Meditation

Practicing mindfulness helps caregivers stay present and reduce emotional reactivity. Techniques like deep breathing, body scans, and mindful observation can be integrated into daily routines.

Regular Physical Activity reduces cortisol levels and boosts endorphins. Activities like yoga, swimming, or even daily walks provide both physical and mental benefits.

Healthful Nutrition

A balanced diet rich in omega-3 fatty acids, whole grains, and antioxidants supports brain health and combats stress. Staying hydrated and avoiding excessive caffeine or alcohol also help regulate mood.

Establishing Boundaries

Setting clear limits on work hours and emotional availability prevents overextension, not only in the worldplace but also at home and at play.

Learning to say "no" when necessary is an act of self-preservation, and it assists others in respecting your boundaries.

Peer-Support Networks

Sharing experiences with colleagues who understand the challenges of caregiving provides validation and camaraderie. Peer groups can also offer practical advice and emotional support.

Professional Supervision

Regular consultation with a supervisor or mentor allows caregivers to process difficult cases and gain perspective. This practice reduces feelings of isolation and builds professional growth.

Scheduled Downtime

Carving out time for hobbies, family, or solitude restores balance. Unstructured relaxation, such as reading or gardening, replenishes energy.

Sleep Hygiene

Prioritizing quality sleep helps the brain recover from daily stressors. Establishing a consistent sleep schedule and creating a calming bedtime routine can improve rest.

Expressive Arts

Creative outlets like journaling, painting, or music allow caregivers to process emotions nonverbally. These activities offer a sense of release and rejuvenation.

Education and Training

Staying informed about trauma care and self-care techniques empowers caregivers to approach their work with confidence. Continuous learning inspires a sense of competence and control.

Gratitude Practices

Focusing on positive moments, whether through a gratitude journal or daily reflections, shifts attention from challenges to achievements. With practice, these reflections become a good habit that produces other good habits.

Seeking Therapy

Caregivers are often reluctant to seek help for themselves, but professional therapy provides a safe space to explore and address their own emotional burdens.

The Role of Organizational Culture

Organizations play a critical role in mitigating burnout by creating an environment that prioritizes caregiver wellbeing. Flexible work schedules are a cornerstone of support, allowing caregivers to balance their professional responsibilities with personal needs. For instance, staggered shifts or part-time options can reduce fatigue while maintaining operational efficiency. Organizations can implement Employee Assistance Programs (EAPs) that provide confidential counseling, financial advice, and wellness coaching. These resources signal a commitment to holistic wellbeing and encourage caregivers to seek help without stigma.

Physical workspace design also matters. Quiet rooms or relaxation areas within healthcare facilities offer caregivers a place to decompress during stressful shifts. Small gestures, such as providing healthful snacks, ergonomic furniture, or on-site fitness options, contribute to an environment that values and nurtures its staff. Regular wellbeing check-ins by supervisors help identify stressors early, creating a culture where mental health conversations are normalized.

Training for Leadership

Leadership is pivotal in shaping organizational culture. Leaders must be trained not only to recognize signs of burnout but also to address them with empathy and action. Comprehensive training programs can include modules on emotional intelligence, active listening, and the impact of secondary trauma. Leaders who understand these dynamics are better equipped to support their teams.

Modeling self-care is equally important. Leaders who prioritize their wellbeing set a powerful example for their staff. This could mean openly discussing their own stress management strategies, setting boundaries on after-hours communication, or taking regular breaks. Encouraging work-life balance through policies and personal behavior creates a culture where caregivers feel permission to prioritize their health.

Clear communication from leadership is essential. Regular team meetings that include discussions about workload distribution, stress levels, and available resources create transparency and trust. Leaders who actively seek feedback and implement suggested changes demonstrate that they value their team's input, enhancing morale and engagement.

Implementing Resilience Programs

Resilience programs are structured initiatives designed to equip caregivers with the tools to manage stress and maintain their effectiveness. Workshops on stress management, for instance, can teach techniques like deep breathing, progressive muscle relaxation, and cognitive reframing. These tools help caregivers navigate high-pressure situations without becoming overwhelmed.

Building resilience also involves building adaptability. Role-playing scenarios or simulations can prepare caregivers for challenging situations, reducing anxiety about the unknown. For instance, disaster response training or de-escalation techniques for handling difficult patients can instill confidence and competence.

Ongoing education is another key element. Offering courses on topics such as the neuroscience of trauma or cultural competence not only enhances professional skills but also reinforces a sense of purpose and mastery. Organizations can partner with universities or professional associations to provide certifications or continuing education credits, ensuring that caregivers feel supported in their career growth.

Promoting Peer Support

Peer-support networks are invaluable for caregivers, providing a sense of connection and shared understanding. Organizations can formalize these networks through mentorship programs, pairing seasoned professionals with those new to the field. These relationships offer guidance, encouragement, and practical advice, helping newer caregivers navigate their roles more effectively.

Regular peer-support groups create safe spaces for caregivers to share their experiences, challenges, and successes. Facilitated by trained moderators, these groups allow for emotional processing and the development of coping strategies. Sharing stories within a trusted circle can alleviate feelings of isolation and normalize the emotional toll of caregiving.

Technology can also enhance peer support. Online forums, apps, or virtual communities allow caregivers to connect regardless of geographic location. These platforms can include features such as moderated discussions, resource libraries, and opportunities for one-on-one mentorship.

Recognizing and celebrating the contributions of caregivers is another way to promote peer solidarity. Organizations can create awards, recognition programs, or appreciation events that highlight the dedication and achievements of their staff. These gestures create a sense of belonging and reinforce the collective mission of caregiving teams.

By integrating these practices, organizations can create a culture that not only supports caregivers but also empowers them to thrive. Addressing burnout at an institutional level ensures that caregivers remain resilient, effective, and fulfilled in their critical roles.

Resources for Healthcare Workers, Caregivers and Healers

There are a variety of resources designed to support caregivers' mental health:

National Center for PTSD: Offers training and resources for mental health professionals. Website: www.ptsd.va.gov.

American Professional Society on the Abuse of Children (APSAC): Provides training for those working with traumatized children. Website: www.apsac.org.

Give an Hour: Connects caregivers with free mental health services. Website: www.giveanhour.org.

National Alliance on Mental Illness (NAMI): Offers peer-led support groups and education programs. Website: www.nami.org.

The Breathe Network: Focuses on trauma-informed care for sexual violence survivors. Website: www.thebreathenetwork.org.

Resilient Minds on the Front Lines: Provides workshops for first responders. Website: www.resilientmindsfrontlines.org.

Healing others is an extraordinary calling, but it requires intentional self-care and support. By recognizing the risks of secondary trauma and implementing strategies to mitigate burnout, caregivers can continue their vital work with strength and resilience. This chapter stands as a tribute to their dedication, reminding them that their wellbeing matters just as much as those they serve.

If-Then Guidance

- If you feel emotionally exhausted after caring for others, then take a step back to evaluate your own needs. Prioritize restorative activities such as mindfulness, journaling, or engaging in a creative hobby. Even short breaks during the day can help replenish your energy and improve your focus.
- If you are experiencing physical symptoms like headaches, fatigue, or muscle tension, then consider how stress may be impacting your body. Physical symptoms are often the first sign of secondary traumatic stress. Integrate stress-relief techniques into your routine, such as yoga, progressive muscle relaxation, or even a brisk walk outdoors. Addressing physical health is a vital part of your emotional recovery.
- If you find it difficult to empathize with those you care for, then recognize this as a potential sign of compassion fatigue. Take time to reflect on why you started this work and reconnect with your sense of purpose. Discussing these feelings with a trusted colleague or mentor can help you regain perspective and restore empathy without feeling overwhelmed.
- If you notice that you are withdrawing from loved ones or social activities, then seek out supportive relationships. Isolation often exacerbates the emotional toll of caregiving. Reach out to a peer support group, attend a social event, or reconnect with friends or

family who understand and appreciate your journey.

- If you feel overwhelmed by the demands of your work or caregiving responsibilities, then set clear boundaries to protect your mental health. Learn to say "no" when necessary and delegate tasks to others when possible. Remember, asking for help is not a sign of weakness—it's a sign of strength and self-awareness.
- If you struggle to process the trauma you witness in your work, then consider seeking professional supervision or therapy. Talking with someone who understands secondary trauma can provide you with tools to process your experiences and reduce emotional burden. Regular supervision is also a way to learn coping strategies and develop resilience.
- If you feel like you are losing your sense of self outside of caregiving, then carve out time for personal passions and activities that bring you joy. Reconnecting with your interests, whether through art, sports, or volunteering in a different capacity, can remind you that you are more than your role as a caregiver. Nurturing your identity outside of work is essential for long-term wellbeing.

Take the Next Step

- Acknowledge your own needs and recognize that caring for others does not mean neglecting yourself. Take the time to assess your physical, emotional, and mental wellbeing. Admitting that you need support or rest is a powerful first step toward sustaining your ability to help others.
- Develop a personalized self-care plan and create a self-care plan tailored to your needs and preferences. Include activities that restore your energy, such as regular exercise, meditation, or creative hobbies.
- Write it down and treat it as a commitment to yourself, revisiting and revising it as needed.
- Set and maintain boundaries by identifying areas in your work or caregiving role where you can set clearer boundaries. Whether it's limiting after-hours communication, delegating tasks, or taking designated breaks, boundaries protect your mental health and

prevent burnout.

- Invest in peer support by connecting with others who understand the challenges of caregiving. Join a support group, participate in peer mentoring, or simply schedule regular check-ins with trusted colleagues. Shared experiences build understanding and provide emotional relief.
- Educate yourself about secondary trauma by learning more about the signs, symptoms, and effects of secondary traumatic stress and burnout. Knowledge empowers you to recognize early warning signs and take proactive measures to address them.
- Seek professional support when needed by consulting a therapist, counselor, or supervisor if you feel overwhelmed. Professionals trained in secondary trauma can provide insights, tools, and strategies to help you navigate your experiences more effectively.
- Advocate for workplace wellness by encouraging your organization to prioritize caregiver wellbeing. Advocate for initiatives such as wellness programs, flexible schedules, and access to mental-health resources. A supportive workplace culture benefits everyone involved.
- Celebrate small victories by taking the time to acknowledge and celebrate your accomplishments, no matter how small. Whether it's successfully setting a boundary or finding a moment of joy in a tough day, recognizing these wins builds confidence and resilience.
- Commit to lifelong resilience practices by viewing resilience as an ongoing journey. Commit to incorporating practices like mindfulness, gratitude journaling, and continuous learning into your daily life. These habits will help you stay grounded and thrive in your role as a caregiver.

Through Their Eyes

Clara, a licensed therapist, had spent over a decade working with survivors of domestic violence. While her work brought her immense satisfaction, it also left her emotionally depleted. Over time, Clara began to notice subtle but concerning changes: restless nights, a persistent feeling of dread before sessions, and a growing sense of detachment from her clients.

She starting questioning her own efficacy, wondering if she was making a meaningful difference. One day, during a team meeting, a colleague noticed Clara's fatigue and encouraged her to seek help. Reluctantly, Clara agreed. Her supervisor helped her identify the signs of secondary traumatic stress and recommended actionable steps to prioritize her mental health.

At the same time, Clara decided to join a local yoga studio, attending weekly classes that emphasized mindfulness and deep breathing. The practice helped her reconnect with her body and emotions, offering a much-needed respite from her demanding role.

As she began implementing these changes, Clara noticed a significant shift. Her energy levels improved, her sleep became more restorative, and she approached her sessions with renewed empathy and patience.

Clara also started journaling, reflecting on moments of progress with her clients and celebrating small victories. These practices not only revitalized her professional life but also strengthened her sense of purpose. Clara now mentors younger therapists, emphasizing the importance of self-care as an integral part of their careers.

Ethan, a firefighter with over 15 years of experience, had seen his share of emergencies. However, one accident—a multi-car pileup on a rainy night—left a lasting scar. The accident claimed several lives, including those of young children, and Ethan found the scene replaying in his mind. He began experiencing intrusive memories, nightmares, and a gnawing sense of guilt, even though he had done everything possible to save lives that day.

Initially, Ethan tried to push through on his own. He threw himself into work, avoiding conversations about the incident and suppressing his emotions. But his coping mechanisms began to fail, and his irritability and detachment started affecting his relationships at home and with his colleagues. Realizing he needed help, Ethan joined a peer support group for first responders. For the first time, he shared his experiences with others who understood the unique challenges of his role.

Ethan also rediscovered his passion for running, an activity he had enjoyed in his youth. Running became his sanctuary—a time to clear his mind, release pent-up energy, and reconnect with his sense of self. Over time, the combination of physical activity and peer support helped Ethan process his emotions and regain a sense of control. He now encourages his colleagues to seek help early and emphasizes the importance of maintaining both physical and mental health.

Priya was assigned to a refugee camp, facing daily exposure to the devastating realities of displacement and loss. Her work involved listening to harrowing stories of survival, finding resources, and advocating for families in dire need. While she was deeply committed to her role, the emotional toll began to manifest in physical exhaustion and frequent headaches. Priya found herself crying without warning and struggling to stay present during meetings.

Determined to reclaim her wellbeing, Priya began exploring mindfulness meditation, dedicating 15 minutes each morning to focused breathing and reflection. She also started journaling, using her entries to process the day's challenges and express gratitude for moments of hope she witnessed in the camp.

However, it was reconnecting with her cultural roots that brought Priya the most solace. She began participating in storytelling circles, a tradition from her homeland, where she shared her experiences and listened to others' tales of resilience and hope.

Priya also introduced cultural rituals into her personal routine, such as lighting candles during evening prayers and reciting affirmations passed down through her family. These practices grounded her, reminding her of the strength and wisdom embedded in her heritage.

Over time, Priya's resilience grew, and she became a resource of stability and compassion for her colleagues and the refugees she served. She now trains other social workers on integrating mindfulness and cultural practices into their self-care routines.

Leo's life changed when his older brother, a veteran diagnosed with severe PTSX, moved in with him. At first, Leo was determined to be everything his brother needed—a companion, advocate and caregiver. However, the demands of caregiving began to weigh heavily on him.

He often found himself waking up in the middle of the night to soothe his brother after nightmares or managing his brother's outbursts during the day. Over time, Leo became isolated, sacrificing his social life and hobbies to focus entirely on his brother's needs.

One evening, after a particularly challenging day, Leo stumbled upon an online caregiver support group. Skeptical but desperate, he decided to join. Hearing the experiences of others who faced similar struggles gave him a sense of validation and relief.

Through the group, Leo learned about the importance of setting boundaries and delegating responsibilities. He began enlisting the help of other family members and seeking professional support for his brother's care.

Leo also carved out time for himself, rediscovering his love for woodworking. Spending an hour in his workshop each evening became his refuge—a time to create, reflect, and recharge. As he regained balance, Leo noticed that his relationship with his brother improved.

He approached caregiving with renewed patience and empathy, and his brother, in turn, responded positively to Leo's calmer demeanor. Today, Leo is an advocate for family caregivers, sharing his journey to inspire others to prioritize their wellbeing.

Claire, an ER nurse, had always thrived in the fast-paced environment of the emergency room. She found meaning in saving lives and comforting patients during their most vulnerable moments. However, exposure to trauma began to take their toll. Claire started feeling emotionally numb, struggling to empathize with her patients and dreading her shifts. She experienced frequent headaches, difficulty sleeping, and a pervasive sense of burnout.

When her hospital implemented a resilience program, Claire was initially hesitant to participate. But after attending the first workshop on stress management, she realized how much she needed support. The program introduced her to mindfulness exercises, such as guided imagery and progressive muscle relaxation, which she began incorporating into her daily routine. Claire also started gratitude journaling, listing three positive moments from each day. This practice helped shift her focus from the challenges of her job to its rewards.

Additionally, Claire developed close bonds with her colleagues through the program's peer support initiatives. Sharing experiences and coping strategies with her team built a sense of camaraderie and mutual understanding. Over time, Claire's perspective on her work transformed. She rediscovered her passion for nursing and became a strong advocate for workplace wellness programs, encouraging her peers to prioritize their mental health as much as their patients'. Today, Claire leads resilience workshops at her hospital, helping others navigate the demands of caregiving with strength and compassion.

52

Navigating the VA: Insider Tips for Veterans and Families

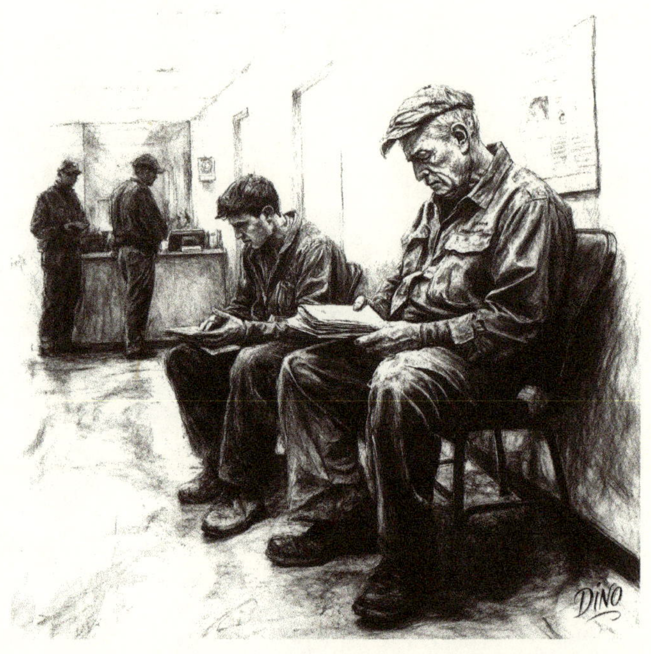

They called it the VA, the place where veterans went to find what was owed to them. It wasn't easy, not by a long shot. The papers stacked high, the forms in triplicate, the men and women behind the counters who barely looked up. But still, veterans came.

Tom had been there three times this month. His knees were shot, and so was his patience. He'd filled out the forms, waited in the lines, answered questions that didn't seem to matter. He had the scars to prove what he'd been through, but still, the system needed more.

"Come back next week," they told him. "We'll have an answer then."

The room smelled of stale coffee and old carpet. He sat there, thinking about the men who didn't make it back, who wouldn't need to wait in lines like this. And then he thought about his wife, holding the bills at the kitchen table, her fingers running over the numbers like they might change if she touched them long enough.

A younger man sat next to him, quiet, shifting in his seat. Tom could see the weight on him, the same weight they all carried. He leaned over, his voice low: "Listen, brother. Don't let them push you off. Be loud if you have to. Be smart. But don't give up. This place owes you, just like it owes me. Don't let them make you feel like you don't deserve it."

The kid nodded, his hands gripping the file in his lap.

When Tom's name was finally called, he stood, his back straight, the old Marine in him still alive. It wasn't just about him. It was about all of them. And he'd keep coming back, as long as it took.

This chapter offers a comprehensive guide to understanding the VA's resources, filing claims effectively, overcoming bureaucratic hurdles, and leveraging insider tips from experts to ensure successful outcomes. The VA is a lifeline for millions of US veterans and their families, offering vital healthcare, benefits, and services designed to support those who have served the nation. From VA disability compensation to education assistance and healthcare, the VA provides resources aimed at improving the quality of life for veterans.

However, navigating the VA system can be a challenging task. Bureaucracy, complex documentation requirements, and long processing times often discourage veterans from accessing the benefits they have earned. Always consult the official VA website, a veterans service organization, or a VA-qualified attorney or law firm for the most up-to-date information on relevant topics.

Stress in the Ranks

Military service is a source of great pride and sacrifice, yet it can also expose personnel to high-intensity stressors that may lead to long-term psychological impacts. When an individual develops PTSX—an extended form of post-traumatic stress that incorporates persistent symptoms affecting personal, social, and occupational functioning—it can complicate the transition from military to civilian life.

The good news is that a structured network of legal protections, disability benefits, and support services exists in the United States to help service members and veterans cope with these challenges. From the earliest stages of medical evaluation in the armed forces, to the intricacies of VA compensation, to workplace accommodations and potential legal recourse, it is crucial for individuals with PTSX and their families to understand these frameworks so they can secure the care and benefits they have earned.

Medical Boards and Fitness for Duty

Active-duty service members experiencing symptoms of PTSX may reach a point where their condition interferes with the performance of their military duties. This situation can trigger the Medical Evaluation Board (MEB) process, which systematically reviews their medical status.

The MEB examines whether a service member meets medical retention standards under branch-specific regulations—such as Army Regulation 40-501 for the Army or similar directives for the Navy, Marine Corps, and Air Force.

Upon gathering documentation from medical professionals and the individual's chain of command, the MEB compiles its findings into a narrative summary. This summary then goes to the Physical Evaluation Board (PEB), which determines whether the service member is fit for continued service.

Throughout these evaluations, individuals have important rights: they can review their medical records, provide personal statements, and consult with assigned counsel or a Physical Evaluation Board Liaison Officer (PEBLO). The legal framework for these boards derives from Title 10 of the US Code, granting the Department of Defense (DoD) authority to assess fitness for duty and determine eligibility for potential separation or medical retirement.

If a PEB concludes that medical conditions including PTSX or its symptoms render the individual unable to fulfill their duties safely and effectively, the member may be medically separated or medically retired, depending on the severity and rating of the condition.

Integrated Disability Evaluation System (IDES)

For many years, the processes for obtaining both DoD and VA disability ratings ran on separate tracks, creating confusion and delays for transitioning service members. To address this, the Integrated Disability Evaluation System (IDES) was created and later fully adopted in 2011.

Under IDES, a service member's fitness for duty (DoD rating) and service-connected disability compensation (VA rating) are evaluated simultaneously. This dual-track approach seeks to ensure that individuals receive a single set of medical examinations and that decisions regarding both retirement eligibility and VA compensation are made more efficiently.

When PTSX is a factor, IDES can be particularly helpful. Often, PTSX involves complex documentation—psychological evaluations, detailed accounts of traumatic exposures, and symptom assessments. By collecting these materials once, rather than duplicating efforts across two separate systems, IDES helps streamline the process.

Upon conclusion, the service member receives a DoD disability rating (used to determine retirement or separation benefits) and a VA disability rating (used for monthly compensation, healthcare enrollment priority, and other benefits). If the service member is found fit for duty, they may continue serving. Otherwise, they depart military service with a better understanding of their future compensation and medical coverage.

Understanding VA Disability Compensation

After separation, the Department of Veterans Affairs becomes the primary agency responsible for supporting former service members dealing with PTSX. The statutory foundation for veterans' benefits rests in Title 38 of the US Code, while specific guidelines for rating disabilities are contained in 38 C.F.R. Part 4, the Schedule for Rating Disabilities.

To initiate this process, a veteran files a disability claim with the VA, typically either online (through VA.gov) or by submitting a paper application. The VA then assists in gathering service treatment records, personnel files, and private medical evidence under the obligations of the Veterans Claims Assistance Act (VCAA). Once the VA has the relevant documentation, the veteran is scheduled for a Compensation and Pension (C&P) examination. During this exam, a licensed mental health professional assesses PTSX symptoms—including re-experiencing, avoidance behaviors, negative alterations in cognition and mood, and heightened arousal and response levels.

The examiner also reviews the nexus between the veteran's condition and their service, determining if there is a direct connection. If the VA finds that PTSX is service-connected, it assigns a disability rating from 0% to 100%, in increments of 10%. The level depends on how significantly symptoms impair daily functioning. Higher percentages translate into larger monthly compensation amounts.

Overview of VA Benefits and Services

The VA offers a wide range of benefits and services that cater to the diverse needs of veterans. Understanding these offerings is the first step toward accessing them effectively:

Disability Compensation

Monthly tax-free payments provided to veterans with service-connected disabilities. These benefits are determined based on the severity of the condition.

Pension Programs

Financial assistance for wartime veterans with limited income, helping them meet basic living expenses.

Healthcare Services

Access to comprehensive medical care, including mental health services, primary care, and specialized treatments at VA facilities.

Educational Benefits

Programs such as the Post-9/11 GI Bill and the Yellow Ribbon Program support higher education and vocational training for veterans and their dependents.

Home Loans

VA-guaranteed home loans help veterans purchase, refinance, or adapt homes to accommodate service-connected disabilities.

Burial and Memorial Benefits

Services include burial allowances, headstones, and markers to honor veterans and their families.

Contact Information

VA Main Website: **va.gov**
VA Customer Service: 1-800-698-2411
Veterans Crisis Line: Dial 988, then press 1 (24/7 support)

Filing Claims for VA Benefits

Filing claims is one of the most critical aspects of accessing VA benefits. Here's a step-by-step guide to clarify the process:

Step 1: Determine Eligibility

- Ensure you have your DD-214 (Certificate of Release or Discharge from Active Duty) as proof of service. This document is crucial for most claims.
- Confirm the existence of a service-connected condition or other qualifying criteria for the benefit you're seeking.

Step 2: Gather Supporting Documentation

- Collect medical records documenting the condition. Include service treatment records and VA or civilian medical evaluations.
- Prepare personal statements describing the impact of the condition on daily life and its connection to your service.

Step 3: Submit the Claim

- Online Submission: Use the VA.gov portal at www.va.gov/disability/how-to-file-claim.
- Paper Submission: Complete VA Form 21-526EZ (Application for Disability Compensation and Related Compensation

Benefits) and mail it to the appropriate VA regional office.

Step 4: VA Review Process

Once submitted, the VA reviews the claim. This includes requesting additional evidence and scheduling Compensation and Pension (C&P) exams to evaluate the condition. Veterans can track progress through the VA Benefits Tracker on **va.gov**.

Step 5: Decision and Next Steps

Upon approval, review your benefits and ratings. In the case of denials, veterans have the option to appeal.

Resources for Filing Claims

- Veterans Service Organizations (VSOs): Groups like the American Legion (legion.org), Disabled American Veterans (**dav.org**), and Veterans of Foreign Wars (**vfw.org**) provide free assistance with claims.
- eBenefits Portal: **ebenefits.va.gov**
- Regional Offices: Locate local offices for in-person help at **va.gov** find-locations.

Navigating the Bureaucratic Process

Navigating the VA's bureaucracy can be overwhelming. Here're some common challenges:

Long Wait Times: Processing claims and appeals can take months or even years.

Confusion Over Documentation: Veterans sometimes struggle to identify what evidence is required.

Inconsistent Communication: Miscommunication or lack of updates can frustrate veterans.

Tips for Overcoming Bureaucratic Hurdles

Stay Organized: Keep copies of all documents, correspondence, and VA notifications. Create a timeline of key events related to your claim.

Be Persistent: Regularly follow up using the VA hotline or the online dashboard. Persistence is often necessary to keep your case moving forward.

Seek Support: Work with a trusted VSO or legal representative to navigate complex issues.

Use Technology: Leverage online tools like the VA mobile app and Benefits Tracker for real-time updates.

Know Your Rights: Familiarize yourself with the appeals process, including supplemental claims, higher-level reviews, and Board of Veterans' Appeals hearings.

Finding Additional Resources

Veterans have access to a wealth of additional resources to complement VA benefits:

Healthcare and Mental Health Support

- VA Health Care: **va.gov/health-care**
- Vet Centers for counseling: **va.gov/find-locations** (filter for Vet Centers).

Educational Resources

- Post-9/11 GI Bill: **va.gov/education**
- Vocational Rehabilitation and Employment (VR&E): **va.gov/careers-employment**

Employment Assistance

- VA Jobs Program: **vaforvets.va.gov**
- USAJobs for federal employment: **usajobs.gov**

Financial Aid and Housing

- Home Loans: **va.gov/housing-assistance**
- VA Pension: **va.gov/pension**

Insider Tips from Experts

Navigating the VA system can be a daunting process, filled with bureaucratic hurdles, detailed documentation requirements, and the potential for delays. However, drawing from the experiences and advice of those who know the system best—VA representatives, veterans, legal advocates, and Board of Veterans' Appeals (BVA) judges—can provide invaluable guidance. Here, we expand on their insights and offer practical and actionable advice to help veterans successfully claim their benefits.

From VA Representatives

VA representatives emphasize the importance of clear and timely communication as a cornerstone of navigating the claims process. Many claims face delays or denials due to missing or incomplete information. Here are their top recommendations:

Respond promptly to VA requests: When the VA requests additional evidence, such as medical records or personal statements, provide the information as soon as possible. Delays in responding can extend the claims process significantly. Keep a checklist of requested items and confirm that all documents are sent to the correct VA office.

Be precise and thorough: Ensure that all submitted forms, such as the VA Form 21-526EZ for disability compensation, are complete and accurate. Double-check for errors or omissions, as these can lead to delays or denials.

Utilize VA resources: Take advantage of the VA's online tools, such as the Benefits Tracker on va.gov, which allows veterans to monitor their claim's progress in real-time. The VA also offers live chat options and phone support for clarifying questions.

Establish a point of contact: Building a relationship with a specific VA representative or caseworker can streamline communication. Consistent contact ensures that your claim remains on track and that any issues are addressed quickly.

From Veterans

Veterans who have successfully navigated the VA system often highlight the importance of early action and seeking external support from trusted organizations. Their firsthand experiences provide critical advice:

File your claim early: Timing is crucial. Filing a claim as soon as possible establishes the "effective date," which determines when benefits begin. Delaying the filing process can mean losing months—or even years—of compensation. Even if all the evidence isn't immediately available, an Intent to File form can secure the effective date while you gather the necessary documentation.

Document everything: Keep detailed records of medical treatments, service-related incidents, and interactions with the VA. Veterans recommend maintaining a physical and digital file containing medical diagnoses, service records, and personal statements. Consistent record-keeping can be the difference between approval and denial.

Seek help from trusted Veterans Service Organizations (VSOs): VSOs, such as the Disabled American Veterans (dav.org) and the Veterans of Foreign Wars (vfw.org), offer free assistance to veterans. These organizations have accredited representatives who are well-versed in VA processes and can help prepare, submit, and monitor claims.

Be persistent: If a claim is denied, don't give up. Many veterans report that persistence and appealing unfavorable decisions eventually led to success. Understand that the process may take time but remain steadfast in advocating for yourself.

From Advocates

Attorneys, legal advocates, and veterans' rights organizations provide additional strategies for navigating complex cases or appealing denied claims. Their insights can help veterans approach the system with greater confidence.

Appeal denials with evidence: Many initial denials occur due to insufficient evidence. When appealing, ensure you provide additional documentation, such as new medical evaluations, expert opinions, or lay statements from family members and friends who can attest to the condition's impact. This supplemental evidence often strengthens the case.

Understand the appeals process: The VA offers three options for challenging a denied claim: a supplemental claim, a higher-level review, or an appeal to the Board of Veterans' Appeals. Each path has its own timeline and requirements, so research which option aligns best with your circumstances. For example, a higher-level review may be appropriate if you believe the VA made an error in reviewing your initial claim.

Hire a qualified, VA-approved attorney: For complex or high-stakes cases, legal representation can be invaluable. Attorneys specializing in VA claims are often familiar with the nuances of the system and can navigate difficult scenarios, such as claims involving secondary conditions or previously denied appeals. They can also represent veterans in hearings before the BVA.

Leverage expert witnesses: In cases involving contested medical diagnoses, enlisting the support of an independent medical expert can be transformative. For example, a physician's detailed report linking your condition to military service can provide compelling evidence for your claim.

From BVA Judges

Judges at the Board of Veterans' Appeals (BVA) play a critical role in adjudicating veterans' claims. Their unique perspective highlights how veterans can present their strongest case:

Prepare for hearings: If your claim reaches the BVA, preparation is key. Judges recommend organizing your evidence chronologically, providing clear explanations of your condition's connection to service, and being ready to answer questions about your military history and symptoms. You can opt for in-person, virtual, or written hearings based on your preference.

Present a cohesive narrative: Judges often stress the importance of telling a consistent and logical story. For example, explain how your injury or condition occurred, how it was treated (or not treated) during service, and how it continues to affect your life today. A clear narrative helps judges understand the case's merits.

Be patient and respectful: BVA judges recognize the frustrations veterans face but advise maintaining professionalism and composure during hearings. Respectful communication can build a positive rapport and ensure that your case is evaluated objectively.

Utilize legal representation: Judges acknowledge that navigating the appellate process can be overwhelming. Accredited attorneys or VSOs can provide essential support, ensuring that your case is presented effectively.

Proactive Planning for Long-Term Success

Build a network of support: Veterans often find that involving family members, fellow veterans, and advocates in their journey provides emotional and logistical assistance. This network can help with record-keeping, attending appointments, or simply offering encouragement.

Stay informed: Regularly review updates to VA policies and benefits programs. Websites like **va.gov** and VSO resources are excellent for staying current on changes that may impact your claim.

Engage in self-care: The claims process can be emotionally taxing. Prioritize mental health by seeking counseling, participating in peer support groups, or engaging in activities that reduce stress.

Empowering Veterans and Families

Navigating the VA system may be complex, but it is achievable with the right knowledge and resources. Veterans and their families deserve the benefits they have earned through their service. By understanding the process, leveraging available tools, and seeking expert guidance, veterans can successfully access critical support. Sharing this knowledge within communities ensures that no veteran is left behind.

The Appeals Process

Not all veterans receive the outcome they expect on the first pass. Perhaps the assigned rating feels too low, or the VA denies service connection for PTSX altogether. Fortunately, the appeals system offers several paths for redress. Under the revamped framework enacted by the Appeals Modernization Act (AMA) of 2017, veterans may choose among three main review lanes:

Higher-Level Review: A senior claims adjudicator re-examines the existing record without new evidence.

Supplemental Claim: The veteran submits additional, "new and relevant" evidence to support the claim.

Appeal to the Board of Veterans' Appeals (BVA): A judge at the BVA reviews the case, and the veteran can request a hearing or submit more evidence. Should the BVA decision still be unfavorable, the veteran may appeal to the US Court of Appeals for Veterans Claims (CAVC), an independent federal court.

At every stage, free or low-cost representation is often available through Veterans Service Organizations (VSOs) like the American Legion, Disabled American Veterans (DAV), or Veterans of Foreign Wars (VFW). Alternatively, the veteran may hire a VA-accredited attorney or claims agent recognized by the VA to help navigate legal complexities. Ask friends and colleagues for referrals.

Workplace Protections and Reemployment Rights

Returning to the civilian workforce can be a significant transition for veterans with PTSX. Some choose to continue serving in the National Guard or Reserves, while others pursue purely civilian roles. In both cases, USERRA (Uniformed Services Employment and Reemployment Rights Act) provides critical safeguards for service members.

USERRA compels employers to reemploy individuals who leave their civilian jobs for military service, ensuring they return to a comparable position, pay grade, and benefits as if they had never left. Veterans must generally meet requirements such as giving prior notice to employers and returning to work within established timelines upon completing service.

For those who have separated from active duty and now seek workplace accommodations for PTSX, the Americans with Disabilities Act (ADA) may come into play. Under the ADA, veterans with documented physical or mental impairments are entitled to "reasonable accommodations" in the workplace, so long as these do not pose an undue hardship on the employer.

Accommodations can include flexible scheduling, remote work, private workspaces, or additional breaks. The key is that the individual's condition must substantially limit one or more major life activities, and the employer must be aware of the need for accommodation.

While privacy about medical conditions is generally protected, it can be beneficial for veterans to disclose the basics of their PTSX diagnosis to Human Resources when seeking accommodations. Doing so typically triggers the employer's legal duty to consider and implement reasonable adjustments.

Confidentiality and Security Clearances

One concern among many service members, especially those on active duty in sensitive roles, is the potential effect of PTSX on security clearances. Contrary to persistent myths, seeking treatment for mental health conditions does not automatically disqualify an individual from holding or obtaining a clearance. US government guidelines typically encourage getting timely mental health care, and an individual's honesty and willingness to manage their condition can be viewed positively.

When it comes to privacy, HIPAA (Health Insurance Portability and Accountability Act) applies in many contexts, but there are instances in which command officials may be notified about a service member's mental health status if it directly impacts fitness for duty or mission readiness. Even then, medical professionals generally safeguard specific therapy notes and sensitive personal details, sharing only what is necessary to maintain operational efficacy.

Discharge Characterization and Upgrades

The characterization of a discharge—whether Honorable, General (Under Honorable Conditions), Other Than Honorable (OTH), Bad Conduct, or Dishonorable—bears profound consequences for post-service life. Most VA benefits require a discharge under conditions other than dishonorable.

Thus, veterans with an OTH or lower often face barriers to receiving healthcare and compensation. However, if a veteran believes that PTSX contributed significantly to misconduct leading to a less favorable discharge, they may apply for a discharge upgrade through their branch's Discharge Review Board (DRB) or Board for Correction of Military Records (BCMR).

These boards review evidence—such as medical documentation verifying that the veteran suffered from undiagnosed or unrecognized mental health conditions at the time of service—which might explain or mitigate the behavior that triggered the discharge. A successful application can change the discharge to a higher characterization, thereby opening the door to benefits.

Indeed, legislation such as the Hagel Memo (2014) and subsequent clarifications have encouraged boards to give "liberal consideration" to cases where mental health issues, including PTSX, were likely factors in the alleged misconduct.

Accessing VA Healthcare and Other Programs

Once separated from the military, veterans with PTSX are often eligible to enroll in the VA Healthcare system. This is not strictly limited to those with high disability ratings. Many veterans qualify, though priority is generally granted to those with service-connected conditions.

VA hospitals and clinics provide a range of specialized mental-health services, including inpatient programs, outpatient counseling, and telehealth for those who cannot easily travel to a facility. These services often feature professionals trained in trauma-specific therapies, such as Cognitive Processing Therapy (CPT) and Prolonged Exposure (PE), which have demonstrated effectiveness in alleviating PTSX symptoms.

In addition to medical care, the VA offers support through the Veteran Readiness and Employment (VR&E) program—formerly known as Vocational Rehabilitation and Employment. Veterans with service-connected disabilities that impede employment may qualify for counseling, training, and job placement services aimed at securing and maintaining suitable work.

For those wishing to pursue further education, the Post-9/11 GI Bill covers tuition, housing allowances, and even tutoring assistance. These benefits can be instrumental in adapting to post-military life, particularly if PTSX makes returning to a previous occupation challenging.

Military Justice Considerations

While active-duty service members remain subject to the Uniform Code of Military Justice (UCMJ), it is worth noting that PTSX by itself does not absolve misconduct. In some cases, however, demonstrating that PTSX symptoms contributed to an individual's behavior can serve as a mitigating factor during sentencing or administrative separation processes.

Commanders and military judges often consider medical evidence, mental-health evaluations, and treatment histories when deciding appropriate disciplinary actions. Certain offenses, especially minor ones, may be diverted to rehabilitative programs or alternative resolutions if the chain of command perceives that untreated mental health conditions are at the core of the conduct. This approach aims to ensure that service members receive help rather than solely punitive measures.

A key piece of advice for anyone in uniform facing legal challenges while managing PTSX is to consult both a military defense counsel—provided at no cost—and a civilian attorney if complexities arise. Early involvement of legal assistance ensures that pertinent medical records and psychological evaluations are introduced into the legal process.

The Importance of Advocacy and Support Networks

Throughout all these administrative and legal proceedings—whether an MEB, VA claim, workplace accommodation request, or discharge upgrade application—having knowledgeable advocates can significantly ease the stress. Veterans Service Organizations (VSOs) are invaluable in this regard.

They employ accredited representatives who understand the intricacies of VA benefits and can offer guidance free of charge. Additionally, legal aid clinics, especially those affiliated with law schools or community nonprofits, often focus on helping veterans with discharge upgrade applications or appeals at no or minimal cost.

Connecting with other veterans who have navigated the same pathways can also reduce the sense of isolation that can accompany PTSX. Peer support groups, mentoring programs and online communities can provide encouragement, tips, and perspectives that might not be available through official channels alone. Such networks help normalize the experience of dealing with stress-related conditions, creating an environment where seeking help is seen as an act of strength rather than weakness.

Special Considerations for Women Veterans

As the number of women serving in the US Armed Forces continues to grow, it is vital to recognize gender-specific contexts that may influence the experience of PTSX. While traditional combat exposure remains a key factor, women may also face additional challenges like military sexual trauma (MST). MST refers to any sexual assault, harassment, or unwanted sexual attention that occurs in a military setting. Survivors of MST often present with heightened psychological distress, which can compound or resemble PTSX.

Legal Protections and MST Reporting

Under Department of Defense Instruction (DoDI) 6495.02, Volume 1, service members who experience sexual assault have the option to file either a Restricted or Unrestricted Report. This policy is part of the DoD's Sexual Assault Prevention and Response (SAPR) Program, which outlines procedures for reporting and responding to sexual assault incidents within the military.

Restricted Reporting: This option allows service members to confidentially disclose a sexual assault to specified individuals, such as Sexual Assault Response Coordinators (SARCs), Sexual Assault Prevention and Response Victim Advocates (SAPR VAs), or healthcare personnel. Under Restricted Reporting, the victim can access medical treatment, counseling and support services without triggering an official investigation or notifying their command.

Unrestricted Reporting: This option involves reporting the sexual assault through normal reporting channels, such as the chain of command, law enforcement, or directly to a SARC or SAPR VA. Unrestricted Reporting initiates an official investigation and allows the victim to receive the same support services as in Restricted Reporting, with the addition of command involvement and potential legal action against the perpetrator.

It's important to note that victims who initially choose Restricted Reporting can later convert to Unrestricted Reporting if they decide to pursue an official investigation. However, once an Unrestricted Report is filed, it cannot be changed to a Restricted Report.

These reporting options are designed to provide victims with choices that best suit their needs and circumstances, ensuring access to care and support while respecting their autonomy.

Survivors who later leave the service may qualify for VA disability benefits if MST led to or aggravated conditions like PTSX. The VA has established MST Coordinators at each medical center to guide survivors through the claims process and ensure that mental health support is trauma-informed.

VA Women's Health Services

The VA Women Veterans Program is designed to provide comprehensive primary care, mental health treatment, and gender-specific services (e.g., mammography, gynecology). Clinics often incorporate trauma-informed approaches sensitive to unique stressors faced by women veterans. Legal recourse and supportive programs for MST survivors are increasing, ensuring that if a woman veteran seeks to document and claim MST-related injuries or stress conditions, the VA and affiliated legal advocates can guide her effectively.

Older Veterans and Long-Term Effects

Although public attention often focuses on younger service members returning from recent conflicts, older veterans—from Vietnam-era to Cold War service—may experience PTSX as well. In many instances, trauma symptoms can remain dormant or unrecognized for decades, only to surface or intensify later in life due to retirement, the loss of a spouse, or emerging health issues.

Statutes of Limitation

While there is no statute of limitations on filing a VA claim for service-connected disability, older veterans may encounter difficulty retrieving complete records if decades have passed. Nonetheless, the duty to assist under the Veterans Claims Assistance Act (VCAA) obligates the VA to help gather any available documentation.

In certain cases, the VA recognizes buddy statements—written testimony from fellow veterans or contemporaries who can attest to the claimant's in-service experiences—as a valid form of evidence when official records are incomplete.

Geriatric Care and VA Programs

The VA offers Geriatric and Extended Care services that integrate mental health support. Community Living Centers, adult day health care, and home-based primary care can all be adapted for veterans with PTSX.

Legal guardianship, advance directives, and estate planning may become pertinent for older veterans with advanced mental or physical health needs. VA social workers and local legal aid clinics can help navigate these issues.

Veteran Homelessness and PTSX

A disheartening reality is that veterans are disproportionately represented among the homeless population in the United States. PTSX, substance use disorders, and the struggle to readjust to civilian life can contribute to housing instability. The VA, in partnership with state and local organizations, has introduced various programs to address these challenges:

Housing and Urban Development-Veterans Affairs Supportive Housing (HUD-VASH) is a collaborative program between the VA and the Department of Housing and Urban Development (HUD). It provides housing choice vouchers (commonly referred to as "Section 8") combined with comprehensive case management to ensure stable housing and access to mental health services.

Homeless veterans working toward recovery from PTSX receive a tailored treatment plan and, once housed, ongoing support to prevent recidivism into homelessness.

Legal Clinics for Homeless Veterans

Many VA medical centers, law schools, and charitable organizations offer Stand Downs and legal aid clinics focused on resolving issues that often keep veterans in a cycle of homelessness—such as outstanding fines, suspended driver's licenses, or minor criminal charges.

These clinics can also connect homeless veterans to VA benefits, including PTSX-related compensation, which may be critical to achieving long-term financial security.

Community-Based Support and Peer Programs

Beyond formal legal structures and federal agencies, community-driven support systems often play an essential role in helping veterans manage PTSX. These options exist both within and outside the VA ecosystem and can be profoundly effective in bridging gaps.

Vet Centers

Operated by the VA but distinct from VA Medical Centers, Vet Centers offer readjustment counseling, outreach, and referral services to combat veterans, survivors of MST, and their families. Because Vet Centers operate under strict confidentiality rules, some veterans feel more comfortable seeking initial support there before engaging with the broader VA system. Vet Center counselors are frequently veterans themselves, providing a peer-based dimension that can help reduce stigma.

Nonprofit Organizations

Groups such as Team Rubicon, which engages veterans in disaster response efforts, or Wounded Warrior Project, which offers a variety of programs and advocacy initiatives, can help veterans maintain a sense of camaraderie and purpose while recovering from PTSX.

Faith-based and community nonprofits frequently organize retreats or workshops focusing on trauma recovery and resilience. They may also connect veterans to legal resources for issues like disability appeals or child custody arrangements impacted by mental health considerations.

Integrating Legal, Medical, and Personal Strategies

One of the fundamental insights for veterans facing PTSX is that a holistic approach—combining legal awareness, effective clinical treatment, and robust personal support—tends to yield the most positive outcomes. The potential for bureaucratic hurdles within the DoD and

VA can be daunting, but preparation and informed advocacy help smooth the path.

Building Your Own Personnel Record File

Maintaining copies of all service treatment records, personnel records, and military awards can streamline an MEB/PEB or VA claim later. Organize private medical records and statements detailing stressor events or symptoms.

If possible, gather "buddy statements" early—testimonials from fellow service members who witnessed a traumatic event or observed behavioral changes.

Staying Engaged in Treatment

Legal processes can be lengthy. While appeals or discharge upgrades are pending, actively continuing mental health treatment ensures wellbeing and demonstrates a commitment to healing.

This consistency can also strengthen a case, as updated treatment records show the VA or review boards that the veteran remains proactive about managing symptoms and improving functionality.

Seeking Expert Guidance

Accredited representatives—whether from a Veterans Service Organization or a specialized law firm—can clarify terminology, explain filing deadlines, and assist in preparing persuasive claim narratives.

Pro bono legal clinics or organizations like the National Veterans Legal Services Program (NVLSP) often undertake complex cases that involve class action lawsuits or systematic challenges within the VA.

Recognizing When to Appeal

Veterans have the right to keep appealing until they reach a satisfactory conclusion or run out of legal avenues. However, it's worth discussing with a legal professional who knows the VA process whether additional evidence or a different review lane (e.g., Supplemental Claim vs. Board hearing) might be a better next step.

Carefully documenting how PTSX impacts relationships, job

performance, and daily functioning can be pivotal in obtaining a higher disability rating or proving a service-connected disability.

Combating Stigma: A Collective Effort

Despite widespread education and high-level policy statements, stigma around mental-health conditions can remain a barrier for both active-duty service members and veterans. Fear of appearing weak or jeopardizing a career might delay seeking care; once in the civilian world, concerns about how employers or peers will react can further deter needed assistance.

Command and Leadership

The DoD, in recent years, has intensified its messaging that seeking help is a sign of strength, not frailty. Leaders at all levels are encouraged to support subordinates who come forward with mental health concerns.

Confidential resource referrals within units—chaplains, Military OneSource, mental health professionals—help ensure that service members get early support, potentially reducing the symptoms of PTSX.

Public Perception

Civilian workplaces increasingly understand that veterans bring unique strengths: discipline, leadership, and teamwork skills. Many also recognize that conditions like PTSX are manageable, especially when appropriate accommodations and support are in place.

Continued outreach by both government agencies and non-government organizations is expanding the dialogue around veteran mental health, aiming to ensure that no one who has served is left to struggle alone with invisible wounds.

Looking Ahead: The Evolving Legal Landscape

The legal frameworks governing US military personnel and veterans' benefits are not static. Congress, the DoD, and the VA routinely refine or update policies to address emerging needs, streamline claims processes, or fill gaps in coverage. For example, legislation over the last decade has encouraged the boards of military departments to consider "liberalizing" standards when reviewing discharge upgrade applications involving mental health. Meanwhile, the VA continuously explores ways to reduce the backlog of claims and appeals.

Legislative Advocacy

Veterans themselves are powerful voices in shaping policy. Many of the improvements in mental health coverage, including expansions in telehealth and support for MST survivors, arose due to grassroots advocacy efforts.

By staying informed through resources like the Federal Register, official VA announcements, and VSO newsletters, veterans can remain aware of new benefits or procedural changes that could directly affect them.

Technological Innovations

The VA has upgraded many of its online platforms, enabling digital submissions of claims and offering telehealth counseling. Emerging tools—such as AI-assisted intake for claims or smartphone apps for symptom tracking—might reduce wait times and facilitate more patient-centered care. Virtual appointments can be especially valuable for those in rural areas or who face mobility challenges, ensuring that no matter where a veteran lives, they can connect with qualified mental health professionals and legal advocates.

A Call to Action

For US service members and veterans, the intersection of PTSX and legal considerations is intricate but not insurmountable. A robust framework of laws and policies—rooted in Titles 10 and 38 of the US Code, the Code of Federal Regulations, and supporting DoD and VA directives—exists to ensure that individuals with service-connected stress conditions receive proper evaluations, fair compensation, and accessible treatment. From the IDES, which streamlines military and VA disability determinations, to the host of VA programs dedicated to medical care, educational assistance, and employment readiness, the system strives to honor the sacrifices made by our nation's defenders.

While none of these processes are without hurdles, awareness is the first step toward effective navigation. Knowing one's rights during MEB and PEB reviews, having a clear grasp of VA claims and appeals procedures, utilizing workplace protections under USERRA and the ADA, and understanding how discharge characterization affects benefit eligibility are all critical components for veterans living with PTSX.

Through diligent documentation, proactive advocacy and willingness to seek help, it is possible to secure the resources and support needed for a productive and fulfilling life beyond military service. Ultimately, the core message is that those who suffer the hidden wounds of trauma are never alone: the law, the VA, and the broader veteran community stand ready to assist in the journey toward healing and stability.

You Are Not Alone

For service personnel and veterans experiencing PTSX, knowledge truly is power. Understanding the interplay of DoD processes like the Medical Evaluation Board or the Integrated Disability Evaluation System, as well as the VA's frameworks for disability compensation, appeals, and healthcare, can significantly reduce anxiety and empower veterans to advocate for themselves. Whether the issue lies in navigating a workplace accommodation under the Americans with Disabilities Act, preventing homelessness through HUD-VASH, or appealing a lower-than-expected VA rating, the critical first step is recognizing that these laws and programs are meant to serve and protect those who have served.

PTSX can be a life-altering condition, but comprehensive legal and medical structures exist to help US service members and veterans manage it effectively. When individuals actively engage with these resources—seeking assistance early, carefully documenting their experiences, and appealing unfavorable decisions when necessary—they stand a far better chance of achieving a stable, fulfilling post-military life. If there is any single piece of advice to carry forward, it is to ask for help and persist. With an informed approach, the path to healing and rightful recognition is firmly within reach.

If-Then Guidance

- If you are a veteran preparing to file a VA benefits claim, then gather all necessary documentation, including your DD-214, service treatment records, and any relevant medical or personal statements. Being well-prepared can significantly streamline the claims process.
- If your initial claim is denied, then file an appeal promptly and consider seeking assistance from a Veterans Service Organization (VSO) such as the American Legion or Disabled American Veterans. Many claims are successfully resolved through the appeals process with the right evidence.
- If you are experiencing long delays or difficulty getting updates on your claim, then utilize online tools like the VA.gov benefits tracker or contact the VA hotline at 1-800-698-2411 for real-time updates and assistance.
- If you find the VA system confusing or overwhelming, then work with a trusted advocate, such as a VSO representative or a certified VA attorney. These professionals can guide you through the process and ensure all paperwork is completed accurately.
- If you need mental health support during the claims process, then reach out to a local Vet Center or call the Veterans Crisis Line at 988 and press 1. The emotional toll of navigating the system is valid, and help is available.
- If you are preparing for a Board of Veterans' Appeals (BVA) hearing, then organize your evidence clearly, rehearse your testimony, and consider enlisting the help of an attorney or VSO to present a cohesive case.
- If you are transitioning from active duty and need to establish benefits, then file an Intent to File form as soon as possible. This establishes your effective date for benefits, giving you time to gather necessary documents without losing eligibility for back pay.
- If you're unsure about the benefits available to you, then explore resources on VA.gov and speak with a VSO to understand your entitlements: healthcare, housing assistance, education programs.

Take The Next Step

- File your claim: Begin the claims process by visiting https://www.va.gov/disability/how-to-file-claim/ to file online or download the necessary forms. Ensure you have all supporting documentation ready.
- Seek assistance: Contact a VSO such as the Disabled American Veterans (DAV) at dav.org or the Veterans of Foreign Wars (VFW) at vfw.org to get free help filing and tracking your claim.
- Track your claim: Use the VA.gov dashboard to monitor your claim's progress and respond promptly to any requests for additional evidence.
- Appeal a denial: If your claim is denied, explore your options for a supplemental claim, higher-level review, or appeal to the BVA. Consult with a certified representative or attorney for guidance.
- Use VA resources: Leverage online tools like the VA Benefits Tracker or mobile apps to stay organized and informed throughout the process.
- Stay connected: Engage with local Vet Centers, peer support groups, or counseling services to navigate the emotional and logistical challenges of the claims process.
- Educate yourself: Familiarize yourself with VA benefits by exploring resources on VA.gov, including the Post-9/11 GI Bill, healthcare services, and housing assistance programs.
- Plan for the future: Regularly review updates to VA policies and benefits. Stay proactive in managing your entitlements to maximize long-term support for you and your family.

Through Their Eyes

"I spent two decades serving as a Counterintelligence Special Agent in the US Army Counterintelligence Command. Over the course of my 20-year career, I was entrusted with some of the highest levels of intelligence, security and safety across multiple theaters of operation, often supporting Special Operations Command.

"I witnessed—and at times, directly experienced—events that would rattle even the toughest among us. These exposures took a serious toll on my emotional and mental wellbeing, although I chose to push through it at the time.

"Looking back, I can pinpoint certain moments that I wish I had handled differently. One in particular stands out: the day I was sexually molested by a fellow servicemember while stationed overseas. I was in an environment where every move was scrutinized, and my own superior—a high-ranking female officer—told me to brush it off if I ever wanted to keep advancing. I believed her, and I stayed silent. Like so many others, I buried my trauma and tried to carry on as if nothing had happened.

"When I finally retired, I thought I'd be stepping into a well-earned life of peace. Instead, all those years of unaddressed stress, trauma, and moral injury came crashing down on me. Depression crept up, slowly at first, then all at once. I found myself in a downward spiral: the once-disciplined soldier in me started partying in Key West and the Bahamas.

"I drank alcohol heavily—something I had almost never done before—and smoked cigarettes to cope. None of it worked. I felt like I was drifting further from my true self, and I had no real plan to make it stop.

"A friend of mine recognized how desperate I had become and suggested I go to the Department of Veterans Affairs (VA). I was skeptical—after all, the military's bureaucracy had already been exhausting, and I was sure the VA would be no different. But she convinced me to enroll and file a disability claim, emphasizing that my years of service and the trauma I had endured might qualify me for both medical and financial assistance.

Starting the Claims Process

"Filing that initial claim was daunting. The forms seemed endless, and the system felt complicated. However, my friend's advice to work with a Veterans Service Organization was a game-changer. My VSO representative walked me through each step, helping me gather all the necessary documents—my DD-214, service treatment records, and statements detailing my in-service stressors and subsequent depression. I learned that timing is critical: submitting the claim early establishes what is known as the 'effective date,' which determines when benefits begin.

"The VA scheduled me for a Compensation and Pension examination, where a licensed mental health professional evaluated my symptoms of depression, anxiety, and PTSX (the extended form of post-traumatic stress). If you're in a similar place, document everything—the more evidence you have, the stronger your claim becomes.

Persistence Pays Off

"My application wasn't approved overnight. In fact, it took me five years of re-submissions and appeals to get the generous disability compensation rating I truly deserved. I often felt discouraged by the long wait times and the VA's requests for additional evidence. Fortunately, my VSO representative kept me on track. Looking back, I realize how important it is to stay organized—keep copies of all correspondence, medical records, and letters from the VA. Be persistent and follow up regularly, either by phone or through the online portal.

Getting Medical Help for Depression

"While my claim inched its way through the VA system, I was also directed to seek medical care. Let me tell you: taking advantage of VA healthcare services changed everything. After enrolling, I got connected with mental health professionals who specialize in trauma-informed care, including therapies specifically designed for veterans. Over time, it became apparent that traditional antidepressants and talk therapy alone were not enough to help me climb out of the darkness.

"My VA care team introduced me to alternative treatments—ketamine infusions and a stellate ganglion block procedure, both of which can be incredibly effective for severe depression and anxiety. It's not a magic cure, but these treatments gave me the first real relief I'd felt in years.

Stepping Into a New Chapter

"Eventually, my disability claim was approved at a level that provided the financial security I needed to focus on my healing. The VA covered the costs of my treatments, which further removed the barriers that had kept me from pursuing comprehensive care. With my mental health improving, I made the choice to pivot my career.

"Today, I work as a consultant to major companies, advising them on intelligence, security, and safety matters. I'm also lucky enough to be invited to speak at events where I share my story—hoping it encourages others to seek help and claim the benefits they rightfully deserve.

"If there's one thing I want fellow veterans to take from my experience, it's this: you are not alone, and help is available. Start with a phone call to the VA or connect with a VSO. Build a support network of peers who've been through it, and seek mental health care. By confronting trauma—through professional help, VA benefits, and a willingness to keep pushing forward—I'm finally reclaiming my peace.

"If you're out there, thinking you're too far gone or that no one will believe you, I promise you: there is a whole community ready to stand alongside you, walk you through the paperwork, and celebrate when you finally come out on the other side.

"You don't have to do this alone."

—Colonel Jennifer E., US Army (ret.)

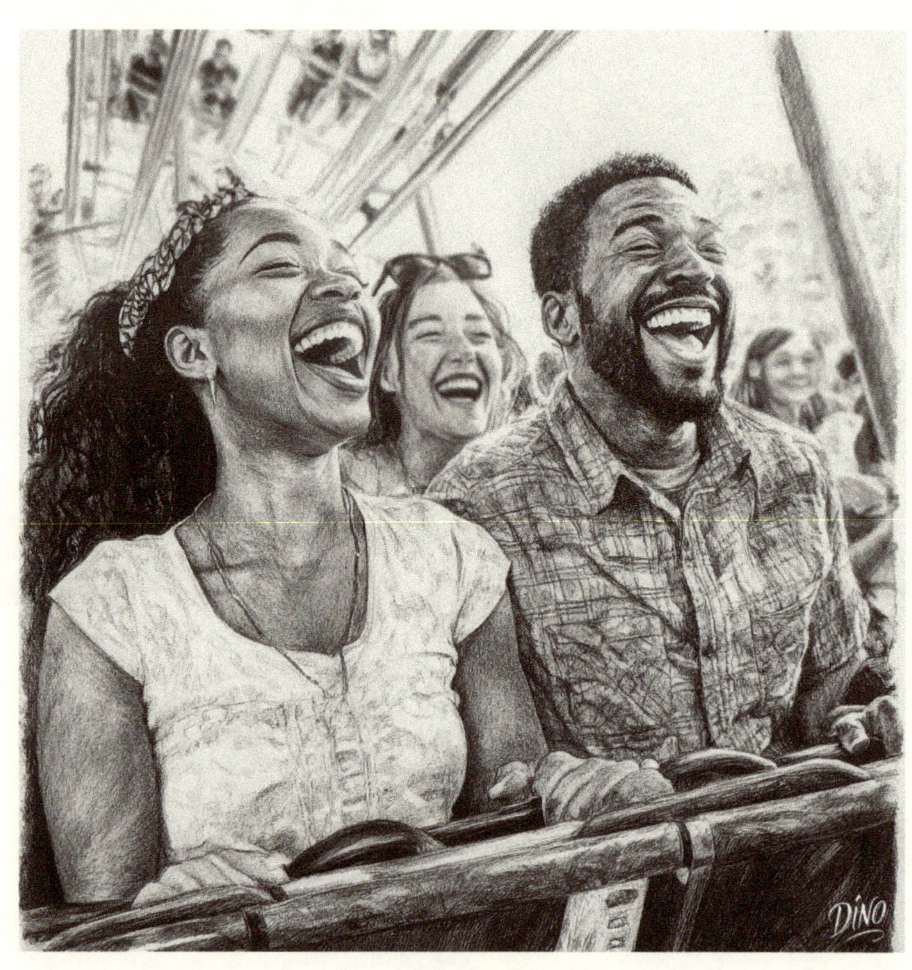
DINO

PART SEVEN

The Molecular Basis of PTSX

53

Deep Molecular Actions Underlie PTSX

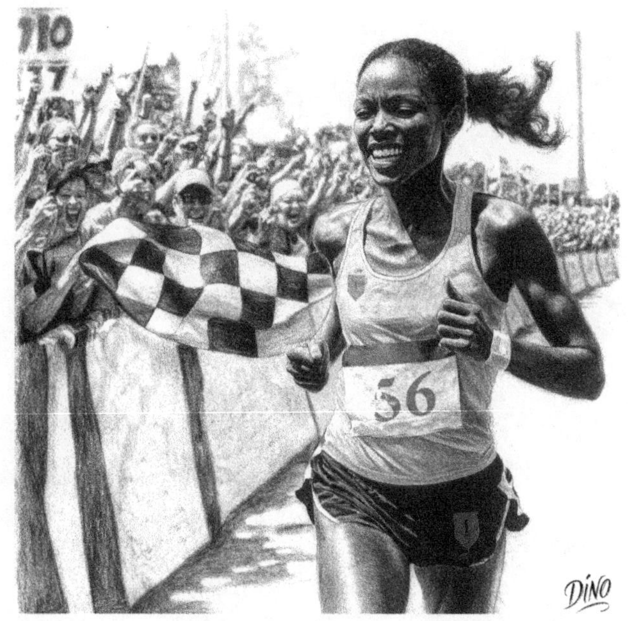

I used to steady my scalpel by humming the cadence we learned at Fort Sam, the rhythm that kept blood and suture in step. At Walter Reed I broke rank, spoke aloud about colleagues who stitched an artery wrong, prescribed benzos like candy, shooed blast-wounded privates out the door with a plastic bag of pills and no scans. The command called me "disruptive." My credentials vanished and now I rent attic office space two blocks from a pawn shop and draft medical opinions for veterans who clutch denial letters in trembling hands.

For too long, we've been told that PTSX is "all in your head," as if it's imagined. That's a lie. Trauma causes a real, physical injury. It sets off a chain reaction that leaves the brain's stress response permanently switched on. The danger outside might be over, but inside, the chemistry doesn't get the memo. Your body is flooded with stress hormones, your natural defenses are burned out, and your brain is literally inflamed. That's why a smell or a sound can throw you right back into the fight. This isn't a theory. This is biology. We need treatments and policies that fix the physical damage, not just talk about the memories. So yes, the injury is in your head. But it's not imagined. It's a deep wound written in our neurochemistry, and it's time we started treating it with hard-core science.

While psychiatry and psychology have told us "it's all your head," we now know the "one pill for every ill" approach is ineffective, especially considering that the underlying nature of all brain injuries and diseases is at the molecular level or below.

These final chapters discuss the molecular basis of PTSX, including the activity of the vagus nerve. The contents do not dismiss any of the traditional therapies discussed in previous chapters. Properly applied, they all have value. It may be years before we can directly treat PTSX by repairing our nerve, neuroimmune and neuroendocrine systems and their cascades of molecules and reactions. Until then, we suggest combining the most helpful care and healing therapies presented previously with the most accurate molecular study and research.

Glutathione: The Body's Protector

For many who live with the weight of post-traumatic stress, the injury feels like more than a memory. It manifests as a heavy physical toll—a persistent brain fog, a bone-deep fatigue, and a general feeling of malaise that can be difficult to describe. Understanding the science of trauma helps us see that these physical symptoms are not just "in your head". They are the very real consequence of a body carrying a silent burden. The key to understanding this connection lies in a remarkable molecule called glutathione.

Inside every cell of our body, a delicate balance is constantly maintained. As our cells produce energy, they also create byproducts called free radicals. These are unstable molecules that, if left unchecked, can cause damage to surrounding cells—a process known as oxidative stress. You can think of it as a form of "cellular rust," a slow and steady wear and tear.

To protect against this, the body produces its own defense: a powerful antioxidant called glutathione. Its primary role is to find and neutralize these free radicals, keeping our cells healthy and functioning properly. It is, in essence, our body's master protector.

"One night, I was so desperate I almost did the unthinkable. My mind was screaming that I had no future—no way out. But just before giving in, I saw a documentary featuring Dr. Mark Gordon. He explained how injuries and trauma can hijack the body at the molecular level, fueling inflammation and messing with the delicate balance of hormones and neurotransmitters."

When Stress Depletes Our Defenses

The state of hypervigilance that defines PTSX—the constant feeling of being "on alert"—places an immense demand on the body's resources. This chronic stress accelerates the production of free radicals, particularly in the brain. To manage this state of emergency, the body draws heavily on its reserves of glutathione.

Over time, with the stress continuing, these reserves can become depleted. The body simply can't produce glutathione fast enough to keep up with the demand. When this happens, the brain and body become more vulnerable to the effects of oxidative stress, which can lead to several scientifically recognized consequences:

- Neuroinflammation: A state of low-grade inflammation in the brain, which research has increasingly linked to symptoms of depression, anxiety, and the cognitive difficulties: "brain fog."

- Mitochondrial Dysfunction: The mitochondria are the tiny power plants within our cells. Oxidative stress can damage them, impairing their ability to produce energy and leading to the profound and lasting fatigue that is so common with PTSX.

This depletion creates a difficult cycle, where the biological stress can amplify the psychological symptoms of the original trauma. Recognizing this connection is a critical step toward healing, as it provides a clear, biological target for intervention. Research into N-acetylcysteine (NAC), a natural compound that helps the body produce more glutathione, has shown significant promise in this area, offering a tangible way to help restore the body's protective balance.

Fractalkine: The Guardian Messenger

Among the key players in maintaining a healthy brain is a substance called fractalkine (CX3CL1). It's produced almost exclusively by neurons in the brain and spinal cord. In its default state, fractalkine is anchored to the outer membrane of those neurons as a long protein stalk. When the brain needs to send a broader signal, enzymes release a soluble form that diffuses through the interstitial space and, in smaller amounts, into the CSF.

The molecule's chief receiver is the microglial cell, which carries a matching receptor called CX3CR1. Under steady conditions, membrane-bound fractalkine provides a "stay calm, monitor silently" message that holds microglia in a surveillance state (often labeled M0). When neurons fire intensely, experience mild injury or encounter learning-related synaptic pruning, they shed soluble fractalkine to fine-tune microglial help without triggering full inflammation.

Trouble arises when chronic stress elevates cortisol or when severe trauma disrupts neuronal metabolism. High glucocorticoid levels down-regulate neuronal CX3CL1 expression, so less fractalkine—both tethered and soluble—reaches the microglia.

Deprived of their calming handshake, microglia are more likely to flip into the pro-inflammatory M1 mode, releasing cytokines that can erode synapses and deepen the neurochemical footprint of PTSX. Thus, fractalkine is not a random by-product in the CSF. It's a neuron-crafted, context-dependent messenger whose availability helps decide whether microglia protect or provoke the stressed brain.

Microglia: Quiet Protectors Turned Stormbringers

Microglia are specialized immune cells that reside permanently in the CNS, including the brain and spinal cord. Unlike peripheral immune cells that patrol the bloodstream, microglia are embedded within brain tissue itself, acting as the first and principal line of defense against infection, injury, and disease. During early embryonic development—around Day 7.5 in mice, with a similar timeline in humans—primitive macrophages emerge in the yolk sac before the body's hematopoietic (blood-forming) system is fully established.

These early immune cells migrate into the developing brain and differentiate into microglia, doing so before the blood-brain barrier forms, allowing them unrestricted access to the central nervous system. Once embedded in brain tissue, microglia become a self-sustaining population, capable of renewing themselves through local proliferation.

Unlike other immune cells, they do not rely on input from bone marrow or circulating monocytes. In a healthy brain, this self-renewal process continues for life, though it can be disrupted by severe trauma, disease or age-related degeneration.

Core Functions of Microglia

1. Surveillance (Sentinel Role)

Microglia are highly dynamic. Even in a "resting" state, their branched processes are constantly moving, scanning the surrounding environment for signs of trouble—such as pathogens, toxins or cellular debris.

2. Phagocytosis (Cellular Cleanup)

When they detect damage, microglia switch into an "activated" state. In this mode, they engulf and digest:

- Dead or dying neurons
- Protein aggregates (e.g., amyloid-beta in Alzheimer's)
- Debris from injured cells

This cleanup helps prevent inflammation and maintain neural health.

3. Synaptic Pruning

During brain development and even into adulthood, microglia shape the brain's wiring by pruning unnecessary synapses. They literally "eat" weak or unused connections, helping sculpt efficient neural circuits. This process is essential for:

- Normal brain development
- Learning and memory
- Neuroplasticity

4. Cytokine and Chemokine Release

Activated microglia release signaling molecules (for example, IL-1Beta, Tumor Necrosis Factor-Alpha) that can:

- Trigger inflammation to fight infection
- Recruit other immune cells (in cases of severe infection)
- Influence neuronal activity and survival

Microglia in Disease and Dysfunction

While microglia are essential for overall brain health, chronic or overactivation can be damaging. They are implicated in a wide range of molecular disorders:

Alzheimer's Disease: Microglia attempt to clear amyloid plaques but may become dysregulated, contributing to sustained inflammation and neuronal damage.

Parkinson's Disease: Overactive microglia release neurotoxic factors that may exacerbate dopaminergic neuron loss.

ALS (Lou Gehrig's Disease): Microglia may contribute to motor neuron degeneration via inflammatory pathways.

Schizophrenia and Autism Spectrum Disorders: Disruptions in microglial synaptic pruning may underlie abnormal brain connectivity.

Depression and PTSX: Chronic stress and trauma can prime microglia toward a pro-inflammatory state, impacting mood regulation and cognitive function.

In traumatic brain injury (TBI) and stroke, microglia respond quickly to physical damage but may perpetuate secondary injury by releasing inflammatory substances and harmful molecules called free radicals. Among the most damaging of these is peroxynitrite, a compound that can break down essential proteins, damage DNA and trigger cellular stress. This chain reaction can have a serious impact on brain health. In fact, results from recent studies highlight how ongoing microglial activation and free-radical production may underlie many persistent, trauma-related symptoms in veterans.

The Double-Edged Sword

In essence, microglia are neuroprotective when balanced but neurotoxic when overactive or dysregulated. Modern neuroscience recognizes that healing the brain—especially after trauma, infection or neurodegeneration—often depends on restoring microglial balance.

Modulating microglial activity is now a promising strategy in treating Alzheimer's, MS, depression, and even long-COVID-related brain fog. Experimental drugs, gene therapies, and lifestyle interventions (like exercise and diet) may recalibrate microglial function, reduce neuroinflammation, and support brain repair.

The Downstream Devastation: Neurotransmission Under Fire

As microglia release peroxynitrite and other reactive chemicals, the production of neurotransmitters—like serotonin, dopamine and GABA—can plummet. Receptors for these crucial brain signals may also get damaged or become less responsive. The result: a decline in cognitive function, mood balance, and emotional regulation. When your brain can't effectively communicate within itself, it's easy to feel trapped in a loop of negative thoughts, hyperarousal and a sense of looming danger.

Despite this bleak-sounding cycle, there is hope. By understanding how chronic cortisol elevation undermines fractalkine signaling and fuels microglial overactivity, we can better grasp the biological underpinnings of PTSX.

Foundations of the HPA Axis and Stress Response

To understand why stress sometimes turns chronic, we need to examine this triad of glands and hormones that orchestrate our stress response. When you encounter a threatening situation, the hypothalamus in your brain releases corticotropin-releasing hormone (CRH). This hormone travels to the pituitary gland, prompting the release of adrenocorticotropic hormone (ACTH). ACTH, in turn, stimulates the adrenal glands (on top of your kidneys) to secrete cortisol. In a healthy, short-term response, this quick surge of cortisol arms you with the energy and focus you need to confront or escape danger.

In theory, the body has a built-in mechanism to prevent the stress response from running wild. Elevated cortisol levels normally feed back to the hypothalamus and pituitary, signaling them to slow down CRH and ACTH production. This negative feedback loop ensures that once you've dealt with the threat, your cortisol levels return to normal and bodily functions like digestion and rest can resume. Research suggests that when this loop functions smoothly, stress is handled efficiently and dissipates relatively quickly.

When the System Goes Off-Key: Chronic or Extreme Stress

Trouble begins when the "safety switch" gets stuck—or, in some cases, fails altogether. In the face of repeated, intense stressors, the HPA axis may remain on high alert, continuously flooding the system with cortisol or keeping it imbalanced at unpredictable times. Think of it like an alarm system that keeps blaring even after the intruder has gone. For military veterans, trauma exposure is often severe and repeated, making this system more likely to break down. The result is a body primed to sense danger, even in situations where true threats no longer exist.

The Fallout: Heightened Inflammation and Altered Brain Chemistry

Excess cortisol doesn't act alone. By diminishing fractalkine, cortisol paves the way for microglial overactivity in the brain. Studies in the last two years confirm that veterans experiencing chronic stress or trauma-related disorders often show evidence of both cortisol dysregulation and neuroinflammation. This one-two punch can damage neurons, lower essential neurotransmitter levels, and alter emotional and cognitive processes.

Veterans and the Unseen Battle

For many servicemembers returning from deployment, the external war is over, but an internal struggle continues. The HPA axis, once an ally on the battlefield, can become a relentless messenger of dread. This biochemical state often manifests as nightmares, flashbacks, flashforwards, mood swings, or an exaggerated startle response.

It can strain relationships, impede daily tasks, and make reintegration into civilian life an uphill battle. The good news is that identifying dysfunction within the HPA axis can guide effective interventions. Certain medications aim to stabilize cortisol levels, while behavioral therapies—from structured exercise routines to mindfulness-based stress reduction—have shown promise in resetting this hormonal rhythm. Results from some studies suggest that improving sleep hygiene also helps the negative feedback loop do its job, preventing an overproduction of cortisol. By addressing the true cause—an overworked stress system—veterans can gradually find relief from PTSX and reclaim a sense of safety in their daily lives.

Cortisol Dysregulation and Its Impact on Fractalkine

Under normal conditions, fractalkine helps maintain a calm and balanced environment by sending signals that keep microglia from overreacting to every minor disturbance. It also supports healthy neuron function, allowing these cells to repair or replace damaged tissue more effectively.

When stress becomes chronic or extreme, high levels of cortisol start to interfere with a variety of biochemical processes. One of the most important discoveries in recent research is that cortisol can reduce the production and effectiveness of fractalkine.

This happens through multiple pathways, including changes in gene expression, in which cortisol essentially "turns down the volume" on the fractalkine signal.

Why is the drop in fractalkine such a problem? Simply put, without adequate fractalkine, microglia lose one of their key regulatory signals. This situation leaves them more prone to jumping into high-alert mode.

With less fractalkine available, veterans with chronic stress or PTSX may experience an exaggerated inflammatory response in the brain—one that isn't easily shut off. This can make the mind feel perpetually under siege.

Connecting the Dots to PTSX

PTSX describes flashbacks, hypervigilance, bodily jolts of fear, symptoms that persist after the original danger is gone and sometimes even when memories are hazy. Much like a phantom limb, the brain keeps replaying threat signals in the absence of an external trigger.

The chain of events—beginning with chronic stress and ending in reduced fractalkine—is a key contributor to PTSX. In military contexts, servicemembers are often under constant threat, which keeps cortisol levels high. Even after returning home, the body may continue overproducing cortisol.

Over time, this hormonal imbalance can gradually chip away at fractalkine's protective influence. The result is an internal battlefield where your own microglia turn hyperactive, potentially fueling the intrusive thoughts, flashbacks, and anxiety that define PTSX.

Scientists are now exploring therapies aimed at restoring or mimicking fractalkine signaling. For instance, experimental drugs that boost fractalkine levels or protect its signaling pathways have shown promise in early rodent studies.

In parallel, integrative approaches—anti-inflammatory diets, regular exercise, and stress-reduction techniques—may also help support fractalkine function. These strategies can be especially beneficial for veterans looking for complementary ways to manage chronic stress. Bringing cortisol levels back to a healthier range is often the first step in preserving fractalkine. Some clinicians use selective steroid receptor antagonists—medications that block excess cortisol effects—to help stabilize hormonal fluctuations.

Also recommended are structured activities like yoga or breathwork, which have been linked to calmer HPA axis activity. Whether through medication or lifestyle changes rebalancing cortisol can clear the path for fractalkine to allow microglia to remain protective, not destructive.

Microglial Activation: From M0 to M1

Under healthy conditions, the brain's first-responders, microglia, quietly patrol the brain in what scientists call the M0 (resting) state. Here, they help clear away cellular debris, watch for invading pathogens, and support neurons by releasing growth factors. It's a crucial job: without microglia, our brains would be far more vulnerable to infections and injuries.

However, these watchful protectors can change dramatically when presented with persistent stress signals, trauma-related chemicals, or infections. Repeated surges of cortisol and reduced fractalkine (the protective chemokine) push microglia to enter a pro-inflammatory mode called M1. In this activated state, microglia begin producing more inflammatory substances, including cytokines, free radicals and reactive nitrogen species.

Reinforcing PTSX

Once in M1 mode, microglia can sustain a feedback loop of heightened reactivity. This loop disrupts neuronal communication, leads to an overproduction of toxic substances such as peroxynitrite, and interferes with normal neurotransmitter levels.

For veterans, these internal dynamics can translate into relentless anxiety, intrusive memories, and difficulty sleeping—common hallmarks of PTSX. Even if the original trauma is no longer present, the brain's microglial cells remain "on guard," contributing to an unending sense of alarm.

Consequences of Chronic Activation

Recent research results demonstrate that long-term microglial activation can accelerate oxidative stress and neuronal damage. Microglia produce not only inflammatory chemicals but also free radicals that damage proteins, cell membranes, and even DNA.

In turn, this damage may exacerbate cognitive issues, emotional regulation problems and heightened stress sensitivity, continuing the cycle of PTSX. Fortunately, interventions targeting microglial activation are an emerging area of scientific exploration. Anti-inflammatory compounds like minocycline have shown promise in reducing overactive microglia. Meanwhile, antioxidant therapies and lifestyle strategies like diets rich in polyphenols (from berries, leafy greens and certain teas)—may offer supportive benefits. Stress-management tools, from mindfulness meditation to structured exercise, can also help modulate the signals that keep microglia stuck in M1 mode.

It's crucial to remember that microglia are not the "enemy." When properly balanced, they protect and nourish neurons, essential for overall brain health. Helping microglia revert to an M0 or more neutral state can yield clear benefits: improved mood, sharper thinking, and relief from the relentless stress signals at the heart of PTSX. With this foundation, we turn our attention later to practical strategies aimed at bringing these cells back into harmony.

Gap Junctions in the Brain: Cellular Communication and Trauma

Gap junctions are microscopic bridges between brain cells, formed by connexin proteins (primarily Cx37, Cx40, and Cx43) that enable direct intercellular communication. These molecular channels allow the rapid exchange of ions, ATP, calcium, and signaling molecules between adjacent cells, particularly in the blood-brain barrier's endothelial network.

Under normal conditions, gap junctions orchestrate vascular tone, immune surveillance, and inflammatory control through precise "whispered" cellular conversations. They maintain the blood-brain barrier's integrity, essential for cognitive protection and neurological stability.

Trauma fundamentally disrupts this cellular communication system. Combat stress, abuse, and other severe stressors trigger inflammatory cascades that release TNF-Alpha, IL-1Beta and cortisol while generating oxidative radicals. This molecular assault causes connexin expression to collapse, severing intercellular dialogue and creating hyperpermeability in brain capillaries.

The consequences manifest as brain fog, executive dysfunction, sleep disturbances, and dysautonomia—symptoms reflecting not visible damage but "missing conversations" in cellular architecture. These represent trauma's most insidious effect: the silencing of cellular coordination rather than direct tissue destruction. Emerging treatments include connexin mimetic peptides, resveratrol, quercetin and vagus nerve stimulation. These restore intercellular dialogue and rebuild the fundamental communication networks that trauma has severed, addressing healing at the deepest molecular level.

Oxidative and Nitrosative Stress: Free Radicals and Peroxynitrite

In a healthy body, reactive molecules like free radicals and reactive nitrogen species serve important functions like fighting off pathogens. However, when there's an excess, these molecules can damage cells and tissues, especially in the brain. This phenomenon is known as oxidative and nitrosative stress and is getting increasing attention in studies of chronic stress and trauma.

When microglia remain stuck in their M1, pro-inflammatory state, they produce large amounts of reactive species. One of the most potent is peroxynitrite—created when superoxide meets nitric oxide. Peroxynitrite is highly reactive, meaning it can "steal" electrons from proteins, lipids and DNA, leading to cellular malfunction or cell death.

Neurotransmitters like serotonin, dopamine and GABA rely on precise chemical reactions and healthy neurons for their production and release. Excess free radicals and peroxynitrite can disrupt the enzymes that synthesize these neurotransmitters, thereby reducing their availability. Damaged receptor sites can further limit how effectively these chemical messengers do their job, causing depression and anxiety.

Bridging the Gap to PTSX

The oxidative onslaught in the brain doesn't just cause physical harm. It can fuel the prolonged stress responses at the core of PTSX. Once neurotransmitter levels are low, mood regulation becomes more difficult. Veterans may find themselves in cycles of persistent irritability, difficulty sleeping, and a heightened sense of threat.

Antioxidant Allies: A Ray of Hope

The good news is that the body has natural defenses against oxidative stress, including antioxidants and detoxification enzymes. Even if those defenses get overwhelmed, we can support them through nutritional and medicinal means. Substances like N-acetylcysteine (NAC) have shown promise in helping the brain clear harmful reactive species. A balanced, antioxidant-rich diet—featuring fruits, vegetables and whole grains—can also bolster the body's ability to counteract oxidative damage.

Multifaceted Interventions: Beyond Diet

While diet and supplements are helpful, they represent only one dimension of a broader approach. Interventions aimed at improving sleep, reducing psychological stress, and modulating the HPA axis can collectively lower the generation of free radicals in the first place. In tandem, certain therapies focus on addressing root causes of trauma and helping veterans develop better coping strategies, thereby diminishing the constant stress signals fueling oxidative damage.

Toward a Healthier Brain Environment

Ultimately, reducing oxidative and nitrosative stress involves striking a balance between the immune system's defensive roles and the preservation of healthy neuronal function. Whether through targeted medications, lifestyle changes, or integrative therapies, the goal is to break the cycle of inflammation, high cortisol, and microglial overactivation. By doing so, a more stable neurochemical environment can be reclaimed.

Downstream Effects on Neurotransmission and Receptor Function

Imagine your brain's communication system as a finely tuned orchestra. Each neurotransmitter (serotonin, dopamine, norepinephrine, glutamate and GABA) plays a unique note, weaving together thoughts, emotions,and behaviors. When microglia become overactive and oxidative stress ramps up, this harmonious interplay starts to fall out of sync. As inflammation continues, vital instruments in this orchestra go silent or produce distorted notes, compromising your overall wellbeing.

Serotonin is often linked to mood, emotional stability, and a sense of wellbeing. Under normal conditions, your brain synthesizes serotonin from tryptophan. However, in a high-stress environment filled with free radicals and peroxynitrite, enzymes necessary for serotonin production can be impaired. This decline in serotonin not only dampens your overall sense of calm but may also worsen symptoms like anxiety, irritability, and sleep disturbances—common complaints among veterans with PTSX.

Dopamine is essential for motivation, reward, and the capacity to experience pleasure. When microglia stay locked in their pro-inflammatory M1 state, they release chemicals that can damage dopamine-producing cells and degrade dopamine transport and receptor sites. The result can feel like an inability to enjoy previously rewarding activities, accompanied by a reduction in drive and a sense of disconnection—feelings frequently reported in chronic stress conditions.

Norepinephrine helps regulate attention, alertness, and the body's "fight-or-flight" response. In a balanced stress system, norepinephrine levels rise temporarily during danger but return to baseline once the threat passes.

However, chronic inflammation can interfere with this reset. If your neurotransmitter system is already strained by oxidative stress, norepinephrine might remain at consistently high levels or fluctuate unpredictably. This state contributes to hyperarousal, making it hard to relax or feel safe—even when you're no longer in a combat zone.

The neurotransmitters GABA and glutamate are like the brain's brake and gas pedals, respectively. Glutamate excites neurons, while GABA dampens overactivity to maintain equilibrium. In chronic stress and inflammatory conditions, microglial activation can lead to an excess of glutamate, which is toxic in large amounts.

Meanwhile, the production of GABA might be compromised by oxidative damage to the enzymes responsible for its synthesis. This imbalance can manifest as heightened anxiety, racing thoughts, and an ongoing sense of restlessness.

Receptor Vulnerabilities in an Oxidative Storm

Even if neurotransmitters are present, their effectiveness depends on healthy receptors—specialized proteins on neurons that recognize and respond to each chemical signal. Under conditions of excessive free-radical production, receptors can become oxidized or dysfunctional, resulting in reduced sensitivity.

This oxidative damage can be especially detrimental in areas of the brain related to memory (the hippocampus) and fear responses (the amygdala), and intensifying trauma-related symptoms.

Healing Pathways: Rebuilding the Orchestra

Restoring balance to neurotransmission and receptor function is a key goal for treating PTSX. Antioxidant therapies like supplements containing NAC or diets rich in polyphenols can help reduce oxidative stress, giving neurons and receptors a better chance at recovery.

Meanwhile, regular exercise, healthy sleep, and stress-reduction techniques like mindfulness can further stabilize neurotransmitter levels. In some cases, prescription medications—SSRIs for serotonin, SNRIs for norepinephrine, or atypical antipsychotics for dopamine regulation—may offer additional support.

Reclaiming Harmony

Think of the brain's chemical disruptions as reversible misalignments rather than permanent failures. By targeting the roots of chronic inflammation and oxidative stress, you can help your neural "orchestra" find its rhythm once again. Interventions that combine both biological and psychological therapies aim to reignite the brain's natural capacity for resilience and recovery. In the next sections, we'll explore treatments that integrate these principles, forming a roadmap to restore harmony where PTSX had once held sway.

Therapeutic and Interventional Perspectives

By the time PTSX symptoms take hold, multiple systems—neuroendocrine, immune, and neurotransmitter pathways—are already affected. Thus, treatment often begins by attempting to restore harmony within the HPA axis.

Certain medications like glucocorticoid-receptor antagonists, are being studied for their potential to stabilize cortisol levels. Additionally, integrative approaches like yoga, acupuncture and guided relaxation have shown promise in reducing the body's stress reactivity, giving veterans more control over runaway stress signals.

Preserving and Boosting Fractalkine

Some experimental compounds aim to enhance fractalkine signaling or mimic its protective effects. While these therapies remain in early clinical trials, they represent an innovative approach: rather than merely suppressing inflammation, they seek to restore the body's innate system for balancing brain immune cells.

Modulating Microglial Activation

Shifting microglia from a pro-inflammatory (M1) state to a more protective mode is a central goal of many new interventions. Minocycline, originally an antibiotic, has shown anti-inflammatory properties that may calm overactive microglia.

Other potential therapeutics include certain flavonoids found in fruits and vegetables, which appear to reduce oxidative damage and encourage microglia to perform normal housekeeping tasks instead of inflammatory functions. Oxidative stress, fueled by the buildup of free radicals and peroxynitrite, can be alleviated by a balanced diet and specific supplements. Compounds like NAC, resveratrol, and vitamins C and E are known for their antioxidant properties. For people dealing with PTSX, combining antioxidant support with stress-management techniques may yield better long-term outcomes than either approach alone.

Replenishing Neurotransmitters

When oxidative and nitrosative stress disrupt neurotransmitter production, symptoms such as anxiety, depression, and cognitive difficulties can worsen. To counter this, some treatment plans include precursors like L-tryptophan or 5-HTP to support serotonin synthesis, or use medications that improve dopamine and norepinephrine availability. In parallel, non-pharmacological interventions like structured exercise help encourage the body's natural regeneration of neurotransmitters, supporting a more stable mood and outlook.

Holistic Pathways to Healing

A purely biological approach, while essential, often works best in tandem with counseling, peer support, or trauma-focused therapy. Veterans frequently benefit from comprehensive care that addresses both the chemical changes in the brain and the psychological aftermath of traumatic experiences. Cognitive behavioral therapy tailored for PTSX, eye movement desensitization and reprocessing, and group support sessions can go a long way in helping individuals process and reframe traumatic memories.

Innovation on the Horizon

Finally, emerging fields such as psychedelic-assisted therapy and transcranial magnetic stimulation are gaining attention for their potential to reset and rewire neural circuits. Early results suggests these methods may offer a breakthrough for individuals whose symptoms persist after traditional treatments. These innovative options add to the growing toolbox available for addressing PTSX at its deepest roots.

Crossing the Finish Line

As we wrap up this chapter, it's clear that PTSX isn't merely a "mental" issue but a whole-body phenomenon fueled by neuroendocrine imbalances and chronic inflammation. Elevated cortisol disrupts fractalkine, leading to microglial overactivation.

This unleashes a storm of free radicals and peroxynitrite, ultimately damaging neurotransmitter systems and keeping stress levels on perpetual high alert. For many veterans, these biological drivers make it feel impossible to shake the grip of past traumas.

Despite the complexity, there is real hope. Understanding the interplay between hormones, microglia, and oxidative stress points us toward multifaceted treatments that target the root causes rather than just managing symptoms. By combining medical interventions to stabilize cortisol or antioxidant treatments to reduce free radical damage, veterans can experience noticeable relief. Coupled with therapy and social support, these measures can pave the way for profound, lasting change.

One of the most powerful aspects of this research is how it validates the real experiences of veterans who feel stuck in "fight or flight" mode. The constant sense of threat, the intrusive memories, and the emotional rollercoaster aren't signs of weakness.

They are expressions of a body and brain adapting—albeit maladaptively—to extreme stress. When veterans realize the biological underpinnings of their struggles, it can reduce stigma and open doors to targeted, effective interventions.

Empowerment Through Education

Education remains a cornerstone of any successful approach. Knowing that PTSX has tangible physiological components can empower veterans and civilian patients (and their healthcare providers) to advocate for comprehensive care. That care might involve integrative strategies such as dietary modifications for antioxidant support, stress-reduction exercises or novel treatments targeting microglial activity. By broadening the scope of options, individuals gain a sense of agency: they're not locked into a single treatment path.

Collaborative Healing: Clinicians, Scientists and Veterans

Real progress requires a team effort. Researchers continue to investigate new interventions, building on the latest findings in neuroendocrinology and immunology. Clinicians translate these discoveries into patient care, adapting therapies to the unique challenges of veterans.

Meanwhile, veterans offer invaluable insights into what truly works in day-to-day life. This cycle of shared knowledge and feedback fuels a more compassionate and effective medical landscape.

The Journey Ahead

Silent scars may not fade overnight, but they need not define a life's path. Bold remedies grounded in scientific understanding—ranging from medication to meditation—can guide veterans toward resilience. The human brain is remarkably plastic, capable of healing when given the right tools and support.

Additional Thoughts

PTSX underscores how deeply trauma can seep into our biology, leaving real, measurable footprints in the brain's cellular and chemical landscapes. Yet, the very mechanisms that perpetuate trauma responses also offer opportunities for targeted interventions.

The journey toward healing can be long, but with ongoing research, innovative care, and unwavering resolve.

If-Then Guidance

- If lingering stress symptoms persist long after trauma, then recognize you may be experiencing PTSX and seek integrative assessments that look at hormone levels, inflammatory markers and neurotransmitter function.
- If cortisol levels remain high or fluctuate wildly, fractalkine (CX3CL1) may be reduced, leading to excessive microglial activation, then consult further with medical professionals .
- If microglia become chronically activated (shifting from M0 to M1), then inflammation and harmful compounds like peroxynitrite can proliferate and perpetuate distress, so inquire about emerging anti-inflammatory therapies that calm overactive microglia.
- If oxidative and nitrosative stress from excess free radicals is unchecked, then neurotransmitter production can decline, damaging emotional and cognitive stability, so incorporate antioxidant approaches (dietary or supplemental) and stress-management routines.
- If neurotransmitter balance is impaired, then intrusive thoughts and hyperarousal can intensify, so explore a combination of prescription options and behavioral therapies to restore mood and cognitive function.
- If you want to address the biology rather than just managing symptoms, then learn about restoring fractalkine levels, reducing chronic cortisol, and calming microglia through physician-guided and integrative methods.
- If you feel isolated with "invisible" injuries, know that biological

processes underlie PTSX, so connect with peer-support or professional groups familiar with trauma's biochemical realities.

Take the Next Step

- Evaluate your *HPA axis* with comprehensive hormone testing from a trauma-informed healthcare professional.
- Consider measuring inflammatory markers (such as CRP) if you suspect chronic inflammation, and pursue anti-inflammatory strategies (diet, exercise or targeted therapeutics).
- Adopt an antioxidant-rich diet that includes whole foods and consider supplements like N-acetylcysteine to mitigate oxidative stress.
- Optimize neurotransmitter support by exploring precursors and discussing therapeutic options with clinicians who understand PTSX at the biological level.
- Incorporate trauma-focused psychotherapy (*EMDR* and CBT for PTSX) or group counseling to address the psychological aftermath alongside physiological interventions.
- Remain open to emerging treatments, such as fractalkine-focused research, TMS, or psychedelic-assisted therapy in approved settings.
- Maintain long-term gains by prioritizing healthy sleep, balanced nutrition, regular exercise, and continued monitoring of hormonal and inflammatory markers.

Through Their Eyes

"I remember the day I felt my life was unraveling. My name is James, Lance Corporal, United States Marine Corps. I had returned from my third deployment and couldn't shake the nightmares, the random bouts of rage, and this unrelenting feeling of being trapped in danger—even when sitting safely at home.

"I tried nearly every therapy the Corps offered: group counseling, prolonged exposure therapy, prescription antidepressants, even some experimental trial that involved VR simulations. I'd attend sessions, follow instructions, and pray for relief. But each success was short-lived.

The hypervigilance always returned, a stubborn guest refusing to leave.

"One night, I was so desperate I almost did the unthinkable. My mind was screaming that I had no future—no way out. But just before giving in, I saw a documentary featuring Dr. Mark Gordon. He explained how injuries and trauma can hijack the body at the molecular level, fueling inflammation and messing with the delicate balance of hormones and neurotransmitters.

"Intrigued, I tracked down Dr. Gordon's work online. I learned of his 'Brain Relief 3' regimen, a program designed to reset the neuroendocrine system. I convinced my commanding officer to let me consult with him, even though it meant a few weeks of testing. Blood draws, hormone panels—I did it all. Then came the custom supplements and dietary changes, all geared toward regulating cortisol, bolstering fractalkine signaling, and calming overactive microglia in my brain.

"At first, I was skeptical. It felt like just another trial. But slowly—maybe three or four weeks in—I noticed something shifting. My mind felt clearer in the mornings. My heart wasn't racing as often. When I closed my eyes at night, the images of combat were still there, but they no longer launched me out of bed sweating profusely.

"Over the following weeks, it became easier to focus at work. My fellow Marines noticed I was less on edge. Dr. Gordon's 'Brain Relief 3' regimen was gradually resetting my system, turning off that internal alarm. My mood improved, the dark thoughts dwindled, and I started truly living again. I still have the occasional rough night—recovery isn't magic, and it doesn't happen overnight.

"I share my story because there are countless others in uniform feeling just as lost as I was. If you're reading this and think you've reached the end of the road, trust me, you haven't. There's a real science behind our suffering—and more importantly, there's real hope."

—Lance Corporal James K., US Marine Corps Veteran

54

The Mechanics of the Mind: Cellular Mechanotransduction

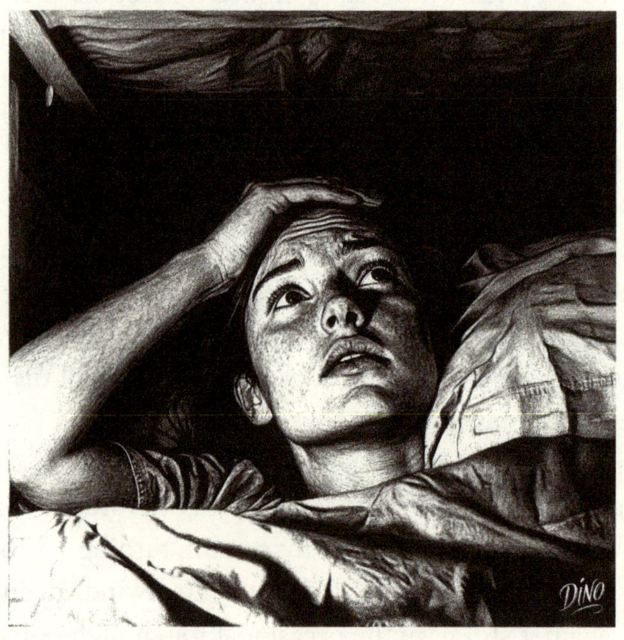

Lena lay awake in her bunk, replaying memories of the roadside blast that had changed everything. She'd been told therapy was the ticket—talk through the trauma, work it out. It helped, but not enough. Then someone mentioned a new angle: the physical mechanics of the brain itself. Something called "mechanotransduction," where tiny parts of cells sense and respond to pressure and tension, igniting cascades of destructive inflammation or the opposite—productive healing.

Yes, it was indeed "all in her head" as some psychiatrists and psychologists told her, but not in some abstract way. It had a true atomic and molecular basis, something very physical that was going wrong. These physical forces led to her behavioral symptoms and manifestations.

At first it sounded too scientific—like an engineer's blueprint, not a path to peace of mind. But the more she read, the more it made sense. The brain wasn't just abstract thoughts and feelings. It was, at a deep molecular level, these subtle fluid shifts and tissue stiffness, each able to trigger a domino effect of stress or repair. The blasts and violent recoil she'd experienced scrambled these signals, leaving behind pockets of constant inflammation that fueled her lingering nightmares.

Lena felt hopeful when she learned about cutting-edge research: scientists targeting specific molecular pathways to reset those wounded mechanics. They spoke of Piezo channels and fluid shear stress, of ways to calm the body's overactive responses, maybe even rewrite the damage done by traumatic brain injury and PTSX.

Neuroinflammation occurs when the brain's immune system gets activated in response to stress, injury or infection. While inflammation can help repair damage in the short term, chronic (long-lasting) neuroinflammation can be harmful. It is a key factor in the development of disorders like TBI and PTSX.

It felt more tangible than simply retracing old memories. It was like diagnosing a broken engine part and learning how to fix it, rather than trying to dampen the loud noise it made. For Lena, it meant another chance at quiet nights and untroubled sleep, fueled by the notion that healing might come as much from the blueprint of our biology as from the stories we tell ourselves.

This chapter explores the intersection of neurobiology, physics, chemistry, molecular biology and mental health. How the push and pull at a subcellular level might clarify why so many veterans endure endless battles in their minds, all the while not knowing that there's another world of tiny mechanical systems at work. And sometimes they are broken and cause untold issues at a higher level like behavior.

If neuroinflammation can be calmed by addressing these deeper mechanics, the mind can finally be healed. Many of these approaches are not yet therapies. They're still in the research stage, and we are learning more and more with each new study. Someday soon, we will be able to heal a damaged brain with highly targeted therapy, including genetic engineering.

The Underlying Mechanics of Traumatic Brain Injury (TBI)

Recent research results increasingly point to mechanotransduction and neuroinflammation as critical factors in understanding the root causes of TBI. This raises a compelling question: could treating neuroinflammation in the brain also lead to healing not only TBI, but also related conditions like PTSX, anxiety and depression?

Ths possibility also shows a profound link between inflammation and a wide range of psychiatric and cognitive disorders, not to mention disorders outside the central nervous system. This chapter does not undermine the insights provided by previous chapters. Instead, it builds on them.

Earlier chapters have been an extensive exploration of the symptoms and effects of TBI and PTSX. Here, we shift focus toward deeper causation, offering new perspectives on the underlying drivers of TBI, PTSX and related brain injuries. By understanding these mechanisms, we open new pathways for potential treatments and therapies that address not only the symptoms but the underlying chemistry and physics of these conditions.

The human brain, much like the rest of the body, operates under a delicate balance of mechanical forces that maintain its function and structure. At the core of this balance is a biological process known as cellular mechanotransduction—the ability of cells to sense mechanical stimuli from their environment and convert them into biochemical and biophysical signals.

This process is critical in various physiological systems, including the brain, where it influences how neurons, glial cells and blood vessels respond to injury, stress and other stimuli.

While mechanotransduction was initially studied in tissues like bone and muscle, it has become evident that this process also plays a pivotal role in the central nervous system. When mechanical forces are altered—whether due to TBI, trauma like PTSX or chronic stress leading to anxiety and depression—cellular mechanotransduction is dysregulated. This dysregulation triggers a cascade of effects, including neuroinflammation, impaired neuroplasticity and metabolic alterations that contribute to the persistence and exacerbation of various issues. By understanding how mechanical cues impact the brain's cellular and molecular processes, researchers can develop new therapeutic strategies to restore function and resilience in individuals with TBI and PTSX.

Hydrostatic Pressure and Brain Function

Hydrostatic pressure (HP), the force exerted by fluids in confined spaces, is an important mechanical cue in the brain. The brain is encased in cerebrospinal fluid (CSF), which helps cushion the delicate neural tissue from injury and maintains fluid balance around neurons.

CSF is also important in collecting and removing various cellular metabolites and toxins from the brain during times of prolonged rest (e.g. sleep). In fact, sleep is one of the most important activities of the day, and allows the body and brain to clear harmful waste products. Under normal conditions, HP regulates key functions like synaptic activity and ion transport across neuronal membranes. However, when HP is elevated, as it often is in TBI, it can cause severe disruptions to neuronal function.

In TBI, mechanical trauma often causes increased intracranial pressure, which can compress brain tissue, disrupt the blood-brain barrier, and alter the conformation of mechanosensitive ion channels such as Piezo1.

These mechanical and subsequent chemical changes initiate a cascade of biochemical signals that culminate in neuroinflammation, characterized by overactive microglia releasing proinflammatory cytokines (e.g., Tumor Necrosis Factor-Alpha IL-1Beta) and dysregulated fractalkine signaling between neurons and microglia. Cytokines impair synaptic function and promote neuronal death, leading to cognitive deficits and emotional disturbances often observed in TBI survivors.

In addition to its role in TBI, abnormal HP can contribute to the development of PTSX, including anxiety and depression. Psychological trauma, particularly when chronic, may lead to increased intracranial pressure through mechanisms like chronic stress-induced neuroinflammation.This sustained increase in HP can activate mechanosensitive pathways that impair synaptic plasticity, the brain's ability to reorganize itself and form new connections. Synaptic plasticity is essential for memory formation and emotional regulation, two functions that are disrupted in PTSX and mood disorders.

Mechanosensitive Ion Channels: Piezo1 and TRPV

Ion channels play a pivotal role in cellular mechanotransduction. Two of the most important mechanosensitive ion channels in the brain are Piezo1 and transient receptor potential vanilloid (TRPV) channels. These channels respond to mechanical stimuli by opening and allowing ions such as calcium (Ca^{2+}) and sodium (Na^{+}) to enter the cell, triggering downstream signaling pathways that influence neuronal activity.

In the context of TBI and psychiatric disorders, Piezo1 and TRPV channels are critical mediators of cellular response to mechanical stress. For example, Piezo1 activation by increased HP or tensile forces leads to calcium influx, which can alter the function of astrocytes (a type of glial cell involved in maintaining the brain's extracellular environment). When astrocytes become activated, they release pro-inflammatory molecules that exacerbate neuroinflammation and contribute to the cognitive and emotional symptoms seen in PTSX.

Similarly, TRPV channels are activated by changes in mechanical forces such as fluid shear stress (FSS) or extracellular matrix (ECM) stiffness. These channels are involved in regulating pain perception and neuroinflammation, both of which are critical factors in the development of mood disorders following trauma.

Targeting these channels with chemical agents could potentially mitigate the effects of mechanical stress on brain function, offering new avenues for treating TBI-related cognitive impairment and PTSX.

Fluid Shear Stress and Vascular Health in the Brain

In the brain, FSS primarily occurs in the cerebrovascular system, where blood flow exerts pressure on the endothelial cells that line blood vessels. This mechanical force is critical for maintaining vascular health, regulating blood-brain barrier (BBB) integrity, and ensuring adequate delivery of oxygen and nutrients to neurons.

In cases of TBI or chronic mental or emotional stress, alterations in FSS can lead to endothelial dysfunction. When FSS is disturbed, endothelial cells activate inflammatory pathways, including the nuclear factor-KappaB (NF-KappaB) pathway, which increases vascular permeability and disrupts the BBB. The breakdown of the BBB allows harmful substances, including inflammatory molecules and immune cells, to enter the brain parenchyma, leading to widespread neuroinflammation. This inflammatory response has been implicated in the development of PTSX, depression and anxiety, as well as the cognitive deficits associated with TBI.

Recent research has shown that mechanotransduction pathways involving FSS play a significant role in regulating the brain's vascular response to injury and stress. For instance, high FSS can promote anti-inflammatory signaling, which protects the brain from ischemic damage and reduces the risk of developing various types of PTSX. However, chronically low FSS, as observed in conditions like cerebrovascular disease or prolonged stress, promotes endothelial dysfunction and neuroinflammation, increasing the likelihood of behavioral correlates like depression and anxiety.

By therapeutically targeting FSS-related mechanotransduction pathways, we may help preserve BBB integrity and reduce inflammation in the brain. For example, pharmacologic agents that enhance endothelial nitric oxide synthase (eNOS) activity—a key mediator of vascular health in response to FSS—could protect against the cognitive and emotional sequelae of TBI and PTSX.

Tensile Force and Axonal Integrity

Tensile force (TF), or stretching force, is another mechanical stimulus that plays a crucial role in the brain. Neurons, particularly axons, are subjected to TF during normal brain activity like head movements or blood flow. However, in TBI, excessive TF can result in axonal injury, a common feature of diffuse brain injuries where axons are stretched or torn due to hyper-mechanical forces. Axonal injury disrupts the transmission of electrical signals among neurons, leading to a range of cognitive and emotional symptoms, including those observed in PTSX. When axons are stretched beyond their physiological limits, mechanosensitive signaling pathways (like the p38 MAPK and ERK1/2 pathways), are activated, triggering neuronal apoptosis (cell death) and promoting neuroinflammation.

While excessive TF is detrimental, moderate levels of TF can promote neuroplasticity, the brain's ability to reorganize itself in response to experience or injury. Mechanical forces can stimulate the release of brain-derived neurotrophic factor (BDNF), a growth factor that supports neuronal survival and synaptic plasticity.

BDNF is essential for recovery from brain injury and for the brain's adaptation to stress and trauma. In conditions like PTSX, in which neuroplasticity is often impaired, targeting TF-related pathways may enhance the brain's ability to recover and adapt.

Integrins, a family of transmembrane receptors that mediate cell-ECM interactions, play a key role in transmitting mechanical signals from the ECM to the cytoskeleton. When activated by TF, integrins trigger downstream signaling cascades like the RhoA/ROCK pathway. This regulates cytoskeletal dynamics and promotes cell survival. By modulating these pathways, researchers hope to improve outcomes for individuals suffering from the long-term effects of TBI and PTSX.

The RhoA/ROCK pathway is a fundamental signaling cascade inside our cells that translates external physical forces into internal biochemical actions. It's a primary way that cells, especially brain cells, respond to their physical environment. The pathway has two main components:

RhoA (Ras homolog gene family, member A): This is a small protein that acts like a molecular switch. When it receives a signal from a receptor on the cell's surface (like the integrins mentioned in your text), it switches to an "on" state.

ROCK (Rho-associated kinase): This is the main "enforcer" protein that RhoA activates when it's switched on. ROCK is a kinase, meaning its job is to activate other proteins by adding a phosphate group to them, which sets off a chain reaction.

The process is a direct chain of command:

Signal Received: A physical force, such as the stretching or shearing from a traumatic brain injury (TBI), is detected by integrin receptors on the cell surface.

Switch Flipped: The integrin receptor activates RhoA, turning its switch "on."

Orders Given: The activated RhoA protein immediately finds and activates its primary target, ROCK.

Action Executed: ROCK then carries out its orders by activating other proteins that directly control the cell's internal skeleton, known as the actin cytoskeleton.

RhoA/ROCK pathway is the master regulator of the cell's physical structure. It primarily controls cell contraction. Think of it as the system that tells a muscle cell to tense up. In brain cells, this "tensing" affects the cell's shape, its connections to other cells, and its ability to move or retract its connections (axons).

The RhoA/ROCK pathway is critical for understanding brain injury because its overactivation is a major source of damage after trauma.

In traumatic brain injury, following a physical impact, the RhoA/ROCK pathway goes into overdrive. This is highly destructive and has been linked to:

Neuronal Death: Excessive and prolonged cell contraction can cause neurons to die.

Failed Neural Repair: It causes the tips of damaged nerve fibers (axons) to collapse and retract, preventing them from reconnecting and healing brain circuits.

Blood-Brain Barrier Damage: It can disrupt the protective barrier around the brain, leading to swelling and inflammation.

In PTSX, while the link is less direct, the same mechanism is relevant. Chronic stress and trauma create maladaptive changes in brain circuits—the fear response gets "stuck." The RhoA/ROCK pathway is a key regulator of this structural plasticity.

An overactive pathway could prevent healthy neural rewiring and reinforce the "stuck" fear circuits, providing a concrete, physical reason why the brain fails to recover.

Extracellular Matrix Stiffness and Mental Health

The ECM is a network of proteins and molecules that provide structural support to tissues, including the brain. In the CNS, the ECM regulates cell migration, differentiation and synaptic plasticity. The mechanical properties of the ECM, particularly its stiffness, play a significant role in determining how cells respond to their environment.

In conditions like TBI, PTSX, anxiety and depression, changes in stiffness of the neuronal extracellular matrix are associated with neuroinflammation and impaired neuroplasticity. Example: mechanical trauma to the brain during TBI can lead to ECM remodeling, where the normal balance of ECM proteins like collagen and elastin is disrupted. This results in increased ECM stiffness, which impairs synaptic plasticity and exacerbates cognitive deficits.

Research has also shown that ECM stiffness plays a role in the development of behavioral disorders. In PTSX and depression, increased ECM stiffness may impair the brain's ability to adapt to new experiences or recover from trauma, leading to persistent symptoms such as emotional dysregulation and cognitive impairment. Targeting these various important pathways, which are activated by changes in ECM stiffness, could provide new therapeutic strategies for promoting synaptic plasticity and improving mental health outcomes.

Neuroinflammation and Mechanotransduction in TBI, PTSX, Anxiety and Depression

While inflammation can help repair damage in the short term, chronic (long-lasting) neuroinflammation can be harmful. It is a key factor in the development of disorders like TBI and PTSX. When the brain experiences physical trauma or psychological stress, certain cells, like microglia and astrocytes, release cytokines that increase inflammation. These molecules disrupt how brain cells function, leading to problems like memory loss, mood swings and difficulty concentrating—common symptoms of these mental-health conditions.

Normally, microglia help keep the brain healthy by cleaning up dead cells and monitoring for infections. However, when the brain is under stress—either from a traumatic injury like TBI or from prolonged psychological stress—microglia become overactive. When this happens, they release pro-inflammatory cytokines, including TNF-alpha, IL-1Beta, and IL-6, which lead to inflammation.

Fractalkine regulates microglia and neuron-glia interactions, and is primarily secreted by neurons. And it can either suppress or activate microglia, depending on the context. This leads to problems with memory, mood and behavior, often seen in PTSX, depression and anxiety. Long-term neuroinflammation has also been linked to neurodegeneration, where brain cells are damaged or lost over time, making it harder for the brain to function properly.

Stress and the Immune System in the Brain

Psychological stress from going through a traumatic experience can also trigger neuroinflammation. Stress has been shown to "prime" the brain's immune system, making it more sensitive to future challenges. For example, if someone experiences a lot of stress and then later gets sick or injured, their brain's immune system might overreact, leading to even more inflammation than normal.

When stress primes the brain's immune system, it can make microglia more reactive. Normally, microglia are in a resting state (M0), but when they are primed by stress, they become more likely to release large amounts of inflammatory molecules when triggered by a secondary challenge (such as an infection or additional stress). This heightened inflammatory response can worsen symptoms of PTSX, anxiety or depression. This process is called "neuroinflammatory priming."

Cytokines and Sickness Behavior

Cytokines—molecules released by microglia—don't just affect brain function. They also trigger something called the "sickness response." This is the body's way of conserving energy so it can focus on fighting infection or healing from injury. When you're sick, you might feel tired, lose interest in activities you usually enjoy, and want to sleep more. These resting behaviors help your body heal.

Interestingly, many of the symptoms of the sickness response are similar to those seen in mood disorders like depression. For example, people with depression often feel tired, lose interest in activities, and experience changes in sleep and appetite—just like in the sickness response. This similarity suggests that inflammation might play a key role in mood disorders. In fact, research has shown that when people are treated with drugs that increase inflammation, they often start to feel symptoms of depression.

Glucocorticoids and Stress-Induced Inflammation

While glucocorticoids (GC) are often thought of as anti-inflammatory, recent research shows that they can sometimes have the opposite effect, especially after prolonged stress. In the brain, GC can prime microglia to become more reactive, increasing the release of pro-inflammatory molecules when triggered by future stressors.

One molecule involved in this process is high mobility group box 1 (HMGB-1), which is released by stressed or damaged cells. HMGB-1 binds to receptors on microglia, activating inflammatory pathways and leading to the release of cytokines like IL-1Beta. This process makes the brain more susceptible to inflammation and the development of psychiatric disorders.

When mechanical forces like HP, FSS and ECM stiffness are altered, they activate pathways that increase inflammation in the brain. Chronic inflammation impairs brain function, contributing to the cognitive and emotional symptoms seen in these conditions.

Understanding how neuroinflammation and mechanotransduction work together opens the door to new treatment possibilities. By targeting the pathways that regulate inflammation, we will be able to reduce the impact of stress and injury on the brain, leading to better outcomes for individuals with psychiatric disorders.

Mechanotransduction and Stem Cell Therapy for Mental Health Disorders

Advances in stem cell research have opened new possibilities for treating psychiatric disorders and brain injuries by harnessing the body's ability to regenerate lost or damaged tissue. Mechanical cues like ECM stiffness and tensile force play a critical role in regulating stem-cell differentiation and migration, making them important targets for stem cell-based therapies.

Recent studies have shown that mechanical stress can modulate stem cell differentiation into cardiovascular cell types, while mechanical forces can improve myocardium regeneration. Moreover, mechanical stretch has been found to promote stem cell migration, offering potential for enhancing recovery following TBI or neurodegenerative conditions.

The relationship between cellular mechanotransduction and stem cells is particularly relevant for regenerative medicine aimed at treating fibrotic diseases. Fibrosis occurs when excess ECM proteins are deposited in tissue, leading to scarring and impaired function. Mechanical cues can drive stem cells toward specific lineages that either exacerbate or mitigate fibrosis. By fine-tuning these mechanical signals, researchers hope to develop therapies that target myofibroblast migration and ECM remodeling, preventing excessive scarring in the brain following trauma.

One promising approach involves the use of adeno-associated virus (AAV)-mediated gene therapy, which has been shown to effectively target specific tissues or organs with minimal immunogenicity. By incorporating designed promoters, AAV can inhibit fibrosis in targeted areas, potentially providing a novel treatment option for fibrotic brain conditions that result from TBI or chronic neuroinflammation.

Mechanosensitive Metabolism and Mental Disorders

Emerging research has also revealed that mechanosensitive metabolism plays a significant role in how cells respond to mechanical cues during migration, differentiation and repair. This metabolic response is particularly important in the context of cancer, where cells dynamically alter their leaders to reduce the thermodynamic costs of invasion.

These findings suggest that cellular mechanotransduction and energy metabolism are intricately linked and have implications for understanding PTSX.

For example, in depression, neuroinflammation and metabolic dysfunction are closely related. The brain's metabolic demands are high, and disruptions in energy metabolism can impair neurotransmitter synthesis and synaptic function. Mechanosensitive pathways may influence how neurons and glial cells adapt to changes in their energy environment, providing insights into how chronic stress and trauma lead to long-term cognitive and emotional deficits.

Conclusions and Perspectives

The role of cellular mechanotransduction in both health and disease is becoming increasingly clear, particularly in the context of mental-health disorders and traumatic brain injury. As we deepen our understanding of the molecular mechanisms by which mechanical cues such as HP, FSS, TF, and ECM stiffness influence brain function, new therapeutic targets are emerging.

Important effectors of mechanotransduction are critical to how the brain responds to mechanical stress and injury. By modulating the signaling pathways associated with these effectors, it may be possible to develop novel treatments for PTSX and cognitive impairments resulting from TBI.

The development of advanced technologies, such as single-cell RNA sequencing, is providing researchers with a more detailed understanding of how different cell types like fibroblasts and stem cells, respond to mechanical cues in specific tissues. This knowledge may lead to precision therapies that target specific cell populations without affecting normal tissue function. For example, targeting myofibroblasts during the wound-healing process could prevent fibrosis without disrupting normal fibroblast activity.

Finally, the use of AAV-mediated gene therapy to modulate mechanical cues in the brain offers a promising avenue for treating fibrotic conditions and other brain disorders. As research continues to explore the intersection of mechanotransduction and neuroinflammation, it is likely that these findings will have broad implications for developing more effective therapies for PTSX and TBI.

By leveraging the insights gained from mechanobiology, we may be able to develop new treatments that not only alleviate symptoms but also promote long-term healing and resilience in individuals affected by trauma and stress.

If-Then Guidance

- If you or someone you know experiences a traumatic brain injury (TBI), then seek early intervention aimed at reducing neuroinflammation, which can help prevent long-term cognitive and emotional deficits. Anti-inflammatory treatments, specific medications, dietary adjustments or lifestyle changes like regular exercise, may reduce the risk of chronic inflammation that contributes to conditions like PTSX, anxiety and depression.
- If you are exposed to chronic psychological stress, then it's important to recognize that this stress can prime your brain's immune system, making it more sensitive to future challenges. Incorporating stress-management techniques like mindfulness, relaxation exercises, or therapy can reduce the likelihood of neuroinflammation and its harmful impact on brain function.
- If you or a loved one suffers from PTSX, anxiety or depression, then explore treatments that target inflammation and the brain's response to mechanical forces may be beneficial. Consult a healthcare provider about anti-inflammatory therapies or treatments that support neuroplasticity: cognitive-behavioral therapy, physical exercise or emerging options like neurofeedback.
- If you are recovering from TBI, then optimizing your body's mechanical and inflammatory responses can aid in healing. Collaborate with your healthcare team to explore options that combine physical rehabilitation (gentle movement and physical therapy) with anti-inflammatory strategies to promote neuroplasticity and reduce long-term damage.
- If you are looking for preventative measures to support brain health, then understanding the role of mechanotransduction can guide your lifestyle choices. Regular exercise, a healthful diet rich in anti-inflammatory foods, and mental-health practices that reduce stress can help maintain brain function and lower the risk of inflammation-driven cognitive decline.
- If you engage in physical activities that carry a risk of head trauma, then taking steps to protect your brain is essential. Wearing proper protective gear and incorporating activities that

enhance resilience, such as balance and coordination exercises, can mitigate mechanical stress on the brain, potentially reducing the chances of inflammation and subsequent brain injuries. The smarter alternative is to avoid these activities altogether.

Take The Next Step

- Take the next step toward deepening your understanding of mechanotransduction and neuroinflammation in the brain by educating yourself on the basic biology of the brain, focusing on how cells respond to mechanical forces and inflammation. This will give you the foundation needed to comprehend more complex processes. Watch the Amazon Prime film *Quiet Explosions*, then contact Dr. Mark Gordon at The Millennium Health Centers to enroll in one of their treatment programs: http://tbimedlegal.com.
- Explore scientific literature and articles that discuss the latest research on brain injuries, stress and mental health. Many studies are now linking these conditions to cellular mechanisms like mechanotransduction, so staying informed will help you connect the dots.
- Consider joining online courses or workshops on neurobiology, neuroscience or related fields. Many educational platforms offer accessible courses on the brain, inflammation and healing mechanisms, giving you a structured learning environment.
- Seek out opportunities to engage with experts or communities focused on mental health, brain injuries or chronic inflammation. Engaging in discussions or attending seminars, whether online or in person, will provide insights from professionals who are actively researching these topics.
- Incorporate the information you learn from your studies into your daily life. Whether it's adopting stress-reduction practices or maintaining a brain-healthy lifestyle, applying what you learn can have a direct positive impact on your cognitive and emotional wellbeing.
- As always, stay curious. Keep asking questions about how the

brain responds to injury and stress. The more you explore, the closer you'll get to understanding the intricate connections between mechanotransduction, neuroinflammation and overall mental health. Remember: the path to healing is a marathon, not a sprint.

Through Their Eyes

"I served as a sniper in the Marine Corps, fighting in some of the most intense battles in Iraq. My days were spent in constant vigilance, scanning for enemies through my scope, and my nights were haunted by the aftermath of the war. But no one prepares you for what happens when the battle is over, when you come home and find that the war inside your mind never stops. After returning to the States, I struggled to adjust. The nightmares were relentless, waking me up in a cold sweat, thinking I was still in the fight. The smallest things would set me off—an argument, a loud noise—and suddenly I was filled with rage.

"I started drinking to numb the pain, but that only made things worse. I became reckless, angry and violent. I was arrested for felony DUIs, and eventually, I lost my family. My wife took the kids and left. I couldn't blame her—I was out of control, spiraling deeper into a darkness I didn't know how to escape. I went through the motions with the VA—therapy sessions, medications, group meetings—but nothing really helped. It felt like the doctors were only treating the symptoms, not the real problem. I was trapped in a cycle of rage, guilt and despair, convinced this was the life I was destined to lead.

"Then one night, after another bout of drinking, I sat down and watched a documentary on Amazon Prime called *Quiet Explosions: Healing the Brain*. It was a moment that changed everything for me. The film was about veterans and athletes who had suffered TBI and were dealing with symptoms just like mine—violent outbursts, memory loss, depression, anxiety. These weren't just guys who'd taken a hard hit on the field or in combat. They were men who were losing their lives, piece by piece, because of the invisible wounds in their brains.

"One of the stars of the film was Dr. Mark Gordon, a pioneer in understanding how brain injuries and trauma lead to neuroinflammation and how that inflammation affects everything from mood to cognitive function. As I watched, something clicked. Dr. Gordon explained that trauma, whether from blasts in combat or repeated concussions, causes some kind of overactive or out-of-control mechanotransduction, a process where the brain's cells are then damaged by mechanical forces. This leads to a state of chronic neuroinflammation—the brain's immune system stays in overdrive, constantly attacking itself. It was like he was describing me exactly and that's when all these lightbulbs exploded in my head. To call it an Aha! moment is an understatement.

"In *Quiet Explosions*, Dr. Gordon showed that these veterans weren't just suffering from psychological issues—they had physical damage in their brains that was treatable. He had developed a method of addressing this inflammation with hormone therapy and supplements to promote brain healing. The stories of patients who had gone through his treatment were incredible. Many of them had been where I was—struggling with anger, depression, substance abuse and broken relationships—and yet, after Dr. Gordon's treatment, they were getting their lives back.

"After the movie ended, I felt something I hadn't felt in a long time: hope. I decided right then that I needed to see Dr. Gordon. I reached out and started the process of working with him, and it changed my life in ways I never thought possible.

"Dr. Gordon didn't treat me like another patient with PTSX. He explained that my brain had been under attack for years, not just from the trauma of war but from the neuroinflammation that followed. He said the root of my violent outbursts, my drinking, and my constant feelings of hopelessness wasn't just psychological—it was biochemical. My brain was stuck in a state of chronic inflammation, and that was affecting everything: my mood, my behavior, my ability to think clearly.

"The treatment plan he put me on was personalized. It wasn't about masking the symptoms. It was about healing the brain at a cellular level. Through a combination of hormone therapy, supplements and a focus on reducing inflammation, I started to notice changes. At first, they were small. Things like sleeping better.

"The constant anger simmering inside me wasn't as intense. Over time, the improvements grew. I wasn't drinking anymore. I felt more in control of my emotions. The nightmares that had plagued me for years began to fade, and for the first time, I could face the memories without drowning in them.

"The more my brain healed, the more I began to heal in other areas of my life. I reached out to my wife, explained the journey I was on, and started the slow process of repairing our relationship. It wasn't easy, but she could see the difference in me. I wasn't the same man who used to fly into rages at the drop of a hat. I was calmer, more focused, more present. I was starting to feel like the person I had been before the war.

"It was the wake-up call I needed. If I hadn't seen that film, I don't know where I'd be today. Dr. Gordon's work gave me a path out of the darkness—a way to understand that the battle wasn't just psychological but biological. Healing the brain isn't just about treating the mind. It's about treating the inflammation that's been causing the mind to suffer in the first place.

"Today, I'm still on that path. The war didn't end when I came home, but with the right treatment, I've learned how to win the battle inside my own head. Thanks to Dr. Gordon and what I learned from *Quiet Explosions*, I've been able to reclaim my life, my family and my future. I'm not just surviving anymore—I'm living. And that's something I never thought possible.

—Gunnery Sergeant Steve D., US Marine Corps (ret.)

55

Traumatic Brain Injury Causes Neuromolecular Dysfunction

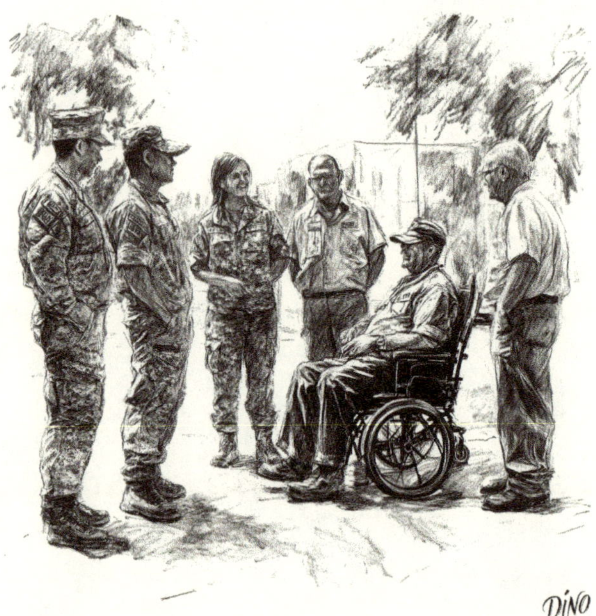

I once flew the US Air Force's F-15E Strike Eagle the way a surgeon wields a scalpel—clean, fast, decisive. Thirty-six combat sorties over Bosnia: bank left, pickle, feel the jet jolt when the bombs release. The roar never frightened me. The silence afterward did. Years later, that silence still follows me into bedrooms and boardrooms, a phantom G-force that yanks my pulse to the redline. They called it PTSD, tossed me a bag of SSRIs, and told me to breathe into a paper sack when the cockpit flashbacks hit. "It's all in your head, Colonel," they said.

This chapter argues otherwise, and I am Exhibit A. Post-traumatic stress injuries—more correctly termed PTSX, Dino Garner's broader and more inclusive name—are chemical ambushes that begin with blast overpressure and end in molecular mutiny. Dr. Mark Gordon's laboratory results show testosterone bottoming out, neurosteroids cratering, cytokines and chemokines spiking. Trauma doesn't just haunt memories. It deranges biophysics, from calcium channel kinetics to mitochondrial ATP yield. Tweak those pathways and the nightmares subside. Ignore them and no amount of talk therapy or medical marijuana can assist.

We have spent decades circling the wrong target, firing counseling and mindfulness flares at symptoms while at least one of the true adversaries—neuroendocrine collapse—flew low under the radar. The future of care is possibly sub-cellular: peptide modulation, gene-edited anti-inflammatories, brain-penetrating hormone precursors calibrated to a patient's physical profile. Dr. Gordon calls it "treating the brain as an organ, not a rumor."

What will it take for the larger medical corps—and Congress, insurers, ivory-tower psychiatrists—to adopt this doctrine? Data, certainly: controlled trials with biomarker endpoints instead of highly subjective self-report scales. Courage, too: a willingness to admit that entire careers were built on an incomplete map. Perhaps it will take more Colonels like me standing up at grand rounds, refusing another psych-med refill until someone draws the labs. Or more families waving coroner reports that list polypharmacy toxicity as the cause of death.

My plea is simple: stop telling us to relax while our cytokines riot. Meet us at the molecular trench line. Give us diagnostics that look beneath the neuron's skin and treatments that recalibrate the circuitry, not just sedate it. I once entrusted my life to the cockpit of a $50M fighter jet at Mach 2. Trusting a prescription should not feel riskier. It's time to file a new flight plan—one plotted in angstroms and millivolts—before another squadron of veterans augers in, unseen by radar that registers only the mind's shadows.

This chapter looks deeper into the molecular basis of TBI. While it doesn't criticize those who still prescribe pills without studying the molecular basis of PTSX, it does suggest focusing more on pure research into deep neuroscience and the true causes of PTSX. To get at the core causes, we must fund research in molecular biology and neuroendocrinology. We also consider another important area of study and treatment: vagus nerve stimulation. It could be that knowing what's going on at the molecular level is highly useful, but "repairing" it may not be the best way to treat PTSX. Still, we offer treatment of neuroendocrine dysfunction as one of the ways to treat PTSX.

Traumatic Brain Injury

TBI has emerged as one of the most pressing healthcare challenges facing US military personnel and veterans, and civilians exposed to repeated trauma, especially in car crashes and contact sports. TBI can lead to both immediate and long-term medical complications like neuroendocrine dysfunction—an often underdiagnosed consequence. It can profoundly shape a person's recovery trajectory and quality of life.

When the body's hormonal regulation systems are disrupted by physical trauma to the brain, a cascade of physiological and psychological symptoms can emerge. It then intertwines with or aggravates PTSX.

TBI in the Military Context

TBI occurs when external forces—such as blasts from improvised explosive devices (IEDs), direct impacts from vehicle accidents, or blunt trauma—jolt or penetrate the brain. Within the US military, particularly among those who have served in overseas deployments (e.g., Iraq, Afghanistan, Syria), TBIs are often associated with explosive devices and high-impact collisions.

From mild concussions to severe penetrating head wounds, these injuries can substantially alter daily functioning and predispose service members to long-term physical challenges. While many forms of TBI present clear immediate effects—loss of consciousness, headaches, blurred vision—some of the injury's most damaging outcomes unfold weeks or months later.

Chronic inflammation and microvascular damage within the brain may disrupt its natural regulatory functions, especially in areas that govern hormone production and distribution. A significant percentage of veterans return home with persistent headaches, sleep disturbances, mood swings and diminished energy, unaware that underlying hormonal imbalances may be exacerbating or even driving their symptoms.

In the civilian population, TBI occurs frequently in people playing contact sports like football and rugby, sometimes leading to chronic traumatic encephalopathy (CTE), which has only been recognized in the past 20 years. This insidious neurodegenerative disease, caused by repetitive head trauma, acts as a silent thief, stealing memories, personality and hope, often decades after the last impact or blast wave.

Primarily associated with contact sports athletes and military veterans, CTE is characterized by a pathological buildup of tau protein in the brain. This protein forms tangles that choke and kill nerve cells, which is different from the plaque and tangle patterns seen in other neurodegenerative diseases like Alzheimer's. Overall, it leads to a decline in neuronal and behavioral function.

The symptoms are an inventory of human suffering: memory loss, profound depression, emotional instability, and impaired judgment that often lead to suicide. CTE leaves families to witness the slow erasure of the person they once knew.

The Neuroendocrine Nexus: Hypothalamus and Pituitary

To understand how TBI produces profound hormonal disturbances, one must look at the "control centers" of the endocrine system: the hypothalamus and pituitary gland. Sitting at the base of the skull, these interconnected structures orchestrate a vast hormonal network that influences metabolism, stress responses, growth, reproduction, and more.

The Hypothalamus

Frequently described as the brain's command post for hormonal regulation, it synthesizes releasing and inhibiting hormones. These substances travel short distances to the adjacent pituitary gland, telling it when to secrete specific hormones into the bloodstream.

The Pituitary Gland

In the context of military TBIs, the hypothalamus and pituitary can be compromised by blast waves, concussive forces, or mechanical impact. The brain's movement inside the skull can stretch, tear, or inflame the delicate pituitary stalk and its vital blood supply.

The result may be hypopituitarism—partial or complete failure of the pituitary to secrete one or more hormones—manifesting in physical and psychological difficulties that can remain hidden beneath other symptoms of TBI or be mistaken for typical post-deployment adjustment challenges.

Mechanisms of Injury: From Blast Forces to Vascular Shear

For US servicemembers deployed in conflict zones, one of the most common sources of TBI is the shockwave emitted by explosive devices. Such a blast wave has considerable kinetic energy to rattle the skull and brain tissues, creating cavitation effects that damage neurons and blood vessels.

Even if a helmet prevents penetrating trauma, the internal movement of the brain can still cause microscopic or subclinical damage to the hypothalamic-pituitary region. Additionally, motor vehicle accidents, helicopter crashes, or training accidents can involve sudden deceleration that exerts similar shearing forces and rotational-acceleration effects.

Following the initial injury, secondary processes such as inflammation and oxidative stress can exacerbate tissue damage. Proinflammatory cytokines and reactive free radicals may harm neurons in the hypothalamic-pituitary region, compounding structural injury with biochemical insult. Small hemorrhages or reduced blood flow in pituitary vessels can set the stage for hormonal deficiencies that might not appear until months or years after the service member's return from deployment.

Recognizing Hormonal Dysfunction in Combat Veterans

In many military and veteran healthcare settings, the focus understandably begins with acute stabilization of wounds and the management of visible functional impairments. However, endocrine issues may be overlooked because their symptoms are often nonspecific—fatigue, weight gain or loss, anxiety, mood instability and poor exercise tolerance.

When layered atop other concerns—post-traumatic stress, chronic pain, sleep problems—these "invisible" complaints can be mistakenly attributed to psychological factors alone.

Key hormonal imbalances seen in TBI-affected veterans include:

Growth Hormone Deficiency: Lethargy, reduced muscle mass, and decreased exercise endurance can occur, accompanied by concentration and memory issues.

Cortisol Dysregulation: This may manifest as constant hyperarousal (elevated cortisol) or chronic fatigue (if cortisol is deficient).

Testosterone or Estrogen Deficiency: In male veterans, low testosterone frequently presents as low libido, weakened physical performance, and even depressive symptoms, while female veterans may notice irregular menstrual cycles or heightened emotional volatility if estrogen or progesterone levels are affected.

Hypothyroidism: This can cause depression-like symptoms—sluggishness, weight changes, and difficulty in regulating body temperature.

For a soldier accustomed to pushing through discomfort, detecting and reporting such symptoms requires considerable awareness and trust in the healthcare system. If these imbalances remain unaddressed, they can magnify the challenges veterans face when readjusting to civilian life or returning to active duty.

Neuroendocrine Dysfunction and Other Symptoms

Combat-related TBI and post-traumatic stress can share overlapping features—hypervigilance, nightmares, irritability and memory lapses. The HPA axis, which modulates cortisol release, is often at the heart of stress-related symptoms.

When a service member encounters life-threatening situations, the HPA axis gears the body for fight-or-flight responses. Under normal conditions, cortisol levels recede once the threat subsides. However, TBI can disrupt this regulatory system, leaving cortisol high or unpredictable long after the combat experience. Alternatively, the system may fail to produce adequate cortisol at all, blunting the individual's ability to handle normal stressors.

Research from veteran-focused studies underscores that dysregulated cortisol not only intensifies anxiety and insomnia but also may worsen depression, cognitive fog, and emotional reactivity. For those with

TBI, these issues are further complicated by the potential for other hormonal deficits or surpluses, forming a complex web of symptoms that resembles or amplifies PTSX. This complexity is why a combination of trauma-focused therapy and thorough endocrine evaluation can be transformative for veterans.

Growth Hormone and the Journey to Recovery

Among the many hormones vulnerable to TBI, growth hormone (GH) stands out for its multifaceted role in tissue repair, metabolism, and brain function. Combat-exposed personnel with moderate-to-severe TBI have relatively high rates of GH deficiency, which can hamper physical rehabilitation and cognitive recovery. Some endocrinologists who treat veterans advocate for GH testing in those who have persistent fatigue, muscle weakness, and a slowed healing process—even if their TBI is classified as "mild."

In controlled settings, GH replacement therapy (for those demonstrably deficient) may boost exercise capacity, muscle tone, and some aspects of cognitive performance. Veterans who undergo GH replacement under a physician's supervision sometimes report a return of energy and improved mood, which can be crucial for engaging in physical therapy, vocational training, or a return-to-duty plan.

However, this type of intervention requires careful assessment, ongoing monitoring, and collaboration among medical professionals, as excessive GH or misuse of hormone treatments can introduce other risks.

Diagnosing TBI-Related Neuroendocrine Dysfunction

Timely, accurate diagnosis is a cornerstone of effective care. Military hospitals and the Department of Veterans Affairs (VA) healthcare system frequently employ standardized screening tools for TBI. Yet endocrine testing is not always routinely included unless there is a high index of suspicion or overt clinical signs. Key elements of a comprehensive diagnostic pathway include:

<u>Detailed History</u>: Clinicians must inquire about the nature of the injury—blast exposure, motor vehicle accidents, falls, or repeated

concussions. It is also vital to track the timeline of symptom development, considering the possibility of delayed hormonal deficiencies.

Physical Examination: This may reveal changes in body composition, hair distribution, blood pressure variability, or other subtle signs of pituitary dysfunction.

Targeted Lab Tests: These can measure morning cortisol, ACTH, thyroid function, gonadal hormones (testosterone or estrogen), and IGF-1 (a marker related to GH production). For borderline results, stimulation tests (like the ACTH stimulation test or growth hormone stimulation tests) can clarify whether a true deficiency is present.

Neuroimaging: MRI scans can identify structural lesions, hemorrhages, or scarring in the hypothalamic-pituitary region. Even so, some microvascular injuries or diffuse axonal damage may not be overt on routine scans.

Given the complexities of military service, an interdisciplinary team approach—combining neurology, endocrinology, mental health and rehabilitation—is often the gold standard.

Integrative Treatment Approaches

Once neuroendocrine dysfunction is confirmed in a combat-exposed veteran, addressing it can yield substantial benefits. However, effective treatment often goes beyond hormone replacement alone. Recommended strategies include:

Hormone Replacement Therapies: Depending on which hormones are deficient, a tailored regimen (e.g., hydrocortisone for adrenal insufficiency, levothyroxine for hypothyroidism, testosterone for male hypogonadism, or recombinant human growth hormone) can stabilize physical and cognitive symptoms.

Stress Reduction and Resilience Training: Yoga, mindfulness-based stress reduction, and breathing techniques can help modulate the stress response at both the psychological and physiological level.

Physical Rehabilitation: Structured exercise programs developed by military-focused physical therapists can help rebuild strength and endurance, which is particularly important if GH or testosterone levels have been low.

Nutrition and Anti-Inflammatory Interventions: A diet rich in whole foods, lean proteins, and antioxidants supports tissue recovery and may mitigate neuroinflammation. Some veterans also benefit from supplements (e.g., omega-3 fatty acids) to enhance neuronal function.

Trauma-Focused Psychotherapy: Cognitive behavioral therapy for PTSX, eye movement desensitization and reprocessing, or group counseling create a framework for processing combat experiences while also addressing the real, physiological aspects of TBI and hormone dysregulation.

Ongoing Monitoring: Hormone levels can shift over time, so regular check-ins with an endocrinologist ensure that therapies remain effective.

By weaving together these various interconnected components, the path to recovery can become more robust and sustainable.

Future Directions and Ongoing Research

Within the broader veteran healthcare community, recognition of TBI-induced neuroendocrine dysfunction continues to grow. Research funded by the Department of Defense and VA is pushing toward more advanced diagnostic tools—such as diffusion tensor imaging and high-resolution MRI—to detect subtle pituitary and hypothalamic changes.

Concurrently, studies examining novel therapies (including anti-inflammatory medications, advanced hormone analogs, and integrative brain-health strategies) aim to improve both acute and long-term outcomes for service members.

A very promising area of study involves the vagus nerve and its actions in PTSX. While we're considering these other promising areas of study and treatment, we still must ask the question: can we possibly treat PTSX and TBI by manipulating the vagus nerve via electrical stimulation? We consider this possibility in the final chapter, "The Vagus Nerve and the Molecular Nature of Neuroinflammation."

Final Thoughts

For US servicemembers, especially those exposed to the harsh realities of combat, traumatic brain injury can represent just the first battle in a prolonged war for overall health and wellbeing. Beyond the overt signs of head trauma, TBI can stealthily undermine endocrine pathways critical for stress regulation, mood stability, energy levels and physical resilience.

As we learn more about these hormonal underpinnings, the importance of comprehensive assessments that include endocrine testing in TBI management becomes ever clearer.

Neuroendocrine dysfunction, often masked by other post-deployment issues, can stall or complicate the recovery process if left unrecognized. When addressed, however, it can open doors to more effective treatments for persistent fatigue, cognitive deficits, depression, anxiety and other maladies plaguing our combat veterans.

Whether a Marine recovering from a roadside bomb in Fallujah or an Air Force servicemember injured in a helicopter crash, identifying and treating TBI-related endocrine damage can be pivotal to restoring not only physical capacity but also hope and direction for the future. For the dedicated men and women who serve in uniform, acknowledging and confronting neuroendocrine dysfunction is a crucial step in transforming silent scars into a pathway for healing.

If-Then Guidance

- If TBI is sustained during combat or training, then consider the possibility of hormonal imbalances that may not appear immediately.
- If headaches, blurred vision or mood swings persist long after the initial injury, then look beyond visible wounds and explore potential endocrine dysfunction.
- If ongoing fatigue, reduced exercise tolerance or lowered libido emerge post-deployment, then investigate deficiencies in growth hormone, testosterone, or other critical hormones.
- If signs of hyperarousal or exhaustion repeatedly appear, then address the possibility of cortisol dysregulation rather than assuming it's just psychological stress.
- If memory lapses, irritability or recurrent anxiety overlap with TBI history, then pursue both trauma-focused therapy and endocrine evaluations.
- If you experience delayed or subtle changes in mood and physical

stamina after returning from service, then request specialized testing for pituitary and hypothalamic function.

- If TBI symptoms complicate your reentry into civilian life or return to active duty, then seek medical professionals who understand neuroendocrine issues, especially in veterans. Dr. Mark Gordon at Millennium Health is an excellent starting point.

Take the Next Step

- Initiate a thorough endocrine assessment if you suspect lingering TBI complications.
- Collaborate with an interdisciplinary team of neurology, endocrinology, and mental-health experts who specialize in military-related injuries.
- Stay alert to hormonal deficiency symptoms and share all relevant concerns with your healthcare provider.
- Incorporate stress-reduction methods like mindfulness or structured breathing exercises, to support your healing process.
- Adopt a balanced, anti-inflammatory diet alongside targeted supplements if recommended by your care team.
- Explore trauma-focused psychotherapy options (for example, EMDR or CBT for PTSX) alongside medical treatment.
- Arrange regular follow-up appointments to ensure any treatment plan remains appropriate and effective.

Through Their Eyes

"I'm Major Joe, United States Air Force fighter pilot, retired. Back in 1991, I was a young fighter pilot flying sorties over the Gulf. Missile alarms and MASTER CAUTIONs were my constant companion. Each time the cockpit blared a launch warning, I'd crank the Viper into evasive maneuvers, snapping my head and neck against the seat. It was the price of survival. I never thought those violent jolts would leave lasting damage, but apparently war's effects don't stop just because you land safely.

"I managed to push through another few years of service before the headaches, dizziness and mood swings got the best of me. I blamed the stress of the job at first. Then it was getting older, or so I told myself. Eventually, I was medically retired, and I learned I'd been fighting something more than just whiplash—traumatic brain injuries that had rattled my pituitary gland. That discovery felt both terrifying and oddly liberating: finally, an explanation for the unexplainable fatigue and unpredictable crashes in my energy.

"These days, I'm on a careful regimen that addresses my hormone imbalances. I also see a therapist to manage my flashbacks. It's a combined approach, and I want every veteran out there to know that there's no shame in seeking help. TBI might be invisible, but the right treatments can bring real relief.

Whether you're dealing with PTSX, persistent headaches, or unexplained exhaustion, don't wait. Ask your doctor to run those extra tests. It took me years to do that, and it made all the difference. We served our country. Now we've got to serve ourselves by getting the care we deserve. I'm living proof that even after the darkest chapters, there's a path forward toward healing and renewed purpose."

—Major Joe, US Air Force (ret.)

56

Rearming Mental Healthcare with Molecular and Biophysical Precision

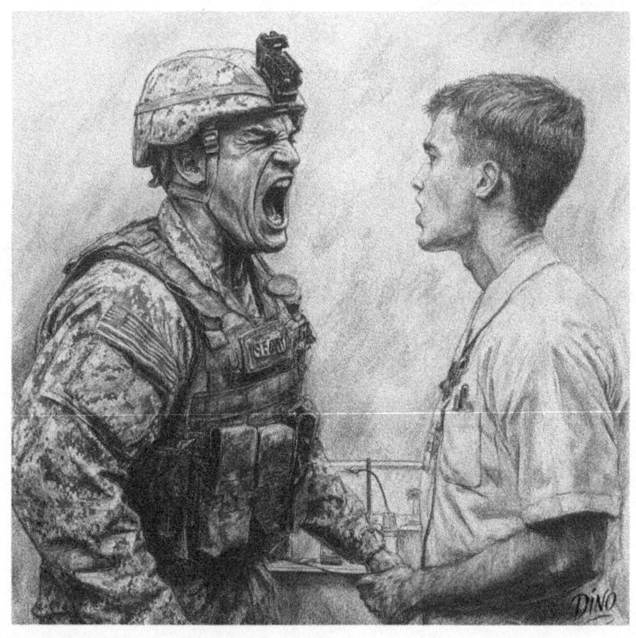

Without ceremony, they threw me out of the clinic the way we toss a flashbang—fast, loud, "don't come back," then they slammed the door. I'm a retired SEAL with twenty-three years, four continents, and more breaching charges than birthdays behind me, and I lost it when the white-coat across the desk handed me a prescription slip before touching a stethoscope, let alone a microscope or centrifuge.

"Selective serotonin reuptake inhibitor," he said, like he was giving away a free patch and paper American flag from the MWR shop.

Man, I was so pissed at this guy, the whole messed-up system that was supposed to take care of us warriors. No blood draw. No hormone panel.

No inflammatory markers. Just pills—again. Even I, with a high school education, knew that PTSX wasn't just some abstract thing inside my mind. Even I knew it had roots right down to my DNA, and it would take a lot more than some head-shrinker to heal my broken brain.

I closed my eyes for a sec, took a deep breath, and imagined I was in full combat uniform, reared my head back, then unleashed a roar right into his smug face. The blast sent him crashing into his chair, then he ran out. Security marched me into the parking lot like I was some detainee I'd interrogated on several missions.

Americans take psychiatric meds the way our Army brothers, the Rangers, downed "Ranger Candy," 800-milligram ibuprofen that did nothing but hide the ache while the march went on. The CDC brags—yes, brags—that 11.4 percent of adults, about 30 million souls, held an antidepressant script as of 2023.

Women carry the load at twice the men's rate. Four in ten citizens over sixty-five juggle five or more bottles a day. Polypharmacy, they call it, like it's a postgraduate degree. Medicaid kids? They're stacking two, three, four psychotropics before they can drive. This, in the self-proclaimed "Country of Bottles and User-Friendly AI."

And that AI? ChatGPT, Claude, Gemini—digital bartenders serving synthetic sympathy to millions who can't find a human ear. The companies crow about "engagement." I see a nation medicated, anxious, lonely, desperate enough to spill secrets to a server rack because it writes prescritions faster than any VA clinic. Suicide curves up. Night terrors still stalk the hall. The pills aren't fixing it. The chatbots sure as hell won't, but they make the statistics at those AI companies look awesome.

I asked the doc for a molecular work-up: neurosteroids, cytokine storm profiles, a full endocrine spread. IED overpressure, breacher's shakes—Dr. Mark Gordon's labs show blast waves slash neurochemistry like shrapnel cuts flesh. Look at glial scarring, mitochondrial choke. Show me the data, then maybe we'll talk about compounds.

So now I sit in my truck, fists still trembling as if a charge is about to blow, and write affidavits for brothers who can't spell half the medicines they swallow. They call at 0200 because the tinnitus won't quit or the dreams turn kinetic. I explain how trauma rewires calcium channels, how cortisol surges wipe out hippocampal circuits, how the fix is chemistry tested, not guessed. I email sixty pages to the VA, line every claim with peer-review citations, and pray some adjudicator sees the sense.

What I want—what we all need—is a reckoning. Stop treating wounded brains like squeaky hinges you drown in WD-40. Draw the blood, run the PET scans, map the endocrine crash. Don't hand a veteran a digital friend and a Zoloft starter pack and call it care.

Until then, I'll keep shouting, clinic or no clinic. Better they escort one furious old frogman to the curb than keep escorting caskets off the tarmac because no one bothered to read the molecules before they wrote the meds.

This chapter seeks to rearm mental healthcare with the molecular tools needed to study, do good research and then treat veterans and civilians for PTSX and all its symptoms. Here we detail all the current scientific disciplines required to do accurate work and diagnose and treat those suffering from PTSX. Using all tools, from neurochemistry to computational neuroscience and bioinformatics, we delve into the underlying nature of post-traumatic stress injuries and how each discipline is or should be used to study and treat all things PTSX.

The Field Guide That Swallowed the Pharmacy

The Diagnostic and Statistical Manual of Mental Disorders—the *DSM*—began life as a wartime triage chart, a quick-reference card for doctors short on time and long on shell-shocked soldiers. Its architects intended it to supply common names, nothing more, so scattered clinicians could speak the same language while they searched for underlying causes.

Since then the booklet has swelled into civic scripture. Insurers deny payment without its codes, and drug reps arrive with color-matched vials for every line item. Even stalwart defenders concede it is "a loose net that catches the worried well" and fattens quarterly sales. What was once a sorting tool has become a blanket license to medicate—breeding a legion of practitioners who reach for the prescription pad before they reach for the laboratory bench.

The Map of Truth: Scientific Disciplines Required for Accurate Diagnoses

If we wish to treat the brain, we need a diagnostic frame built on molecules, circuits and reliable metrics. That frame is wide. It must rest on many beams:

Neurochemistry

Why It Matters: Abnormal fluctuations in neurotransmitters (e.g., glutamate, GABA, dopamine, serotonin) can drive or exacerbate hyperarousal, intrusive memories, and mood dysregulation characteristic of PTSX.

Research Applications: Real-time microdialysis and fast-scan cyclic voltammetry help identify acute vs. chronic chemical changes that may mark transitions from acute stress responses to persistent trauma-related states.

Therapeutic Implications: By pinpointing the spatiotemporal profiles of these neurochemicals, clinicians can optimize timing and dosing of pharmacotherapies (e.g., SSRIs, NMDA receptor modulators). This precision improves outcomes over static, one-size-fits-all protocols.

Molecular Neurobiology

Why It Matters: Trauma can trigger gene expression shifts that alter synaptic plasticity. Epigenetic modifications can lock in or perpetuate maladaptive stress responses.

Research Applications: Studying RNA editing and alternative splicing helps us see how a single gene can produce multiple isoforms influencing neuronal responsiveness to stress. Single-cell multi-omics can reveal distinct cell populations particularly vulnerable to traumatic insult.

Therapeutic Implications: Identifying precisely which gene networks become dysregulated after trauma may lead to targeted interventions—e.g., small molecules or biologics that correct faulty protein–protein or protein–RNA interactions implicated in prolonged stress states.

Biophysics

Why It Matters: The behavior of ion channels, membrane potentials, and sub-membrane domains can shift in the wake of traumatic stress, changing how neurons fire or become sensitized to stimuli.

Research Applications: Combining true intracellular recording with molecular-dynamics simulations can reveal subtle changes in channel conductance after repeated stress or injury. Understanding these at an Ångström-to-millisecond scale is essential for designing drugs that precisely modulate channel activity.

> "So I speak to anyone who will lend an ear: do not let a DSM and a fast pen decide your fate. Demand the scans, the bloodwork, the molecular truth. We would never send a sailor into a hot zone without a map. Your brain deserves the same reconnaissance."

Therapeutic Implications: Many of the medications used for trauma-related disorders target ion channels or receptor conformations (e.g., calcium-channel blockers for hyperarousal, NMDA modulators for dissociative symptoms). Refining these compounds through biophysical insights can yield therapies with fewer side effects and greater efficacy.

Neurophysiology

Why It Matters: The patterns and rhythms of neuronal firing underlie core symptoms—hypervigilance or disrupted sleep—common in PTSX.

Research Applications: Techniques like two-photon calcium imaging and magnetoencephalography (MEG) enable researchers to visualize and quantify how neural circuits respond to stress or re-exposure to trauma cues. Optogenetic tagging can test whether specific circuit nodes are causally involved in the generation of anxiety or flashbacks.

Therapeutic Implications: Neurophysiological data guide interventions such as transcranial magnetic stimulation (TMS) or deep brain stimulation (DBS). These modalities restore normal firing patterns or disrupt pathological synchrony that perpetuate trauma symptoms.

Neurogenomics & Epigenetics

Why It Matters: Individual genetic and epigenetic profiles modulate susceptibility to, or resilience against, traumatic stress. Changes in 3D genome architecture may cause long-term shifts in gene expression tied to PTSX-like syndromes.

Research Applications: Hi-C assays reveal how chromatin loops reorganize under stress, potentially "tuning up" proinflammatory genes or "silencing" neuroprotective pathways. Cut&Run can pinpoint the exact locations where transcription factors (proteins that control gene activity) bind to DNA in response to high cortisol or cytokine exposure.

Therapeutic Implications: Since trauma physically rewires how our genes work, targeted drugs (like HDAC inhibitors) could potentially reset those genes back to a healthier state. We can also use large-scale genome-wide association studies (GWAS) to identify specific genetic variants that predict who is most at risk for PTSX.

Neuroimmunology

Why It Matters: Inflammatory processes are increasingly recognized in prolonged stress and trauma responses. Excessive or dysregulated inflammation can exacerbate neuronal damage and promote persistent stress circuitry activation.

Research Applications: Studies focus on how peripheral immune factors (gut microbiome metabolites, circulating cytokines and chemokines) cross the blood–brain barrier or signal through the vagus nerve, priming microglia to adopt proinflammatory phenotypes.

Therapeutic Implications: Anti-inflammatory agents (e.g., IL-1 or IL-6 blockers) and interventions that modulate the gut–brain axis (e.g., probiotics, vagal nerve stimulation) may help manage or even prevent long-term sequelae of traumatic stress. Integrating T- and B-lymphocyte activity in trauma care could illuminate immune-mediated mechanisms of chronic stress syndromes.

Neuroendocrinology

Why It Matters: Hormonal dysregulation—beyond cortisol—impacts emotional reactivity, fear, memory consolidation, and recovery from stress. Agents like allopregnanolone or oxytocin can modulate threat processing.

Research Applications: Investigating circadian patterns in hormone release (cortisol awakening response, pulsatile oxytocin secretion) can help pinpoint when an individual is most vulnerable or most amenable to therapy.

Therapeutic Implications: Chrono-endocrine insights guide interventions like timed medication administration or bright-light therapy to realign circadian rhythms. Hormone-based therapies (e.g., progesterone analogs) may help stabilize mood and stress reactivity in PTSX.

Pharmacogenomics

Why It Matters: Individuals with certain genetic backgrounds (e.g., specific CYP450 polymorphisms) may metabolize psychiatric medications differently, affecting drug efficacy and side effects.

Research Applications: Complex polygenic risk scores and pharmacometabonomics help predict how an individual might respond to SSRIs, benzodiazepines, or newer interventions. This enables fine-tuned therapy that accounts for both genetic and environmental factors.

Therapeutic Implications: Personalized medicine strategies could reduce trial-and-error prescribing. Patients with high-risk genotypes for adverse effects might receive alternative treatments earlier, leading to faster, more sustained remission of trauma-related symptoms.

Connectomics & Systems Neuroscience

Why It Matters: Trauma can alter large-scale brain networks, from structural connectivity (e.g., reduced white-matter integrity in the uncinate fasciculus) to functional network dynamics (heightened amygdala–prefrontal coupling).

Research Applications: Mesoscale connectomics dissects how particular neuron types communicate across brain regions important for memory, fear response, and emotional regulation. Graph-theoretic analyses of functional MRI data help visualize how network "hubs" become hyper- or hypo-connected post-trauma.

Therapeutic Implications: Network-level insights can guide neuromodulatory therapies. For instance, real-time functional MRI neurofeedback might teach patients to regulate overactive threat circuits. Understanding systems-level disruptions also aids the design of targeted cognitive therapies that restore normal oscillatory synchrony.

AI Computational Neuroscience & Bioinformatics

Why It Matters: PTSX research generates massive datasets (e.g. imaging, genomics, wearables). Extracting meaningful patterns via AI apps requires advanced computational approaches that can identify causal pathways rather than mere correlations.

Research Applications: Bayesian inference and deep generative models can integrate multi-omics with clinical phenotypes to predict resilience vs. persistent stress. Causal discovery algorithms test potential pathways for how a molecular change triggers circuit alterations and, ultimately, behavioral outcomes.

Therapeutic Implications: Explainable AI can help clinicians tailor interventions based on individual data patterns. Avoiding "black-box" models ensures results can be translated into actionable strategies, improving engagement and trust in precision mental health solutions for trauma survivors.

Clinical Pharmacology & Trial Design

Why It Matters: Traditional clinical trials might overlook key subgroups or biomarkers indicative of who responds best to a given treatment. Adaptive designs can optimize interventions faster and more effectively.

Research Applications: By grouping trial participants based on their biology (using PET scans), researchers can prove who a drug truly benefits and confirm how it is physically changing the brain. Data from wearables, like smartwatches, can then validate if these improvements actually hold up in the real world.

Therapeutic Implications: More agile, data-driven trials shorten the development pipeline for new PTSX interventions, from repurposed drugs to novel molecular entities. Personalized dosing schedules can be established by integrating dynamic monitoring (heart rate variability, sleep patterns) to adjust therapy in real time.

Overall Significance for PTSX

Bringing these disciplines together creates a multi-layered view—from molecular switches to large-scale networks—of how traumatic experiences can encode lasting physiological and psychological changes. By leveraging the tools and insights from each field, researchers and clinicians can develop precision strategies to prevent, diagnose and treat PTSX more effectively.

Further Observations

Integration over Isolation – Each discipline samples a different axis of the same system. No single axis is sufficient. Precision diagnosing demands multimodal pipelines in which neurochemistry informs molecular neurobiology, which feeds biophysical models tested in vivo by neurophysiology, and so on.

Temporal Resolution – Many definitions imply static measurement. Disease processes like PTSX unfold over minutes (catecholamine bursts), hours (gene transcription), and years (circuit re-wiring). Diagnostic platforms must capture trajectory, not snapshots.

Translational Loop – Clinical pharmacology should not sit at the terminus. Insights must loop back to refine mechanistic understanding, driving iterative biomarker validation.

Skill-Set Implications – A diagnostician competent across these domains must command statistics, benchwork, *in vivo* physiology, and regulatory science—an expertise profile rare in current training pathways. Universities and residency programs must therefore re-engineer curricula toward integrated neuroscientist-clinicians. An accurate diagnosis of any

CNS injury demands proficiency across these frontiers, not a weekend seminar or continuing-education short course for credit.

Changes Are Coming

History shows that guilds like the American Psychiatric Association, American Psychological Association and the American Medical Association yield only when pressed from outside. They all have had decades to write the rules and lobby Congress to make laws to enforce those rules. The average psychiatrist receives no bench training in proteomics, few hours in electrophysiology, and scant drills in coding neural data.

Most clinical psychologists see even less. They learn the *DSM*, the psychometric tests and the liability forms—and then step into clinics where pharmaceutical algorithms whisper that every riddle has a chemical key. The gap between clinic and lab continues to widen. In it grow polypharmacy, side-effects and despair.

And an epidemic of suicide, especially among veterans and active-duty personnel, continues unabated. It's time for a change: the current adminstrators must yield to a new way of doing things, using proven molecular tools that treat more than just symptoms. A sea change is coming, as more and more ordinary veterans and citizens demand better and smarter healthcare.

Veterans: On the Front Lines

No group feels that gap more than the men and women who returned from war with invisible wounds. Congress, alarmed by rising veteran suicides, has ordered studies into whether overmedication inside the Department of Veterans Affairs feeds the death count.

A recent report profiles a Marine who left the Corps with six prescriptions and no clear plan. He dropped them one by one and lived, then began to study the system that almost killed him. Veterans know firefights. They can smell friendly fire, even when it comes in capsule form—from the very institution that promised to care for them and their loved ones.

Toward Precision Molecular Diagnosing

Research is moving—but very slowly. Precision-diagnosing trials now weave genomics, proteomics, imaging and environment to predict which agent fits which patient. The VA is spending $40 million in research on esketamine for treatment-resistant depression, even without biomarker detection. Critics argue that more rigorous biomarker-based approaches would accelerate progress and ensure funding is used as efficiently as possible.

Reviewers in 2024 call the biomarker field for major depression "hampered" and lament the absence of any test a family doctor could order. So far, many tests exist only in the laboratory, and are slow to be used routinely in hospital and clinic settings.

While poetic, "the science is young, the need is old, and the clinic writes scripts while it waits" this passage is also heartbreaking. It underscores how organizations get entrenched in old ways of doing things, dismissing new ideas, while those with PTSX continue to suffer.

PTSX: A Case Study in the Need for Depth

The new term PTSX, while more inclusive than PTSD, is still too general and fails to demonstrate the true underlying causes of post-traumatic stress injuries. Scan ten survivors of the same blast: some bear night-flashes, others numb estrangement, still others rage. *DSM* assigns them a common label and code, and often a common drug.

Yet rodent studies reveal at least four molecular subtypes by hippocampal gene expression. Human post-mortem tissue shows divergent BDNF signatures. And fMRI work spots network breaks that predict who will respond to exposure therapy and who will not. Until clinicians can read those signatures the way an internist reads a troponin level, medication will stay a game of chance.

Building that capacity is not impossible, but it faces an uphill battle against the traditional model of medicine and pharmacy. Cardiology once groped in the dark too. Then came electro-cardiography, coronary angiography, troponin assays, and now genomic risk panels.

The practices of psychiatry and psychology must follow the same arc: observe, measure, classify by mechanism, then treat with precision.

That arc bends through the disciplines named above, through training programs that marry scalpels and sequences, through databases that combine million-patient genotypes with stress maps and drug outcomes.

Revolution in White Paper and Waiting Room

Veterans harmed by toxic prescription cocktails, adolescents handed black-box drugs with tiny-print suicide warnings, and families devastated by the spiraling costs of lifetime polypharmacy have united in a clarion call for reform. Their demands are unmistakable:

Use the *DSM* for Initial Triage

The *DSM* was never intended to be the final word on the complexity of mental-health conditions, yet it has become a gatekeeper for insurance billing and patient categorization. While assigning codes can secure coverage for essential services, these codes fail to capture the deep biological underpinnings of mental health challenges—particularly trauma-related conditions such as PTSX.

A purely code-based approach overlooks the crucial interplay of neurochemistry, receptor dynamics and biophysical factors that shape an individual's response to trauma. To address this gap, diagnostic decisions must be overseen by professionals who understand the intricate biology of stress responses—experts fluent in neurotransmitter flux, receptor conformational states, and the cascading effects of inflammatory cytokines on the brain.

Such specialized knowledge ensures that each diagnosis, even when assigned a *DSM* code for administrative purposes, is grounded in real molecular processes. Ultimately, the *DSM* should serve only as an initial sorting mechanism: a means to open doors to care, not serve as the ultimate guide to healing. It has proven itself to be far short of that.

Mandate Multidisciplinary Panels

Treating trauma-related conditions demands an integrated approach that unites multiple domains of expertise. No single title—be it psychiatrist, psychologist or neurologist—can address the layered effects of biochemical imbalances, genetic predispositions, and environmental stressors. Too often, a clinician with specialized letters after their name prescribes a medication regimen without comprehensive input from experts in immunology, molecular biology, or advanced imaging techniques.

A patient with PTSX might need anti-inflammatory strategies for neuroinflammation, hormone regulation for endocrine imbalances, and cognitive-behavioral therapies for maladaptive thought patterns. By mandating multidisciplinary panels, we hold ourselves accountable to evidence-based rigor—pooling insights from psychiatrists, neurologists, molecular scientists, and experts in computational biology and AI diagnosing.

This cross-functional practice could ensure that any long-term medication plan is not just a reflexive prescription but a carefully considered strategy, mapped to each patient's biological markers and life circumstances.

Fund Bench-to-Bedside Fellowships

One reason for the disconnect between cutting-edge laboratory discoveries and clinical practice is the siloed nature of medical education. While surgeons historically trained by dissecting cadavers and observing procedures firsthand, many psychiatrists and prescribing professionals rarely step foot in a research lab after their initial schooling.

A bench-to-bedside fellowship could remedy this, immersing clinicians in molecular research environments where they can witness live-cell imaging, genomic assays, or real-time analyses of synaptic behavior. This proximity to scientific discovery enriches their decision-making back in the clinic and supports a culture that focuses on continuous learning. We also suggest that this level of learning be certified in the same way as board certifications are awarded following extensive education and proven studies.

When clinicians observe how certain stress hormones can alter gene expression or how neuroinflammatory signals propagate, they become more adept at tailoring treatments that address root causes instead of merely managing symptoms.

Enforce Biomarker Baselines

In the era of personalized medicine, guesswork has no place in prescribing potentially life-altering psychiatric drugs. Establishing biomarker baselines—measuring hormone levels, inflammatory markers, or neuroimaging readouts—before initiating treatment provides a data-driven foundation.

Rather than prescribing a medication blindly and hoping for the best, clinicians can track molecular changes over time, adjusting dosages or exploring different therapeutic avenues when a specific biomarker veers off course. For instance, if an individual displays elevated inflammatory cytokines or abnormal cortisol rhythms, treatments could target these disruptions directly.

This approach respects the heterogeneity of PTSX by recognizing that one patient's neuroendocrine imbalance may differ substantially from another's. Continuous monitoring ensures that interventions adapt to a patient's evolving physiological state, creating a feedback loop of evidence-based care.

Tie Federal Reimbursement to Integrated, Data-Driven Care

Real reform is unlikely to take root without concrete financial incentives or penalties. Tying federal reimbursement to the use of integrated, data-driven care compels healthcare providers to adopt the best practices of multidisciplinary collaboration, biomarker monitoring, and ongoing evaluation of treatment efficacy. If legislatures fail to pass laws mandating these standards, the judicial system may step in. Civil suits for psychiatric malpractice become increasingly plausible as patients and attorneys recognize the gulf between what is currently provided under the "standard of care" and what modern science knows about molecular interventions, genomics, and immune-mediated pathology.

The tort bar is beginning to notice this discrepancy, suggesting that accountability—whether through legislation or legal action—will emerge as a powerful catalyst for change. If the various groups that currently control the mental healthcare field don't evolve, they may face more and more civil litigation and jury trials.

More Than Policy—A Moral Imperative

This movement toward integration transcends bureaucracy or debates about reimbursement codes. It is a push to protect the vulnerable: veterans suffering from toxic polypharmacy, adolescents endangered by black-box warnings, and families who are collapsing under the financial and emotional strain of misguided long-term prescriptions.

An outdated system that obscures vital information, narrows diagnoses to shorthand codes, and prizes profit over patient welfare must be overhauled from the ground up. If we fail to act, we risk allowing countless individuals with PTSX and related conditions to slip through the cracks—casualties not just of trauma itself, but of a broken healthcare model.

We owe it to every patient, every family, and every community to build a truly integrated, ethically sound, and scientifically informed approach to healing PTSX. It goes without saying that we should take this same approach to all diseases and medical issues.

Closing with a Simple Truth

I have watched people bleed in the dirt and watched others sink in a chair, eyes open, mind replaying a blast that never ends. The first wound we know how to sew. The second we cover with labels and pills because it is quicker than tracing the broken wires.

But the men and women who carry that wound have earned better work from all of all of us, especially the psychiatrists, psychologists and neurologists. They have earned the full weight of neurochemistry, biophysics, molecular biology, and every science we possess.

If-Then Guidance

- If your provider reaches for a prescription pad after fewer than fifteen minutes of discussion, then request a full diagnostic work-up that includes blood panels, neuro-imaging, and a review by a multidisciplinary team.
- If your symptoms began after a definable trauma—blast, collision, or assault—then insist on a physical evaluation for traumatic brain injury before accepting a psychiatric label.

- If you have been given three or more psychotropic medications simultaneously, then ask for a medication-reconciliation conference to assess necessity, interactions, and molecular rationale.
- If your insurer refuses coverage for biomarker testing, then file an appeal citing parity laws and emerging standards of precision care.
- If you feel pressured to rely on a chatbot for primary emotional support, then schedule face-to-face time with a trained clinician and at least one trusted human companion.
- If your clinician dismisses questions about molecular tests as unnecessary, then request written justification that cites peer-reviewed evidence. If he actually dismiss you, then find another clinician.
- If new or worsening symptoms are brushed off as "normal side-effects," then demand a taper plan and thorough differential diagnosis.
- If dosage changes are made without parallel lifestyle or therapy recommendations, then ask for integrated care that includes CBT and physical activity.
- If the pharmacy substitutes a new generic that alters your response, then request brand exemption or bioequivalence documentation.
- If your chart labels you "treatment-resistant" without biomarker confirmation, then seek referral to a precision-neurodiagnostic center.

Take the Next Step

- Gather your complete medical and medication records.
- Schedule a second-opinion consult with a clinician trained in neurobiology, molecular biology and pharmacogenomics.
- Request baseline cognitive and endocrine testing before you accept any new prescription.
- Enroll in a vetted support group—veteran, caregiver or trauma-survivor—within the next week.
- Start a daily log tracking sleep, mood, and any side-effects to

share with your care team.

- Download a reputable symptom-tracking app that syncs with your wearable to capture heart-rate variability and sleep cycles.
- Identify a nearby academic center running molecular neurobiology trials to test for PTSX, and check eligibility within 30 days.
- Draft a concise health timeline—traumas, medication shifts, environmental exposures—and share it with upcoming specialists.
- Set aside daily time for neuro-regenerative practices like aerobic exercise or mindfulness, beginning this week.
- Circulate a one-page advocacy letter among peers affected by overmedication and invite them to co-sign policy-reform petitions that you send to your congressional representative, demanding positive action.
- Contact elected representatives and demand for all veterans a proper, across-the-board testing for PTSX from a knowledgable mental healthcare provider, not simply a psychiatrist, psychologist or neurologist.

Through Their Eyes

"Like my SEAL buddies, I used to count blasts like reps on a pull-up bar. Two frag grenades in Anbar. Three stacked breachers on a steel door in Tikrit. An IED that lifted our convoy truck high enough for daylight to wedge under the tires. The ringing always faded, so I wrote "ALL OK" in my log and fell back in with the platoon. SEALs finish the mission. They do not fill sick-call chits.

"Years later the static stayed. Words jammed on my tongue. I would walk into a room and forget why I was there. A swim-buddy cracked a joke about "too many lightning flashes in that skull," and I laughed, but my chest tightened. The Navy doctor called it depression, scribbled sertraline on a pad, and sent me back to work. Sertraline became bupropion, then topiramate when the migraines hit.

"Still, the ground kept tilting. I missed rappelling cues during a VBSS drill and a junior operator grabbed my harness before I pitched over the rail. Pride is a heavy rucksack. It finally split. I checked myself into Balboa, where a young neurologist ordered diffusion-tensor imaging. The scans lit up like tracer fire: micro-tears running along the white-matter highways that carry memory, balance, mood. Traumatic brain injury—blast-wave etchings carved deeper with every breach that I had logged as routine.

"They told me that my head got shot back and forth then twisted in a gnarly rotational acceleration that sheared my nerves small increments at a time. They also said my brain's wiring was resilient. But not that resilient.

"Knowing did not heal me, but knowledge aimed the treatment. They drew blood for inflammatory markers, mapped my hormone drift, genotyped my liver enzymes so the next medication fit rather than fought my chemistry. The cocktail shrank from five scripts to one. Physical therapy rewired gait, vestibular drills steadied the horizon, cognitive rehab taught me to pace tasks before the tasks drowned me. Most of all, the team listened. They spoke of circuits, not character flaws, and left room for questions the way a good dive officer leaves air in the tanks.

"I still drop words. My wife keeps a chalkboard by the fridge where I can sketch the missing nouns. Some nights the tinnitus plays its high E-string and won't let go, but I know why it sings and what quiets it. I know the blast line etched into my brain is injury, not destiny, and injury can be treated when science is allowed to march beside valor.

"So I speak to anyone who will lend an ear: do not let a *DSM* and a fast pen decide your fate. Demand the scans, the bloodwork, the molecular truth. We would never send a sailor into a hot zone without a map. Your brain deserves the same reconnaissance."

—Master Chief Brad, US Navy (ret.)

57

The Vagus Nerve and the Molecular Nature of Neuroinflammation

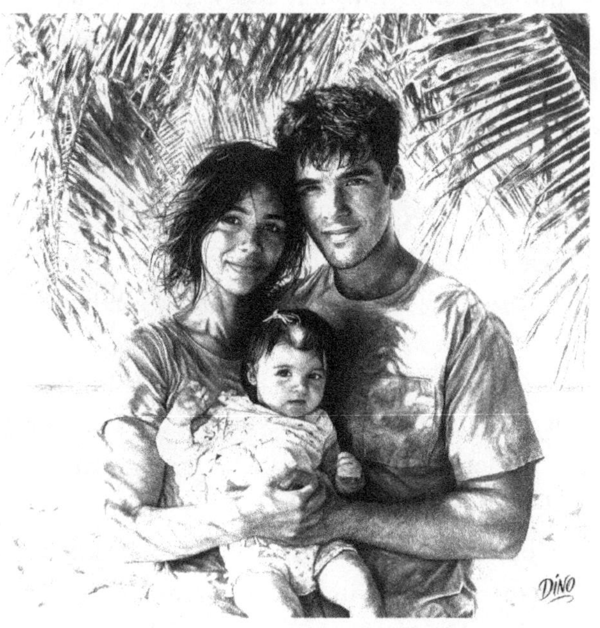

I was twenty-three when the first IED lifted our MRAP like a carnival ride gone wrong. The second—six months later on the same dusty highway north of Ramadi—snapped my helmet against the radio rack hard enough to blur the world into static. I chalked it up to "getting my bell rung" and stayed on mission, but the headaches, vertigo, and a creeping sadness followed me home.

At the VA they called it major depression. The psychiatrist never asked about blast overpressure or ringing ears. He simply wrote a script for sertraline, 100 mg, and nodded toward the pharmacy window. For a year I swallowed those little blue tablets and floated through shift work at a warehouse, half-awake. Half-alive, if even that.

One sleepless night my scrolling thumb landed on a magazine article about veterans using an external vagus-nerve stimulator—just twenty minutes a day pressed to the skin below the left ear. It spoke of cooling the brain's inflammation instead of dimming it with meds. I ordered a device with my own money, set the timer, and felt a gentle pulse under my jaw.

By week three the morning fog began to thin. A month in, I laughed—really laughed—during a movie date with my husband, who had stood by my side through the medicated haze. The protocol then shifted to once-a-week sessions for six months. Migraines faded, night terrors quieted, and I rediscovered the thrill of planning a future.

Today I manage a big-box home-improvement store in Pensacola, Florida. Our daughter, Luna, was born last spring. When she grips my finger her stare is desert-sun bright, but the heat no longer burns. The blasts marked me, yes—but a humming little device helped me claim the rest of my story.

This chapter concentrates on one highway that touches every organ system in the human body: the vagus nerve. Acting as both messenger and circuit breaker, it senses the gut microbiome, steadies heartbeat, and tells immune cells when to stand down. Emerging evidence shows that purposeful modulation of vagal tone—through targeted stimulation, precise breath work, diet-driven microbiome shifts, and closed-loop bioelectronic devices—can reach deep enough to influence ion channels, cytokine cascades, and neuroinflammation at the root of PTSX.

Keep in mind, though, that any stimulator—external or implanted—will target a large number of vagal nerve fibers and the cells they innervate. It is not meant to zero in on one specific area of the vagal nervous system. Therefore, it will stimulate areas not necessarily intended. For example, if you are attempting to assuage depression or anxiety, using a vagus nerve stimulator on the neck will affect a large region of this great nerve. It will hopefully decrease the molecular affects of depression, anxiety, etc. and it may also have other effects.

Finally, in the section "Where the Science of Vagal Healing Stands—and Where It Still Needs to Go," we survey the established science and emerging frontiers of vagus nerve stimulation, highlighting its potential to reduce inflammation, stabilize mood and support recovery from trauma.

When a blast wave, a childhood trauma, or a decade of sleepless nights leaves its mark, the wound seldom stops at memory. It echoes in aching joints, irritable bowels, and bloodwork that flags perpetual low-grade inflammation. Modern science has traced much of that echo to one roaming ribbon of nerve tissue: the vagus.

While clinical trials, FDA clearances, and biomarker research affirm that enhancing parasympathetic tone can help manage conditions like PTSX, TBI, and chronic stress gaps persist. The section also raises vital questions about precision dosing, organ-specific targeting, therapy sequencing, and synergy with other interventions.

It also points to practical strategies—tracking heart rate variability, adopting fiber-rich diets, and integrating noninvasive devices—while urging broader collaboration among clinicians, engineers and policymakers to further refine and expand vagal healing approaches.

Threshold: Why This Nerve, Why Now?

Running from brain-stem to gut, from heartbeat to spleen, it is both a messenger and a thermostat. Strengthen its signal and inflammation cools. Neglect it and molecular fires rage. Veterans and civilians alike stand to benefit from understanding—and tuning—this quiet guardian.

Trauma—an explosion or blast, a verbal assault or prolonged high alert—does not end at the moment of impact. It initiates a biochemical and molecular cascade. Within milliseconds, electrical and chemical signals spread through body and brain. Ion-channels allow calcium and sodium to enter neurons and alter membrane voltage, setting off phosphorylation pathways, gene-expression switches and inflammatory mediators. This process extends the influence of the original stressor well beyond the first shock.

A Quiet Giant: Meeting Your Vagus

The great vagus (Latin for "wanderer") nerve is cranial nerve X (ten), and laces through the neck, chest and abdomen. Roughly eighty percent of its fibers carry information upward, letting the brain know what the heart, lungs and gut are experiencing. The remaining fibers carry orders downward, slowing the pulse, deepening breath, releasing digestive enzymes, and—crucially—dialing back the immune system's artillery shells of cytokines.

Researchers christened that dialogue the "inflammatory reflex," a feedback loop in which the vagus detects rising cytokines and replies with an acetylcholine-coded command—stand down—to macrophages and microglia. Healthy vagal tone therefore resembles a well-trained fire brigade: vigilant, swift and proportionate.

Firefighters in the Brain: Neuroinflammation 101

Inflammation is indispensable when we scrape a knee, but in the brain it can overstay its welcome. Traumatic brain injury unleashes microglia—the brain's immune cells—whose good intent can degrade into chronic release of tumor-necrosis factor, interleukins and reactive oxygen species.

Months later, patients may struggle with brain fog, migraines and dark moods once chalked up to "just stress." We now know better: persistent neuroinflammation can prune synapses, impair neurogenesis, and sabotage mood circuitry.

The War Zone Within: Trauma, Autonomic Imbalance and Flames Lingering

Combat enventually ends, yet the body's fight-or-flight circuitry can loop on repeat. Studies measuring heart-rate variability—an electrocardiographic fingerprint of vagal tone—have found that service members with lower baseline variability before deployment were far more likely to develop severe PTSX after combat stress.

Similar patterns appear in civilians after car crashes or domestic abuse. When the sympathetic accelerator sticks and the parasympathetic brake fails, cortisol surges, gut barriers leak, and the inflammatory reflex loses power. The result is a body-wide alarm state that feels like anxiety but behaves like chemical warfare on tissue.

From Sparks to Storms: How Gut Microbes Dial the Vagus

Your gut microbiome—trillions of bacteria, fungi, and other tiny organisms—manufactures metabolites that act like text messages to the vagus. Short-chain fatty acids like butyrate send a calm note to vagal endings, lowering systemic cytokines. Conversely, dysbiosis can shout "all is lost" and flood the nerve with distress calls.

Germ-free mouse experiments have proven causality: implant a healthy microbiota and vagal tone rises. Cut the vagus and the behavioral benefits of probiotics vanish. Veteran cohorts, those with the lowest gut-species diversity, also show the weakest heart-rate variability and highest inflammatory markers—a three-way link among microbes, vagus and inflammation.

Listening to the Static: Diagnostics and Biomarkers

Heart-rate variability (HRV): The term HRV refers to the subtle differences in time, measured in milliseconds (ms), between each of your heartbeats, and it's measured by looking at how much that interval varies over a fixed period—commonly five minutes. For instance, if your heart beats at a rate of 60 beats per minute, you might assume there is exactly one second between each beat, but in a healthy person that spacing actually varies slightly (e.g., 0.9 seconds, then 1.1 seconds, and so on). That natural fluctuation is the "variability" being measured.

HRV is closely tied to the activity of your autonomic nervous system. When the parasympathetic branch—governed largely by the vagus nerve—is strong and active, your heart rate can slow quickly and respond flexibly to changing needs. As a result, you'll see more variation in the intervals between beats.

A higher HRV is thus commonly interpreted as a sign of good cardiovascular fitness, better stress resilience, and overall calmness in the body. Conversely, a lower HRV suggests reduced flexibility in heart rate adjustments, often linked to higher stress levels or possible health concerns.

Consumer wearables and five-minute electrocardiograms make it easy to detect these beat-to-beat changes. By tracking HRV over time, you gain insight into how one's nervous system responds to daily pressures, exercise and recovery. Essentially, the higher your HRV, the stronger your body's "rest-and-recover" signal (parasympathetic tone), indicating a healthier balance between stress response and relaxation.

Inflammatory panels: High-sensitivity C-reactive protein, interleukin-6, tumor-necrosis factor, and neurofilament light now form the VA Neuro-Immune Index, guiding triage to vagal therapies within a seventy-two hour period.

Portable PET/MRI helmets: Deployed medics can image microgliosis at the bedside and wirelessly program a vagus stimulator before the patient boards a med-evac flight—technology proven in 2025 field drills.

Flipping the Switch: Implanted Vagus Nerve Stimulation

The medical field stumbled onto vagus nerve stimulation through epilepsy surgery. Electrodes wrapped around the left cervical vagus send tiny pulses that, over months, remodeled brain circuits. Patients reported not only fewer seizures but brighter moods and stronger immunity. In rheumatoid arthritis, implanted stimulation halved joint pain and systemic cytokines.

PTSX breakthrough: A recent multi-center trial pairing implanted stimulation with trauma-focused therapy produced a clinically meaningful drop in symptom scores that persisted through a twelve-month period. Most participants no longer met diagnostic criteria for PTSX.

TBI neuroprotection: Animal and early human studies report reduced blood-brain-barrier leakage, smaller lesion volumes, and improved cognition when stimulation is applied within days of head injury.

Safety: Serious device-related side effects remain below three percent, typically minor voice hoarseness or transient cough.

Handheld Hope: Non-Invasive Devices

Not everyone needs—or wants—surgery. An alternative is transcutaneous auricular stimulation that clips onto the ear, where a branch of the vagus surfaces. A single fifteen-minute session can lower heart rate, dampen sympathetic tone, and trim circulating cytokines for hours.

Portable, FDA-cleared devices are already issued through VA programs for PTSX and long-COVID autonomic dysfunction. A parallel neck-based option, the GammaCore Sapphire® nVNS, has secured FDA clearances for cluster headache (2017) and migraine (2018) and is now supplied in many VA clinics.

Early adopters report minimal side-effects—transient throat flutter or mild skin tingling—and welcome the autonomy of a pocket-sized "rescue switch." Patients also report greatly improved sleep patterns and a restful state upon awakening.

Whole-Body Vibration Therapy: Frequencies That Move Trauma Out

Trauma is not only held in memory but in immobility—in the fascia, the interoceptive maps, and the underused core of the body. Top-of-the-line, tri-motor vibration therapy platforms were not designed for trauma per se, but their therapeutic effect is unmistakable.

By applying simultaneous oscillatory, linear, and pulsating vibration, these devices stimulate mechanoreceptors in the feet, spine, and postural chain. This stimulation travels through the connective tissue network, baroreceptors, and lymphatic vessels—supporting interoception, proprioception, and parasympathetic tone.

Whole-body vibration has been shown to improve HRV (heart rate variability), promote fascia hydration and circulation, and gently activate the vagal-adjacent baroreceptors of the feet and spine.

For trauma survivors who feel frozen, flat or dissociated, vibration becomes not agitation—but safe movement. The body begins to move itself again, rhythmically, without fear.

Breath, Cold, and Song: Everyday Vagal Tonics

The following are a number of everyday practices that can tone down the vagus nerve:

<u>4:5:6 breathing</u>: inhale four counts, hold five counts, exhale six while

This is the molecular basis of PTSX: a storm of ions, free radicals, and immune signals that, if left unchecked, rewires perception into permanent alarm.

Enter the vagus nerve—the body's master circuit breaker. In calm times its parasympathetic pulses slow the heart, deepen breath and, through the "inflammatory reflex," instruct immune cells to stand down once threats are neutralized.

pursing your lips and slowly forcing air from your lungs. Prolonged exhalation tugs the vagal brake and raises HRV within minutes.

Cold-water rinses and facials: rapid facial cooling engages the dive reflex, a vagus-mediated drop in heart rate.

Humming and singing: vocal-cord vibration massages vagal branches and eases social anxiety.

Simple, cost-free, and easily layered with medical treatments, these practices train the nervous system the way push-ups train muscles.

The Civilian Front: Barracks Science in Living Rooms

Level-I trauma centers in Boston, Denver, and Houston now pair auricular vagus-nerve stimulation with eight-week mindfulness-based stress-reduction (MBSR) classes. Preliminary data show a 12-ms rise in the Root Mean Square of Successive Differences (RMSSD) and a 40% drop in intrusive-memory scores compared with MBSR alone. RMSSD is one of the most widely used time-domain metrics of HRV. It captures how much the intervals between consecutive heartbeats—called R-R intervals—fluctuate on a beat-to-beat basis.

Why RMSSD matters

Parasympathetic proxy – RMSSD is highly sensitive to vagal (parasympathetic) activity and minimally influenced by sympathetic tone, making it a reliable surrogate for "vagal tone."

Health correlations – Higher RMSSD is linked to better emotional regulation, lower systemic inflammation, improved insulin sensitivity, and reduced mortality risk after cardiac events.

Typical ranges

Elite endurance athletes: 80–120 ms

Healthy adults: 40–70 ms

Chronic stress / PTSX cohorts: often <40 ms

Values vary by age, time of day, and posture, so tracking readings over time is more informative than single readings.

Practical use in *Silent Scars* protocols

Breathwork goal – An 8–10 ms rise after a week of coherent-breathing drills signals successful vagal engagement.

Device titration – taVNS or cervical VNS sessions are adjusted upward or downward based on RMSSD change in the first 30 min post-stimulation.

Insurance justification – Reimbursement pilots accept ≥8 ms sustained RMSSD increase as a marker of clinically meaningful autonomic improvement.

In short, RMSSD is the heartbeat-to-heartbeat "fingerprint" of the vagus nerve, translating invisible autonomic shifts into a single, actionable number.

Private insurers like Horizon and Anthem cite these HRV-linked outcome curves in newly published coverage bulletins, reimbursing device rentals when patients document a ≥8-ms RMSSD improvement. This is a clear signal that parasympathetic medicine is no longer confined to military protocols but is reshaping civilian standards of care, as well.

Closed-Loop Futures and Bioelectronic Harmonies

Next-generation stimulators sense HRV dips or cytokine spikes and adjust output in real time. A recent scientific article showed that closed-loop systems enhanced spinal-cord-injury recovery while using sixty percent less energy. Trials for PTSX are slated for 2026. Meanwhile, researchers are continuing to explore bacteriophage cocktails to delete pro-inflammatory gut strains, with vagal metrics as endpoints.

Field Guide: Your First Steps Toward Vagal Balance

Check your pulse: Request an HRV reading. Numbers under forty milliseconds suggest poor parasympathetic tone.

Choose a daily practice: 4:5:6 breathing twice a day or a cold-water face or whole-body rinse. Track mood and HRV weekly.

Feed your microbes: Aim for thirty different plant foods each week, and add kefir or kimchi if tolerated.

Discuss neuromodulation: If symptoms remain severe, discusses implanted or auricular stimulation with your provider—this chapter can provide findings that stimulate a conversation.

Team up: Healing accelerates in community. HRV rises when we feel safe with others. Find your tribe, contribute meaningfully, and you'll soon discover that you are actively studying your own and healing yourself.

Chicken, Egg, and Exploding Circuitry: How Trauma Unravels Molecules—and How the Vagus Rescues Them

Trauma is rarely a single event. Rather it's a biochemical chain reaction. At the flashpoint—an IED blast, a humiliating interrogation, years of hyper-alert caregiving—forces ripple through body and brain in milliseconds. Ion channels embedded in neuronal membranes stretch open like sprung trapdoors. Calcium and sodium rush inside, triggering waves of electrical disarray.

Within minutes, microglia transform from caretakers into combatants, spraying cytokines meant to sterilize injury but equally capable of eroding healthy synapses. Cortisol spikes, mitochondrial pores leak, and DNA repair enzymes scramble to keep pace with oxidative damage.

This is the molecular basis of PTSX: a storm of ions, free radicals, and immune signals that, if left unchecked, rewires perception into permanent alarm.

Enter the vagus nerve—the body's master circuit breaker. In calm times its parasympathetic pulses slow the heart, deepen breath, and, through the "inflammatory reflex," instruct immune cells to stand down once threats are neutralized. But trauma can cripple this brake in two distinct ways.

Bottom-Up Breakdown

Mechanical or biochemical forces strike first. Blast pressure waves, repeated concussive forces, or surges of glutamate shear axonal cytoskeletons and pepper membranes with micro-tears. Damaged neurons leak ATP, a distress flare that rouses microglia into chronic vigilance. These same inflammatory mediators—tumor-necrosis factor, interleukins, reactive oxygen species—bathe the medulla where vagal nuclei reside, corroding receptor sensitivity and reducing acetylcholine output. The vagus, soaked in its own cytokine bath, begins to misfire.

What started as tissue damage cascades into autonomic collapse: heart-rate variability sinks, digestion stalls, nightmares flourish.

Top-Down Failure

Sometimes the sequence flips. A prolonged siege of psychological stress or moral injury shoves the autonomic balance toward perpetual "fight-or-flight." The sympathetic system throttles up and the vagus idles in low gear.

Decreased vagal tone lifts the immune system's leash, allowing even mundane infections or dietary irritants to initiate exaggerated inflammatory responses. Leaky-gut by-products slip into circulation, breach the blood–brain barrier, and activate microglia exactly as a blast would. In this version, the weak brake comes first, molecular wreckage second.

The Vicious Spiral

Whether bottom-up or top-down, each pathway accelerates the other. Initial cytokine surges make the vagus less responsive. A sluggish vagus, in turn, permits further cytokine escalation. Over weeks, neurosteroids that normally soothe limbic circuits decline, while excitatory amino acids remain high.

Ion channels responsible for mechanotransduction—Piezo1, TRPV4—become hypersensitive, converting everyday vibrations or sudden noises into pain and panic. Astrocytes, star-shaped support cells, swell and release S100B protein, a signal to tighten scar tissue around neurons, resulting in emotional flexibility, converting to rigid fear responses.

Therapeutic Leverage

The spiral's two-lane path is encouraging, however, allowing interventions to enter at multiple junctures. Bioelectronic stimulators or deep, slow breathing can jack up vagal tone, re-engaging the inflammatory reflex even while molecular fires still burn.

Conversely, omega-3 fatty acids, antioxidant polyphenols, or short-chain-fatty-acid-rich fermented foods can dampen cytokine production, giving the vagus a cleaner signal environment in which to reboot. By recognizing that vagal dysfunction and molecular mayhem are co-authors of PTSX, the leverage doubles πfor rewriting the story of recovery.

Anatomy of Hope

Trauma robs control by rewiring alarms and lighting hidden fires. The vagus nerve is extinguisher and architect, cooling inflammation while rebuilding trust between the brain, gut and heart. Strengthening it will not erase the past, nor guarantee a life without sorrow. It simply restores the body's forgotten capacity to down-shift, digest and heal.

Whether you are a veteran who still startles at fireworks or a civilian whose childhood still harbors emotional mines, the tools described here—electrodes, breath, fiber and friendship—offer hope grounded in peer-reviewed, published facts.

Where the Science of Vagal Healing Stands—and Where It Still Needs to Go

The moment you pick up a vagus-nerve stimulator, put on an HRV-tracking watch, or swallow a synbiotic (probiotic + prebiotic in one capsule), you stand at the intersection of two landscapes. One terrain is paved and well-lit: dozens of clinical trials, FDA clearances, and biomarker tables tell us how and why parasympathetic signaling calms inflammation and steadies mood.

The other terrain is still sketched in pencil: bold theories, early animal data, and passionate advocacy hint that the vagus may be the keystone in conditions we have long treated piecemeal. To close this book, we turn to twenty questions that chart the boundary between proven fact and promising speculation.

For each, you will see first what years of peer-reviewed evidence already confirm—solid ground on which to plant your next step—and then the open-ended inquiries that invite curious clinicians, inventive engineers, and determined policymakers to keep walking.

1. Master Regulator or Supporting Actor?

What we know – Clamp the cervical vagus in an operating room and heart rate drops. Stimulate it and the tumor-necrosis factor plummets. Low vagal tone predicts higher mortality across cardiovascular, metabolic, and psychiatric cohorts. These findings stretch back two decades and have been replicated around the globe.

What we're still asking – Even an orchestra led by the finest conductor falls flat if the violins are untuned. Mitochondrial distress, micronutrient deficits, and circadian misalignment can all sabotage recovery despite perfect vagal pulses. The next wave of studies must reveal whether routine parasympathetic "tuning" can override these parallel failures or whether comprehensive molecular housekeeping remains essential.

2. Molecular Dominoes—Which Falls First?

What we know – Blast overpressure and blunt concussion shear axonal components, flood neurons with calcium, and ignite microglial cytokine storms. Chronic emotional alarm depletes heart-rate variability, loosens the vagus's grip on immunity, and permits low-grade inflammation to smolder. Both sequences are real.

What we're still asking – No human study has yet traced the minute-by-minute choreography of injury, vagal collapse or systemic fallout. Would an hour-zero vagus pulse after blast blunt the molecular avalanche, or would antioxidants deployed first make later stimulation more effective? Longitudinal human "black-box" data paired with wearable vagal metrics could finally map causality.

3. Precision Dosing vs. Blanket Stimulation

What we know – Cervical implants approved for epilepsy run 20-30 Hz bursts, 30 s on / 5 min off. Auricular devices for migraine favor 25 Hz at 250 μs. Side-effects climb sharply at higher amperage or continuous duty.

What we're still asking – Post-traumatic stress injuries differ by gender, age, hormone milieu and trauma load. Closed-loop stimulators that throttle output to real-time HRV or cytokine telemetry may personalize therapy the way smart insulin pumps revolutionized diabetes care. Large comparative trials will decide whether adaptive dosing beats best-guess presets.

4. Anatomical Targeting

What we know – Cardiac fibers run heavy in the left cervical trunk, explaining occasional bradycardia during high-amplitude cervical stimulation. Auricular branches bypass the heart, making ear-clip devices safer for self-administration. Early, promising metabolic trials show that laparoscopic cuffs on abdominal vagal trunks improve insulin sensitivity and reduce body weight.

What we're still asking – Can multi-contact cuffs steer current specifically to splenic or hepatic fibers, dampening rheumatoid arthritis without lowering heart rate? Will we one day prescribe "pancreas-sparing vagus bursts" or "spleen-targeted cycles" the way oncologists order organ-specific radiation fields? Engineers and neurophysiologists are striving to give clinicians that level of granularity.

5. Biomarker Benchmarks

What we know – In rheumatoid arthritis and depression studies, a 10 ms rise in RMSSD HRV and a 30 % fall in IL-6 correlated with clinical remission. Those numbers appear again and again, suggesting practical if provisional targets.

What we're still asking – Are those same cut-points meaningful for blast TBI, moral injury, or long-COVID brain fog? Should we add neurosteroid panels or vagus-evoked EEG potentials to confirm central engagement? Standardized "success signatures" would let researchers meaningfully compare protocols and speed regulatory approvals.

6. Microbiome Feedback Loop

What we know – Short-chain fatty acids produced by dietary fiber-loving gut bacteria activate vagal afferents, lowering systemic inflammation. Conversely, vagal outflow strengthens gut-barrier tight junctions and dampens pathogenic overgrowth.

What we're still asking – Does a diet-only strategy raise vagal tone enough to quell severe PTSX, or must electrical or breath-based stimulation be layered in? A factorial trial—synbiotic alone, taVNS alone, combination, and placebo—could answer whether one modality alone can close the feedback loop or that synergy rules.

7. Personalized Autonomics

What we know – HRV declines with age and chronic stress, and women's stronger baseline parasympathetic tone shifts during perimenopause. Blast loading reduces vagal tone in direct proportion to concussive events.

What we're still asking – Do gene variants in acetylcholine receptors or ion-channel polymorphisms predict whose HRV rebounds fastest? Could saliva or cheek-swab tests tell clinicians whether to aim for auricular versus cervical leads? The personalized-medicine revolution that has reshaped oncology may soon enter neuromodulation.

8. Therapy Sequencing

What we know – Pilot PTSX trials show exposure therapy coupled with simultaneous cervical VNS more than doubles remission rates relative to exposure alone.

What we're still asking – What is the optimal order for complex cases? Should antioxidant infusions precede neuromodulation, should taVNS prime the brain for psychotherapy, or is a three-phase protocol required? Trial designs that randomize sequence, not just treatment vs. placebo, will refine clinical playbooks.

9. Safety and Contraindications

What we know – The largest safety database (epilepsy implants) shows serious adverse events below three percent, with hoarseness and cough leading the list. Arrhythmias are rare, but documented.

What we're still asking – Will decades-long suppression of pro-inflammatory cytokines weaken cancer surveillance or infection clearance? Post-market vigilance and national device registries must monitor immune outcomes across the lifespan.

10. Bench to Barracks and Beyond

What we know – The VA, DARPA, and NIH are funding multi-site trials on taVNS for PTSX and cognitive deficits after TBI. Reimbursement lags. Only migraine and depression codes exist for auricular devices.

What we're still asking – Can value-based purchasing models spread devices to rural veterans and low-income civilians? Evidence must demonstrate cost savings in hospital admissions and medication burden.

11. Causal Proof vs. Correlation

What we know – Historic vagotomy surgeries for ulcers correlated with later autoimmune flare-ups, suggesting the cut nerve removes an anti-inflammatory brake. Animal models confirm vagal knockouts suffer exaggerated cytokine storms.

What we're still asking – Human Mendelian-randomization using genetic proxies for low cholinergic tone would provide quasi-randomized evidence. Trials are in design. Meanwhile, fully closed-loop RCTs—device off vs. adaptive on—could reveal causal weight.

12. Organ-Specific Signatures

What we know – In rodents, splenic fiber stimulation lowers TNF, whereas pancreatic bursts modulate insulin release. Compound action potentials differ by branch.

What we're still asking – Human translation will require ultra-thin cuff arrays that read and write signals without neuropraxia. If successful, clinicians could dial therapy to whichever organ system needs relief, sparing side tissues.

13. Circadian Synchrony

What we know – HRV and glucocorticoid rhythms dance daily. Inflammatory gene expression peaks mid-afternoon.

What we're still asking – Trials aligning taVNS sessions with individual cortisol spikes could prove chronotherapy's value. Wearables tracking HRV and cortisol via sweat sensors may automate precision timing.

14. Placebo or Neuroplasticity?

What we know – Sham-controlled fMRI studies find nucleus tractus solitarius activation only during true taVNS. Sham arms still record modest symptom gains, highlighting subject's expectancy's influence.

What we're still asking – How can clinicians ethically harness expectancy without overselling? Transparent education, ritualized device use, and objective biomarker tracking may blend belief with biology.

15. Dual-Path Targets

What we know – Ion-channel stabilizers like beta-hydroxybutyrate limit membrane micro-damage. taVNS quells inflammatory spillover.

What we're still asking – Phase-II trials combining both for blast TBI are underway. Additive benefits remain to be proven. Positive results could spawn combination "neuro-macro packs" similar to chemo-radiation pairings in oncology.

16. Endocrine Echoes

What we know – Acute VNS lowers cortisol and modestly raises oxytocin. Chronic stimulation can normalize DHEA levels in some PTSX cohorts.

What we're still asking – Should quarterly hormone panels guide dosing? Could oxytocin spikes serve as bedside markers for therapeutic engagement? No protocol yet mandates endocrine monitoring, but emerging data urge consideration.

17. Childhood Trauma Imprint

What we know – High Adverse Childhood Experience (ACE) scores correlate with life-long low HRV and high inflammation.

What we're still asking – Small mindfulness-plus-taVNS trials in adults with high ACE show HRV gains but unclear whether they match never-traumatized baselines. Multi-year follow-ups will reveal the ceiling of adult reversal.

18. Longevity and All-Cause Mortality

What we know – Epidemiological studies show HRV predicts death more accurately than cholesterol or BMI.

What we're still asking – Government health economists model savings if vagal training becomes common, but no randomized community study has confirmed reduced mortality. Such large-scale trials would carry significant logistical hurdles but promise historic insights.

19. Device-Free Modulation

What we know – Slow diaphragmatic breathing, cold-water immersion, and chanting or humming or singing reliably raise HRV by 5–10 ms in laboratory settings—a modest but meaningful shift.

What we're still asking – Can behavioral "stacks" replace devices in severe PTSX? So far, test groups outperform behavioral-only groups in head-to-head comparisons, but maintenance phases may rely on behavior once acute crises subside.

20. Ethical and Equity Dimensions

What we know – Implantable generators cost several thousand dollars. Ear-clip devices and consumable device costs add up for low-income users. Data from closed-loop stimulators include sensitive biometrics, raising patient privacy questions.

What we're still asking – Could public "neuromodulation libraries" modeled on CPAP rental programs bridge gaps? How do we ensure cultural competence so that instructions, apps, and coaching meet diverse veteran populations? Policymakers must ensure user affordability, privacy, and respect issues are addressed.

Converging Paths, Shared Horizon

The North-Star truths—parasympathetic tone matters, vagal pulses can calm inflammation, gut microbes and heart rhythms dance in synchrony—give immediate direction. The uncharted stretches—personalized dosing, chrono-adaptive loops, organ-specific fiber maps—define where the next expeditions must head.

For readers still carrying silent scars, the compass points to actionable ground that includes tracking HRV, adopting dietary fiber-rich diets, experimenting with breath drills or supervised taVNS, pushing for biomarker testing, and demanding competent clinicians who speak the dual languages of nerves and molecules.

For clinicians, it's a frontier: incorporate autonomic metrics into every trauma intake, design trials that test sequence and specificity, and partner with engineers to make neuromodulation precise and affordable. Above all, the vagus narrative reframes trauma from a one-way slide into chronic degeneration to a bidirectional system that can be re-tuned. Healing need not wait for the next blockbuster drug or brain implant. It can begin with a measured breath, a cup of fermented vegetables, or a 25-Hz whisper of current under the ear. Every trauma survivor can walk toward a horizon where circuitry, chemistry and character converge in quiet strength.

Your next step is neither heroic nor complicated: breathe, measure, adjust, repeat. Each deliberate exhale nudges your vagus nerve toward steadier tone. Each steady beat calms inflammatory circuits that once kept you on alert. Track the numbers, because numbers cut through doubt.

Ask for help, because precision medicine is now a team sport. Feed the microbes that signal serenity, move enough to remind mitochondria they matter, sleep as though it were a prescription. Use devices when breath and food are not enough. Set them down when competence returns.

Progress will not arrive as a single revelation but as a collection of small, verifiable gains. When setbacks appear, treat them as data along your recovery path, not destiny written in solid granite. The science you have read is real, the tools are available, and your agency is intact.

If-Then Guidance

- If your resting heart-rate variability (HRV) sits below 40 ms for two consecutive weeks, then request a referral for autonomic testing and a vagus-nerve evaluation, not just an antidepressant refill.
- If you experience sudden digestive trouble, migraines or tinnitus after a major stress event, then ask your clinician to screen for low vagal tone and hidden neuroinflammation. It's not normal aging.
- If an explosion or blast, high-G flight, or repeated concussions are part of your history, then insist on blood panels for interleukin-6, Tumor Necrosis Factor, and neurofilament light before accepting a purely psychiatric label.
- If your provider recommends implanted vagus-nerve stimulation without trying non-invasive auricular or cervical devices first, then seek a second opinion on step-wise therapy.

- If a taVNS unit is prescribed, then verify if the stimulation protocol is paired with breath-training or exposure therapy—evidence shows combined care amplifies results.
- If lab results confirm dysbiosis—low short-chain-fatty-acid–producing bacteria—then integrate fiber-rich fermented foods or a targeted synbiotic into your plan, because gut metabolites directly modulate vagal signaling.
- If an insurance reviewer denies coverage for neuromodulation on grounds of "experimental," then cite FDA clearances for migraine and depression plus published veteran trials showing durable PTSX remission.
- If you notice HRV improves but brain fog lingers, then request endocrine labwork. Vagal repair often unmasks treatable hormone deficits.
- If a wearable or ECG shows large HRV swings after coffee, alcohol, or high-sugar meals, then treat diet as dosage—reduce the offending trigger before adjusting device parameters.
- If two months of daily stimulation yield no change in HRV or inflammation markers, then re-assess lead placement, stimulation dose, and microbiome status before declaring the therapy a failure.

Take the Next Step

- Print your last month of HRV data and bring it to your next appointment.
- Schedule vagus-focused breathwork—six-beat cycles—five minutes, twice daily, starting tomorrow.
- Order a synbiotic with L. plantarum and inulin, and log gut or mood changes for thirty days.
- Download the manufacturer's taVNS app and set reminders for the prescribed stimulation windows.
- Track migraines, tinnitus, or GI symptoms in parallel with HRV to reveal and understand cause-effect patterns and relationships.
- Locate a certified bioelectronic-therapy clinic, ideally within driving distance, and book an information session within two weeks.

- Prepare an insurance appeal template citing peer-reviewed VNS evidence. Keep it ready should claims be denied.
- Assign a "vagal buddy"—spouse, friend, or wingman—to check in on device adherence and daily breathing drills.
- Draft a one-page personal timeline linking key traumas, symptom flares, and biomarker data. Share it with every new clinician.
- Celebrate micro-wins: each five-millisecond rise in HRV or one-point drop in C-reactive protein is proof your biology is movable.

Through Their Eyes

"I logged more than four thousand hours in fighters—first the F-15C, later the F-22A—pulling eight and nine Gs until the horizon bent like heated glass. Each sortie was a razor-edge dance: SAM warnings wailing in my headset, wingmen breathing through oxygen masks that smelled of rubber and adrenaline.

"We skimmed ridgelines over Iraq, stitched contrails above Afghanistan, dodged missiles in Syria that burned into the night like angry comets. I tagged the victories on my kneeboard, but the shock waves tagged me back.

"Retirement wasn't gentle. Twenty years after my last combat sortie, panic would ambush me in the cereal aisle when a rattling shopping cart mimicked rotor wash.

"My hands, once steady enough to flip a jet on its back at Mach 1.8, trembled on conference-hall lecterns. Night sweats soaked flight-suit dreams that never ended with 'gear down, locked, three green.' My wife learned to wake me with a soft whistle instead of a touch. Fingertips felt too much like hot shrapnel.

"A VA neurologist finally ordered cytokine panels and an HRV trace instead of another psych questionnaire. Vagal tone in the basement, Interleukin-6 redlined—slow-burn neuro-inflammation fueled by thousands of G-loads and a decade of unfiled fear reports. He handed me a thumb-sized auricular vagus-nerve stimulator and said, 'Two sessions, fifteen minutes a day. Breathe five in, seven out. Let the current do the rest.' The first week felt like soda bubbles under my ear—nothing heroic—but by day ten the grocery store was just fluorescent light and tile, not a kill zone of rattling carts. At one month my HRV climbed from twenty-eight to forty-two milliseconds. The sweat-soaked dreams cooled to a damp forehead. I started lifting again, light at first, then the old iron. My granddaughter calls the device my 'ear engine.' She thinks it powers my stories. Maybe she's right.

"I had commanded wings, air-expeditionary task forces, even briefed presidents, yet I couldn't brief my own physician on invisible pain. Two tiny electrodes and a disciplined breath finally did what rank and resolve could not: they gave the ground back its stillness and the sky its invitation. I'm flying again—this time in a world that no longer tilts beneath my feet.

"Last week I stood in front of new pilots at Sheppard and told them the same checklist I follow every dawn: coherent breathing, ten minutes of ear-clip pulses, a glass of kefir for the gut-brain treaty. I show them my before-and-after HRV graph. The green line rises like a runway flare.

"They ask if the stimulator hurts. I smile and tell them it feels like the hum of hydraulics when the gear locks—a quiet signal that every system is ready for takeoff. The mission now is mentorship, not missiles, but the objective hasn't changed: bring everyone home, including ourselves."

—Lt Gen T., US Air Force (ret.)

58

A Gentle Revolution: Rewiring Healthcare Without Tearing Down the House

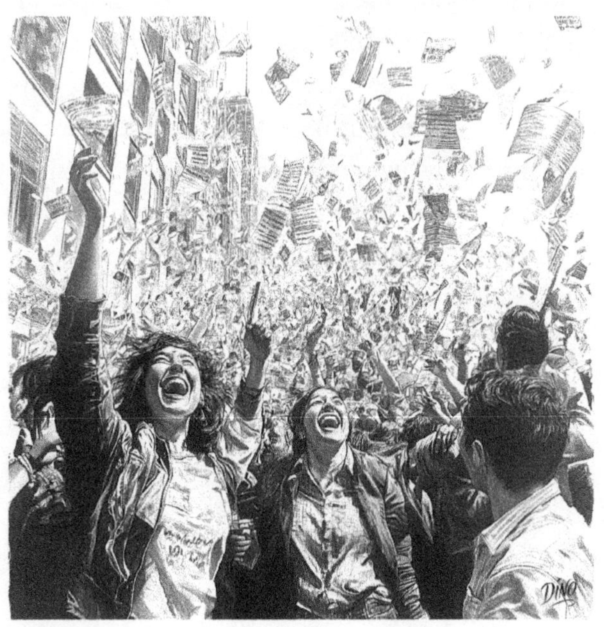

No system built over a century can—nor should—be revolutionized overnight. The pharmaceutical industry, the American Psychiatric Association, the American Medical Association, the American Psychological Association, and other medical and health and healthcare guilds around the globe have improved millions of lives. Antibiotics cured sepsis. Selective-serotonin re-uptake inhibitors pulled countless people back from the cliff. And ketamine-infusing therapy is now greatly assisting veterans and others reclaiming their lives.

Yet in the realm of PTSX, major depressive episodes, and traumatic brain injury, outcomes have plateaued. Polypharmacy climbs, disability rolls swell, suicide numbers refuse to budge. We stand at an inflection point: not a call to abandon pharmacology, but an invitation to evolve from symptom-treatment toward root-level healing—biochemical, molecular and autonomic.

Silent Scars, Bold Remedies invites readers to look beneath familiar psychiatric labels and recognize the associated biology: chronic inflammation, neurosteroid depletion, gut-microbiome imbalances, and—linking them all—a weakened vagal signal. Recognizing these layers does not diminish the value of existing treatrments and medications; rather, it expands our therapeutic toolkit. Medication remains an essential lane, now joined by others: ear-clip taVNS that strengthens heart-rate variability, synbiotic programs that restore gut integrity, and personalized neuromodulators that fine-tune immune tone.

In such a future, pharmaceutical innovators, professional guilds, and insurers can succeed by championing precision bio-electronic devices, microbiome-based therapies, and rapid molecular diagnostics—solutions that complement, and sometimes shorten, traditional pharmacologic courses.

Revenue would flow from demonstrable outcomes instead of indefinite refills, aligning financial health with patient well-being. Achieving this vision is not wishful thinking. It's within reach when scientists, clinicians, industry leaders, and policymakers collaborate toward shared, evidence-based goals.

How do we shift a system of this magnitude without breaking it? The answer is a concerted, cross-sector moonshot—a collaborative re-orientation that rewards discovery, safeguards patients, and keeps the economic engine humming. We suggest the following eight major changes:

A Congressional "Bio-Electric & Biome" Act

Just as the Cancer Moonshot galvanized oncology, Congress can launch a five-year, $5-billion initiative that funds NIH, DARPA and VA trials on vagus-nerve stimulation, gut-brain therapies and inflammatory-reflex mapping to find cures for the invisible wounds afflicting millions of our citizens. Stipulate public-private partnerships so device makers,

The next pages in medical history could read like this:

"In 2028, the first closed-loop vagus-synbiotic combo won FDA clearance, slashing veteran suicide rates by 90%. By 2030, primary-care clinics performed fingertip HRV during vital-sign checks, and insurers defaulted to neuromodulation bundles before escalating to lifelong polypharmacy."

Such sentences will never write themselves. They require persistent action—letters to legislators, CME proposals, venture funding pitched with both profitability and human flourishing on the slide deck.

Silent Scars, Bold Remedies provides the map and safe routes.

pharmaceutical giants and university labs share intellectual property, thus reducing silos and accelerating translation.

FDA Pathways for Bio-Electronic Medicines

Current FDA lanes—drug, device, biologic—do not cleanly fit closed-loop VNS or engineered probiotics. A new "Electro-Biotic Therapeutic" designation would streamline approval, combining pharmacokinetic rigor with real-time telemetry requirements. Guideline clarity invites industry investment the same way the Orphan Drug Act catalyzed rare-disease research.

Reimbursement that Rewards Outcomes

CMS and private insurers can pilot value-based bundles: if taVNS plus synbiotic therapy cuts CAPS-5 scores ≥50 % for one year, providers receive a bonus equal to a year of polypharmacy savings. The model flips incentives from pill counts to durable remission.

Industry-Led Curriculum Shifts

The various pharmaceutical, medical, health and healthcare industries control accreditation and continuing-education credits. Their seal can legitimize the new science overnight. Mandate at least 10 CME hours per cycle on autonomic diagnostics, microbiome interventions, and bio-electronic therapeutics. Residency programs would follow suit, graduating a workforce fluent in both SSRIs and RMSSD graphs.

Pharmaceutical Pivot, Not Retreat

Big-pharma R&D divisions can co-develop peptide-coupled VNS leads that release anti-inflammatory micro-doses precisely when the nerve fires, or license microbiome strains that up-regulate vagal afferents. Revenue flows through patentable adjuncts rather than ever-longer medication lists.

Integrated Autonomic Clinics

Seed grants can help VA Medical Centers and academic hospitals open "Autonomic Recovery Units" where psychiatrists, gastroenterologists, neurologists, and rehabilitation specialists share dashboards: HRV traces, cytokine panels, microbiome sequencing, sleep-stage metrics. Patients receive one synchronized plan instead of five disconnected prescriptions.

National Registry & Real-World Data

An opt-in registry that logs HRV, flare dates, stimulator settings, medication doses, and genomic overlays will generate the big-data backbone needed for AI-guided care. Pharma and device firms can mine anonymized trends to design next-gen interventions, while patients gain dashboards that translate biomarkers into everyday choices.

Public Communication—From Stigma to Stewardship

Guilds and industry associations can co-sponsor campaigns that reframe autonomic testing as routine as blood pressure checks. When civilians see a CEO and an Army officer comparing HRV scores on morning news shows, curiosity replaces stigma. Demand rises organically for clinics that offer breath coaching, taVNS, and synbiotic consults.

A Ladder Everyone Can Climb

Our proposed sea change challenges entrenched powers to trade a comfortable shoreline for deeper water—but not without life vests. Pharmaceutical companies gain fresh IP territory. Organizations like the American Psychiatric Association expand authority into autonomic science. Lawmakers score bipartisan wins by cutting long-term disability costs. Most important, patients inherit a system that no longer manages decline but engineers a recovery for all who face trauma.

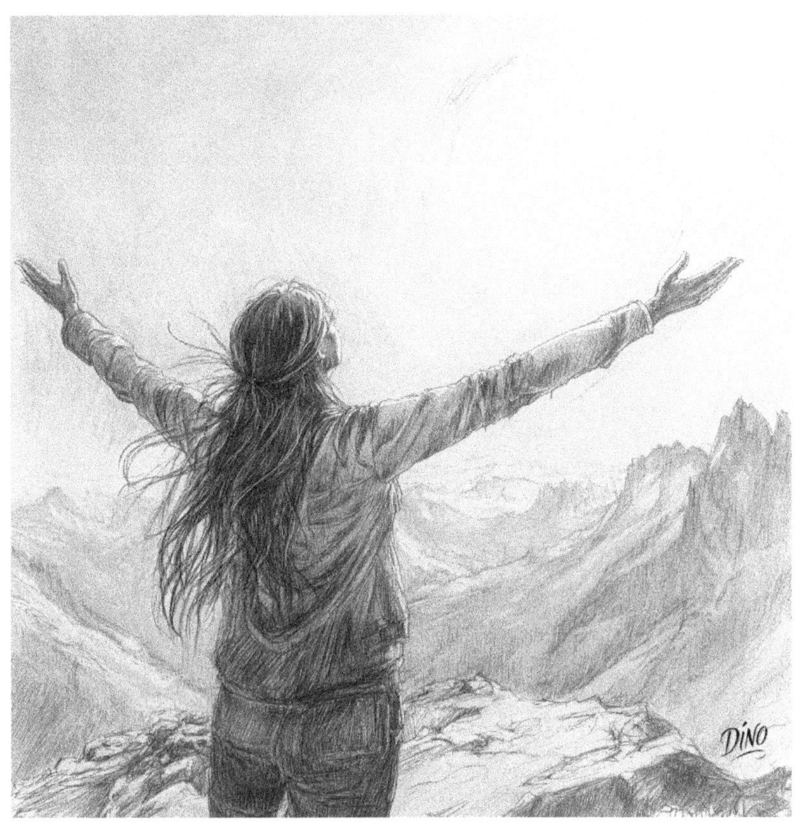

Summits

I stood where ragged summits kiss the sun,
My breath a hymn that mingled sky and stone,
The storms that chased me here are silent now,
Their thunder only memories half-blown.
From fractured nights and valleys strewn with fear
I climbed toward dawn beyond the hush of tears,
And met a laughing wind that stirred my chest.
O Joy, bright insurgent of the burdened soul,
Your banner lifts where weary pilgrims rise,
Painting new dawns across forgiving skies,
Let scars be maps,
steep paths still sing of grace,
for hope, once claimed, can never be erased.

DINO

Afterword

Walking Each Other Home

The last page of a book is never the end. It is a threshold. If *Silent Scars, Bold Remedies* has taught us anything, it is that every threshold contains two imperatives: look back with unflinching honesty and step forward with hope. For more than one thousand pages, we have followed warfighters, clinicians, scientists and families into the hidden interiors of Post-Traumatic Stress Injuries and then back out toward daylight. Dino and Liz call it the all-encompassing "PTSX," and I refer to it as the more-targeted "PTSI."

The journey has wound through laboratories humming with centrifuges, living-rooms heavy with unspoken sorrow, and combat zones where fear and loyalty mingle in equal measure. If, when you close the book, you feel both humbled by the weight of suffering and buoyed by the breadth of possibility, these pages have done their work.

And if you feel moved to place a gentler hand on your own scars—or on the shoulder of someone still bleeding invisibly—then the authors, Dino Garner and Liz Fetter, along with the storytellers and the researchers whose voices speak inside these chapters, will have fulfilled their deeper mission.

A New Language for Invisible Wounds

Words build worlds. They also build clinics, policies, and self-concepts. Early in this volume the authors went beyond the term PTSD and replaced it with "PTSX." A single consonant shift—from the finality of "disorder" to the unfinished openness of "X"—can reposition trauma from a life sentence to an injury capable of healing. The more-inclusive "X" stands for the unknown variables of injury and recovery: neuroinflammation, traumatic brain injury, depression, moral injury, endocrine collapse—all facets of one multifaceted wound.

A kinder taxonomy naturally seeds kinder science and medicine. Researchers who once designed studies to manage "chronic disorders" now design protocols to accelerate tissue repair, modulate cytokine cascades, and restore synaptic harmony. Clinicians who once expected incremental gains now anticipate full recovery. Most of all, survivors who once whispered, "Something is wrong with me," can now declare, "Something happened to me—and it can be mended." Uncertainty is now a scalpel, cutting shame away from biology.

The ripple effect can be profound: grant panels reword calls for proposals, insurance codes update diagnostic rubrics, and families shift from judgment to curiosity. One letter widens the aperture through which further curiosity and compassion, research and funding, and innovation must pass.

Eight Movements, One Arc

A journey of recovery unfolds in eight movements, mirroring the spiral path by which trauma first wounds and then, through painstaking work, relinquishes its grip.

Part I – Foundations maps the biology, psychology and sociology of trauma. They prove that childhood adversity, combat stress and domestic violence leave molecular signatures long after bruises fade. Micro-RNA strands curl differently, cortisol pulses misfire, and dendritic spines withdraw in silent retreat. To acknowledge those interior changes is not to surrender. It is to see the battlefield clearly.

Part II – Challenges confront the hard ground: suicide risk, systemic barriers, substance misuse and family fallout. Statistics—as many as 30 veterans dying by their own hand each day—become faces and names. Policy acronyms reveal unintended cruelty. Waiting lists are measured not in days but in funerals. Yet even here the journey of recovery refuses despair: within every challenge emerges an opportunity for intervention.

Part III – Therapies walks us through a vault of treatment options that would have sounded like science fiction a decade ago. Stellate ganglion block calms adrenal sirens in fifteen minutes. Low-dose ketamine elbows depression off its throne. MDMA-assisted psychotherapy teaches the amygdala that terror can coexist with tenderness. Psychedelics, once dismissed as counter-culture curiosities, step forward wearing white coats and carrying peer-review data. Innovation and compassion, this book insists, are not rivals but siblings.

Part IV – Foundational Healing reminds us that recovery is neither exclusively high-tech nor high-cost. Nutrition laden with omega-3 fatty acids, circadian-honoring sleep, service animals, faith traditions and community rituals belong beside PET scanners and peptide panels. A mother gardening with her son is executing neurorehabilitation just as surely as any neurosurgeon removes a brain tumor.

Part V – Emerging Science peers into the frontier: gut microbiome therapies, quantum mechanotransduction, AI-augmented care, closed-loop vagal stimulation. Here the authors stretch imagination without breaking credibility, grounding each vision in early data and ethical guardrails.

Part VI – Stories & Guidance hands the microphone to veterans and clinicians who have learned to convert scars into roadmaps. The prose, punctuated by "If–Then Guidance" and "Take the Next Step" boxes, translate theory into actionable practice. If nightmares spike, then lower evening caffeine. If isolation grows fangs, then call the peer network before midnight. All sections include tactics and so become a usable tool for healing and recovery.

Part VII – Molecular Basis shrinks the lens to the nanometer, revealing cytokine storms, neurosteroid droughts, and ion-channel tremors. Recovery, this part argues, will ultimately be as bespoke as a fingerprint: biomarker-driven and precision-timed.

Enhancing every section is the gentle charcoal artwork: a mechanic haunted by IED echoes, a nurse practitioner healing with stillness, children molding castles in fragile sand. The artwork softens what science exposes.

Part VIII – A comprehensive library of references, including popular and scientific/technical books, review papers, and scientific and medical articles on the latest developments in care and healing from PTSX and associated injuries.

Integration over Isolation

Science alone cannot vanquish an amygdala's nightmares, and empathy alone cannot tame a runaway named Neurotropic Factor. *Silent Scars* advances a radical yet ancient theorem: healing demands integration. Pair molecular diagnostics with psychotherapy. Couple psychedelics with meaning-making. Braid warrior stoicism with vulnerable storytelling. The body keeps the score, yes, but the soul writes the margin notes, and the community supplies the annotations. Even the speculative VAL™ chapter—where an empathetic robot calibrates VR landscapes to a veteran's heartbeat—illustrates the integration principle. Silicone sensors track micro-tremors. A soft-voiced avatar offers breathing cues.

A human therapist reviews biometric readouts and tailors the next session. Silicon precision meets soul-attuned presence. The future will not ask us to choose between circuit boards and compassion. It will insist we wield both.

Agency Restored

Across testimonies, survivors reclaim authorship. Jason trades beer-numbed nights for balanced therapy and learns that courage sometimes wears pajamas and shows up to 0900 appointments. Sofia, once haunted by severe trauma that splintered her timeline, watches neuroplasticity lace new dendrites across old abscesses. Colonel Josh, conditioned to outrun exhaustion, discovers that eight hours of sleep is not indulgence but strategy.

Agency here is not hollow bootstrap advice. It is a biologically plausible outcome. When inflammatory cytokines retreat, prefrontal circuits re-engage, and oxytocin trickles back into social synapses, choice emerges and expands further. The veteran who once lunged for the exit seat in every restaurant can now linger by a window, sunlight warming coffee, mission orders softened in the quiet language of safety.

From Stigma to Stewardship

Stigma, this book argues, is a public-health emergency. Silence kills just as surely as shrapnel. By exposing mis-tied arteries in military hospitals, pill-pushing shortcuts, and denial letters that reduce biochemistry to "lack of moral fiber," the authors transform blame into stewardship.

Commanders can learn to spot hypervigilance not as insubordination but as injury. Employers will discover that workplace accommodations cost pennies compared to turnover. Faith communities re-examine sermons that once equated depression with spiritual failure.

Future Directions — Twelve Vistas on the Horizon

Precision Molecular Biology & Neurobiology – Within a decade, finger-prick assays will map cytokine constellations, neurosteroid tides, and mRNA signatures in under an hour. Treatment plans will resemble custom orchestral scores, each medication, nutrient and therapy timed to the patient's biochemical rhythm.

Portable Neuroimaging – Picture a helmet much lighter than an eight-pound Kevlar, capable of simultaneous PET/MRI imaging. Medics in forward zones will scan blast-exposed soldiers before the dust settles, differentiating concussion from cerebral bleed, triaging with unprecedented clarity.

Bio-Electronic Resets – Next-generation stellate-ganglion stimulators and trans-auricular vagus paddles will act as dimmers for sympathetic overdrive. Adjustable, reversible and programmable from a smartphone, they will render panic as modifiable as volume on a radio.

Psychedelic-Assisted Integration – MDMA, psilocybin and 3-MEO-DMT, paired with trauma-trained guides, will migrate from Phase III trials to frontline clinics. Expect group protocols for unit cohesion, micro-dosing regimens for moral injury, and AI-curated playlists that sync music with neural oscillations.

Microbiome-Mind Pharmaco-nutrition – Precision pre-, pro-, and post-biotics will coax gut flora into anti-inflammatory alliances. Veterans with intractable depression will find relief in a spoonful of spore-based therapeutics rather than another SSRI.

Quantum-Level Mechanotransduction Repair – Nanocarriers loaded with antioxidant enzymes will patrol axonal membranes, patching micro-shears invisible to surgical microscopes. Physics and biology will sign an armistice in the nanoscopic trenches.

Compassionate AI – VAL™-class systems will live in rural clinics and urban shelters alike, triaging symptom spikes, scheduling follow-up, and nudging users toward hydration or breathwork. They will not replace human bond. They will widen its reach.

Trauma-Informed Governance – Policies will soon require biomarker corroboration before dismissing disability claims. "It's all in your head" will be struck from bureaucratic vocabulary, replaced by data-anchored research results, compassion and empathy. We will then be in a new era of healthcare, rooted in a molecular basis.

Trans-Generational Epigenetic Reversal – Advanced molecular biology and CRISPR-guided methylation edits may one day soften the inheritance of hypervigilance passed from combat veteran to newborn. History will still echo. It will no longer imprison.

Restorative Justice Containers – Courtrooms will weigh neurobiological evidence of trauma, offering rehabilitation pods where therapy, education and community service replace punitive isolation. Justice will pivot from retribution to repair.

Community Purpose Platforms – Veteran-led disaster-relief teams, regenerative farms and maker-spaces will channel residual adrenaline into craftsmanship. Post-deployment identities will be forged not in shadows but in shared sunlight.

Global Lexicon Shift – As PTSX becomes *lingua franca*, cultures across continents will adopt injury-not-disorder frameworks. Funding formulas will expand, stigma will contract, and the language of healing will sound less like diagnosis and more like invitation.

A Hand on Your Shoulder

Dear Reader—perhaps you are a medic still smelling diesel and dust, a survivor of childhood chaos, a clinician bone-tired of fifteen-minute appointments, or a family member scanning faces for sparks of the person you love. This section is written as a quiet hand resting on your shoulder, neither pushing nor pulling, simply reminding you that weight shared is weight diminished.

To those suffering: You are not broken glass. You are stained-glass—trauma made you both fragile and luminous. Rotate your life even a few degrees and observe how fractures refract sunrise into unexpected colors.

To clinicians: Develop your double-helix stethoscope: one ear for cytokines, the other for stories. Do not permit genomes to drown out anecdotes, nor anecdotes to eclipse lab values. Healing is a duet.

To policymakers: Budgets are moral documents. A shot of lidocaine in the neck can prevent a funeral. Audit not just the dollars spent but also the lives saved and relationships preserved.

To researchers: Publish in high-impact journals, yes, but also in kitchens, barbershops, and barracks. Translate P values into plain English so hope scales faster than hypotheses.

To families: Your patience is medicine. Your laughter is medicine. Your boundaries are medicine. Remember that secondary trauma is a real diagnosis, not a footnote Seek your own rest, support groups and therapy.

And to every reader who feels unseen: know that these pages have been written with a seat reserved just for you. You are the reason for this book and all its contents.

Closing Benediction

Across these chapters, charcoal sketches rendered in black and white, yet each vignette hinted at in saturated color. Likewise, science may diagram neurons in grayscale, but living neurons fire in technicolor gradients of possibility. This final takeaway is neither facile optimism nor sterile empiricism. It is reverent pragmatism—the conviction that rigorous knowledge wedded to radical kindness can transmute silent scars into bold remedies.

So as you close the cover of this book, resist the urge to shelve this volume under "Reference." Keep it on your desk, spill coffee on its margins, return to the "If–Then" lists when symptoms spike, screenshoot the self-assessment and text it to a friend who may be afraid to ask, and let the call-out quotes echo like chapel bells on an air base at dawn. Carry the ribbon that marks your favorite chapter the way a medic carries gauze: both field dressing and compass.

We heal in spirals—wider with each revolution. We move from trigger to tool, from wound to wisdom. And we do it together, walking each other home, one deliberate, hope-filled step after another.

—Dr. Eugene Lipov, MD
Inventor/Practitioner of Stellate Ganglion Block & Dual Sympathetic Reset Therapies
The Stella Center
Oak Park, Illinois

Resilient Souls

Amid the trials of war's fierce night,
Our soldiers stand, hearts bold, souls bright.
Through pain and shadows, fear and fight,
They bear the weight, yet seek love's light.
For those who serve, with scars unseen,
Whose minds still battle fields between—
Though wounds run deep, their spirits keen,
To heal, to rise, to become serene.
In honor of each valiant soul,
Who seeks once more to feel made whole—
May strength and peace, their lives enfold,
Our heroes brave, beautiful and bold.

—Dino Garner

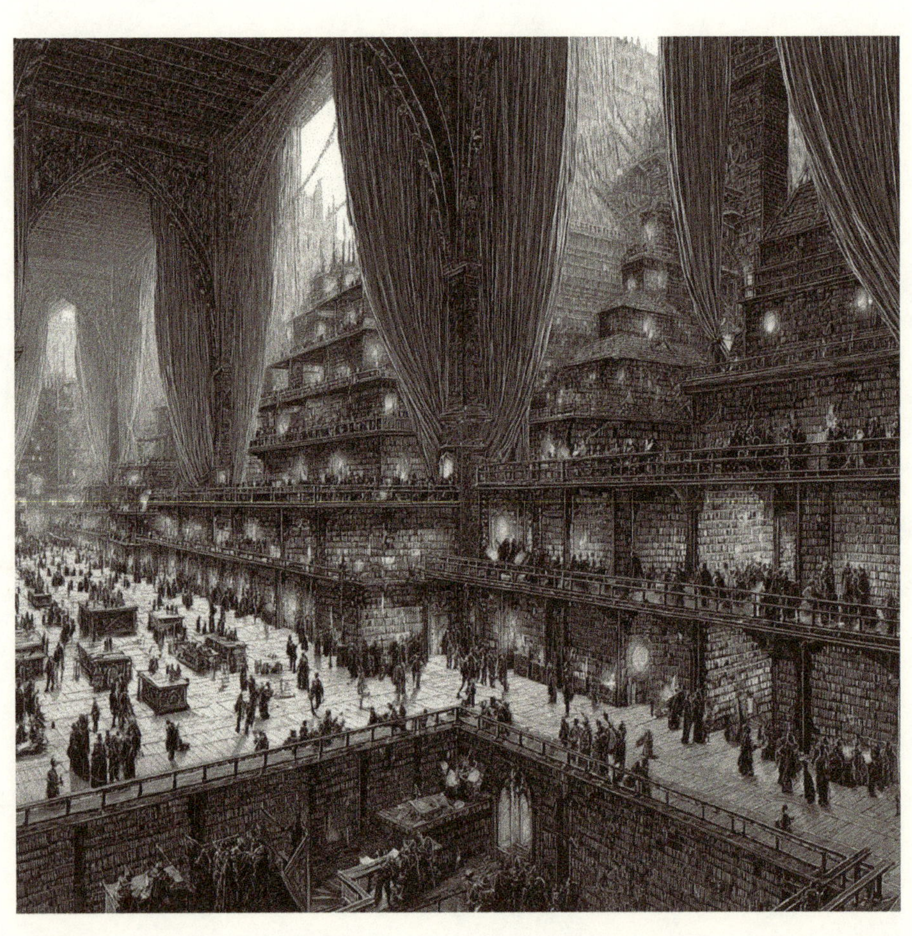

PART EIGHT

A Curated Library

Books on PTSX: Scientific, Medical and Mainstream

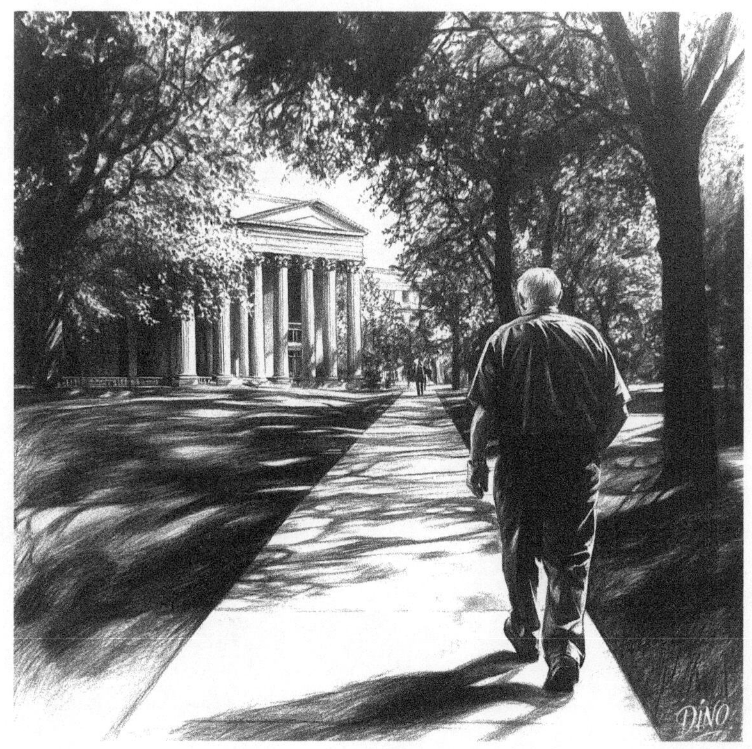

We categorized these representative books and included a brief summary of each one. This list is not complete and should be used only as a starting point for personal research. Most books are available on online bookstores.

The word **Summary** is in bold for easy reference. As you turn each page, the summaries literally jump from the page and invite you to explore before you actually consult a book at your library or purchase one from your local bookstore.

Advances in PTSX Treatments and Interventions

Forbes D, Bisson JI et al. (eds.) (2020). *Effective Treatments for PTSD: Practice Guidelines from the International Society for Traumatic Stress Studies*, 3rd ed. The Guilford Press. **Summary**: Offers comprehensive guidance on evidence-based assessments and interventions for PTSX (formerly PTSD), including novel approaches and updated recommendations for clinicians.

Friedman MJ, Keane TM and Resick PA (eds.) (2014). *Handbook of PTSD: Science and Practice* (2nd ed.) The Guilford Press. **Summary**: Provides an extensive overview of PTSX research, covering diagnosis, risk factors, neurobiology, and diverse treatment modalities.

Body-Based and Somatic Approaches

Biggs QM, Vance MC et al. (2022). The epidemiology of acute stress disorder and other early responses to trauma in adults. In J. G. Beck & D. M. Sloan (eds.), *The Oxford handbook of traumatic stress disorders* (2nd ed., pp. 97–125). Oxford University Press. **Summary**: Reviews acute stress disorder epidemiology, detailing its prevalence, risk factors and initial trauma responses among adults following traumatic exposure.

Block SH and Block CB (2010). *Mind-Body Workbook for PTSX: A 10-Week Program for Healing After Trauma*. Oakland, CA: New Harbinger Publications. **Summary**: A structured 10-week program offering a holistic approach to healing PTSX through mindfulness and cognitive techniques.

Emerson D and Hopper E (2011). *Overcoming Trauma through Yoga: Reclaiming Your Body*. Berkeley, CA: North Atlantic Books. **Summary**: Provides a guide to trauma-informed yoga practices designed to help individuals heal.

Fisher J (2021). *Transforming the Living Legacy of Trauma: A Workbook for Survivors and Therapists*. PESI Publishing. **Summary**: A practical guide combining somatic approaches with therapeutic techniques for trauma healing.

Levine, PA and Frederick A (1997). *Waking the Tiger: Healing Trauma*. North Atlantic Books. **Summary**: Introduces Somatic Experiencing (SE), a body-oriented approach to healing trauma. Emphasizes how trauma is stored in the body and how releasing it can aid PTSX recovery. Though not veteran-specific, the principles apply broadly.

Levine PA (2008). *Healing Trauma: A Pioneering Program for Restoring the Wisdom of Your Body*. Boulder, CO: Sounds True. **Summary**: Explores somatic-based trauma healing, emphasizing the body's innate ability to recover from trauma.

Levine PA (2010). *In an Unspoken Voice: How the Body Releases Trauma and Restores Goodness*. Berkeley, CA: North Atlantic Books. **Summary**: Delves into how trauma affects the body and how physical healing can lead to emotional recovery.

Levine PA (2015). *Trauma and Memory: Brain and Body in a Search for the Living Past: A Practical Guide for Understanding and Working with Traumatic Memory*. Berkeley, CA: North Atlantic Books. **Summary**: Examines the complex relationship between trauma and memory, focusing on how traumatic memories are stored and healed.

Ogden P and Fisher J (2015). *Sensorimotor Psychotherapy: Interventions for Trauma and Attachment.* WW Norton and Company. **Summary**: Although not exclusively focused on neuroception, this book incorporates the concept of body-based trauma therapy, working with neuroceptive processes to help clients regulate their autonomic responses.

Ogden P, Minton K et al. (2006). *Trauma and the Body: A Sensorimotor Approach to Psychotherapy.* New York: WW Norton and Company. **Summary**: Explores the role of sensory and motor experiences in trauma therapy, focusing on the body-centered approach to healing.

Rothschild B (2000). *The Body Remembers: The Psychophysiology of Trauma and Trauma Treatment.* New York: WW Norton and Company. **Summary**: Explains how trauma affects the body and how physical responses play a crucial role in healing PTSX.

Rothschild B (2003). *The Body Remembers Casebook: Unifying Methods and Models in the Treatment of Trauma and PTSD.* New York: WW Norton and Company. **Summary**: Provides practical examples and case studies for applying trauma therapy techniques in clinical settings.

Scaer R (2005). *The Trauma Spectrum: Hidden wounds and human resiliency.* New York: WW Norton and Company. **Summary**: Explores how trauma manifests in both mind and body, includes discussions relevant to veterans and military personnel, focuses on the holistic healing approach, integrating somatic therapy into PTSX treatment.

Neuroimaging and Brain Structure

Bremner, JD (2005). *Does Stress Damage the Brain?: Understanding Trauma-Related Disorders from a Mind-Body Perspective.* WW Norton and Company. **Summary**: Explores how chronic stress and trauma can lead to structural and functional brain changes, with implications for PTSX.

Bremner, JD (2005). *Brain Imaging Handbook.* WW Norton and Company. **Summary**: A practical guide to brain imaging techniques, focusing on their applications in PTSX research.

Saigh PA and Bremner JD (eds.). (1998). *Posttraumatic Stress Disorder: A Comprehensive Text.* Allyn & Bacon. **Summary**: Provides a detailed overview of PTSX, encompassing neurobiology, diagnosis, and therapeutic approaches.

van der Kolk BA (2015). *The Body Keeps the Score: Brain, Mind, and Body in the Healing of Trauma.* Penguin Books. **Summary**: Examines how trauma reshapes the body and brain, offering innovative strategies for recovery.

Childhood Trauma

Barrett D (2001). *Trauma and Dreams.* Harvard University Press. **Summary**: This compilation explores the profound impact of trauma on dreaming, featuring contributions from various experts who discuss how traumatic experiences manifest in dreams and the therapeutic potential of dream analysis.

Briere, JN and Scott C (2014). *Principles of Trauma Therapy: A Guide to Symptoms, Evaluation, and Treatment*. SAGE Publications. **Summary**: This comprehensive guide offers an in-depth look at trauma therapy, detailing symptomatology, assessment methods, and evidence-based treatment approaches for trauma-related disorders.

Courtois CA (2020). *It's Not You, It's What Happened to You: Complex Trauma and Treatment*. Telemachus Press, LLC. **Summary**: Provides insights into complex trauma, emphasizing that individuals' responses are normal reactions to abnormal situations, and discusses therapeutic strategies for healing.

Courtois CA and Ford JD (2015). *Treatment of Complex Trauma: A Sequenced, Relationship-Based Approach*.. The Guilford Press. **Summary**: Focuses on developmental and relational impacts of early trauma, providing empirically based treatment frameworks and emphasizing the importance of addressing dissociation and attachment disruptions.

Fisher J (2017). *Healing the Fragmented Selves of Trauma Survivors: Overcoming Internal Self-Alienation*. Routledge. **Summary**: Internal fragmentation experienced by trauma survivors, offering therapeutic techniques to help clients integrate dissociated parts of themselves.

Foo S (2022). *What My Bones Know: A Memoir of Healing from Complex Trauma*. Ballantine Books. **Summary**: Chronicles the author's journey with complex PTSX, exploring the effects of childhood trauma, the challenges of recovery, and the transformative insights gained through therapy and personal resilience.

Goodyear-Brown P (ed.) (2011). *Handbook of Child Sexual Abuse: Identification Assessment and Treatment*. Wiley. **Summary**: A multi-author resource focusing on best practices for assessing and treating childhood sexual abuse, covering evidence-based interventions and specialized approaches for survivors.

McConnaughey J (2017). *BRAVE: A Personal Story of Healing Childhood Trauma*. WestBow Press. **Summary**: The author recounts her personal journey of recovering from severe childhood trauma, emphasizing the importance of recognizing dissociation and seeking therapy tailored to individual experiences.

Mindwell L (2023). *Reclaiming Innocence: Healing the Wounds of Childhood Trauma through Creative Expression*. North Atlantic Books. **Summary**: Explores how expressive arts therapies can stimulate emotional healing and self-discovery in survivors of childhood trauma, featuring personal narratives and practical applications.

Perry BD and Szalavitz M (2007). *The Boy Who Was Raised as a Dog: And Other Stories from a Child Psychiatrist's Notebook*. Basic Books. **Summary**: Shares clinical vignettes illustrating how severe childhood trauma shapes the developing brain, highlighting treatment approaches that prioritize safety, attachment, and emotional regulation.

van der Hart, O Nijenhuis ER and Steele K (2006). *The Haunted Self: Structural Dissociation and the Treatment of Chronic Traumatization*. WW Norton and Company. **Summary**: Provides a theoretical model of structural dissociation for repeated childhood trauma, offering guidelines to address complex dissociation patterns and restore integration.

van der Kolk BA (2014). *The Body Keeps the Score: Brain, Mind, and Body in the Healing of Trauma*. Viking. **Summary**: Examines how trauma reshapes the body and brain, offering innovative strategies for recovery.

Walker P (2013). *Complex PTSD: From Surviving to Thriving*. Azure Coyote Press. **Summary**: A self-help guide addressing the long-term aftermath of prolonged childhood trauma, offering tools for building emotional regulation, healthy boundaries, and self-compassion.

Clinical Applications

Shapiro F (2017). *Eye Movement Desensitization and Reprocessing (EMDR): Basic principles, protocols, and procedures*. The Guilford Press. **Summary**: Though not traditionally somatic therapy, EMDR incorporates body awareness and has been highly effective in trauma recovery, including among veterans with PTSX.

Sloan DM and Marx BP (2019). *Written Exposure Therapy for PTSD: A brief treatment approach for mental health professionals*. American Psychological Association Press. http://dx.doi.org/10.1037/0000139-001. **Summary**: Presents a concise, evidence-based guide for mental health professionals on implementing Written Exposure Therapy as an effective and accessible treatment for individuals with post-traumatic stress-related challenges.

Clinical and Treatment Guides

Banitt SP (2018). *Wisdom, Attachment, and Love in Trauma Therapy: Beyond Evidence-Based Practice*. Routledge. **Summary**: A holistic guide to trauma therapy that integrates wisdom traditions with modern therapeutic practices.

Briere JN and Scott C (2012). *Principles of Trauma Therapy: A Guide to Symptoms, Evaluation, and Treatment*. Thousand Oaks, CA: SAGE Publications. **Summary**: A comprehensive manual for clinicians offering integrative approaches to trauma treatment.

Bremner JD and Marmar CR (1998). *Trauma, Memory, and Dissociation*. Washington, DC: American Psychiatric Association Publishing. **Summary**: Explores the intersection of trauma, attachment and dissociation.

Herman J (1997). *Trauma and Recovery: The Aftermath of Violence—From Domestic Abuse to Political Terror*. New York: Basic Books. **Summary**: A seminal work that redefined the understanding of trauma and recovery, focusing on both individual and societal implications.

Muller RT (2018). *Trauma and the Struggle to Open Up: From Avoidance to Recovery and Growth*. New York: WW Norton and Company. **Summary**: Examines the challenges of opening up about trauma and the importance of vulnerability in the healing process.

Steele K, Boon S and van der Hart O (2016). *Treating Trauma-Related Dissociation: A Practical, Integrative Approach*. New York: WW Norton and Company. **Summary**: Provides strategies for clinicians working with dissociative disorders related to trauma.

Comorbidities With PTSX

Brady KT, Back SE and Greenfield SF (eds.) (2009). *Women and Addiction: A Comprehensive Handbook.* The Guilford Press. **Summary**: Although not exclusively on PTSX, many chapters address the intersection of trauma and substance use in female populations.

Gordon M (2015). *Traumatic Brain Injury: A Clinical Approach to Brain Health.* Millennium Health Press. **Summary**: Discusses the endocrinological and neurological implications of traumatic brain injury, offering a functional medicine approach for restoring cognitive and emotional health.

Jakupcak M, Wagner AW et al. (2020). *The PTSD Behavioral Activation Workbook: Activities to Help You Rebuild Your Life from Post-Traumatic Stress Disorder.* New Harbinger Publications. **Summary**: Offers practical activities based on behavioral activation techniques to help individuals with PTSX re-engage in meaningful life activities, aiming to reduce avoidance behaviors and improve mood.

Najavits LM (2001). *Seeking Safety: A Treatment Manual for PTSD and Substance Abuse.* The Guilford Press. **Summary**: Present-focused therapy designed to simultaneously address PTSX and substance-use disorders, emphasizing safe coping skills and psychoeducation.

Epigenetics

Carey N (2013). *The Epigenetics Revolution: How Modern Biology is Rewriting Our Understanding of Genetics, Disease, and Inheritance*. Columbia University Press. **Summary**: Explores the foundational concepts of epigenetics and its implications for health, disease, and human behavior.

Francis RC (2012). *Epigenetics: How Environment Shapes Our Genes*. WW Norton and Company. **Summary**: Examines how environmental factors influence gene expression and the broader implications for health and society.

Sapolsky RM (2017). *Behave: The Biology of Humans at Our Best and Worst*. Penguin Press. **Summary**: Discusses the complex interplay between genetics, environment, and behavior, providing insights into how these factors contribute to stress and trauma-related conditions.

Emerging and Established Therapies for PTSX

Resick PA, Monson CM and Chard KM (2024). *Cognitive Processing Therapy for PTSD: A Comprehensive Manual*. The Guilford Press. **Summary**: Presents a proven, structured protocol for treating PTSX, detailing session-by-session interventions and guidance for addressing stuck points.

Schnyder U and Cloitre M (eds.) (2022). *Evidence Based Treatments for Trauma-Related Psychological Disorders: A Practical Guide for Clinicians*. Springer. **Summary**: Offers a variety of established and emerging interventions, including EMDR, prolonged exposure, and other innovative treatments, supported by empirical evidence.

Exercise as Medicine

Block SH (2010). *Mind-Body Workbook for PTSX: A 10-Week Program for Healing After Trauma*. Oakland, CA: New Harbinger Publications. **Summary**: A structured program offering a holistic approach to healing PTSX through cognitive techniques.

Carless D and Douglas K (2010). *Sport and Physical Activity for Mental Health*. Wiley-Blackwell. **Summary**: Investigates how structured physical activities can alleviate depression, anxiety, and PTSX symptoms, with case examples demonstrating the therapeutic benefits of exercise.

Emerson D and Hopper E (2011). *Overcoming Trauma through Yoga: Reclaiming Your Body*. Berkeley, CA: North Atlantic Books. **Summary**: Provides a guide to trauma-informed yoga practices designed to help individuals heal from PTSX.

Ratey JJ and Hagerman E (2013). *Spark: The Revolutionary New Science of Exercise and the Brain*. New York, NY: Little, Brown Spark. **Summary**: Explores how physical exercise benefits the brain, and its role in improving mood, cognition and resilience to stress.

van der Kolk BA (2014). *The Body Keeps the Score: Brain, Mind, and Body in the Healing of Trauma*. Viking. **Summary**: Examines how trauma reshapes the body and brain, offering innovative strategies for recovery.

General Topics & Epidemiology

Biggs QM, Vance MC et al. (2022). The epidemiology of acute stress disorder and other early responses to trauma in adults. In J. G. Beck & D. M. Sloan (Eds.), *The Oxford handbook of traumatic stress disorders* (2nd ed., pp. 97–125). Oxford University Press. **Summary**: Reviews acute stress disorder epidemiology, detailing its prevalence, risk factors and initial trauma responses among adults following traumatic exposure.

Friedman MJ (2008). *After the War Zone: A Practical Guide for Returning Troops and Their Families.* Balance. **Summary**: Examines the historical development and epidemiology of PTSX in military populations, offering insight into screening practices and public health approaches.

Hyperbaric Oxygen Therapy for PTSX

Harch PG and McCullough V (2010). *The Oxygen Revolution: Hyperbaric Oxygen Therapy and the Healing of Trauma*. Hatherleigh Press. **Summary**: Discusses the theoretical basis of hyperbaric oxygen therapy for PTSX and presents clinical experiences showing symptom improvement and neurocognitive benefits.

McCabe E (2011). *Flood Your Body With Oxygen: Therapy for Our Polluted World*. Energy Publications LLC. **Summary**: Advocates for oxygen-based therapies to counteract environmental toxins, suggesting protocols that may bolster overall health and resilience to stress.

Mindfulness and Meditation

Brach T (2004). *Radical Acceptance: Embracing Your Life With the Heart of a Buddha*. Bantam. **Summary**: Guides readers in applying mindfulness and acceptance to heal emotional wounds and foster self-compassion after trauma.

Brach T (2013). *True Refuge: Finding Peace and Freedom in Your Own Awakened Heart*. Bantam. **Summary**: Continues the exploration of mindfulness-based strategies for coping with trauma, focusing on compassion practices and emotional healing.

Follett VM, Briere J et al. (2017). *Mindfulness-Based Interventions for Trauma: Integrating Contemplative Practices*. The Guilford Press. **Summary**: Provides theoretical foundations and practical applications of mindfulness-based therapies for trauma survivors, including those with PTSX.

Germer CK Siegel RD and Fulton PR (eds.) (2013). *Mindfulness and Psychotherapy* (2nd ed). The Guilford Press. **Summary**: Presents a collection of essays and research on integrating mindfulness into clinical practice, including strategies for addressing trauma-related symptoms.

Kabat-Zinn J (2013). *Full Catastrophe Living: Using the Wisdom of Your Body and Mind to Face Stress Pain and Illness*. Bantam Books. **Summary**: Introduces mindfulness-based stress reduction (MBSR) for managing stress, pain and trauma, offering techniques for cultivating resilience.

Kornfield J (2009). *The Wise Heart: A Guide to the Universal Teachings of Buddhist Psychology*. Bantam. **Summary**: Explores how Buddhist principles and mindfulness-based practices can support emotional resilience and recovery from trauma.

Treleaven DA (2018). *Trauma-Sensitive Mindfulness: Practices for Safe and Transformative Healing*. New York: WW Norton and Company. **Summary**: Offers practical techniques for integrating mindfulness safely in trauma therapy to promote transformative healing.

Novel Treatment Approaches

Sloan M (2018). *Red Light Therapy: Miracle Medicine*. Lulu Press. **Summary**: Explores the science behind red and near-infrared light therapy, highlighting its potential to reduce inflammation, boost cellular health, and complement trauma recovery protocols.

Personal Growth and Recovery

Burke Harris N (2018). *The Deepest Well: Healing the Long-Term Effects of Childhood Adversity*. New York: Houghton Mifflin Harcourt. **Summary**: Examines how childhood trauma impacts long-term health and offers strategies for healing adverse childhood experiences.

Tedeschi RG, Park CL and Calhoun LG (1998). *Post-Traumatic Growth: Positive Changes in the Aftermath of Crisis*. Mahwah, NJ: Lawrence Erlbaum Associates. **Summary**: Discusses the phenomenon of post-traumatic growth and how individuals can experience positive psychological changes following trauma.

Epstein M (2014). *The Trauma of Everyday Life*. New York: Penguin Press. **Summary**: Blends Buddhist philosophy and psychotherapy to explore how trauma is an inherent part of life and offers insights into emotional healing.

Frankl VE (1959). *Man's Search for Meaning*. Boston: Beacon Press. **Summary**: A classic exploration of how individuals find meaning after traumatic experiences, offering insights into resilience and survival.

Lee D (2012). *The Compassionate Mind Approach to Recovering from Trauma*. London: Robinson Publishing. **Summary**: Integrates compassion-focused therapy with trauma recovery, offering strategies for building emotional resilience.

Nakazawa DJ (2016). *Childhood Disrupted: How Your Biography Becomes Your Biology, and How You Can Heal.* New York: Atria Books. **Summary**: Explores how adverse childhood experiences (ACEs) can impact long-term health and offers pathways for healing.

Walker P (2013). *Complex PTSX: From Surviving to Thriving*. New York: Azure Coyote Press. **Summary**: A self-help guide that offers strategies for healing from prolonged trauma and focuses on Complex PTSX.

Polyvagal Theory and Nervous System

Dana D (2020). *Polyvagal Exercises for Safety and Connection: 50 Client-Centered Practices.* WW Norton and Company. **Summary**: A practical guide with exercises designed for therapists to help individuals apply Polyvagal Theory principles in therapy sessions for better safety and connection.

Dana D (2020). *Polyvagal Flip Chart: Understanding the Science of Safety*. WW Norton and Company. **Summary**: A visual aid that helps therapists explain Polyvagal Theory concepts to clients, making complex neurophysiological ideas more understandable.

Dana D (2021). *Anchored: How to Befriend Your Nervous System Using Polyvagal Theory*. Sounds True. **Summary**: Offers a guide for individuals to understand and apply Polyvagal Theory in their everyday lives, focusing on emotional and physical regulation.

Dana D and Porges SW (2018). *The Polyvagal Theory in Therapy: Engaging the Rhythm of Regulation*. WW Norton and Company. **Summary**: Provides practical applications of neuroception in therapy, guiding therapists on how to work with clients' autonomic states and improve their capacity for detecting safety.

Porges SW (2011). *The Polyvagal Theory: Neurophysiological Foundations of Emotions, Attachment, Communication, and Self-Regulation*. New York: WW Norton and Company. **Summary**: Introduces Polyvagal Theory and neuroception, explaining how the nervous system responds to trauma and its implications for therapy.

Porges SW (2017). *The Pocket Guide to the Polyvagal Theory: The Transformative Power of Feeling Safe*. Norton. **Summary**: A more accessible version of the original text, aimed at helping clinicians and therapists understand and apply Polyvagal Theory in their practice.

Porges SW (2021). *Polyvagal Safety: Attachment, Communication, Self-Regulation*. WW Norton and Company. **Summary**: Expands on the role of safety in human behavior, and how it applies to therapeutic and clinical settings.

Porges SW (2024). *Polyvagal Perspectives Interventions, Practices and Strategies*. WW Norton and Company. **Summary**: Polyvagal Theory applications specifically for trauma recovery and PTSX treatment.

Porges SW and Dana D (2018). *Clinical Applications of the Polyvagal Theory: The Emergence of Polyvagal-Informed Therapies*. WW Norton and Company. **Summary**: Discusses how neuroception and other concepts from Polyvagal Theory are applied in clinical settings to treat trauma, anxiety, and other disorders.

PTSX and the Gut Microbiome

Anderson SC, Cryan JF and Dinan T (2017). *The Psychobiotic Revolution: Mood, Food, and the New Science of the Gut-Brain Connection*. Harper Wave. **Summary**: Explores the emerging science of psychobiotics, emphasizing how gut bacteria influence mood and mental health and providing strategies for improving emotional resilience through gut health.

Enders, G (2018). *Gut: The Inside Story of Our Body's Most Underrated Organ*. Greystone Books. **Summary**: Provides a comprehensive and accessible overview of the gut's functions, including its microbiome, and its impact on physical and mental health.

Mayer E (2016). *The Mind-Gut Connection: How the Hidden Conversation Within Our Bodies Impacts Our Mood, Our Choices, and Our Overall Health*. Harper Wave. **Summary**: Investigates the intricate communication between the gut and brain, emphasizing its implications for mental health and emotional wellbeing.

Perlmutter D (2015). *Brain Maker: The Power of Gut Microbes to Heal and Protect Your Brain—For Life*. Little, Brown Spark. **Summary**: Examines the critical role of the gut microbiome in neurological and mental health, advocating for dietary and lifestyle changes to optimize gut-brain communication.

PTSX and Substance Use Disorder Comorbidity

Brady KT, Back SE and Greenfield SF (eds.) (2009). *Women and Addiction: A Comprehensive Handbook*. The Guilford Press. **Summary**: Although broader in scope, contains key chapters on the intersection of trauma and addiction, focusing on PTSX risk factors and gender-specific treatment approaches.

PTSX and the Whole Body

Dana D (2018). *The Polyvagal Theory in Therapy: Engaging the Rhythm of Regulation*. WW Norton and Company. **Summary**: Provides practical applications of Polyvagal Theory, helping therapists work with clients' autonomic states to promote safety and emotional regulation.

Emerson D and Hopper E (2017). *Overcoming Trauma through Yoga: Reclaiming Your Body*. Read How You Want Books. **Summary**: Offers a guide to trauma-informed yoga practices designed to support individuals in healing from PTSX.

Lilley J (2019). *Heavy Metals Detox*. Independent Publishing. **Summary**: Examines the impacts of heavy-metal accumulation on the human body and outlines detoxification strategies for improved health and vitality.

Rothschild B (2000). *The Body Remembers: The Psychophysiology of Trauma and Trauma Treatment*. WW Norton and Company. **Summary**: Examines the body's involuntary responses to trauma, detailing how body-centered interventions can effectively address PTSX symptoms.

Somerville J (2018). *The Optimal Dose: Restore Your Health With the Power of Vitamin D3*. Independently Published. **Summary**: Investigates the therapeutic benefits of high-dose vitamin D3 supplementation, proposing protocols to enhance immune function and potentially mitigate stress-related disorders.

van der Kolk BA (2015). *The Body Keeps the Score: Brain, Mind, and Body in the Healing of Trauma*. Penguin Books. **Summary**: Explores how trauma affects the body and mind and provides innovative methods for healing, including movement, EMDR, and neurofeedback.

Walker P (2013). *Complex PTSD: From Surviving to Thriving*. Azure Coyote Publishing. **Summary**: A practical guide for understanding and recovering from complex trauma, focusing on emotional healing and personal growth.

Resilience Social Support and Post-Traumatic Growth in PTSX

Calhoun LG and Tedeschi RG (1999). *Facilitating Posttraumatic Growth: A Clinician's Guide.* Mahwah, NJ: Lawrence Erlbaum Associates. **Summary**: Clinician's manual explaining theoretical foundations, assessment techniques, and therapeutic interventions that help trauma survivors achieve positive psychological change, meaning, and enhanced relationships after adversity.

Calhoun LG and Tedeschi RG (eds.) (2006). *The Handbook of Posttraumatic Growth: Research and Practice.* Mahwah, NJ: Lawrence Erlbaum Associates. **Summary**: Comprehensive reference compiling empirical findings, theoretical models, measurement issues, and applied approaches across diverse populations, illuminating mechanisms and practical considerations for building posttraumatic growth.

Calhoun LG and Tedeschi RG (2012). *Posttraumatic Growth in Clinical Practice.* New York, NY: Routledge. **Summary**: Upcoming volume translating posttraumatic growth research into actionable clinical techniques, presenting case studies, assessment tools, and integrative treatment protocols for various trauma-affected populations.

Tedeschi RG and Calhoun LG (1995). *Trauma and Transformation: Growing in the Aftermath of Suffering.* Thousand Oaks, CA: Sage. **Summary**: Seminal text introducing concept of growth through trauma, presenting qualitative research and survivor narratives demonstrating new perspectives, personal strength, and relational depth after suffering.

Tedeschi RG, Park CL and Calhoun LG (eds.) (1998). *Posttraumatic Growth: Positive Changes in the Aftermath of Crisis*. Mahwah, NJ: Lawrence Erlbaum Associates. **Summary**: Edited collection surveying theoretical frameworks, methodological challenges, and empirical studies highlighting positive psychological changes following crises, with cross-cultural perspectives and practical clinical implications.

Stellate Ganglion Block

Lipov E and Ungeldi L (2026). *The God Shot: Healing Trauma's Legacy: The Science, the Stories, the Solution*. Post Hill Press. **Summary**: In *The God Shot*, Dr. Eugene Lipov reframes trauma as a visible, treatable brain injury. He introduces a revolutionary nerve block procedures, Stellate Ganglion Block and Dual Sympathetic Reset, that reset the body's stuck fight-or-flight response. Based on verified neuroscience, these treatments offers instant calm and a biology-based blueprint for lasting recovery from invisible wounds.

Savastano S (ed.) (2025). *Percutaneous Stellate Ganglion Block for Electrical Storm.* Springer. **Summary**: Comprehensive manual outlines autonomic-driven ventricular arrhythmias and details rationale, evidence, and step-by-step technique for life-saving percutaneous stellate ganglion block in electrical storm.

Traditional Therapeutic Approaches

Herman JL (2022). *Trauma and Recovery: The Aftermath of Violence—From Domestic Abuse to Political Terror*. Basic Books. **Summary**: A seminal text that redefined trauma treatment, outlining phased recovery (safety, remembrance, reconnection) and its relevance to both individual and collective healing.

Trauma Science and Research

Shaili J (2019). *The Unspeakable Mind: Stories of Trauma and Healing from the Frontlines of PTSD Science*. Harper Wave. **Summary**: Combines cutting-edge research with patient stories to explore PTSX treatment advances.

Lewis MD (2016). *When Brains Collide: What Every Athlete and Parent Should Know About the Treatment of Concussions and Head Injuries*. Austin: Lioncrest Publishing. **Summary**: Provides an overview of concussion science, offering actionable strategies to identify, manage, and treat head injuries while mitigating long-term risks.

Morris DJ (2015). *The Evil Hours: A Biography of Post-Traumatic Stress Disorder*. Boston: Eamon Dolan/Houghton Mifflin Harcourt. **Summary**: A deeply personal exploration of PTSX, blending history, science and personal experience to examine its effects and treatment.

van der Kolk, Bessel A et al. (eds.) (1996). *Traumatic stress: The effects of overwhelming experience on mind, body, and society*. The Guilford Press. **Summary**: Explores long-term trauma effects and various treatment approaches, including somatic therapies. Focuses on trauma in military and veteran populations with evidence-based support for body-oriented treatments.

van der Kolk and Bessel A (2015). *The Body Keeps the Score: Brain, Mind, and Body in the Healing of Trauma*. Viking. **Summary**: Examines how trauma affects both the mind and body, emphasizing somatic methods such as yoga, EMDR, and body awareness for PTSX treatment. Specific discussions on veterans and military trauma.

The Vagus Nerve

Rosenberg S (2017). *Accessing the healing power of the vagus nerve: self-help exercises for anxiety, depression, trauma, and autism.* Berkeley, CA: North Atlantic Books. **Summary**: Offers gentle craniosacral, breathing, and movement exercises that stimulate vagus nerve tone, easing anxiety, depression, trauma symptoms, and enhancing social engagement in autism spectrum conditions.

Tracey, KJ (2025). *The Great Nerve*. Avery. **Summary**: Distills neurosurgeon Dr. Kevin J. Tracey's pioneering work on bioelectronic medicine, showing how precisely timed electrical stimulation of the vagus nerve can trigger the body's anti-inflammatory reflex and dramatically improve—or even reverse—chronic conditions such as rheumatoid arthritis, inflammatory bowel disease, lupus, diabetes, depression, Alzheimer's and Parkinson's, all illustrated through compelling patient recoveries and rigorous clinical evidence.

Workbooks and Professional Resources

Lipsky L (2009). *Trauma Stewardship: An Everyday Guide to Caring for Self While Caring for Others*. San Francisco: Berrett-Koehler Publishers. **Summary**: A guide for caregivers and trauma professionals to manage secondary trauma and maintain personal wellbeing while helping others.

Naparstek B (2005). *The Invisible Heroes: Survivors of Trauma and How They Heal*. New York: Random House. **Summary**: Focuses on how survivors of trauma can heal, with an emphasis on the use of guided imagery as a recovery tool.

Perry BD and Szalavitz M (2007). *The Boy Who Was Raised as a Dog: And Other Stories from a Child Psychiatrist's Notebook*. New York: Basic Books. **Summary**: Uses real-life cases to illustrate the profound impact of childhood trauma and offers insights into effective healing methods.

Schiraldi GR (2009). *The Post-Traumatic Stress Disorder Sourcebook*. New York: McGraw-Hill Education. **Summary**: A comprehensive guide offering a variety of treatment options and strategies for understanding and overcoming PTSX.

Shapiro F and Forrest MS (2016). *EMDR: The Breakthrough Therapy for Overcoming Anxiety, Stress, and Trauma*. New York: Basic Books. **Summary**: A key text on EMDR therapy, offering insights into this breakthrough treatment for anxiety, stress, and trauma.

Williams MB and Soili P (2016). *The PTSX Workbook: Simple, Effective Techniques for Overcoming Traumatic Stress Symptoms*. Oakland, CA: New Harbinger Publications. **Summary**: A self-help workbook filled with practical exercises for individuals coping with PTSX symptoms.

Wolynn M (2017). *It Didn't Start with You: How Inherited Family Trauma Shapes Who We Are and How to End the Cycle*. New York: Penguin Life. **Summary**: The intergenerational transmission of trauma and offers techniques for breaking the cycle of inherited trauma.

State of the Art in PTSX: Annotated Review Articles

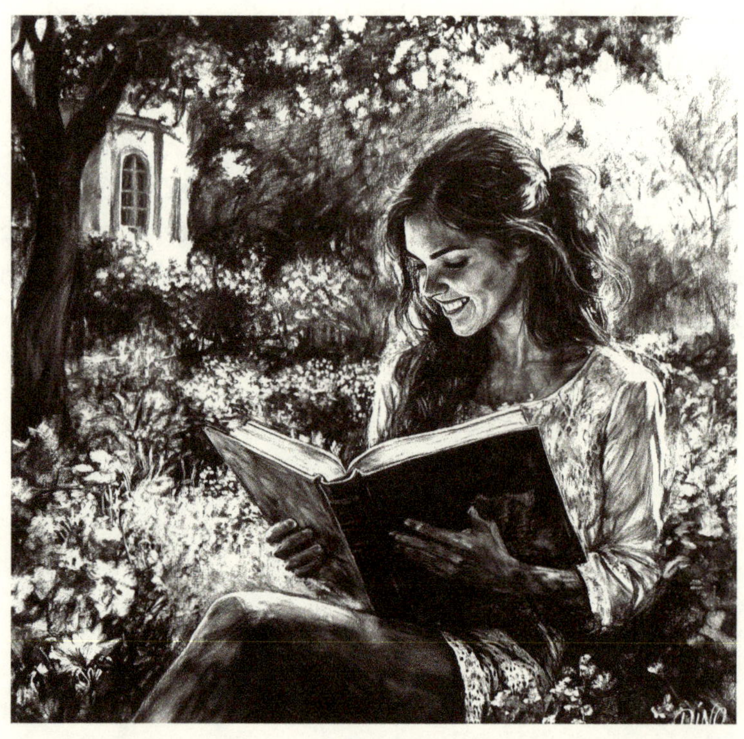

Review articles provide a general overview or "state of the art" of a particular subject. They typically survey a number of scientific and medical articles, then summarize them in general terms. All are categorized for easy reference, and the names of all journals spelled out completely.

We also include a brief **Summary** of each article. The word **Summary** is in bold for easy reference. As you turn each page, the summaries literally jump from the page and invite you to explore before you actually consult an article.

Advances in PTSX Treatments and Interventions

Belsher BE, Beech EH et al. (2024). Internet and Mobile Interventions for Adults with PTSX and Their Family Members: A Systematic Review. Department of Veterans Affairs (US). PMID: 39167690. **Summary**: Evaluates online and mobile tools for managing PTSX in veterans and their families, noting limited but evolving evidence.

Resnik J, Miller CJ et al. (2024). A Systematic Review of the Department of Veterans Affairs Mental Health-Care Access Interventions for Veterans With PTSX. *Military Medicine* 189(5–6), 1303–1311. doi: 10.1093/milmed/usad376. **Summary**: Reviews VA mental health-care interventions aimed at improving access for veterans with PTSX.

Shalev AY, Liberzon I and Marmar C (2017). Post-Traumatic Stress Disorder. *The New England Journal of Medicine* Jun 22;376(25):2459-2469. doi: 10.1056/NEJMra1612499. **Summary**: This comprehensive review provides an overview of PTSX, including its etiology, clinical features, and evidence-based treatment approaches.

Challenges and Impacts

Almeida TM, Lacerda da Silva UR et al. (2024). Effectiveness of Ketamine for the Treatment of Post-Traumatic Stress Disorder - A Systematic Review and Meta-Analysis. *Clinical Neuropsychiatry* 21(1):22-31. doi: 10.36131/cnfioritieditore20240102. **Summary**: Summarizes state of the art for using ketamine as therapy for, and to manage, PTSX.

IsHak WW, Meyer A et al. (2024). Overview of Psychiatric Medications in the Pipeline in Phase III Trials as of June 1, 2024: A Systematic Review. *Innovations in Clinical Neuroscience* 21(7–9), 27–47. PMID: 39329027. **Summary**: Summarizes emerging pharmacological treatments for psychiatric conditions currently in advanced clinical trials, discussing potential implications for practice and research.

Hashimoto K. (2019). Rapid-acting antidepressant ketamine, its metabolites and other candidates: A historical overview and future perspective. *Psychiatry Clinical Neuroscience* 73(10):613-627. doi: 10.1111/pcn.12902. **Summary**: Explores rapid-acting antidepressants, including ketamine, as innovative treatments for types of PTSX including major depressive disorder.

Liu JJW, Ein N et al. (2024). Ketamine in the effective management of chronic pain, depression, and PTSX for Veterans: A meta-analysis and systematic review. *Frontiers in Psychiatry* 15. doi: 10.3389/fpsyt.2024.1338581. **Summary**: Finds ketamine shows promise in addressing co-occurring pain, depression, and PTSX in military populations.

Ragnhildstveit A, Roscoe J et al. (2023). The potential of ketamine for posttraumatic stress disorder: a review of clinical evidence. *Therapeutic Advances in Psychopharmacology* 13. doi: 10.1177/20451253231154125. **Summary**: Evaluates clinical evidence suggesting ketamine shows promising rapid antidepressant and anti-anxiety effects for treating posttraumatic stress disorder, warranting further robust clinical investigation.

Childhood Trauma

Karimov-Zwienenberg M, Symphor W et al. (2024). Childhood trauma, PTSD/CPTSD and chronic pain: A systematic review. *PLOS* (Public Library of Science) *One* 19(8), e0309332. https://doi.org/10.1371/journal.pone.0309332. **Summary**: This systematic review examines the associations between childhood trauma, PTSX/CPTSX, and chronic pain in adults, highlighting the complex interplay between early adverse experiences and long-term physical health outcomes.

Sweeney A, Filson B et al. (2018). A paradigm shift: Relationships in trauma-informed mental health services. *British Journal of Psychology Advances* 24(5), 319–333. doi: 10.1192/bja.2018.29. **Summary**: This review discusses the importance of adopting trauma-informed approaches in mental health services, emphasizing the need for relational safety and collaborative practices to support recovery.

Comorbidities with PTSX

Bisson JI, Olff M (2020). Prevention and treatment of PTSD: the current evidence base. *European Journal of Psychotraumatology* 11(1), 1824381. doi: 10.1080/20008198.2020.1824381. **Summary**: Provides a comprehensive review of the current evidence base for the prevention and treatment of PTSX, discussing various therapeutic approaches and their efficacy.

Jimenez-Labaig P, Aymerich C et al. (2024). A comprehensive examination of mental health in patients with head and neck cancer: systematic review and meta-analysis. *Journal of the National Cancer Institute Cancer Spectrum* 8(3), pkae031. doi: 10.1093/jncics/pkae031. **Summary**: Details the prevalence of depression, anxiety, and PTSX in head and neck cancer patients.

Passos IC, Vasconcelos-Moreno MP et al. (2015). Inflammatory markers in post-traumatic stress disorder: a systematic review, meta-analysis, and meta-regression. *Lancet Psychiatry* 2(11):1002-12. doi: 10.1016/S2215-0366(15)00309-0. **Summary**: Investigates the presence of neuroinflammatory markers in PTSX, providing robust evidence for heightened inflammatory signaling as a contributor to trauma-related symptoms and potential intervention targets.

Qassem T, Aly-ElGabry D et al. (2021). Psychiatric Co-Morbidities in Post-Traumatic Stress Disorder: Detailed Findings from the Adult Psychiatric Morbidity Survey in the English Population. *Psychiatric Quarterly* 92(1):321-330. doi: 10.1007/s11126-020-09797-4. **Summary**: Investigates the frequency and impact of psychiatric comorbidities in individuals with PTSX, highlighting the challenges in diagnosis and treatment due to overlapping symptoms.

Emerging Science and Innovation

Andrews SR and Harch PG (2024). Systematic review and dosage analysis: hyperbaric oxygen therapy efficacy in the treatment of posttraumatic stress disorder. *Frontiers in Neurology* 15:1360311. doi: 10.3389/fneur.2024.1360311. **Summary**: This systematic review and meta-analysis evaluates the efficacy of hyperbaric oxygen therapy (HOT) in controlled trials for treating PTSX.

Antos Z, Zackiewicz K et al. (2024). Beyond Pharmacology: A Narrative Review of Alternative Therapies for Anxiety Disorders. *Diseases* 12(9), 216. doi: 10.3390/diseases12090216. Epub 2024 Sep 16. **Summary**: Discusses a range of non-pharmacological therapies—including mindfulness, yoga, and other integrative approaches—for effectively managing anxiety disorders.

Barch D and Liston C (2024) Neuroimaging in psychiatry: toward mechanistic insights and clinical utility. *Neuropsychopharmacology* 50, 1–2. https://doi.org/10.1038/s41386-024-01984-2. **Summary**: Reviews current imaging in psychiatric disorders.

Damsa C, Kosel M and Moussally J (2009). Current status of brain imaging in anxiety disorders. *Current Opinions in Psychiatry* 22(1):96-110. doi: 10.1097/YCO.0b013e328319bd10. **Summary**: Reviews neuroimaging findings in anxiety disorders, focusing on structural and functional brain changes associated with the disorder.

Liberzon I and Abelson JL (2016). Context processing and the neurobiology of PTSD. *Neuron* 92(1), 14-30. doi: 10.1016/j.neuron.2016.09.039 **Summary**: Highlights impaired context processing in PTSX, emphasizing its relationship to amygdala hyperactivity and other neurobiological features.

Peter H. (2025). Neuroimaging Findings in Psychiatric Disorders. Researchgate.net/publication/392392560_Neuroimaging_Findings_in_Psychiatric_Disorders. **Summary**: Discusses the latest neuroimaging findings, offering insights into the structural and functional alterations in PTSX.

Epigenetics

Bale TL and Epperson CN (2015). Sex differences and stress across the lifespan. *Nature Neuroscience* 18(10):1413-20. doi: 10.1038/nn.4112. **Summary**: Reviews how genetic and epigenetic mechanisms underlie sex differences in stress responses and their implications for disorders like PTSX.

Klengel T and Binder EB (2015). Epigenetics of stress-related psychiatric disorders and gene-environment interactions. *Neuron* 86(6), 1343-1357. doi: 10.1016/j.neuron.2015.05.036. **Summary**: Summarizes research on the role of epigenetics in stress-related disorders, including the impact of environmental influences on genetic predispositions.

Nestler EJ (2014). Epigenetic mechanisms of depression. *Journal of the American Medical Association Psychiatry* 71(4), 454-456. doi: 10.1001/jamapsychiatry.2013.4291. **Summary**: Discusses the role of epigenetic changes in the development and progression of depression, highlighting parallels with PTSX.

Smith KV and Johnson EM (2022). The role of genetic and epigenetic factors in the development of PTSD: A review. *Psychological Medicine* 52(7), 1234-1243. doi: 10.31887/DCNS.2019.21.4/kressler. **Summary**: This review examines the contributions of genetic and epigenetic factors to PTSX development, shedding light on biological underpinnings and potential personalized interventions.

Turecki G and Meaney MJ (2016). Effects of the social environment and stress on glucocorticoid receptor gene methylation: A systematic review. *Biological Psychiatry* 79(2), 87-96. doi: 10.1016/j.biopsych.2014.11.022. **Summary**: Explores the impact of stress and environment on glucocorticoid receptor methylation and its relevance to stress disorders like PTSX.

Exercise as Medicine

Bisson JI, Roberts NP and Andrew M (2013). Psychological therapies for chronic PTSX in adults. *The Cochrane Database of Systematic Reviews* 2013(12):CD003388. doi: 10.1002/14651858.CD003388.pub4. **Summary**: Evaluates the efficacy of various psychological therapies for chronic PTSX in adults.

Fetzner MG and Asmundson GJG (2015). Aerobic exercise reduces symptoms of posttraumatic stress disorder: A randomized controlled trial. *Cognitive Behaviour Therapy* 44(4), 301-313. doi: 10.1080/16506073.2015.1012. **Summary**: Aerobic exercise significantly reduces PTSX symptoms, providing evidence for its therapeutic efficacy.

Rosenbaum S, Tiedemann A and Sherrington C (2014). Physical activity interventions for people with mental illness: a systematic review and meta-analysis. *Journal of Clinical Psychiatry* 75(9):964-74. doi: 10.4088/JCP.13r08765. **Summary**: Reviews the effectiveness of exercise interventions for mental disorders, emphasizing their benefits for conditions like PTSX and depression.

Tsatsoulis A and Fountoulakis S (2006). The protective role of exercise on stress system dysregulation and comorbidities. *Annals of the New York Academy of Sciences* 1083, 196-213. doi: 10.1196/annals.1367.020. **Summary**: Examines how exercise mitigates stress-related disorders by regulating the hypothalamic-pituitary-adrenal axis (HPA axis).

Zhao F, Liu C and Lin Z (2025). A narrative review of exercise intervention mechanisms for PTSX in veterans. *Frontiers in Public Health* 12. doi: 10.3389/fpubh.2024.1483077. **Summary**: Examines how structured exercise protocols might reduce PTSX symptom burden in military service members.

Foundational Healing Approaches

Payne P, Levine PA and Crane-Godreau MA (2015). Somatic experiencing: Using interoception and proprioception as core elements of trauma therapy. *Frontiers in Psychology* 6, 93. doi: 10.3389/fpsyg.2015.00093. **Summary**: Explores somatic experiencing as a therapeutic approach.

Psychedelic-Assisted Therapy

Aicher HD, Müller F and Gasser P (2025). Further education in psychedelic-assisted therapy – experiences from Switzerland. *BioMed Central Medical Education* 25(1), 341. doi: 10.1186/s12909-025-06871-y. **Summary**: Reviews specialized training programs in Switzerland for psychedelic-assisted therapy, addressing the growing demand for treatments targeting depression, PTSX, and anxiety with psychedelic substances.

Barnett BS, Mauney EE and King F (2025). Psychedelic-assisted therapy: An overview for the internist. *Cleveland Clinic Journal of Medicine* 92(3), 171–180. doi: 10.3949/ccjm.92a.24032. **Summary**: Introduces psychedelic-assisted therapy to internists, summarizing evidence for treating depression, PTSX, and substance-use disorders with psychedelics like MDMA and psilocybin.

Halman A, Conyers R et al. (2025). Harnessing pharmacogenomics in clinical research on psychedelic-assisted therapy. *Clinical Pharmacology & Therapeutics* 117(1), 106–115. doi: 10.1002/cpt.3459. **Summary**: Examines optimizing personalized medicine in psychedelic research and treatment.

Li JR, Chiang KT et al. (2025). The association between study design and antidepressant effects in psychedelic-assisted therapy: A meta-analysis. *Journal of Affective Disorders* 369, 421–428. doi: 10.1016/j.jad.2024.10.016. **Summary**: Meta-analysis demonstrating how different study designs impact antidepressant outcomes in psychedelic-assisted therapy, highlighting effective methodologies for enhancing therapeutic benefits of psychedelics.

Miller M, Meyers M et al. (2025). A rapid review of psychedelic-assisted therapy in the context of palliative care. *Journal of Hospice and Palliative Nursing* 27(2), 67–73. doi: 10.1097/NJH.0000000000001096. **Summary**: Provides an overview of psychedelic-assisted therapy's application in palliative care settings, highlighting its potential benefits in managing psychological distress and existential concerns.

Nicol GE, Adams DR et al. (2025). Shrinking the know-do gap in psychedelic-assisted therapy. *Nature Human Behaviour* 9(4), 665–672. doi:10.1038/s41562-025-02103-x. **Summary**: Investigates barriers between research knowledge and clinical implementation in psychedelic-assisted therapy, proposing strategies to accelerate the translation of evidence into practical treatment approaches.

PTSX Therapies and Treatments

American Psychological Association (2025). Clinical practice guideline for the treatment of post-traumatic stress disorder. *American Psychological Association* https://www.apa.org/ptsd-guideline/ptsd.pdf. **Summary**: Provides updated treatment guidelines, focusing on the efficacy of psychological and pharmacological interventions for adults with PTSX.

Bisson JI, Roberts NP and Andrew M (2013). Psychological therapies for chronic PTSX in adults: A state-of-the-art review of efficacy and guidelines. *The Cochrane Database of Systematic Reviews* 2013(12):CD003388. doi: 10.1002/14651858.CD003388.pub4. **Summary**: Evaluates the effectiveness of psychological therapies for chronic PTSX and offers evidence-based treatment recommendations.

Charuvastra A and Cloitre M (2008). Social Bonds and Posttraumatic Stress Disorder. *Annual Review of Psychology* 59:301-28. doi: 10.1146/annurev.psych.58.110405.085650. **Summary**: Reviews the role of social support and attachment in mitigating PTSX, underscoring the importance of relational approaches in therapy.

Clauss K, Cheney T et al. (2024). When the attention control condition works: A systematic review of attention control training for PTSX. *Journal of Traumatic Stress* 38(1):16-28. doi: 10.1002/jts.23104. **Summary**: Explores attention control training as a means of reducing PTSX symptoms by improving cognitive regulation.

Ganesh A, Al-Shamli S et al. (2024). The Frequency of Neuropsychiatric Sequelae After Traumatic Brain Injury in the Global South: A systematic review and meta-analysis. *Sultan Qaboos University Medical Journal* 24(2), 161–176. doi: 10.18295/squmj.12.2023.088. **Summary**: Highlights the prevalence and spectrum of TBI-induced neuropsychiatric conditions in low- and middle-income nations, detailing socioeconomic factors that influence prognosis.

Higgins KS, Nolan D et al. (2024). Current Research on Matching Trauma-Focused Therapies to Veterans: A Scoping Review. *Military Medicine* 189(7–8), e1479–e1487. doi: 10.1093/milmed/usae229. **Summary**: Investigates how matching therapy type to veteran characteristics may improve trauma-focused treatment outcomes in PTSX.

Markowitz JC (2024). Interpersonal Psychotherapy for Posttraumatic Stress Disorder: A Critical Review of the Evidence. *The Journal of Clinical Psychiatry* 85(2), 23nr15172. doi: 10.4088/JCP.23nr15172. **Summary**: Critically assesses Interpersonal Psychotherapy's application to PTSX, weighing current findings and suggesting future research.

Minen MT, Mahmood N et al. (2024). Treatment Options for Posttraumatic Headache: A Current Review of the Literature. *Current Pain and Headache Reports* 28(4). doi: 10.1007/s11916-023-01199-y. **Summary**: Summarizes pharmacologic and behavioral approaches addressing headache linked to PTSX and TBI.

McLean CP and Foa E (2024). State of the Science: Prolonged exposure therapy for the treatment of posttraumatic stress disorder. *Journal of Traumatic Stress* 37, 535–550. https://doi.org/10.1002/jts.23046. **Summary**: Delineates mechanisms, addresses barriers.

Orme-Johnson DW, Barnes VA et al. (2024). Effectiveness of Meditation Techniques in Treating Post-Traumatic Stress: A Systematic Review and Meta-Analysis. *Medicina* 60(12), 2050. doi: 10.3390/medicina60122050. **Summary**: Concludes that various meditation practices may alleviate PTSX symptoms and support long-term healing.

Ostacher MJ (2024). What Does a Systematic Review of Cannabis and PTSX Tell Us? That We Need to Learn More. *Journal of Clinical Psychiatry* 85(1). doi: 10.4088/JCP.23com15279. **Summary**: Concludes that current cannabis research for PTSX remains inadequate and calls for further rigorous study.

Palmisano AN, Meshberg-Cohen S et al. (2024). A systematic review evaluating PTSD treatment effects on intermediate phenotypes of PTSD. *Psychological Trauma* 16(5), 768–783. doi: 10.1037/tra0001410. **Summary**: Analyzes changes in neurobiological, cognitive, and behavioral markers following PTSX interventions, offering insights into precise therapeutic targets.

Reisman M (2016). PTSD Treatment for Veterans: What's Working, What's New, and What's Next. *Pharmacy and Therapeutics* 41(10), 623-634. PMID: 27757001. **Summary**: Reviews effective and emerging treatments for PTSX among military veterans, highlights current research findings, and explores forthcoming therapeutic innovations.

Sippel LM, Hamblen JL et al. (2024). Novel Pharmacologic and Other Somatic Treatment Approaches for Posttraumatic Stress Disorder in Adults: State of the Evidence. *American Journal of Psychiatry* 181(12), 1045–1058. doi: 10.1176/appi.ajp.20230950. **Summary**: Treatments for PTSX in adults, outlining crucial gaps and recommending robust pathways.

Sullivan GM and Neria Y (2023). State-of-the-art review: Trauma-focused psychotherapy for PTSX. *Psychiatric Clinics of North America* 46(1), 119-131. doi: 10.1016/j.psc.2022.12.003. **Summary**: This article outlines trauma-focused psychotherapies, including cognitive behavioral therapy and prolonged exposure, for treating PTSX well.

Summers MR and Nevin RL (2017). Stellate Ganglion Block in the Treatment of Post-traumatic Stress Disorder: A Review of Historical and Recent Literature. *Pain Practice* 17(4):546-553. doi: 10.1111/papr.12503. **Summary**: Reviews historical and contemporary literature on stellate ganglion block for PTSX, evaluating evidence of its clinical effectiveness, safety, evolving therapeutic indications, and underlying biological mechanisms.

Williams T, Phillips NJ et al. (2022) Pharmacotherapy for post traumatic stress disorder (PTSD). *Cochrane Database of Systematic Reviews* 3(3):CD002795. doi: 10.1002/14651858. CD002795.pub3. **Summary**: Assesses the use of SSRIs in managing PTSX symptoms.

Zaretsky TG, Jagodnik KM (2024). The Psychedelic Future of Post-Traumatic Stress Disorder Treatment. *Current Neuropharmacology* 2024;22(4):636-735. doi: 10.2174/1570 159X22666231027111147. **Summary**: Reviews psychiatric applications of psychedelics in PTSX.

Virtual Reality for PTSX Therapy

Gausemel Å and Filkuková P (2024). Virtual realities, real recoveries: exploring the efficacy of 3MDR therapy for treatment-resistant PTSD. *Frontiers in Psychology* 15, 1291961. doi: 10.3389/fpsyg.2024.1291961. **Summary**: Highlights the success of 3MDR (multi-modular motion-assisted memory desensitization and reconsolidation) within a virtual reality setting.

Liu Q, Zhang Y et al. (2025). Efficacy of virtual reality in alleviating post-ICU syndrome symptoms: A systematic review and meta-analysis. *Nursing in Critical Care* 30(2), e70004. doi: 10.1111/nicc.70004. **Summary**: Analyzes multiple studies to confirm the effectiveness of VR interventions in mitigating symptoms of post-intensive care syndrome, significantly improving patients' recovery experiences.

Lu S, Ji Y et al. (2025). Effectiveness of virtual reality on anxiety, pain, sleep quality, and post-traumatic stress disorder for critically ill patients in intensive care units: A systematic review and meta-analysis of randomized controlled trials. *Australian Critical Care* 38(4), 101233. doi: 10.1016/j.aucc.2025.101233. **Summary**: Reviews randomized controlled trials showing VR significantly reduces anxiety, pain, PTSX, and improves sleep quality in critically ill ICU patients.

Miltiadis I, Skarlis A and Burko P (2025). The role of virtual reality in personalized medicine: Advancing prediction, prevention, and participation. *Journal of Medical Systems* 49(1), 56. doi: 10.1007/s10916-025-02191-2. **Summary**: Discusses VR's transformative impact on personalized medicine, emphasizing its role in enhancing predictive diagnostics, preventive strategies, and patient participation through immersive technology.

Wankhede NL, Koppula S et al. (2025). Virtual reality modulating dynamics of neuroplasticity: Innovations in neuro-motor rehabilitation. *Neuroscience* 566, 97–111. doi: 10.1016/j.neuroscience.2024.12.040. **Summary**: Reviews advancements in VR as a revolutionary tool for neuro-motor rehabilitation, emphasizing its unique ability to modulate neuroplasticity and improve recovery outcomes in neurological conditions.

Scientific and Medical Papers on PTSX

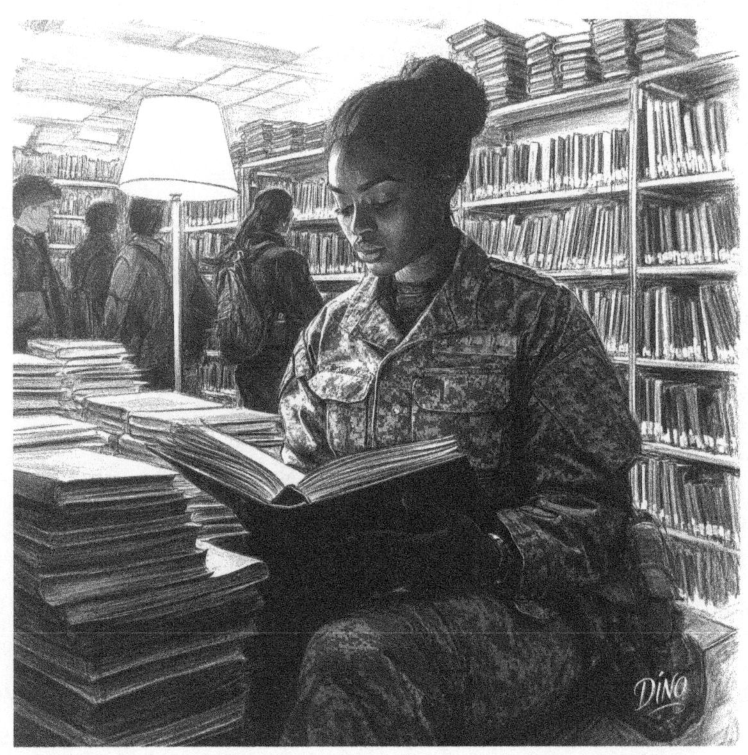

The following scientific and medical papers and some highly relevant reviews provide a snapshot of the state of the art in PTSX research and treatments, mostly from 2022 to present. We acknowledge that there are more than 1,500 other relevant papers in the field of PTSX. We chose to include this representative sample as a starting point for your own research.

Papers are categorized for easy reference, with the names of all scientific and medical journals spelled out completely. We also include a brief summary of each article and paper. The word **Summary** is in bold for easy reference. As you turn each page, the summaries literally jump from the page and invite you to explore before you actually consult an article or paper.

Advances in PTSX Treatments and Interventions

Kitaj M and Goff DC (2024). Why Do Veterans Not Respond as Well as Civilians to Trauma-Focused Therapies for PTSX? *Harvard Review of Psychiatry* 32(4), 160–163. 10.1097/HRP.0000000000000400. **Summary**: Explores why veterans often have poorer outcomes than civilians when undergoing trauma-focused therapies for PTSX.

Li WW, Nannestad J et al. (2024). The effectiveness of mindfulness-based stress reduction (MBSR) on depression, PTSX, and mindfulness among military veterans: A systematic review and meta-analysis. *Health Psychology Open* 11. doi: 10.1177/20551029241302969. **Summary**: Demonstrates MBSR's efficacy in reducing depressive and PTSX symptoms and in enhancing mindfulness for veterans.

Liu JJW, Nazarov A et al. (2025). Treating Posttraumatic Stress Disorder in Military Populations: A Meta-Analysis. *Journal of Clinical Psychiatry* 86(2):24r15571. doi: 10.4088/JCP.24r15571. **Summary**: Provides robust evidence on the efficacy of therapeutic interventions for PTSX in military settings, emphasizing treatment heterogeneity.

Malhotra B, Jones LC et al. (2024). A conceptual framework for a neurophysiological basis of art therapy for PTSX. *Frontiers in Human Neuroscience* 18. doi: 10.3389/fnhum.2024.1351757. **Summary**: Explores how art therapy could modulate neurophysiological processes underlying PTSX in civilian and military groups.

McMahon B, Guindalini C and Mellor R (2024). Computerised health interventions targeting Australian veterans and their families: A scoping review. *Health Promotion Journal of Australia* 35(4), 875–890. 10.1002/hpja.832. **Summary**: Surveys digital interventions to mitigate PTSX symptoms in Australian veterans and their families.

Milligan T, Smolenski D et al. (2025). Loss of PTSD Diagnosis in Response to Evidence-Based Treatments: A Systematic Review and Meta-Analysis. *Journal of the American Medical Association Psychiatry* doi: 10.1001/jamapsychiatry.2025.0695. **Summary**: Meta-analysis of 126 trials reveals 38 percent diagnostic remission after evidence-based care, with cognitive therapies outperforming others, setting benchmarks and urging broader dissemination of validated PTSX interventions.

Norred MA, Zuschlag ZD and Hamner MB (2024). A Neuroanatomic and Pathophysiologic Framework for Novel Pharmacological Approaches to the Treatment of Post-traumatic Stress Disorder (PTSD). *Drugs* 84(2), 149–164. doi:10.1007/s40265-023-01983-5. **Summary**: Proposes new pharmacological targets beyond serotonergic pathways for managing PTSX.

Provan M, Ahmed Z et al. (2024). Are equine-assisted services beneficial for military veterans with post-traumatic stress injuries? A systematic review and meta-analysis. *BioMed Central Psychiatry* 24(1).doi:10.1186/s12888-024-05984-w. **Summary**: Assesses how equine-assisted programs may improve psychological outcomes for veterans with PTSX.

Shalev AY, Liberzon I and Marmar C (2017). Post-Traumatic Stress Disorder. *The New England Journal of Medicine* 376(25):2459-2469. doi: 10.1056/NEJMra1612499. **Summary**: Provides an overview of PTSX, including its etiology, clinical features, and evidence-based treatment approaches.

Wolfgang AS, Fonzo GA et al. (2025). MDMA and MDMA-Assisted Therapy. *American Journal of Psychiatry* 182(1),79–103. 10.1176/appi.ajp.20230681. **Summary**: Reviews the history, regulatory status, and therapeutic potential of MDMA for PTSX. Discusses ongoing phase 3 trials, mechanistic underpinnings, safety considerations, and the FDA's "Breakthrough Therapy" designation.

Body-Based and Somatic Approaches

Krauss BJ (2024). To Calm and to Commend: Veterans' Musical Preferences Anticipating End of Life. *Military Medicine* 189(11–12):e2332–e2339. 10.1093/milmed/usae216. **Summary**: Investigates end-of-life music preferences among veterans and reveals how song selection reflects values, identity and spiritual readiness.

Levy CE, Uomoto JM et al. (2025). Creative Arts Therapies in Rehabilitation. *Archives of Physical Medicine and Rehabilitation* 106(1), 153–157. doi: 10.1016/j.apmr.2024.07.008. **Summary**: Reviews evidence for music, dance, and visual arts therapies enhancing mood, cognition, and motor function and suggests creative-arts integration within rehabilitation for veterans recovering from trauma and neurologic injury.

Niles BL, Kaiser AP et al. (2024). Tai Chi and Wellness Interventions for Veterans with Gulf War Illness: A Randomized Controlled Feasibility Trial. *International Journal of Behavioral Medicine* doi: 10.1007/s12529-024-10338-7. **Summary**: Shows that Tai Chi may improve somatic and emotional symptoms in veterans with Gulf War I illness, offering a mind-body adjunct to standard care.

Provan M, Ahmed Z et al. (2024). Are equine-assisted services beneficial for military veterans with post-traumatic stress disorder? A systematic review and meta-analysis. *BioMed Central Psychiatry* 24(1):544. doi: 10.1186/s12888-024-05984-w. **Summary**: Assesses efficacy of equine-assisted therapies in treating PTSX, supporting their role in holistic rehabilitation for trauma-affected veterans.

Sun S, Singer A et al. (2025). Promoting Psychological Health and Overall Wellness in Female Veterans With Military Sexual Trauma Through Complementary Health Interventions: A Quality Improvement Project. *Military Medicine* 190(5-6), e1326–e1332. doi: 10.1093/milmed/usae547. **Summary**: Implements yoga, acupuncture, and mindfulness protocols, demonstrating feasible somatic-based enhancements in mood, sleep and pain for women veterans with MST-related PTSX within VA-settings programs.

Childhood Trauma

Alisic E and Jongmans M (2011). Children's perspectives on Dealing with traumatic events. *Journal of Child Psychology and Psychiatry* 16(6). doi: 10.1080/15325024.2011.576979. **Summary**: Examines trauma recovery in children from a developmental perspective, emphasizing age-related factors influencing PTSX symptoms and treatment approaches.

Barazzone N, Santos I et al. (2019). The links between adult attachment and post-traumatic stress: A systematic review. *Psychology and Psychotherapy* 92(1):131-147. doi: 10.1111/papt.12181. **Summary**: Explores how attachment styles and the quality of interpersonal relationships can affect work-related stress, providing insights into the broader implications of attachment theory in adult functioning.

Cloitre M, Stovall-McClough KC et al. (2010). Treatment for PTSD Related to Childhood Abuse: A Randomized Controlled Trial. *American Journal of Psychiatry* 167(8). doi: 10.1176/appi.ajp.2010.09081247. **Summary**: Explores the lasting effects of childhood trauma on adult functioning, highlighting its implications for PTSX diagnosis and therapeutic interventions.

Invitto S and Moselli P (2024). Exploring Embodied and Bioenergetic Approaches in Trauma Therapy: Observing Somatic Experience and Olfactory Memory. *Brain Science* 14(4), 385. 10.3390/brainsci14040385. **Summary**: Investigates how integrating body-centered techniques and olfactory cues into trauma therapy can enhance somatic awareness, potentially enriching the therapeutic process and facilitating deeper healing.

Karatzias T, Shevlin M et al. (2022). Childhood trauma, attachment orientation, and complex PTSD (CPTSD) symptoms in a clinical sample: Implications for treatment. *Development and Psychopathology* 34(3):1192-1197. 10.1017/S0954579420001509. **Summary**: Investigates the relationship between childhood trauma, attachment orientations, and CPTSX symptoms, suggesting that attachment-focused interventions may be beneficial in treatments.

Karatzias T, Shevlin M et al. (2016). An initial psychometric assessment of an ICD-11 based measure of PTSD and complex PTSD (ICD-TQ): Evidence of construct validity. *Journal of Anxiety Disorders* 44:73-79. 10.1016/j.janxdis.2016.10.009. **Summary**: Presents the development and validation of a measure for assessing PTSX and CPTSX as defined in the ICD-11, contributing to the accurate diagnosis and differentiation of these disorders.

Karimov-Zwienenberg M, Symphor W et al. (2024). Childhood trauma, PTSD/CPTSD and chronic pain: A systematic review. *PLOS* (Public Library of Science) *One* 19(8), e0309332. **Summary**: Examines the associations between childhood trauma, PTSX/CPTSX, and chronic pain in adults, highlighting the complex interplay between early adverse experiences and long-term physical health outcomes.

Medeiros GC, Demo I et al. (2024). Personalized use of ketamine and esketamine for treatment-resistant depression. *Translational Psychiatry* 14(1), 481. 10.1038/s41398-024-03180-8. **Summary**: Discusses how patient-specific factors can guide ketamine or esketamine therapy for severe depression, reviewing biomarkers, genetic markers, and clinical profiles to enhance treatment precision.

Sweeney A, Filson B et al. (2018). A paradigm shift: Relationships in trauma-informed mental health services. *British Journal of Psychiatry Advances* 24(5), 319–333. **Summary**: Discusses the importance of adopting trauma-informed approaches in mental health services, emphasizing the need for relational safety and collaborative practices to support recovery.

Vannini MBN, Xu B et al. (2025). A Network Analysis of Post-Traumatic Stress, Depression, and Alcohol Use in US Veterans: Exploring Differences by Childhood Maltreatment Exposure. *Journal of Affective Disorders* 389, 119662. doi: 10.1016/j.jad.2025.119662. **Summary**: Childhood maltreatment intensifies connectivity among PTSX, depressive and alcohol-use nodes, pinpointing trauma-specific intervention targets to reduce cascading psychopathology.

Woodhouse S, Ayers S and Field AP (2015). The relationship between adult attachment style and post-traumatic stress symptoms: A meta-analysis. *Journal of Anxiety Disorders* 35, 103–117. **Summary**: Examines the association between adult attachment styles and post-traumatic stress symptoms.

Clinical Applications

Aikins DE, Wargo Aikins J et al. (2025). Rethinking Stigma: Prejudicial Beliefs Impact Psychiatric Treatment in US Soldiers. *Psychological Services* 22(2), 337–341. doi: 10.1037/ser0000912. **Summary**: Survey of active-duty soldiers reveals internalized prejudicial beliefs significantly predict psychotherapy avoidance, indicating stigma reduction campaigns remain critical for improving mental-health engagement in military populations.

Brenner LA, Capaldi V et al. (2025). Assessment and Management of Patients at Risk for Suicide: Synopsis of the 2024 US Department of Veterans Affairs and US Department of Defense Clinical Practice Guidelines. *Annals of Internal Medicine* 178(3), 416–425. doi: 10.7326/ANNALS-24-01938. **Summary**: Details evidence-based screening, risk stratification, lethal-means counseling, and follow-up protocols, offering clinicians concise recommendations to reduce suicide among at-risk veterans and servicemembers.

Chang CJ, Fischer IC et al. (2025). Sexual Orientation Moderates the Association Between Health Care Utilization-Related Factors and Mental Health Service Nonutilization Among United States Military Veterans. *Psychological Services* 22(2), 383–394. doi: 10.1037/ser0000907. **Summary**: Among veterans, sexual minority status moderates how logistical barriers, perceived stigma, and symptom severity deter mental-health utilization, highlighting the need for orientation-sensitive outreach and tailored service delivery.

Gomes KD, Moore BA et al. (2024). Identifying Predictors of Positive and Negative Affect at Mid-Deployment Among Military Medical Personnel. *Military Medicine* 189(Suppl 3):142–148. doi: 10.1093/milmed/usae062. **Summary**: Examines emotional responses among deployed military medical staff, identifying key predictors of affective states in combat environments.

Manzo LL, Dindinger RA et al. (2024). The Impact of Military Trauma Exposures on Servicewomen's Pregnancy Outcomes: A Scoping Review. *Journal of Midwifery & Women's Health* 69(5):634–646. doi: 10.1111/jmwh.13620. **Summary**: Investigates how trauma histories among servicewomen affect prenatal and perinatal health outcomes, revealing a range of psychosocial risks.

Murphy JW, Shotwell-Tabke C et al. (2025). Evaluating Self-Efficacy as a Treatment Mechanism During an Intensive Treatment Program for Posttraumatic Stress Disorder. *Psychological Trauma* doi: 10.1037/tra0001836. **Summary**: Demonstrates that increases in trauma-coping self-efficacy mediate posttreatment symptom reduction, underscoring self-belief enhancement as a key mechanism driving intensive program effectiveness.

Murphy JW, Smith DL et al. (2025). Examining Treatment Outcomes for Military Service Members in an Intensive Treatment Program for Posttraumatic Stress Disorder. *Military Psychology* doi: 10.1080/08995605.2025.2521951. **Summary**: Reports significant symptom and functional gains after a two-week multidisciplinary intensive program, supporting brief, concentrated treatment delivery in military behavioral-health settings.

Havermans DCD, Coeur EMN et al. (2025). The Diagnostic Accuracy of PTSD Assessment Instruments Used in Older Adults: A Systematic Review. European *Journal of Psychotraumatology* 16(1), 2498191. doi: 10.1080/20008066.2025.2498191. **Summary**: Finds high sensitivity but variable specificity across instruments, recommending age-adapted thresholds and multimethod assessment to improve diagnostic precision in geriatric populations.

Ranney RM, Bernhard PA et al. (2025). Gender as a Moderator of Associations Between Military Sexual Trauma and Post-Traumatic Stress Disorder Treatment Utilization. *Psychological Services* 22(2), 395–401. doi: 10.1037/ser0000886. **Summary**: Finds that female gender amplifies the relationship between MST exposure and mental-health service use, guiding gender-sensitive outreach strategies to improve PTSX treatment engagement across care systems.

Touponse SC, Guo Q et al. (2025). Effect of Agreement Between Clinician-Rated and Patient-Reported PTSD Symptoms on Intensive Outpatient Treatment Outcomes. *Psychiatry Research* 343, 116287. doi: 10.1016/j.psychres.2024.116287. **Summary**: Shows that concordance between clinician and patient symptom ratings predicts greater symptom reduction and completion rates, advocating shared assessment frameworks to optimize PTSX intensive outpatient programs.

Comorbidities with PTSX

Back SE, Jarnecke AM et al. (2024). State of the Science: Treatment of comorbid posttraumatic stress disorder and substance use disorders. *Journal of Traumatic Stress* 37(6), 803–813. 10.1002/jts.23049. **Summary**: Surveys integrated interventions and underscores the complexities in addressing high comorbidity rates of PTSX and substance use disorders.

Bennett DC, Goodkind MS et al. (2025). Associations Between Interpersonal Trauma Histories, Perpetrator Characteristics, and Mental Health Symptom Profiles Among Veterans Seeking Treatment Associated with Military Sexual Trauma. *Violence and Victims* 40(2), 179–198. doi: 10.1891/VV-2023-0154. **Summary**: Treatment-seeking veterans with differing military sexual trauma perpetrator characteristics display distinct symptom constellations, guiding individualized assessment and therapeutic planning for complex interpersonal trauma recovery within VA clinical settings.

Brown R, Cherian K et al. (2024). Repetitive transcranial magnetic stimulation for post-traumatic stress disorder in adults. *Cochrane Database of Systematic Reviews* 8(8), CD015040. 10.1002/14651858.CD015040.pub2. **Summary**: Systematically evaluates repetitive transcranial magnetic stimulation (rTMS) in adult PTSX, synthesizing current evidence on efficacy and tolerability.

Buccellato KH, Peterson AL (2024). The role of cortisol in development and treatment of PTSX among service members: A narrative review. *Psychoneuroendocrinology* 169. 10.1016/j.psyneuen.2024.107152. **Summary**: Examines how cortisol dysregulation may contribute to the onset and therapeutic response of PTSX in military populations.

Ghassemi AE (2022). Reliable and comprehensive assessment of post-traumatic stress disorder is required to provide population-based prevention and treatment of PTSD during the COVID-19 pandemic. *Evidence-Based Nursing* 25(3), 102. **Summary**: Argues for thorough assessment methods for PTSX, particularly in the context of the increased psychological distress observed during the COVID-19 pandemic.

Gordon ML, Agee B (2023). Addressing the dual burden: Treatment outcomes for traumatic brain injury (TBI) and post-traumatic stress disorder (PTSD). The Millennium Health Centers Inc Veterans-TBI Project 1-10. **Summary**: Presents findings from the Veterans-TBI Project, focusing on treatment outcomes for the dual burden of TBI and PTSX in veterans.

Hargrave AS, Cohen BE et al. (2025). Sexual Trauma, Suicide, and Overdose in a National Cohort of Older Veterans. *Annals of Internal Medicine* 178(6), 775–787. doi: 10.7326/ANNALS-24-01145. **Summary**: National analysis shows sexual-trauma history markedly elevates suicide attempts and overdose deaths, underscoring integrated screening and prevention across aging veteran care.

Larach DB, Waljee JF et al. (2024). Perioperative opioid prescribing and iatrogenic opioid use disorder and overdose: a state-of-the-art narrative review. *Regional Anesthesia and Pain Medicine* 49(8), 602–608. 10.1136/rapm-2023-104944. **Summary**: Examines how perioperative opioid prescribing may increase risks of iatrogenic use disorder and overdose, calling for refined strategies to mitigate long-term harms.

Lawrence S and Scofield RH (2024). Post traumatic stress disorder associated hypothalamic-pituitary-adrenal axis dysregulation and physical illness. *Brain Behavior and Immunity Health* 41, 100849. 10.1016/j.bbih.2024.100849. **Summary**: Explores how PTSX-induced HPA axis disturbances can compromise immune function and heighten susceptibility to diverse physical health conditions.

Livingston WS, Blais RK et al. (2025). Recent Intimate Partner Violence Is Associated with Worse Sexual Function Among Women Veterans. *Psychological Trauma* doi: 10.1037/tra0001877. **Summary**: Finds recent partner violence correlates with diminished desire, arousal, and satisfaction, indicating trauma-informed interventions must address relational and sexual-health domains.

Mei P, Cotiga D et al. (2025). Cardiovascular Care in Women Veterans: An Updated Profile. *Current Cardiology Reports* 27(1):93. doi: 10.1007/s11886-025-02247-2. **Summary**: Outlines cardiovascular health risks and care gaps specific to female veterans, emphasizing trauma-related etiologies and gender-based disparities.

Mitchell KS, Serier KN et al. (2025). Eating Disorder Screening Measures in Post-9/11 Veteran Men and Women. *Psychological Assessment* 37(4), 172–179. doi: 10.1037/pas0001369. **Summary**: Validates multiple brief instruments for detecting eating disorders in veterans, establishing psychometric reliability and gender invariance to facilitate early identification of disordered eating comorbid with PTSX.

Nichter B, Hill ML et al. (2025). Intimate Partner Violence Perpetration and Firearm Ownership and Storage Practices Among US Military Veterans. *Journal of Psychiatric Research* 185, 177–185. doi: 10.1016/j.jpsychires.2025.03.033. **Summary**: Links intimate-partner violence perpetration to firearm ownership and unsafe storage, highlighting lethal risk intersections and informing prevention strategies for veterans with trauma histories.

Nilaweera D, Phyo AZZ, Teshale AB et al. (2023). Lifetime posttraumatic stress disorder as a predictor of mortality: A systematic review and meta-analysis. *Biomed Central Psychiatry* 23, Article 229. **Summary**: Examines the association between lifetime PTSX and increased mortality risk, emphasizing the long-term health implications of PTSX.

Ray TN, Esquivel AP et al. (2025). Risk and Protective Factors of Probable Binge Eating Disorder in US Military Spouses: Findings from the Millennium Cohort Family Study. *American Journal of Epidemiology* 194(6), 1631–1641. doi: 10.1093/aje/kwae206. **Summary**: Identifies deployment-related stress, spousal PTSX symptoms, and social support deficits as predictors of binge eating, informing family-centered prevention efforts within military communities, worldwide health promotion.

Serier KN, Burns HM et al. (2025). Functioning and Disability Consequences of Comorbid Post-Traumatic Stress Disorder and Diabetes in Vietnam Era Men and Women Veterans. *Health Psychology* doi: 10.1037/hea0001516. **Summary**: Demonstrates additive impact of PTSX and diabetes on physical limitations, work impairment, and healthcare utilization, underscoring need for integrated behavioral-medical management strategies for aging veterans.

Serier KN, Knutson EK et al. (2025). Examining the Factor Structure of the Nine-Item Avoidant/Restrictive Food Intake Disorder Screen in a National US Military Veteran Sample. *Psychological Assessment* 37(3), 123–128. doi: 10.1037/pas0001362. **Summary**: Enables identification of disordered eating patterns that often co-occur with PTSX among veterans.

Strigo IA, Craig ADB, Simmons AN (2024). Expectation of pain and relief: A dynamical model of the neural basis for pain-trauma co-morbidity. *Neuroscience and Biobehavioral Reviews* 163, 105750. 10.1016/j.neubiorev.2024.105750. **Summary**: Proposes a dynamic neural framework connecting pain anticipation and trauma, elucidating mechanisms for how perceived relief or ongoing distress modulates both pain and PTSX symptoms.

Swannell M, Bradlow RCJ et al. (2024). Pharmacological treatments for co-occurring PTSD and substance use disorders: A systematic review. *Journal of Substance Use and Addiction Treatment* 169. 10.1016/j.josat.2024.209601. **Summary**: Reviews medications targeting both PTSX and substance use, highlighting integrated treatment needs.

Vyas KJ, Marconi VC et al. (2025). Post-Traumatic Stress Disorder and Its Associations with Morbidity and Mortality Among Veterans with HIV. *AIDS* doi: 10.1097/QAD.0000000000004241. **Summary**: Links PTSX diagnoses to elevated multimorbidity burden and all-cause mortality in HIV-positive veterans, emphasizing integrated mental-infectious disease care to mitigate compounded health risks over time.

Vyas KJ, Marconi VC et al. (2025). Post-Traumatic Stress Disorder and Its Associations with Antiretroviral Therapy Among Veterans with HIV. *AIDS* 39(5), 597–608. doi: 10.1097/QAD.0000000000004105. **Summary**: Reveals that PTSX is linked to delayed Antiretroviral Therapy initiation, reduced adherence, and viremia, indicating mental-health-driven obstacles to viral suppression within veteran HIV-care programs, significantly undermining outcomes.

Emerging and Established Therapies for PTSX

Back SE, Jarnecke AM et al. (2024). State of the Science: Treatment of comorbid posttraumatic stress disorder and substance use disorders. *Journal of Traumatic Stress* 37(6), 803–813. 10.1002/jts.23049. **Summary**: Evaluates leading interventions for managing PTSX and substance use together.

Brown R, Cherian K et al. (2024). Repetitive transcranial magnetic stimulation for post-traumatic stress disorder in adults. *Cochrane Database of Systematic Reviews* 8(8). 10.1002/14651858.CD015040.pub2. **Summary**: Evaluates rTMS as an innovative, non-pharmacological intervention for PTSX based on randomized trials.

Haderlein TP, Guzman-Clark J et al. (2024). Improving Veteran Engagement with Virtual Care Technologies: a Veterans Health Administration State of the Art Conference Research Agenda. *Journal of General Internal Medicine* 39(Suppl 1), 21–28. 10.1007/s11606-023-08488-7. **Summary**: Highlights telehealth strategies to enhance veteran participation in PTSX treatments across the VA system.

Liu JJW, Nazarov A et al. (2025). Treating Posttraumatic Stress Disorder in Military Populations: A Meta-Analysis. *Journal of Clinical Psychiatry* 86(2), 24r15571. doi: 10.4088/JCP.24r15571. **Summary**: Confirms efficacy of pharmacologic, psychotherapeutic, and combined modalities in service members, highlighting moderators and evidence gaps to steer future therapy research.

Leichsenring F, Rabung S and Leibing E (2004). The efficacy of short-term psychodynamic psychotherapy in specific psychiatric disorders: a meta-analysis. *Archives of General Psychiatry* 61(12):1208-16. 10.1001/archpsyc.61.12.1208. **Summary**: Evaluates the efficacy of short-term psychodynamic psychotherapy for PTSX, providing robust support for its therapeutic benefits.

Nieforth LO, Leighton SC (2024). Animal-assisted interventions for military families: a systematic review. *Frontiers in Public Health* 12. 10.3389/fpubh.2024.1372189. **Summary**: Reviews the impact of equine or canine-assisted therapies on PTSX outcomes for veterans and their family members.

Norred MA, Zuschlag ZD and Hamner MB (2024). A Neuroanatomic and Pathophysiologic Framework for Novel Pharmacological Approaches to the Treatment of Post-traumatic Stress Disorder. *Drugs* 84(2), 149–164. 10.1007/s40265-023-01983-5. **Summary**: Proposes a detailed neuroanatomic model to guide next-generation PTSX pharmacotherapies, focusing on emerging non-serotonergic drug targets that may alleviate core symptoms more effectively.

Quintanilla B, Zarate CA Jr, Pillai A (2024). Ketamine's mechanism of action with an emphasis on neuroimmune regulation: can the complement system complement ketamine's antidepressant effects? *Molecular Psychiatry* 29(9):2849-2858. 10.1038/s41380-024-02507-7. **Summary**: Ketamine's antidepressant effects involve neuroimmune modulation, particularly through interactions with the complement system, suggesting therapeutic benefits via immune pathways in depressive disorders.

Sippel LM, Hamblen JL et al. (2024). Novel Pharmacologic and Other Somatic Treatment Approaches for PTSX in Adults: State of the Evidence. *American Journal of Psychiatry* 181(12), 1045–1058. 10.1176/appi.ajp.20230950. **Summary**: Reviews emerging therapies—medications and somatic interventions—for adults with PTSX who do not respond to standard care.

Tseng PT, Zeng BY et al. (2024). Efficacy and acceptability of noninvasive brain stimulation for treating posttraumatic stress symptoms: A network meta-analysis of randomized controlled trials. *Acta Psychiatrica Scandinavica* 150(1), 5–21. 10.1111/acps.13688. **Summary**: Compares multiple noninvasive brain stimulation methods for alleviating PTSX symptom severity.

Epigenetics

Baghaei A, Zoshk MY et al. (2024). Prominent genetic variants and epigenetic changes in post-traumatic stress eXtended among combat veterans. *Molecular Biology Reports* 51(1). 10.1007/s11033-024-09276-0. **Summary**: Identifies key genetic and epigenetic factors underpinning PTSX in combat-exposed veterans.

Bailo P, Piccinini A et al. (2024). Epigenetics of violence against women: a systematic review of the literature. *Environmental Epigenetics* 10(1). 10.1093/eep/dvae012. **Summary**: Explores epigenetic modifications stemming from violent trauma, including PTSX-related outcomes in women.

Katrinli S, Wani AH et a. (2024). Epigenome-wide association studies identify novel DNA methylation sites associated with PTSD: a meta-analysis of 23 military and civilian cohorts. *Genome Medicine* 16(1):147. 10.1186/s13073-024-01417-1. **Summary**: Reveals specific DNA methylation markers associated with PTSX, offering new insight into biological signatures of trauma across diverse populations.

Yang R, Kannan S et al. (2025). Long-Term miRNA Changes Predicting Resiliency Factors of Post-Traumatic Stress Disorder in a Large Military Cohort–Millennium Cohort Study. *International Journal of Molecular Sciences* 26(11), 5195. doi: 10.3390/ijms26115195. **Summary**: Identifies persistent microRNA expression patterns linked to resilience against PTSX, suggesting epigenetic biomarkers that could forecast long-term adaptation and guide personalized preventive strategies in military populations.

Yehuda R, Daskalakis NP, Lehrner A (2018). Intergenerational trauma effects: A review of epigenetic transmission and clinical implications. *World Psychiatry* 17(3):243–257. 10.1002/wps.20568. **Summary**: Reviews evidence for the transmission of trauma through epigenetic mechanisms and its impact on subsequent generations.

Zannas AS, Chrousos GP (2017). Epigenetic programming by stress and glucocorticoids along the human lifespan. *Molecular Psychiatry* 22(5), 640-646. **Summary**: Investigates how stress and glucocorticoids induce epigenetic changes over the lifespan and their implications for disorders like PTSX.

Exercise as Medicine

Haderlein TP, Guzman-Clark J et al. (2024). Improving Veteran Engagement with Virtual Care Technologies: a Veterans Health Administration State of the Art Conference Research Agenda. *Journal of General Internal Medicine*, 39(Suppl 1), 21–28. 10.1007/s11606-023-08488-7. **Summary**: Highlights telehealth-focused strategies and research imperatives aimed at bolstering veteran participation and outcomes in virtual healthcare platforms.

Hegberg NJ, Tone EB (2014). Physical activity and stress resilience: Considering those At-Risk for developing mental health problems. *Mental Health and Physical Activity* 8(4). 10.1016/j.mhpa.2014.10.001. **Summary**: Explores the neurobiological mechanisms through which exercise enhances resilience and aids in recovery from trauma.

Kolassa IT, Elbert T (2007). Structural and Functional Neuroplasticity in Relation to Traumatic Stress. *Current Directions in Psychological Science* 16(6), 321-325. https://doi.org/10.1111/j.1467-8721.2007.00529.x. **Summary**: Reviews structural brain changes in PTSX patients, emphasizing neuroplasticity and potential interventions like exercise.

Walton SR, Fraser JJ et al. (2025). Aerobic Exercise and Brain Structure Among Military Service Members and Veterans with Varying Histories of Mild Traumatic Brain Injury: A LIMBIC-CENC Exploratory Investigation. *Public Library of Science ONE* 20(3), e0320004. doi: 10.1371/journal.pone.0320004. **Summary**: Demonstrates that higher aerobic fitness correlates with increased cortical thickness and white-matter integrity following mTBI, suggesting exercise-driven neuroprotection and a non-pharmacologic rehabilitation avenue for PTSX-affected personnel.

Yuan Z, Peng C et al. (2025). Effects of physical activity on patients with posttraumatic stress disorder: A systematic review and meta-analysis of randomized controlled trials. *Medicine* (Baltimore) 104(3), e41139. 10.1097/MD.0000000000041139. **Summary**: Evaluates randomized trial data to demonstrate how structured exercise interventions can alleviate PTSX symptom severity and improve patient wellbeing.

Gap Junctions in the Brain

Chadjichristos, CE, Matter CM et al. (2006). Reduced Connexin43 Expression Limits Neointima Formation after Balloon Distension Injury in Hypercholesterolemic Mice. *Circulation* 113 (24): 2835–2843. https://doi.org/10.1161/circulationaha.106.627703. **Summary**: Demonstrates a protective role in post-injury vascular remodeling through modulation of cell communication and inflammatory response.

De Bock M, Wang N et al. (2013). Endothelial Calcium Dynamics, Connexin Channels and Blood–Brain Barrier Function. *Progress in Neurobiology* 108 (1): 1–20. https://doi.org/10.1016/j.pneurobio.2013.06.001. **Summary**: Connexin-mediated calcium signaling critically regulates blood-brain barrier integrity, linking endothelial calcium dynamics to barrier function and highlighting connexin channels as therapeutic targets in neurovascular disorders.

Orellana JA, Hernández DE et al. (2011). ATP and Glutamate Released via Astroglial Connexin43 Hemichannels Mediate Neuronal Death through Activation of Pannexin1 Hemichannels. *Journal of Neurochemistry* 118 (5): 826–840. https://doi.org/10.1111/j.1471-4159.2011.07210.x. **Summary**: Astroglial Connexin43 hemichannels release ATP and glutamate, triggering neuronal death via Pannexin1 activation, revealing a key astrocyte–neuron interaction pathway in neuroinflammatory and neurodegenerative damage.

Retamal, MA, Froger N et al. (2007). Cx43 Hemichannels and Gap Junction Channels in Astrocytes Are Regulated Oppositely by Proinflammatory Cytokines Released from Activated Microglia. *Journal of Neuroscience* 27 (50): 13781–13792. https://doi.org/10.1523/jneurosci.2042-07.2007. **Summary**: Proinflammatory cytokines from microglia oppositely regulate astrocytic Connexin43 hemichannels and gap junctions, showing divergent channel responses during neuroinflammation and identifying potential therapeutic modulation sites.

Wong CW, Christen T et al. (2006). Connexin37 Protects against Atherosclerosis by Regulating Monocyte Adhesion. *Nature Medicine* 12 (8): 950–954. https://doi.org/10.1038/nm1441. **Summary**: Connexin37 expression reduces atherosclerosis by inhibiting monocyte adhesion to the endothelium, uncovering a protective mechanism involving gap junction proteins in vascular inflammation and plaque formation.

General Topics and Epidemiology

Akiki TJ, Jubeir J et al. (2025). Neural circuit basis of pathological anxiety. *Nature Reviews Neuroscience* 26(1), 5–22. 10.1038/s41583-024-00880-4. **Summary**: Overview of anxiety disorders' neurocircuitry, offering insights relevant to understanding PTSX etiology.

Breslau N, Wilcox HC et al. (2004). Trauma exposure and posttraumatic stress disorder: a study of youths in urban America. *Journal of Urban Health* 81(4):530-44. 10.1093/jurban/jth138. **Summary**: Provides an updated analysis of trauma exposure prevalence and PTSX rates in the general population, emphasizing demographic and contextual variations.

Bruce MJ, Pagán AF and Acierno R (2025). State of the Science: Evidence-based treatments for postraumatic stress disorder delivered via telehealth. *Journal of Traumatic Stress* 38(1):5-15. 10.1002/jts.23074. **Summary**: Summarizes current knowledge on telehealth's effectiveness in delivering PTSX interventions.

Edwards ER, Geraci JC et al. (2025). Improving Explainability of Post-Separation Suicide Attempt Prediction Models for Transitioning Service Members: Insights from the Army Study to Assess Risk and Resilience in Servicemembers – Longitudinal Study. *Translational Psychiatry* 15(1), 37. doi: 10.1038/s41398-025-03248-z. **Summary**: Machine-learning model interpretation techniques reveal the most salient demographic, deployment, and clinical predictors of post-separation suicide attempts, enhancing transparency and guiding personalized prevention strategies for transitioning service members.

Forehand JA et al. (2022). Association between post-traumatic stress disorder severity and death by suicide in US military veterans: retrospective cohort study. *British Journal of Psychiatry* 1-7. 10.1192/bjp.2022.110. **Summary**: Examines the correlation between the severity of PTSX symptoms and elevated suicide risk in a large sample of US veterans, highlighting the need for targeted interventions based on symptom intensity.

Gjerstad SF, Nordin L et al. (2024). How is trauma-focused therapy experienced by adults with PTSX? A systematic review of qualitative studies. *Biomed Central Psychology* 12:135. doi.org/10.1186/s40359-024-01588-x. **Summary**: Analyzes firsthand patient perspectives on trauma-focused therapy, highlighting perceived benefits and risks.

Havermans DCD, Coeur EMN et al. (2025). The diagnostic accuracy of PTSD assessment instruments used in older adults: A systematic review. *European Journal of Psychotraumatology* 16(1):2498191. doi: 10.1080/20008066.2025.2498191. **Summary**: Reviews PTSX diagnostic tools for older adults, highlighting discrepancies in sensitivity and specificity among military and civilian populations.

Howard JT, Stewart IJ and Pugh MJ (2025). Suicide Rate Trends for Post–September 11, 2001, US Military Veterans. *JAMA Network Open* ;8(9):e2530216. doi:10.1001/jamanetworkopen.2025.30216. **Summary**: Suicide rates among US veterans who served after 11 September 2001 significantly increased between 2006 and 2022. The rise was most pronounced in younger veterans and those with a history of combat deployment, highlighting an urgent public health crisis.

Humphreys K, Korthuis P et al. (2025). Therapeutic Potential of Psychedelic Drugs: Navigating High Hopes, Strong Claims, Weak Evidence, and Big Money. *Annual Review of Psychology* 76(1), 143–165. 10.1146/annurev-psych-020124-023532. **Summary**: Evaluates MDMA and psilocybin for PTSX amid concerns about insufficient data and commercial motivations in selfish interests.

Kessler RC, McLaughlin KA, and Green JG (2005). Lifetime prevalence and age-of-onset distributions of DSM-IV disorders in the National Comorbidity Survey Replication. *Archives of General Psychiatry* 62(6):593-602. 10.1001/archpsyc.62.6.593. **Summary**: Analyzes the lifetime prevalence and age-of-onset distributions of DSM-IV disorders, with specific attention to PTSX patterns in the National Comorbidity Survey Replication.

Larach DB, Waljee JF et al. (2024). Perioperative opioid prescribing and iatrogenic opioid use disorder and overdose: A state-of-the-art narrative review. *Regional Anesthesia and Pain Medicine* 49(8), 602–608. 10.1136/rapm-2023-104944. **Summary**: Explores how perioperative opioid use may heighten misuse risk in populations that can include PTSX patients.

LeBeau K, Lopez J et al. (2025). Understanding the Intersectionality of the Rural Hispanic/Latino Veteran Population: A Scoping Review of Health-Related Challenges. *Ethnicity & Health* doi: 10.1080/13557858.2025.2486413. **Summary**: Identifies socioeconomic, cultural, and geographic barriers shaping health outcomes for rural Hispanic/Latino veterans, calling for intersectional policies to improve trauma care access.

Moore MJ, Shawler E et al. (2025). Veteran and Military Mental Health Issues. In: *StatPearls* [Internet]. Treasure Island, FL: StatPearls Publishing. doi: n/a. **Summary**: Comprehensive overview of psychiatric disorders, risk factors, and evidence-based interventions among servicemembers and veterans.

Pugach CP, Adams SW et al. (2025). Identifying Transdiagnostic Traumatic Stress Reactions in US Military Veterans: A Nationally Representative Study. *Journal of Traumatic Stress* 38(2), 259–271. doi: 10.1002/jts.23119. **Summary**: Delineates overlapping PTSX, depression,and anxiety symptom profiles, and suggests transdiagnostic assessment and tailored interventions.

Roscoe RA. (2025). Narrating the Sociocultural Experience and Management of Stigma Related to Military Caregiving. *Health Communication* 40(4), 642–653. doi: 10.1080/10410236.2024.2360177. **Summary**: Qualitative analysis reveals strategies caregivers employ to resist stigmatizing narratives, highlighting cultural contexts that shape support-seeking behaviors for families dealing with PTSX-related injuries over time.

Wolfgang AS, Fonzo GA et al. (2025). MDMA and MDMA-Assisted Therapy. *American Journal of Psychiatry* 182(1), 79–103. 10.1176/appi.ajp.20230681. **Summary**: Reviews clinical trial evidence supporting MDMA-assisted therapy for PTSX treatment and potential FDA approval pathways.

Wright S, Karyotaki E et al. (2024). Predictors of study dropout in cognitive-behavioural therapy with a trauma focus for PTSX in adults: An individual participant data meta-analysis. *British Medical Journal Mental Health* 27(1). doi:10.1136/bmjment-2024-301159. **Summary**: Identifies factors leading to dropout from CBT-based trauma treatments, emphasizing the need for personalized strategies.

Webermann AR, Coppola EC et al. (2025). Association of Psychiatric Diagnoses and Military Sexual Trauma Type with Denied Post-Traumatic Stress Disorder Service Connection. *Journal of Affective Disorders* 381, 69–76. doi: 10.1016/j.jad.2025.03.171. **Summary**: Analyzes Veterans Affairs claims, revealing how specific psychiatric comorbidities and assault types predict denial of PTSX benefits, highlighting systemic barriers and informing equitable adjudication policies.

Yancey JR, Carson CN et al. (2024). A Literature Review of Mental Health Symptom Outcomes in US Veterans and Servicemembers Following Combat Exposure and Military Sexual Trauma. *Trauma, Violence, and Abuse* 25(2), 1431–1447. 10.1177/15248380231178764. **Summary**: Surveys mental health issues stemming from two prevalent military traumas—combat and military sexual trauma—outlining their distinct and overlapping psychological impacts, as well as current treatment gaps.

Glutathione, N-Acetylcysteine and PTSX

Brady KT and Kalivas PW (2016). A Double-Blind, Randomized, Controlled Pilot Trial of N-Acetylcysteine in Veterans With Posttraumatic Stress Disorder and Substance Use Disorders. *Journal of Clinical Psychiatry* Nov;77(11):e1439-e1446. doi: 10.4088/JCP.15m10239. **Summary**: Tested N-acetylcysteine (NAC) in veterans with both PTSX and substance use disorders. Compared to a placebo, the eight-week NAC treatment significantly reduced symptoms of PTSX, depression, and substance cravings, identifying it as a promising, well-tolerated pharmacological therapy for this challenging dual diagnosis.

Eakin K, Baratz-Goldstein R et al. (2014). Efficacy of N-acetylcysteine in traumatic brain injury. *Public Library of Science One*. Apr 16;9(4):e90617. doi: 10.1371/journal.pone.0090617. **Summary**: Early post-injury treatment with N-Acetylcysteine (NAC) reversed behavioral deficits associated with the TBI in mice.

Marazziti D, Caruso V et al. (2025). The Emerging Role of N-Acetylcysteine in Psychiatry: A Narrative Review of Available Data. *Current Medicinal Chemistry* Sep 23. doi: 10.2174/0109298673365458250901115725. **Summary**: Examines the efficacy of NAC in treating psychiatric conditions, including mood disorders, schizophrenia, anxiety disorders, post-traumatic stress injuries (PTSX), obsessive-compulsive disorder (OCD), substance-use disorders (SUDs), and neurodevelopmental disorders.

Zhou Y, Yuan X and Guo M (2025). Unlocking NAC's potential ATF4 and m6A dynamics in rescuing cognitive impairments in PTSD. *Metabolic Brain Disease* Feb 15;40(2):129. doi: 10.1007/s11011-024-01485-7. **Summary**: Reveals how N-acetylcysteine (NAC) may reverse cognitive deficits in PTSX. The study shows NAC's therapeutic effects are linked to its ability to regulate a stress pathway and modulate certain RNA modifications. This molecular mechanism appears key to rescuing cognitive functions impaired by trauma.

Hyperbaric Oxygen Therapy for PTSX

Doenyas-Barak K, Kutz I et al. (2023). Memory surfacing among veterans with PTSD receiving hyperbaric oxygen therapy. U*ndersea and Hyperbaric Medicine* 50(4), 395–401. **Summary**: Explores how hyperbaric oxygen therapy may trigger the re-emergence of trauma memories in veterans undergoing treatment for PTSX symptoms.

Doenyas-Barak K, Kutz I et al. (2023). Hyperbaric Oxygen Therapy for Veterans With Treatment-resistant PTSD: A Longitudinal Follow-up Study. *Military Medicine* 188(7–8), e2227–e2233. doi: 10.1093/milmed/usac360. **Summary**: Evaluates the longer-term effects of hyperbaric oxygen therapy on veterans with persistent PTSX, noting sustained improvements in symptom severity and daily functioning.

Ketamine and Combined Therapies for PTSX

Feder A, Parides MK et al.(2014). Efficacy of intravenous ketamine for treatment of chronic posttraumatic stress disorder: a randomized clinical trial. *Journal of the American Medical Association Psychiatry* Jun;71(6):681-8. doi:10.1001/jamapsychiatry.2014.62. **Summary**: This double-blind, placebo-controlled trial demonstrates ketamine's efficacy in significantly reducing PTSX symptoms compared to placebo.

Dadabayev AR, Joshi SA et al. (2020). Low Dose Ketamine Infusion for Comorbid Posttraumatic Stress Disorder and Chronic Pain: A Randomized Double-Blind Clinical Trial. *Chronic Stress* (Thousand Oaks) 4:2470547020981670. 10.1177/2470547020981670. **Summary**: Investigates optimized low-dose ketamine infusion protocols for PTSX, highlighting their efficacy and tolerability in clinical practice.

Krystal JH, Abdallah CG et al. (2019). Ketamine: A Paradigm Shift for Depression Research and Treatment. Neuron 101, 774–778. https://doi.org/10.1016/j.neuron.2019.02.005. **Summary**: Highlights ketamine's transformative role in depression research and therapy, emphasizing its rapid antidepressant effects and potential to revolutionize current psychiatric treatment paradigms.

Lasic E, Lisjak M et al. (2019). Astrocyte Specific Remodeling of Plasmalemmal Cholesterol Composition by Ketamine Indicates a New Mechanism of Antidepressant Action. *Scientific Reports* 9, 10957. https://doi.org/10.1038/s41598-019-47459-z. **Summary**: Demonstrates ketamine-induced remodeling of cholesterol composition in astrocyte membranes, suggesting a novel cellular mechanism underlying its rapid antidepressant effects.

Villega F, Fernandes A et al. (2024). Ketamine alleviates NMDA receptor hypofunction through synaptic trapping. *Neuron* 112, 1–18 https://doi.org/10.1016/j.neuron.2024.06.028. **Summary**: Ketamine and other NMDAR blockers enhance receptor trapping at excitatory synapses via scaffolding protein interactions, reversing synaptic and behavioral impairments induced by anti-NMDAR encephalitis patient autoantibodies.

Wolfgang AS, Fonzo GA et al. (2025). MDMA and MDMA-Assisted Therapy. *American Journal of Psychiatry* 182(1), 79–103. 10.1176/appi.ajp.20230681. **Summary**: Reviews the therapeutic potential of MDMA-assisted psychotherapy for PTSX, examining clinical trial outcomes, neurobiological mechanisms, and regulatory considerations shaping its future in psychiatric care.

Zhang Y, Ye F et al. (2021). Structural basis of ketamine action on human NMDA receptors. *Nature* 596, 301-305. doi: 10.1038/s41586-021-03769-9. **Summary**: Elucidates ketamine's molecular interactions with human NMDA receptors through structural analysis, revealing specific binding sites that explain its rapid anesthetic and antidepressant effects.

Mechanotransduction and Neural Pathways

Ahmadzadeh H, Smith DH and Shenoy VB (2015). Mechanical Effects of Dynamic Binding between Tau Proteins on Microtubules during Axonal Injury. *Biophysical Journal* 109(11), 2328–2337. doi: 10.1016/j.bpj.2015.09.010. **Summary**: Shows how dynamic binding between tau proteins and microtubules mechanically impacts axonal integrity during injury, influencing axonal damage outcomes.

Bazarian JJ, Zhong J et al. (2007). Diffusion tensor imaging detects clinically important axonal damage after mild traumatic brain injury: a pilot study. *Journal of Neurotrauma* 24(9), 1447–1459. doi: 10.1089/neu.2007.0241. **Summary**: Demonstrates diffusion tensor imaging effectively identifies significant axonal injury after mild traumatic brain injury, providing sensitive detection beyond standard clinical assessments.

Keating CE and Cullen DK (2021). Mechanosensation in traumatic brain injury. *Neurobiology of Disease* 148:105210. doi: 10.1016/j.nbd.2020.105210. **Summary**: Mechanosensation in traumatic brain injury, highlighting how mechanical forces disrupt neural cells and networks, triggering cellular dysfunction and neurological impairment.

Neurobiological Mechanisms and Biomarkers

Grove AB, Green BA et al. (2024). A Narrative Commentary on the Use of a Rational Emotive Behavior Therapy-Informed Group to Address Irrational Beliefs, Posttraumatic Stress, and Comorbidities. *Brain Sciences* 14(2), 129. doi: 10.3390/brainsci14020129. **Summary**: Explores how REBT-based group therapy can alter negative cognitions and related neurocognitive patterns in PTSX.

Invitto S and Moselli P (2024). Exploring Embodied and Bioenergetic Approaches in Trauma Therapy: Observing Somatic Experience and Olfactory Memory. *Brain Sciences* 14(4), 385. doi: 10.3390/brainsci14040385. **Summary**: Investigates how sensory-based therapies might affect brain processes central to PTSX healing.

Michopoulos V, Norrholm SD and Jovanovic T (2015). Diagnostic Biomarkers for Posttraumatic Stress Disorder: Promising Horizons from Translational Neuroscience Research. *Biological Psychiatry* 78(5), 344–353. doi: 10.1016/j.biopsych.2015.01.005. **Summary**: Reviews emerging biomarkers that may aid in the accurate diagnosis of PTSX, highlighting translational neuroscience findings with potential clinical applications for early detection and targeted treatment.

Neuroendocrine Dysfunction

Araki T, Ikegaya Y et al. (2021). The effects of microglia- and astrocyte-derived factors on neurogenesis in health and disease. *European Journal of Neuroscience* 54(5):5880–5901. doi: 10.1111/ejn.14969. **Summary**: Explores how molecules secreted by microglia and astrocytes regulate neurogenesis under different conditions.

Banks WA (2009). The blood-brain barrier in psychoneuroimmunology. *Neurobiology of Stress* 29(2):223-8. doi: 10.1016/j.iac.2009.02.001. **Summary**: Discusses how the blood-brain barrier modulates the interplay between the immune and nervous systems, particularly under stress conditions.

Fang S, Wu Z et al. (2023). Roles of microglia in adult hippocampal neurogenesis in depression and their therapeutics. *Frontiers in Immunology* 14. doi.org/10.3389/fimmu.2023.1193053. **Summary**: Examines how microglia influence the generation of new neurons in the hippocampus, focusing on depression-related changes.

Malcangio M (2019). Role of the immune system in neuropathic pain. *Scandinavian Journal of Pain* 20(1):33–37. doi: 10.1515/sjpain-2019-0138. **Summary**: Provides a concise overview of how immune cells, including microglia, contribute to the onset and persistence of neuropathic pain.

Mecca C, Giambanco I et al. (2018). Microglia and Aging: The Role of the TREM2-DAP12 and CX3CL1-CX3CR1 Axes. *International Journal of Molecular Sciences* 19(1):318. doi: 10.3390/ijms19010318. **Summary**: Explores how microglial receptors change with age, influencing the inflammatory landscape in the brain.

Norden DM and Godbout JP (2013). Microglia of the aged brain: primed to be activated and resistant to regulation. *Neuropathology and Applied Neurobiology* 39(1), 19–34. doi: 10.1111/j.1365-2990.2012.01306.x. **Summary**: Shows that aging primes microglia to adopt a reactive state that can exacerbate inflammation and neurodegenerative processes.

Pawelec P, Ziemka-Nalecz M et al. (2020). The Impact of the CX3CL1/CX3CR1 Axis in Neurological Disorders. *Cells* 9(10):2277. doi: 10.3390/cells9102277. **Summary**: Examines the critical role in neuron-microglia communication, and how dysregulation of this axis may lead to exacerbated inflammation in various neurological conditions, making it a promising target for therapeutic intervention.

Perry VH and Holmes C (2014). Microglial priming in neurodegenerative disease. *Nature Reviews Neurology* 10(4), 217–224. doi: 10.1038/nrneurol.2014.38. **Summary**: Explores how "primed" microglia respond more aggressively to stimuli, potentially accelerating the progression of neurodegenerative disorders.

Ransohoff RM and Cardona AE (2010). The myeloid cells of the central nervous system parenchyma. *Nature* 468(7321), 253–262. doi.org/10.1038/nature09615. **Summary**: Provides an overview of CNS myeloid cells (including microglia), detailing their roles in homeostasis and disease pathogenesis.

Smith SM and Vale WW (2006). The role of the hypothalamic-pituitary-adrenal axis in neuroendocrine responses to stress. *Dialogues in Clinical Neuroscience* 8(4), 383–395. doi: 10.31887/DCNS.2006.8.4/ssmith. **Summary**: Examines how the HPA axis orchestrates hormonal and physiological responses to stress, influencing both mental and physical health outcomes.

Subbarayan MS, Joly-Amado A et al. (2022). CX3CL1/CX3CR1 signaling targets for the treatment of neurodegenerative diseases. *Pharmacology and Therapeutics* 231:107989. doi: 10.1016/j.pharmthera.2021.107989. **Summary**: Reviews emerging drugs and biological interventions that modulate the fractalkine signaling pathway (CX3CL1/CX3CR1), with a particular focus on preventing or slowing neurodegeneration.

Vecchiarelli HA, Lopes LT et al. (2024). Synapse Regulation. *Advances in Neurobiology* 37:179–208. doi: 10.1007/978-3-031-55529-9_11. **Summary**: Explores how microglia and other glial cells influence synapse formation and elimination.

Wang M, Pan W et al. (2022). Microglia-Mediated Neuroinflammation: A Potential Target for the Treatment of Cardiovascular Diseases. *Journal of Inflammation Research* 15:3083–3094. doi: 10.2147/JIR.S350109. **Summary**: Shows the systemic nature of inflammation about how microglial activation influences CNS and cardiac functioning.

Wang MJ, Kang L et al. (2022). Microglia in motor neuron disease: Signaling evidence from last 10 years. *Developmental Neurobiology* 82(7-8):625–638. doi: 10.1002/dneu.22905. **Summary**: Summarizes research from the past decade on how microglial signaling pathways contribute to motor neuron diseases like ALS.

Wilkinson ST and Sanacora G (2018). A new generation of antidepressants: an update on the pharmaceutical pipeline for novel and rapid-acting therapeutics in mood disorders based on glutamate/GABA neurotransmitter systems. *Drug Discovery Today* 24(2):606–615. doi: 10.1016/j.drudis.2018.11.007. **Summary**: Surveys emerging antidepressant therapies and novel mechanisms of action and potential benefits for treatment-resistant depression.

Zhou R, Ji B etal (2021). PET Imaging of Neuroinflammation in Alzheimer's Disease. *Frontiers in Immunology* 12:739130. doi: 10.3389/fimmu.2021.739130. **Summary**: Addresses the utility of positron emission tomography (PET) scans in detecting and mapping neuroinflammation in Alzheimer's disease.

Neuroimaging and Brain Structure

Akiki TJ, Jubeir J et al.(2025). Neural circuit basis of pathological anxiety. *Nature Reviews Neuroscience* 26(1), 5–22. doi: 10.1038/s41583-024-00880-4. **Summary**: Reviews the neurobiological circuits implicated in pathological anxiety, emphasizing how these insights may refine therapeutic approaches.

Ben-Zion Z, Korem N et al. (2023). Structural Neuroimaging of Hippocampus and Amygdala Subregions in Posttraumatic Stress Disorder: A Scoping Review. *Biological Psychiatry Global Open Science* 4(1), 120–134. doi: 10.1016/j.bpsgos.2023.07.001. eCollection 2024 Jan. **Summary**: Reviews the structural integrity of specific hippocampal and amygdala subregions in PTSX and discusses implications for diagnostic and therapeutic strategies.

Disner SG, Marquardt CA et al. (2017). Spontaneous neural activity differences in posttraumatic stress disorder: A quantitative resting-state meta-analysis and fMRI validation. *Human Brain Mapping* 39(2), 837–850. doi: 10.1002/hbm.23886. **Summary**: Presents meta-analytic evidence of altered resting-state brain activity in PTSX, reinforcing the role of aberrant intrinsic connectivity in symptom manifestation.

Ely SL, Zundel CG et al. (2023).Attention, attention! Posttraumatic stress disorder is associated with altered attention-related brain function. *Frontiers in Behavioral Neuroscience* 17, 1244685. doi: 10.3389/fnbeh.2023.1244685. **Summary**: Demonstrates that individuals with PTSX show significant deviations in neural processes supporting attention, suggesting a new biomarker for this dysfunction.

Flory JD, Yehuda R (2015). Comorbidity between post-traumatic stress disorder and major depressive disorder: alternative explanations and treatment considerations. *Dialogues in Clinical Neuroscience* 17(2), 141–150. doi: 10.31887/DCNS.2015.17.2/jflory. **Summary**: Examines the relationship between PTSX and MDD, highlighting overlapping etiological factors, differential diagnoses, and integrated therapeutic approaches.

Hinojosa CA, George GC and Ben-Zion Z (2024). Neuroimaging of posttraumatic stress disorder in adults and youth: progress over the last decade on three leading questions of the field. *Molecular Psychiatry* 29(10), 3223–3244. doi.org/10.1038/s41380-024-02558-w. **Summary**: Highlights major neuroimaging findings in PTSX across different age groups, synthesizing results from the past decade and proposing priorities for future research.

Huang M, Lewine JD, Lee RR (2020). Magnetoencephalography for Mild Traumatic Brain Injury and Posttraumatic Stress Disorder. *Neuroimaging Clinics of North America* 30(2), 175–192. doi: 10.1016/j.nic.2020.02.003. **Summary**: Examines the utility of magnetoencephalography in detecting subtle brain dysfunction in patients with mild TBI and PTSX, discussing its value for both diagnosis and intervention planning.

Joshi SA, Duval ER et al. (2020). A review of hippocampal activation in post-traumatic stress disorder. *Psychophysiology* 57(1), e13357. doi: 10.1111/psyp.13357. **Summary**: Surveys hippocampal function and activation patterns in PTSX, addressing methodological issues and potential implications for targeted treatments.

Ju Y, Ou W et al. (2020). White matter microstructural alterations in posttraumatic stress disorder: An ROI and whole-brain based meta-analysis. *Journal of Affective Disorders* 266, 655–670. doi: 10.1016/j.jad.2020.01.047. **Summary**: Synthesizes ROI- and whole-brain analyses that reveal consistent white matter disruptions in individuals with PTSX, suggesting altered connectivity as a core feature.

Kitaj M and Goff DC (2024). Why Do Veterans Not Respond as Well as Civilians to Trauma-Focused Therapies for PTSD? *Harvard Review of Psychiatry* 32(4), 160–163. doi: 10.1097/HRP.0000000000000400. **Summary**: Examines the factors contributing to reduced treatment efficacy in veterans compared to civilians and highlights the unique stressors and complexities often faced by servicemembers that impedes therapy outcomes.

Landsteiner A, Ullman K et al. (2022). Neuroimaging and Neurophysiologic Biomarkers for Mental Health: An Evidence Map. Washington (DC): Evidence Synthesis Program, Health Services Research and Development Service, Office of Research and Development, Department of Veterans Affairs. VA ESP Project #09-009. **Summary**: Provides a comprehensive overview of current neuroimaging and neurophysiological markers for mental health diagnoses, with a focus on PTSX and other psychiatric conditions.

Landvater J, Kim S, Caswell K et al. (2024). Traumatic brain injury and sleep in military and veteran populations: A literature review. *NeuroRehabilitation* 55(3), 245–270. doi: 10.3233/NRE-230380. **Summary**: Summarizes research on the intersection of TBI and sleep disturbances in servicemembers and veterans, outlining clinical implications and gaps in current knowledge.

McLean SA, Ressler K et al. (2020). The AURORA Study: a longitudinal, multimodal library of brain biology and function after traumatic stress exposure. *Molecular Psychiatry* 25(2), 283–296. doi: 10.1038/s41380-019-0581-3. **Summary**: Describes a large-scale, longitudinal project on the biological and functional outcomes following traumatic stress, integrating neuroimaging, genomic, and behavioral data.

Medeiros GC, Matheson M et al. (2023). Brain-based correlates of antidepressant response to ketamine: a comprehensive systematic review of neuroimaging studies. *Lancet Psychiatry* 10(10), 790–800. doi: 10.1016/S2215-0366(23)00183-9. **Summary**: Reviews neuroimaging findings related to ketamine's rapid antidepressant action.

Pitman RK, Rasmusson AM et al. (2012). Biological studies of post-traumatic stress disorder. *Nature Reviews Neuroscience* 13(11), 769–787. doi: 10.1038/nrn3339. **Summary**: Examines biological underpinnings of PTSX, focusing on findings from neuroimaging and biochemical research.

Polimanti R and Wendt FR (2021). Posttraumatic stress disorder: from gene discovery to disease biology. *Psychological Medicine* 51(13), 2178–2188. doi: 10.1017/S0033291721000210. **Summary**: Summarizes how genetic findings are reshaping the biological understanding of PTSX, outlining new avenues for research and potential precision therapeutics.

Salat DH, Robinson ME et al. (2017). Neuroimaging of deployment-associated traumatic brain injury (TBI) with a focus on mild TBI (mTBI) since 2009. *Brain Injury* 31(9), 1204–1219. doi: 10.1080/02699052.2017.1327672. **Summary**: Synthesizes key imaging findings on TBI in deployed military populations, emphasizing mild TBI and post-concussive symptoms.

Schmaal L, van Harmelen AL et al. (2020). Imaging suicidal thoughts and behaviors: a comprehensive review of 2 decades of neuroimaging studies. *Molecular Psychiatry* 25(2), 408–427. doi: 10.1038/s41380-019-0587-x. **Summary**: Surveys two decades of neuroimaging literature on suicidality, identifying key brain regions and networks associated with suicidal ideation and behaviors.

Stevens KL, Marquardt CA et al. (2025). Post-Traumatic Stress Symptomatology Rather Than Mild Traumatic Brain Injury Is Related to Atypical Early Neural Processing During Cognitive Control. *Neuropsychology* doi: 10.1037/neu0001008. **Summary**: Event-related potential analyses indicate that PTSX, not mTBI, drives early mediofrontal abnormalities during conflict monitoring, refining neuroimaging biomarkers for differential diagnosis and targeted interventions in veteran populations.

Strigo IA, Craig ADB and Simmons AN (2024). Expectation of pain and relief: A dynamical model of the neural basis for pain-trauma co-morbidity. *Neuroscience and Biobehavioral Reviews* 163, 105750. doi: 10.1016/j.neubiorev.2024.105750. **Summary**: Proposes a neural mechanism by which expectations of pain and subsequent relief may exacerbate or maintain co-occurring pain and trauma-related conditions.

Thompson PM, Jahanshad N et al. (2020). ENIGMA and global neuroscience: A decade of large-scale studies of the brain in health and disease across more than 40 countries. *Translational Psychiatry* 10(1), 100. doi: 10.1038/s41398-020-0705-1. **Summary**: Highlights the collaborative efforts of the ENIGMA consortium in pooling neuroimaging data globally, offering major insights into brain structure and function in numerous psychiatric and neurological conditions.

van Rooij SJH and Jovanovic T (2019). Impaired inhibition as an intermediate phenotype for PTSD risk and treatment response. *Progress in Neuropsychopharmacology and Biological Psychiatry*, 89:435–445. doi: 10.1016/j.pnpbp.2018.10.014 **Summary**: Discusses how imaging studies reveal inhibition deficits in PTSX, linking these to treatment outcomes.

van Rooij SJH, Sippel LM et al. (2021). Defining focal brain stimulation targets for PTSD using neuroimaging. *Depression and Anxiety* 20:10.1002. doi: 10.1002/da.23159. **Summary**: Addresses the use of neuroimaging modalities to pinpoint precise targets for neuromodulation in PTSX, underscoring methodological complexities and clinical implications.

Wilde EA, Bouix S et al. (2015). Advanced neuroimaging applied to veterans and service personnel with traumatic brain injury: state of the art and potential benefits. *Brain Imaging and Behavior* 9(3), 367–402. doi: 10.1007/s11682-015-9444-y. **Summary**: Reviews cutting-edge neuroimaging methods for assessing TBI in military populations and focuses on clinical utility, diagnostic refinement, and improved patient outcomes.

Yue JK, Burke JF et al. (2017). Selective Serotonin Reuptake Inhibitors for Treating Neurocognitive and Neuropsychiatric Disorders Following Traumatic Brain Injury: An Evaluation of Current Evidence. *Brain Sciences* 7(8), 93. doi: 10.3390/brainsci7080093. **Summary**: Evaluates the therapeutic role of SSRIs in managing post-TBI neurocognitive and neuropsychiatric sequelae, discussing efficacy data, dosing considerations, and the potential for improving long-term functional outcomes.

Zhu X, Helpman L et al. (2017). Altered resting state functional connectivity of fear and reward circuitry in comorbid PTSD and major depression. *Depression and Anxiety* 34(7):641-650. doi: 10.1002/da.22594. **Summary**: Reveals altered connectivity between fear and reward networks in PTSX using resting-state fMRI.

Neuroinflammation and Immune Response

Beumer W, Gibney SM et al. (2012). The immune theory of psychiatric diseases: a key role for activated microglia and circulating monocytes. *Journal of Leukocyte Biology* 92(5):959-75. doi: 10.1189/jlb.0212100. **Summary**: Highlights the role of activated microglia and circulating monocytes in the immune mechanisms underlying psychiatric disorders.

Block ML, Zecca L and Hong JS (2007). Microglia-mediated neurotoxicity: uncovering the molecular mechanisms. *Nature Reviews Neuroscience* 8(1), 57-69. doi: 10.1038/nrn2038. **Summary**: Explores the molecular pathways of microglia-mediated neurotoxicity and its implications for neurodegenerative diseases.

Dantzer R, OConnor JC et al. (2008). From inflammation to sickness and depression: when the immune system subjugates the brain. *Nature Reviews Neuroscience* 9(1), 46-56. doi.org/10.1038/nrn2297. **Summary**: The paper discusses how systemic inflammation can induce sickness behavior and depression by impacting brain function.

Felger JC and Miller AH (2012). Cytokine effects on the basal ganglia and dopamine function: the subcortical source of inflammatory malaise. *Frontiers in Neuroendocrinology* 33(3), 315-327. doi: 10.1016/j.yfrne.2012.09.003. **Summary**: Links cytokine-induced inflammation to basal ganglia dysfunction and depressive symptoms via altered signaling.

Madison AA, Wallander SE et al. (2025). C-Reactive Protein as a Possible Indicator of PTSD Prognosis and Comorbid Anhedonia. *Brain, Behavior, and Immunity* 125, 178–183. doi: 10.1016/j.bbi.2025.01.001. **Summary**: Elevated baseline C-reactive protein predicts poorer PTSX recovery and greater anhedonia, implicating systemic inflammation as a prognostic biomarker and potential treatment target.

Miller AH and Raison CL (2016). The role of inflammation in depression: from evolutionary imperative to modern treatment target. *Nature Reviews Immunology* 16(1), 22-34. doi.org/10.1038/nri.2015.5. **Summary**: Connects inflammation's evolutionary roots to its modern implications in depression and outlines potential treatment approaches.

Wohleb ES, Franklin T et al. (2016). Integrating neuroimmune systems in the neurobiology of depression. *Nature Reviews Neuroscience* 17(8), 497-511. doiorg/10.1038/nrn.2016.69. **Summary**: Integrates neuroimmune interactions to elucidate their contributions to the pathophysiology of depression.

Psychedelic-Assisted Therapy

Ellis S, Bostian C et al. (2025). Single-Dose Psilocybin for US Military Veterans with Severe Treatment-Resistant Depression—A First-in-Kind Open-Label Pilot Study. *Journal of Affective Disorders* 369, 381–389. doi: 10.1016/j.jad.2024.09.133. **Summary**: Single 25-mg psilocybin dose rapidly alleviates severe depression in veterans, sustaining mood improvements for eight weeks and supporting further trials of psychedelic-assisted interventions.

Lasic E, Lisjak M, et al. (2019). Astrocyte specific remodeling of plasmalemmal cholesterol composition by ketamine indicates a new mechanism of antidepressant action. *Scientific Reports* 9, 10957. doi:10.1038/s41598-019-47459-z. **Summary**: Identifies ketamine-induced cholesterol remodeling in astrocyte membranes, suggesting a novel cellular mechanism that explains ketamine's rapid antidepressant effects via astrocyte functionality.

Mauney E, King F et al. (2025). Psychedelic-assisted therapy as a promising treatment for irritable bowel syndrome. *Journal of Clinical Gastroenterology* 59(5), 385–392. doi:10.1097/MCG.0000000000002149. **Summary**: Examines the therapeutic potential of psychedelic-assisted therapy, specifically psilocybin, in managing refractory irritable bowel syndrome unresponsive to traditional medical and behavioral treatments.

Neitzke-Spruill L, Beit C et al. (2025). Supportive touch in psychedelic-assisted therapy. *American Journal of Bioethics* 25(1), 29–39. doi:10.1080/15265161.2024.2433428. **Summary**: Discusses ethical considerations and therapeutic benefits of supportive touch in psychedelic-assisted therapy.

Ram AV, Abraham KL and Storch EA (2025). Evidence-based therapy models in a new age of psychedelic-assisted psychotherapy. *Journal of Cognitive Psychotherapy* Advance online publication. doi:10.1891/JCP-2025-0005. **Summary**: Evaluates evidence-based therapy models integrated into psychedelic-assisted psychotherapy, providing guidance for clinicians on effectively utilizing psychedelics to enhance therapeutic outcomes.

Rieser NM, Bitar R et al. (2025). Psilocybin-assisted therapy for relapse prevention in alcohol use disorder: A phase 2 randomized clinical trial. *EClinicalMedicine* 82, 103149. doi:10.1016/j.eclinm.2025.103149. **Summary**: Phase 2 clinical trial showing psilocybin-assisted therapy's efficacy in reducing relapse rates in individuals with alcohol use disorder, highlighting its therapeutic potential.

Wolfgang AS, Fonzo GA et al. (2025). MDMA and MDMA-Assisted Therapy. *American Journal of Psychiatry* 182(1),79–103. doi: 10.1176/appi.ajp.20230681. **Summary**: Reviews the history, regulatory status and therapeutic potential of MDMA for PTSX.

Polyvagal Theory

Porges SW (2025). Disorders of gut-brain interaction through the lens of polyvagal theory. *Neurogastroenterology & Motility* 37(3):e14926. 10.1111/nmo.14926. **Summary**: Applies polyvagal theory to disorders of gut-brain interaction, illuminating the physiological basis of trauma responses and their somatic manifestations in military and civilian populations.

Porges SW (2023). The vagal paradox: A polyvagal solution. *Comprehensive Psychoneuroendocrinology* 16:100200. 10.1016/j.cpnec.2023.100200. **Summary**: Introduces the "vagal paradox" and explains how polyvagal theory can resolve apparent contradictions in trauma-related autonomic responses, offering a new lens for understanding dysregulation in PTSX.

PTSX and Chronic Pain

Anderson J, Parr NJ and Vela K (2020). Evidence Brief: Transcranial Magnetic Stimulation (TMS) for Chronic Pain, PTSD, TBI, Opioid Addiction, and Sexual Trauma. Washington (DC): Department of Veterans Affairs (US). Available from: https://www.ncbi.nlm.nih.gov/books/NBK566938/. **Summary**: Reviews the current evidence for TMS across several conditions common in veteran populations, evaluating safety, effectiveness and clinical applications.

Baria AM, Pangarkar S et al. (2019). Adaption of the Biopsychosocial Model of Chronic Noncancer Pain in Veterans. *Pain Medicine* 20(1), 14–27. doi: 10.1093/pm/pny058. **Summary**: Proposes a veteran-focused adaptation of the biopsychosocial model to address unique risk factors and comorbidities in chronic pain management.

Beech EH, Rahman B et al. (2021). Evidence Brief: Treatment of Comorbid Conditions. Washington (DC): Department of Veterans Affairs (US). Available from: https://www.ncbi.nlm.nih.gov/books/NBK576985/. **Summary**: Summarizes up-to-date research and best practices for treating comorbid mental and physical health disorders, focusing on the needs of veteran populations.

Benedict TM, Keenan PG et al. (2020). Post-Traumatic Stress Disorder Symptoms Contribute to Worse Pain and Health Outcomes in Veterans With PTSD Compared to Those Without: A Systematic Review With Meta-Analysis. *Military Medicine* 185(9–10), e1481–e1491. doi: 10.1093/milmed/usaa052. **Summary**: Quantitatively demonstrates that PTSX severity correlates with heightened pain levels and poorer overall health in veteran populations.

Bradlow RCJ, Berk M et al. (2022). The Potential of N-Acetyl-L-Cysteine (NAC) in the Treatment of Psychiatric Disorders. *CNS Drugs* 36(5), 451–482. doi: 10.1007/s40263-022-00907-3. **Summary**: Evaluates NAC's antioxidant and glutamatergic properties and reviews its potential benefits in PTSX, substance use and mood disorders.

de C Williams AC and Baird E (2016). Special Considerations for the Treatment of Pain from Torture and War. *Current Anesthesiology Reports* 6(4), 319–326. doi: 10.1007/s40140-016-0187-0. **Summary**: Discusses the unique clinical, ethical and psychosocial challenges involved in managing chronic pain arising from torture and war-related injuries.

Fishbein JN, Malaktaris A et al. (2025). Multisite Pain Among United States Veterans with Posttraumatic Stress Disorder: Prevalence, Predictors, and Associations with Symptom Clusters. *Journal of Pain* 28, 104763. doi: 10.1016/j.jpain.2024.104763. **Summary**: Reports 63 percent multisite pain prevalence; higher pain relates to hyperarousal and avoidance, emphasizing need for integrated pain management within PTSX care plans.

Fishbain DA, Pulikal A et al. (2017). Chronic Pain Types Differ in Their Reported Prevalence of Post-Traumatic Stress Disorder (PTSD) and There Is Consistent Evidence That Chronic Pain Is Associated with PTSD: An Evidence-Based Structured Systematic Review. *Pain Medicine* 18(4), 711–735. doi: 10.1093/pm/pnw065. **Summary**: Consolidates evidence linking chronic pain to PTSX and reveals variable prevalence rates across different pain conditions but consistently showing higher PTSX risk.

Glynn H, Möller SP et al. (2021). Prevalence and Impact of Post-traumatic Stress Disorder in Gastrointestinal Conditions: A Systematic Review. *Digestive Diseases and Sciences* 66(12), 4109–4119. doi: 10.1007/s10620-020-06798-y. **Summary**: Examines the frequency and consequences of PTSX among individuals with various GI disorders and highlights biobehavioral mechanisms and gaps in treatment.

Goldsmith E, Koffel E et al. (2021). Implementation of Psychotherapies and Mindfulness-based Stress Reduction for Chronic Pain and Chronic Mental Health Conditions: A Systematic Review. Washington (DC): Department of Veterans Affairs (US). PMID: 35239290. **Summary**: Evaluates the evidence supporting psychotherapies and mindfulness-based interventions for pain and mental health disorders and shows implementation barriers and facilitators in clinical settings.

Hass NC, Wachen JS et al. (2025). Changes in Pain and Related Health Outcomes After Cognitive Processing Therapy in an Active-Duty Military Sample. *Journal of Traumatic Stress* doi: 10.1002/jts.23143. **Summary**: Cognitive processing therapy significantly reduces pain severity and interference.

Higgins DM, Martin AM et al. (2018). The Relationship Between Chronic Pain and Neurocognitive Function: A Systematic Review. *Clinical Journal of Pain* 34(3), 262–275. doi: 10.1097/AJP.0000000000000536. **Summary**: Synthesizes findings on chronic pain-related deficits in memory, attention, and executive functions, underscoring the clinical implications for treatment.

Highland JN, Zanos P et al. (2021). Hydroxynorketamines: Pharmacology and Potential Therapeutic Applications. *Pharmacological Reviews* 73(2), 763–791. doi: 10.1124/pharmrev.120.000149. **Summary**: Investigates ketamine metabolites and their distinct glutamatergic mechanisms, exploring therapeutic possibilities for mood and stress-related disorders.

Invitto S, Moselli P (2024). Exploring Embodied and Bioenergetic Approaches in Trauma Therapy: Observing Somatic Experience and Olfactory Memory. *Brain Sciences* 14(4), 385. doi: 10.3390/brainsci14040385. **Summary**: Investigates how integrating body-centered and olfactory-based methods can enhance trauma therapy.

Johnson JM and Capehart BP (2019). Psychiatric Care of the Post-September 11 Combat Veteran: A Review. *Psychosomatics* 60(2), 121–128. doi: 10.1016/j.psym.2018.11.008. **Summary**: Addresses psychiatric challenges facing post-9/11 veterans, emphasizing integrated treatment approaches for PTSX, depression and comorbid conditions.

Kansagara D, O'Neil M et al. (2017). Benefits and Harms of Cannabis in Chronic Pain or Post-traumatic Stress Disorder: A Systematic Review. Washington (DC): Department of Veterans Affairs (US). Available from: https://www.hsrd.research.va.gov/publications/esp/cannabis.pdf. PMID: 29369568. **Summary**: Reviews existing data on the efficacy and risks of cannabis in managing chronic pain and PTSX and identifies crucial gaps and future research priorities.

Kelly MR, Robbins R and Martin JL (2019). Delivering Cognitive Behavioral Therapy for Insomnia in Military Personnel and Veterans. *Sleep Medicine Clinics* 14(2), 199–208. doi: 10.1016/j.jsmc.2019.01.003. **Summary**: Reviews tailored strategies for applying CBT-Insomnia protocols to military personnel and veterans, identifying unique barriers and key adaptations.

Kent M, Rivers CT and Wrenn G (2015). Goal-Directed Resilience in Training (GRIT): A Biopsychosocial Model of Self-Regulation, Executive Functions, and Personal Growth (Eudaimonia) in Evocative Contexts of PTSD, Obesity, and Chronic Pain. *Behavioral Sciences* (Basel), 5(2), 264–304. doi: 10.3390/bs5020264. **Summary**: Proposes a resilience-promoting framework that harnesses self-regulation and executive function skills to create psychological growth across multiple chronic conditions.

Kim DJ, Mirmina J et al. (2022). Altered physical pain processing in different psychiatric conditions. *Neuroscience and Biobehavioral Reviews* 133, 104510. doi: 10.1016/j.neubiorev.2021.12.033. **Summary**: Summarizes how psychiatric conditions—including PTSX—can modulate the perception and processing of physical pain, underscoring unique neural pathways in each disorder.

Kind S, Otis JD (2019). The Interaction Between Chronic Pain and PTSD. *Current Pain and Headache Reports* 23(12), 91. 10.1007/s11916-019-0828-3. **Summary**: Explores how PTSX and chronic pain can exacerbate one another through shared neurobiological pathways, highlighting the need for collaborative treatment.

Levander XA, Overland MK (2015). Care of women veterans. *Medical Clinics of North America* 99(3), 651–662. doi: 10.1016/j.mcna.2015.01.013. **Summary**: Explores healthcare needs specific to women veterans, highlights reproductive health, mental health and socioeconomic factors impacting care.

Li Y and Loshak H (2021). Stellate ganglionb lock for the treatment of post-traumatic stress disorder, depression, and anxiety. *Ottawa (ON): Canadian Agency for Drugs and Technologies in Health* PMID: 34255448. **Summary**: Summarizes emerging evidence on stellate ganglion block as a therapeutic intervention for PTSX, depression and anxiety, with emphasis on safety and outcomes.

Liang JJ and Rasmusson AM (2018). Overview of the Molecular Steps in Steroidogenesis of the GABAergic Neurosteroids Allopregnanolone and Pregnanolone. *Chronic Stress* (Thousand Oaks), 2, 2470547018818555. doi: 10.1177/2470547018818555. **Summary**: Describes the biochemical pathways for synthesizing allopregnanolone and pregnanolone and discusses their potential relevance to PTSX pathophysiology and treatment.

McCarthy MJ, Wicker A et al. (2024). Feasibility and utility of mobile health interventions for depression and anxiety in rural populations: A scoping review. *Internet Interventions* 35, 100724. doi: 10.1016/j.invent.2024.100724. **Summary**: Synthesizes available data on mHealth solutions for depression and anxiety in rural settings and discusses their potential benefits, barriers and future directions.

Madsen C, Vaughan M and Koehlmoos TP (2017). Use of Integrative Medicine in the United States Military Health System. *Evidence-Based Complementary and Alternative Medicine* 2017:9529257. doi: 10.1155/2017/9529257. **Summary**: Examines the prevalence, types and outcomes of integrative health services in the US military healthcare System, along with policy implications and patient satisfaction.

Mehalick ML and Glueck AC (2018). Examining the relationship and clinical management between traumatic brain injury and pain in military and civilian populations. *Brain Injury* 32(11), 1307–1314. doi: 10.1080/02699052.2018.1495339. **Summary**: Reviews overlapping mechanisms of TBI and pain across diverse populations, with targeted interventions and interdisciplinary care models.

Minervini G, Franco R et al. (2023). Post-traumatic stress, prevalence of temporomandibular disorders in war veterans: Systematic review with meta-analysis. *Journal of Oral Rehabilitation* 50(10), 1101–1109. doi: 10.1111/joor.13535. **Summary**: Offers meta-analytic evidence linking PTSX to increased rates of temporomandibular disorders in war veterans, and gives diagnostic considerations and treatment options.

Nguyen KT, Beauchamp DW and O'Hara RB (2024). A Pathophysiological Approach for Selecting Medications to Treat Nociceptive and Neuropathic Pain in Servicemembers. *Military Medicine* 189(9–10):e1879–e1889. doi: 10.1093/milmed/usad506. **Summary**: Proposes a stepwise, mechanism-based model for treating various types of pain in military personnel, for individualized pharmacotherapy to optimize service-related pain management.

Kaiser A, Cook JM et al. (2019). Posttraumatic stress injuries in older adults: a conceptual review. *Clinical Gerontologist* 42(4), 359–376. doi: 10.1080/07317115.2018.1539801. **Summary**: Examines how PTSX manifests and is managed in older adults, featuring life-course factors, comorbidity profiles and tailored interventions.

Rasmusson AM, Marx CE et al. (2017). Neuroactive steroids and PTSD treatment. *Neuroscience Letters* 649, 156–163. doi: 10.1016/j.neulet.2017.01.054. **Summary**: Explores the therapeutic role of neuroactive steroids in PTSX, focusing on their potential to modulate neurobiological stress circuits and alleviate symptoms.

Reid KF, Bannuru RR et al. (2019). The effects of tai chi mind-body approach on the mechanisms of Gulf War Illness: an umbrella review. *Integrative Medicine Research* 8(3), 167–172. 10.1016/j.imr.2019.05.003. **Summary**: Analyzes existing evidence on tai chi's effects in Gulf War I illness, and discusses its role in modifying symptoms through mind-body pathways.

Reid MW and Velez CS (2015). Discriminating military and civilian traumatic brain injuries. *Molecular and Cellular Neuroscience*, 66(Pt B), 123–128. doi: 10.1016/j.mcn.2015.03.014. **Summary**: Contrasts the underlying pathophysiology of TBI sustained in military settings with that seen in civilian populations, with implications for diagnosis and treatment.

Ruben MA, Blanch-Hartigan D and Shipherd JC (2018). To Know another's pain: A meta-analysis of caregivers' and healthcare providers' pain assessment accuracy. *Annals of Behavioral Medicine* 52(8), 662–685. doi: 10.1093/abm/kax036. **Summary**: Meta-analysis of how well caregivers and clinicians evaluate patient pain levels.

Saconi B, Polomano RC et al. (2021). The influence of sleep disturbances and sleep disorders on pain outcomes among veterans: A systematic scoping review. *Sleep Medicine Reviews* 56, 101411. doi: 10.1016/j.smrv.2020.101411. **Summary**: Examines the relationship between poor sleep quality and worsened chronic pain in veteran populations, advocating integrated strategies to address co-occurring issues.

Santini A, Petruzzo A et al. (2021). Management of chronic musculoskeletal pain in veterans: a systematic review. *Acta Biomed* 92(S2), e2021011. doi: 10.23750/abm.v92iS2.11352. **Summary**: Addresses tailored approaches for chronic musculoskeletal pain in veterans, emphasizing interdisciplinary strategies and psychosocial interventions.

Schoneboom BA, Perry SM et al. (2016). Answering the call to address chronic pain in military service members and veterans: Progress in improving pain care and restoring health. *Nursing Outlook* 64(5), 459–484. doi: 10.1016/j.outlook.2016.05.010. **Summary**: Chronicles advancements in pain care policy and practice for military and veteran populations.

Strigo IA, Craig ADB and Simmons AN (2024). Expectation of pain and relief: A dynamical model of the neural basis for pain-trauma co-morbidity. *Neuroscience and Biobehavioral Reviews* 163, 105750. doi: 10.1016/j.neubiorev.2024.105750. **Summary**: Proposes a computational model illustrating how anticipation of pain and subsequent relief might drive the interplay between chronic pain and PTSX symptoms.

PTSX and the Gut Microbiome

Bercik P, Denou E et al. (2011). The intestinal microbiota affect central levels of brain-derived neurotrophic factor and behavior in mice. *Gastroenterology* 141(2), 599-609. doi: 10.1053/j.gastro.2011.04.052. **Summary**: Highlights the impact of gut microbiota on brain-derived neurotrophic factor (BDNF), influencing behavior and stress responses in animal models.

Clarke G, Grenham S et al. (2013). The microbiome-gut-brain axis during early life regulates the hippocampal serotonergic system in a sex-dependent manner. *Molecular Psychiatry* 18(6), 666-673. doi.org/10.1038/mp.2012.77. **Summary**: Examines how early-life microbiome changes affect serotonin regulation in the hippocampus, with implications for mood disorders and PTSX.

Hoban AE, Stilling RM et al. (2016). Regulation of prefrontal cortex myelination by the microbiota. *Translational Psychiatry* 6(10), e891. doi.org/10.1038/tp.2016.42. **Summary**: Investigates how gut microbiota influence myelination in the prefrontal cortex, a region implicated in emotional regulation and PTSX.

Kalisch R, Russo SJ, Müller MB (2024). Neurobiology and systems biology of stress resilience. *Physiological Reviews* 104(3), 1205–1263. doi: 10.1152/physrev.00042.2023. **Summary**: Synthesizes key molecular, neural, and network-level mechanisms that underpin resilience to stress, offering a systems biology perspective on potential therapeutic targets.

Kelly JR, Borre Y et al. (2016). Transferring the blues: Depression-associated gut microbiota induces neurobehavioural changes in the rat. *Journal of Psychiatric Research* 82, 109-118. doi: 10.1016/j.jpsychires.2016.07.019. **Summary**: Demonstrates that gut microbiota from depressed individuals induces depressive-like behaviors in animal models, thus supporting the gut-brain axis hypothesis.

Petakh P, Duve K et al. (2024). Molecular mechanisms and therapeutic possibilities of short-chain fatty acids in posttraumatic stress disorder patients: a mini-review. *Frontiers in Neuroscience* 18, 1394953. doi: 10.3389/fnins.2024.1394953. **Summary**: Discusses how short-chain fatty acids influence neuroimmune processes in PTSX and examines emerging therapeutic strategies targeting the gut microbiota.

Petakh P, Oksenych V et al. (2024). Exploring the interplay between posttraumatic stress disorder, gut microbiota, and inflammatory biomarkers: a comprehensive meta-analysis. *Frontiers in Immunology* 15, 1349883. doi: 10.3389/fimmu.2024.1349883. **Summary**: Meta-analysis of associations between dysregulated gut microbiota, heightened inflammatory markers and PTSX pathophysiology.

Porges SW (2025). Disorders of gut-brain interaction through the lens of polyvagal theory. *Neurogastroenterology & Motility* 37(3):e14926. 10.1111/nmo.14926. **Summary**: Applies polyvagal theory to disorders of gut-brain interaction, illuminating the physiological basis of trauma responses and their somatic manifestations in military and civilian populations.

Ribera C, Sánchez-Ortí JV et al. (2024). Probiotic, prebiotic, synbiotic and fermented food supplementation in psychiatric disorders: A systematic review of clinical trials. *Neuroscience and Biobehavioral Reviews* 158, 105561. doi: 10.1016/j.neubiorev.2024.105561. **Summary**: Critically reviews clinical trial findings on the efficacy of gut-targeted nutritional interventions in mental health settings and suggests emerging psychobiotic strategies.

Schenck CH (2025). REM sleep behaviour disorder (RBD): Personal perspectives and research priorities. *Journal of Sleep Research* e14228. 34(2):e14228. doi: 10.1111/jsr.14228. **Summary**: Presents firsthand observations on RBD, delineates current research gaps, and proposes future directions to deepen understanding and improve clinical management.

Strandwitz P (2018). Neurotransmitter modulation by the gut microbiota. *Brain Research* 1693, 128-133. doi: 10.1016/j.brainres.2018.03.015. **Summary**: Explores how gut bacteria produce neurotransmitters like serotonin and GABA, which affect mood and cognitive processes central to PTSX.

Verma A, Inslicht SS and Bhargava A (2024). Gut-Brain Axis: Role of Microbiome, Metabolomics, Hormones, and Stress in Mental Health Disorders. *Cells* 13(17), 1436. doi: 10.3390/cells13171436. **Summary**: Highlights the multifaceted influence of gut microbiota, metabolic byproducts, and endocrine responses on mental health, underscoring the promise of microbiome-based interventions.

PTSX and Psychotherapy and Cognitive Behavioral Treatments

Acierno R, Jaffe AE et al. (2021). A randomized clinical trial of in-person vs. home-based telemedicine delivery of prolonged exposure for PTSD in military sexual trauma survivors. *Journal of Anxiety Disorders* 83:102461. doi.org/10.1016/j.janxdis.2021.102461. **Summary**: Women veterans with MST-related PTSX were randomized to in-person or home-based telemedicine prolonged exposure. Both reduced PTSX/depression similarly. Session dose was linked to greater symptom improvement.

Acierno R, Knapp R et al. (2017). A non-inferiority trial of prolonged exposure for posttraumatic stress disorder: In-person versus home-based telehealth. *Behaviour Research and Therapy* 89, 57–65. doi.org/10.1016/j.brat.2016.11.009. **Summary**: Telehealth-delivered prolonged exposure reduced PTSX symptoms as effectively as clinic sessions.

Back SE, Killeen T et al. (2019). Concurrent treatment of substance use disorders and PTSD using prolonged exposure: A randomized clinical trial in military veterans. *Addictive Behaviors* 90, 369–377. doi.org/10.1016/j.addbeh.2018.11.032. **Summary**: Integrating prolonged exposure within substance-use treatment significantly lowered PTSX severity and alcohol or drug use in veterans, supporting concurrent therapy's safety and efficacy.

DeJesus CR, Trendel SL and Sloan DM (2024). A systematic review of written exposure therapy for the treatment of posttraumatic stress symptoms. *Psychological Trauma* 16(Suppl 3):S620-S626. doi: 10.1037/tra0001659. **Summary**: Synthesizes findings on written exposure therapy's effectiveness for PTSX-related symptoms.

Dell L, Sbisa AM et al. (2023). Massed v. standard prolonged exposure therapy for PTSD in military personnel and veterans: 12-month follow-up of a non-inferiority randomised controlled trial. *Psychological Medicine* 53(15), 7070-7077. doi: 10.1017/S0033291723000405. **Summary**: Compares massed versus standard prolonged exposure therapy for PTSX in military personnel and veterans, demonstrating non-inferiority at a 12-month follow-up.

Fredman SJ, Gamaldo AA et al. (2025). An Initial Examination of Couple Therapy for PTSD Outcomes Among Black/African American Adults: Findings from an Uncontrolled Trial with Military Dyads. *Behavioral Sciences* 15(4), 537. doi: 10.3390/bs15040537. **Summary**: Culturally adapted couple therapy yields moderate PTSX and relationship improvements, spotlighting the importance of inclusive, relationship-based interventions for underserved groups.

Levis M, Dimambro M et al. (2025). Evaluating Evidence-Based Psychotherapy Utilization Patterns Among Suicide-Risk-Stratified Veterans Diagnosed with Posttraumatic Stress Disorder. *Clinical Psychology & Psychotherapy* 32(1), e70041. doi: 10.1002/cpp.70041. **Summary**: VA database analysis shows lowest psychotherapy uptake among highest suicide-risk veterans, underscoring systemic barriers and urging targeted outreach to enhance treatment equity.

Peterson AL, Blount TH et al. (2023). Massed vs Intensive Outpatient Prolonged Exposure for Combat-Related Posttraumatic Stress Disorder: A Randomized Clinical Trial. *Journal of the American Medical Association Network Open* 6;(1):e2249422. doi:10.1001/jamanetworkopen.2022.49422. **Summary**: Compares massed and intensive outpatient prolonged exposure therapy for combat-related PTSX.

PTSX and Sleep Disturbances

Al-Khalil Z, Attarian H et al. (2024). Sleep health inequities in vulnerable populations: Beyond sleep deserts. *Sleep Medicine* X 7:100110. doi: 10.1016/j.sleepx.2024.100110. **Summary**: Analyzes structural, socioeconomic and environmental barriers that controbute to poor sleep health in underserved populations, and suggests strategies to address these inequities.

Atwood ME (2024). Effects of Sleep Deficiency on Risk, Course, and Treatment of Psychopathology. *Sleep Medicine Clinics* 19(4), 639–652. doi: 10.1016/j.jsmc.2024.07.010. **Summary**: Reviews the clinical impact of inadequate sleep on the onset, progression and management of various psychiatric disorders, integrating sleep assessments into standard mental healthcare.

Barone DA (2024). Trauma-Associated Sleep Disorder. *Sleep Medicine Clinics* 19(1), 93–99. doi: 10.1016/j.jsmc.2023.10.005. **Summary**: Defines the criteria and pathophysiology of trauma-associated sleep disorder, highlighting its distinct features and potential interventions for affected individuals.

Boyle JT, Fischer I et al. (2025). Negative Aging Stereotypes and Clinical Insomnia in Older US Military Veterans. *Gerontologist* 65(4), gnaf036. doi: 10.1093/geront/gnaf036. **Summary**: Older veterans endorsing negative aging stereotypes exhibit greater insomnia severity independent of demographics and comorbidity, suggesting cognitive-belief interventions may complement sleep treatments to improve late-life mental health.

Bryant BJ (2024). Trauma Exposure in Migrant Children: Impact on Sleep and Acute Treatment Interventions. *Child and Adolescent Psychiatric Clinics of North America* 33(2), 193–205. doi: 10.1016/j.chc.2023.08.001. **Summary**: Identifies how traumatic experiences in migrant children disrupt sleep patterns.

Contractor AA, Almeida IM et al. (2024). Posttraumatic Stress Disorder Symptoms and Sleep Disturbances Among Asian Indians: A Systematic Review. *Trauma, Violence, and Abuse* 25(2), 1468–1483. doi: 10.1177/15248380231184207. **Summary**: Summarizes literature on PTSX symptomatology and co-occurring sleep problems in Asian Indian populations.

Efstathiou M, Kakaidi V et al. (2025). The prevalence of mental health issues among nursing students: An umbrella review synthesis of meta-analytic evidence. *International Journal of Nursing Studies* 163:104993. doi: 10.1016/j.ijnurstu.2025.104993. **Summary**: Synthesizes multiple meta-analyses documenting elevated rates of anxiety, depression and stress among nursing students, and suggests structural and educational reforms.

Fellman V, Heppell PJ and Rao S (2021). Afraid and Awake: The Interaction Between Trauma and Sleep in Children and Adolescents. *Psychiatric Clinics of North America* 30(1):225-249. doi: 10.1016/j.chc.2020.09.002. **Summary**: Explores how trauma disrupts sleep architecture in young people.

Georgescu MF, Fischer IC et al. (2025). Posttraumatic Stress Disorder and Insomnia in US Military Veterans: Prevalence, Correlates, and Psychiatric and Functional Burden. *Journal of Sleep Research* 34(1), e14269. doi: 10.1111/jsr.14269. **Summary**: National cohort shows PTSX strongly associated with chronic insomnia, compounding psychiatric comorbidity and functional impairment, underscoring the need to integrate sleep interventions into trauma care.

Germain A (2013). Sleep Disturbances as the Hallmark of PTSD: Clinical Challenges and Advanced Therapies. American *Journal of Psychiatry* 170(4):372-82. 10.1176/appi.ajp.2012.12040432. **Summary**: Highlights the severe disruption of sleep and nightmares in PTSX, and discusses advanced therapeutic approaches.

Giannotta G, Ruggiero M and Trabacca A (2024). Chronobiology in Paediatric Neurological and Neuropsychiatric Disorders: Harmonizing Care with Biological Clocks. *Journal of Clinical Medicine* 13(24), 7737. 10.3390/jcm13247737. **Summary**: Examines how disruptions in circadian rhythms affect pediatric neurologic and psychiatric outcomes, and proposes chronotherapeutic approaches to align treatments with inherent biological cycles.

Goldstein LA, Bernhard PA et al. (2025). Prevalence of Obstructive Sleep Apnea Among Veterans and Nonveterans. *American Journal of Health Promotion* 39(2), 215–223. doi: 10.1177/08901171241273443. **Summary**: Large survey estimates higher obstructive sleep apnea prevalence in veterans versus civilians, indicating military-service factors warrant routine sleep-disordered breathing evaluation in VA systems.

Herring TE, Chopra A et al. (2024). Post traumatic stress and sleep disorders in long COVID: Patient management and treatment. *Life Sciences* 357,123081. doi: 10.1016/j.lfs.2024.123081. **Summary**: Reviews emerging evidence on PTSX-like symptoms and sleep disturbances in long COVID patients, offering insights into diagnostic strategies and integrated care models.

Huang CY, Zhao YF et al. (2024). Psychotherapeutic and pharmacological agents for post-traumatic stress disorder with sleep disorder: network meta-analysis. *Annals of Medicine* 56(1), 2381696. doi: 10.1080/07853890.2024.2381696. **Summary**: Compares multiple therapies for PTSX with concurrent sleep disturbances.

Kalra A, Kang JK et al. (2024). Long-Term Neuropsychiatric, Neurocognitive, and Functional Outcomes of Patients Receiving ECMO: A Systematic Review and Meta-Analysis. *Neurology* 102(3), e208081. doi: 10.1212/WNL.0000000000208081. **Summary**: Consolidates data on post-ECMO survivors' prolonged mental health, cognitive and functional challenges, demonstrating the need for targeted follow-up care.

Lappas AS, Glarou E et al. (2024). Pharmacotherapy for sleep disturbances in post-traumatic stress disorder (PTSD): A network meta-analysis. *Sleep Medicine* 119, 467–479. doi: 10.1016/j.sleep.2024.05.032. **Summary**: Evaluates and ranks diverse pharmacologic agents in sleep disruptions in PTSX, and guides clinical decision-making based on comparative effectiveness.

Mehta MM, Johnson AE et al. (2024). Climate Change and Aging: Implications for Psychiatric Care. *Current Psychiatry Reports* 26(10), 499–513. doi: 10.1007/s11920-024-01525-0. **Summary**: Discusses how climate-related stressors disproportionately affect older adults' mental health.

Mendes TP, Pereira BG et al. (2025). Factors impacting prazosin efficacy for nightmares and insomnia in PTSD patients – a systematic review and meta-regression analysis. *Progress in Neuro-Psychopharmacology and Biological Psychiatry* 136, 111253. doi: 10.1016/j.pnpbp.2025.111253. **Summary**: Investigates prazosin's mixed efficacy on PTSX-related sleep disruptions, and identifies patient- and study-level factors influencing treatment response.

Mendoza Alvarez M, Balthasar Y et al. (2025). Systematic review: REM sleep, dysphoric dreams and nightmares as transdiagnostic features of psychiatric disorders with emotion dysregulation – Clinical implications. *Sleep Medicine* 127, 1–15. doi: 10.1016/j.sleep.2024.12.037. **Summary**: Provides a transdiagnostic perspective on disturbed REM sleep and nightmares across psychiatric illnesses, and proposes novel interventions targeting nightmare-related emotion dysregulation.

Todd RC 3rd (2024). A Dynamic Foundation: Aberrations of Sleep Architecture and Its Association With Clinical and Sub-clinical Psychopathology. *Cureus* 16(2), e55262. doi: 10.7759/cureus.55262. **Summary**: Discusses how deviations in sleep stages and transitions might exacerbate both full-blown and borderline psychiatric conditions, and suggests avenues for diagnostic enhancement and early intervention.

Worley CB, Meshberg-Cohen S et al. (2025). Trauma-Related Nightmares Among US Veterans: Findings from a Nationally Representative Study. *Sleep Medicine* 126, 159–166. doi: 10.1016/j.sleep.2024.11.031. **Summary**: Quantifies prevalence, frequency, and clinical correlates of distressing nightmares, highlighting their independent association with PTSX severity and underscoring the need for targeted sleep-focused interventions in veterans.

PTSX and Substance Use Disorder Comorbidity

Back SE, Jarnecke AM et al. (2024). State of the Science: Treatment of comorbid posttraumatic stress and substance use disorders. *Journal of Traumatic Stress* 37(6), 803–813. doi: 10.1002/jts.23049. **Summary**: Surveys integrated interventions addressing both PTSX and SUD, noting high co-occurrence and complex treatment challenges.

Rawls E, Marquardt CA et al. (2025). Post-Traumatic Reexperiencing and Alcohol Use: Mediofrontal Theta as a Neural Mechanism for Negative Reinforcement. *Journal of Psychopathology and Clinical Science* 134(3), 308–318. doi: 10.1037/abn0000925. **Summary**: Demonstrates that heightened mediofrontal theta power bridges PTSX intrusions and alcohol craving, proposing a neurophysiological target to disrupt maladaptive self-medication cycles in veterans with comorbidity.

Kaye JT, Betts JM et al. (2025). Behavioral Activation for Smoking Cessation in Veterans with Posttraumatic Stress Disorder: A Randomized Clinical Trial. *Nicotine & Tobacco Research* Published online March 12. doi: 10.1093/ntr/ntaf054. **Summary**: Behavioral activation markedly increases biochemically verified quit rates, demonstrating an effective adjunct for addressing nicotine addiction and reinforcing positive mood among smoking veterans with PTSX.

PTSX and the Whole Body

Beumer W, Gibney SM, Drexhage RC, et al. (2012). The immune theory of psychiatric diseases: A key role for activated microglia and circulating monocytes. *Journal of Leukocyte Biology* 92(5), 959-975. doi: 10.1189/jlb.0212100. **Summary**: Highlights the role of immune activation, particularly microglia, in the pathology of psychiatric disorders, including PTSX.

LeBeau K, Lopez J et al. (2025). Understanding the intersectionality of the rural Hispanic/Latino Veteran population: A scoping review of health-related challenges. *Ethnicity & Health* 10.1080/13557858.2025.2486413. **Summary**: Synthesizes health disparities faced by rural Hispanic/Latino veterans.

Manzo LL, Dindinger RA et al. (2024). The Impact of Military Trauma Exposures on Servicewomen's Pregnancy Outcomes: A Scoping Review. *Journal of Midwifery and Women's Health* 69(5), 634–646. doi: 10.1111/jmwh.13620. **Summary**: Synthesizes data on how combat and military sexual trauma can influence reproductive health among servicewomen, with implications for prenatal care and the potential need for trauma-informed obstetrics support.

McCarthy KJ, Morgan NR et al. (2025). The Impact of Adversity on Body Mass Index as Veterans Transition to Civilian Life. *Military Medicine* 190(5-6), e1121–e1131. doi: 10.1093/milmed/usae433. **Summary**: Military adversity experiences predict higher BMI trajectories during civilian reintegration, highlighting need for trauma-sensitive weight-management programs addressing stress-eating and metabolic dysregulation.

Mei P, Cotiga D et al. (2025). Cardiovascular Care in Women Veterans: An Updated Profile. *Current Cardiology Reports* 27(1), 93. doi: 10.1007/s11886-025-02247-2. **Summary**: Reviews cardiovascular disease burden, sex-specific risk factors, and screening gaps in women veterans, advocating integrated cardiology-mental-health approaches that account for PTSX's contributions to heart disease.

Morse JL, Fishbein JN et al. (2025). Posttraumatic Stress Disorder and Weight Loss in Male and Female Active-Duty Service Members: A Weight Management Study. *Military Medicine* doi: 10.1093/milmed/usae561. **Summary**: Predicts less weight loss during standardized lifestyle intervention, indicating trauma-linked behavioral and physiological barriers.

Zucker TL, Samuelson KW et al. (2009). The effects of respiratory sinus arrhythmia biofeedback on heart rate variability and posttraumatic stress disorder symptoms: a pilot study. *Applied Psychophysiology and Biofeedback* 34(2):135-43. doi: 10.1007/s10484-009-9085-2. **Summary**: Provides evidence for the effectiveness of heart-rate variability biofeedback in improving emotional regulation and reducing PTSX symptoms.

Resilience, Social Support and Post-Traumatic Growth in PTSX

Borowski S, Caine ED et al. (2025). Well-Being and Suicidal Ideation in US Veterans: Age Cohort Effects During Military-to-Civilian Transition. *American Journal of Preventive Medicine* 68(5), 944–953. doi: 10.1016/j.amepre.2025.01.023. **Summary**: Age-cohort analysis shows declining psychological wellbeing and increasing suicidal ideation during military-to-civilian transition, especially among younger veterans, informing age-specific prevention and resilience-building initiatives programs nationwide.

Brennan CJ, Roberts C and Cole JC (2024). Prevalence of occupational moral injury and post-traumatic embitterment disorder: a systematic review and meta-analysis. *British Medical Journal Open* 14(2), e071776. doi: 10.1136/bmjopen-2023-071776. **Summary**: Identifies moral injury as a workplace stressor leading to PTSX-like distress across various professional settings.

Danon A, Dekel R et al. (2025). Between Mourning and Hope: A Mixed-Methods Study of Ambiguous Loss and Post-Traumatic Stress Symptoms Among Partners of Israel Defence Force Veterans. *Psychological Trauma* 17(4), 795–804. doi: 10.1037/tra0001794. **Summary**: Quantitative and qualitative findings show ambiguous loss intensifies post-traumatic stress while hope and relational support mitigate distress.

D'Antoni F, Matiz A, Crescentini C (2025). Mindfulness-Oriented Professional Resilience (MOPR) Training to Reduce Compassion Fatigue in Healthcare Workers: A Pilot Study. *Healthcare* (Basel) 13(2):92. 10.3390/healthcare13020092. **Summary**: Presents a pilot study demonstrating how MOPR training can reduce compassion fatigue in healthcare workers, with implications for trauma recovery and resilience-building in high-stress environments.

Farzandipour M, Sharif R and Anvari S (2025). Effects of mhealth applications on military personnel's physical and mental health: A systematic review. *Military Psychology* 37(3):199-207. doi: 10.1080/08995605.2024.2336640. **Summary**: Smartphone-based interventions promote resilience and reduce PTSX symptoms in military cohorts.

Fortney JC, Garcia N et al. (2024). A Systematic Review of Social Support Instruments for Measurement-Based Care in Posttraumatic Stress Issues. *Current Psychology* 43(22). doi: 10.1007/s12144-024-05799-8. **Summary**: Reviews validated tools for assessing social support, reinforcing its relevance to PTSX recovery.

Grover LE, Williamson C et al. (2024). Level of perceived social support, and associated factors, in combat-exposed (ex-)military personnel: a systematic review and meta-analysis. *Social Psychiatry and Psychiatric Epidemiology* 59(12), 2119–2143. doi: 10.1007/s00127-024-02685-3. **Summary**: Reviews how perceived social support correlates with mental-health outcomes in combat-exposed personnel.

Grubbs KM, Knopp KC et al. (2025). Discrepancies in Perceptions of PTSD Symptoms Among Veteran Couples: Links to Poorer Relationship and Individual Functioning. *Family Process* 64(1), e13041. doi: 10.1111/famp.13041. **Summary**: Symptom-perception gaps within couples correlate with reduced relationship satisfaction and higher distress, suggesting dyadic assessment should foster mutual understanding to support recovery.

Hinojosa CA, George GC and Ben-Zion Z (2024). Neuroimaging of posttraumatic stress disorder in adults and youth: progress over the last decade on three leading questions of the field. *Molecular Psychiatry* 29(10), 3223–3244. 10.1038/s41380-024-02558-w. **Summary**: Discusses new imaging data that shows resilience factors and neural plasticity in PTSX across lifespan.

Irrgang M, Boyd MR et al. (2025). Patterns of Psychosocial Functioning of Treatment-Seeking Veterans Following Military Sexual Trauma: The Differential Association of Functioning and Identity. *Psychological Services* 22(2), 369–376. doi: 10.1037/ser0000919. **Summary**: Latent profile analysis reveals distinct post-MST functioning patterns; identity disruption predicts poorer outcomes, guiding tailored rehabilitation to support self-concept and social reintegration nationwide.

McCarthy MJ, Wicker A et al. (2024). Feasibility and utility of mobile health interventions for depression and anxiety in rural populations: A scoping review. *Internet Interventions* 35, 100724. doi: 10.1016/j.invent.2024.100724. **Summary**: Shows how digital tools can enhance access to care and bolster resilience for rural individuals with PTSX or other mental-health conditions.

Manzo LL, Dindinger RA et al. (2024). The Impact of Military Trauma Exposures on Servicewomen's Pregnancy Outcomes: A Scoping Review. *Journal of Midwifery and Women's Health* 69(5), 634–646. doi: 10.1111/jmwh.13620. **Summary**: Investigates how PTSX from military trauma influences pregnancy experiences among servicewomen.

Metts A, Mendoza C et al. (2025). Longitudinal Associations Among Resilience, Social Isolation, and Gender in US Iraq and Afghanistan-Era Veterans. *Journal of Traumatic Stress* 38(1), 146–157. doi: 10.1002/jts.23111. **Summary**: Resilience buffers deleterious effects of social isolation differently by gender, suggesting targeted community-building strategies to sustain psychological health among Iraq-Afghanistan era veterans over time.

Shin J, Fischer IC et al. (2025). Successful Aging in US Veterans with Mental Disorders: Results from the National Health and Resilience in Veterans Study. *American Journal of Geriatric Psychiatry* 33(1), 85–91. doi: 10.1016/j.jagp.2024.07.018. **Summary**: Identifies psychological resilience, purpose, and social connectedness as key predictors of successful aging despite PTSX, offering modifiable targets to promote late-life wellbeing in veteran communities.

Vigilante K, Batten SV et al. (2025). Camaraderie Among US Veterans and Their Preferences for Health Care Systems and Practitioners. *Journal of the American Medical Association Network Open* 8(4), e255253. doi: 10.1001/jamanetworkopen.2025.5253. **Summary**: Finds that strong veteran camaraderie predicts preference for peer-inclusive, military-competent providers, suggesting that social connection can guide service design and enhance engagement in PTSX treatment.

Wan R, Wan R et al. (2025). Current Status and Future Directions of Artificial Intelligence in Post-Traumatic Stress: A Literature Measurement Analysis. *Behavioral Sciences* (Basel) 15(1), 27. doi: 10.3390/bs15010027. **Summary**: Examines how AI can enhance diagnosis, personalized treatment, and research innovation in PTSX care.

Wells SY, Patel TA et al. (2024). The impact of trauma-focused psychotherapies on anger: A systematic review and meta-analysis. *Psychological Trauma* 10.1037/tra0001697. doi: 10.1037/tra0001697. **Summary**: Demonstrates that reducing core PTSX symptoms often yields concurrent reductions in anger.

Yancey JR, Carson CN et al. (2024). A Literature Review of Mental Health Symptom Outcomes in US Veterans and Servicemembers Following Combat Exposure and Military Sexual Trauma. *Trauma, Violence, and Abuse* 25(2), 1431–1447. doi: 10.1177/15248380231178764. **Summary**: Reviews how personal strengths and coping resources influence post-traumatic growth in PTSX-affected servicemembers.

Yuan Z, Peng C et al. (2025). Effects of physical activity on patients with posttraumatic stress: A systematic review and meta-analysis of randomized controlled trials. *Medicine* 104(3), e41139.doi: 10.1097/MD.0000000000041139. **Summary**: Reveals structured exercise programs can reduce PTSX symptom severity and improve coping.

Yang R, Fischer IC et al. (2025). Psychosocial Correlates of Optimism Among US Military Veterans. *Journal of Clinical Psychiatry* 86(2), 25br15791. doi: 10.4088/JCP.25br15791. **Summary**: Examines veterans' various service-related predictors of dispositional optimism and reveals key social and mental health factors.

Stellate Ganglion Block and Combined Therapies

Hanling SR, Hickey A and Lesnik I (2016). Stellate ganglion block for the treatment of posttraumatic stress disorder: a randomized, double-blind, controlled trial. *Regional Anesthesia and Pain Medicine* 41(4), 494-500. doi: 10.1097/AAP.0000000000000402. **Summary**: Double-blind controlled trial investigates the effectiveness of SGB in treating PTSX, offering evidence on its clinical utility.

Hasoon J, Sultana S et al. (2024). Stellate Ganglion Blocks for Post-Traumatic Stress Disorder: A Review of Mechanisms, Efficacy, and Complications. *Psychopharmacol Bulletin* 54(4), 106–118. PMID: 39263203. **Summary**: Explores the rationale and physiological underpinnings of stellate ganglion blocks in PTSX, assessing clinical effectiveness, safety profile, and potential complications.

Hickey A, Hanling S et al. (2012). Stellate ganglion block for PTSD. *American Journal of Psychiatry* 169(7), 760. doi.org/10.1176/appi.ajp.2012.1111172. **Summary**: Discusses the application of SGB in PTSX treatment, highlighting clinical observations and potential benefits.

Lipov EG (2024). Comments on "A Comprehensive Overview of the Stellate Ganglion Block Throughout the Past Three Decades: A Bibliometric Analysis." *Pain Physician* 27(7):E795-E801. PMID: 39353132. **Summary**: Commentary on a bibliometric analysis of stellate ganglion block, emphasizing its evolution, research trends and clinical relevance over the past three decades.

Lipov EG, Candido K and Ritchie EC. (2017). Possible Reversal of PTSD-Related DNA Methylation by Sympathetic Blockade. *Journal of Molecular Neuroscience* 62(1):67-72. doi: 10.1007/s12031-017-0911-3. **Summary**: Explores how sympathetic blockade may reverse PTSX-related DNA-methylation changes.

Lipov EG, Faber JA. (2023). Efficacy of cervical sympathetic blockade in the treatment of primary and secondary PTSD symptoms: A case series. *Heliyon* 9(6):e17008. doi: 10.1016/j.heliyon.2023.e17008. **Summary**: Evaluates cervical sympathetic blockade's efficacy in treating primary and secondary PTSX symptoms, and shows notable symptom reduction.

Lipov EG, Jacobs R et al. (2022). Utility of Cervical Sympathetic Block in Treating Post-Traumatic Stress Disorder in Multiple Cohorts: A Retrospective Analysis. *Pain Physician* 25(1):77-85. PMID: 35051147. **Summary**: Cervical sympathetic block is effective in reducing PTSX symptoms across diverse patient groups.

Lipov E, Ritchie EC (2015). A review of the use of stellate ganglion block in the treatment of PTSD. *Current Psychiatry Reports* 17(8), 599. doi: 10.1007/s11920-015-0599-4. **Summary**: Discusses the potential mechanisms and clinical outcomes of using stellate ganglion block as a treatment modality for PTSX.

Mulvaney SW, McLean B and de Leeuw J (2010). The use of stellate ganglion block in the treatment of panic/anxiety symptoms with combat-related post-traumatic stress disorder; preliminary results of long-term follow-up: a case series. *Pain Practice* 10(4):359-65. 10.1111/j.1533-2500.2010.00373.x. **Summary**: Stellate ganglion block effectively reduces panic and anxiety symptoms in combat-related PTSX patients.

Mulvaney SW, Lynch JH and Hickey MJ (2014). Stellate ganglion block used to treat symptoms of post-traumatic stress disorder: a case series of 166 patients. *Military Medicine* 179(10), 1133-1140. 10.7205/MILMED-D-14-00151. **Summary**: Examines the use of stellate ganglion block in treating PTSX symptoms among military personnel and provides insights into its therapeutic potential.

Mulvaney SW, McLean B and De Leeuw J (2010). The use of stellate ganglion block in the treatment of panic/anxiety symptoms with combat-related post-traumatic stress disorder: preliminary results of long-term follow-up: a case series. *Pain Practice* 10(4), 359-365. 10.1111/j.1533-2500.2010.00373.x. **Summary**: Examines the long-term efficacy of stellate ganglion block in alleviating panic and anxiety symptoms in combat-related PTSX patients.

Navaie M, Keefe MS et al. (2014). Use of stellate ganglion block for refractory post-traumatic stress disorder: a review of published cases. *Journal of Anesthesia and Clinical Research* 5(4), 403. doi.org/10.4172/2155-6148.1000403. **Summary**: Examines the use of SGB for refractory PTSX, evaluating its effectiveness as a treatment option.

Olmsted KLR, Bartoszek M et al. (2020). Effect of stellate ganglion block treatment on posttraumatic stress disorder symptoms: a randomized clinical trial. *Journal of the American Medical Association Psychiatry* 77(2), 130-138. 10.1001/jamapsychiatry.2019.3474. **Summary**: Assesses the impact of stellate ganglion block treatment on PTSX symptoms and its role in PTSX management.

Singh H and Rajarathinam M (2024). Stellate ganglion block beyond chronic pain: A literature review on its application in painful and non-painful conditions. *Journal of Anaesthesiology and Clinical Pharmacology* 40(2), 185–191. 10.4103/joacp.joacp_304_22. **Summary**: Reviews the growing indications for stellate ganglion block therapy.

Sippel LM, Hamblen JL et al. (2024). Novel Pharmacologic and Other Somatic Treatment Approaches for Posttraumatic Stress Disorder in Adults: State of the Evidence. *American Journal of Psychiatry* 181(12), 1045–1058. 10.1176/appi.ajp.20230950. **Summary**: Examines emerging pharmacological and somatic interventions, ranging from novel medications to brain stimulation techniques, and emphasizes research gaps and future directions for PTSX treatment.

Telehealth Therapies for PTSX

Blackie M, De Boer K et al. (2024). Digital-Based Interventions for Complex Post-Traumatic Stress Disorder: A Systematic Literature Review. *Trauma, Violence, and Abuse* 25(4), 3115–3130. 10.1177/15248380241238760. **Summary**: Examines the effectiveness of digital modalities (e.g., smartphone apps, online programs) in mitigating CPTSX symptomatology.

Bruce MJ, Pagán AF and Acierno R (2024). State of the Science: Evidence-based treatments for posttraumatic stress disorder delivered via telehealth. *Journal of Traumatic Stress* 38(1):5-15. doi: 10.1002/jts.23074. **Summary**: Reviews current telehealth modalities used to treat PTSX, showing that various internet and telephone-based interventions maintain comparable efficacy to in-person therapy while improving access.

El-Refaay SMM, Toivanen-Atilla K and Crego N (2024). Efficacy of technology-based mental health interventions in minimizing mental health symptoms among immigrants, asylum seekers or refugees; systematic review. *Archives of Psychiatric Nursing* 51, 38–47. doi: 10.1016/j.apnu.2024.04.002. **Summary**: Reports promising outcomes of digital mental-health tools for vulnerable immigrant communities, showing that culturally adapted approaches may enhance engagement and symptom reduction.

Haderlein TP, Guzman-Clark J et al. (2024). Improving Veteran Engagement with Virtual Care Technologies: a Veterans Health Administration State of the Art Conference Research Agenda. *Journal of General Internal Medicine* 39(Suppl 1), 21–28. doi: 10.1007/s11606-023-08488-7. **Summary**: Identifies how to bolster telehealth services.

McLean CP and Foa EB (2024). State of the Science: Prolonged exposure therapy for the treatment of posttraumatic stress disorder. *Journal of Traumatic Stress* 37(4), 535–550. doi: 10.1002/jts.23046. **Summary**: Overview of prolonged exposure therapy's efficacy, core principles and recent adaptations, affirming it as a first-line PTSX intervention with robust empirical support.

Taylor LS, Caloudas SG et al. (2024). Asynchronous assessment with the PCL-5: Practice considerations and recommendations. *Psychological Services* 21(3), 552–559. doi: 10.1037/ser0000824. **Summary**: Addresses best practices for administering the PTSD Checklist for *DSM-5* (PCL-5) asynchronously, discussing benefits and caveats in tele-assessment contexts.

Tng GYQ, Koh J et al. (2024). Efficacy of digital mental health interventions for PTSD symptoms: A systematic review of meta-analyses. *Journal of Affective Disorders* 357, 23–36. 10.1016/j.jad.2024.04.074. **Summary**: Demonstrating that digital platforms like e-therapy and mobile apps provide a viable and often cost-effective approach to PTSX symptom reduction.

Yoshikawa M, Narita Z and Kim Y (2024). Digital health-based exposure therapies for patients with posttraumatic stress disorder: A systematic review of randomized controlled trials. *Journal of Traumatic Stress* 37(6), 814–824. doi: 10.1002/jts.23052. **Summary**: Reviews RCTs assessing digital exposure therapies for PTSX, indicating that internet-delivered and VR-based exposure can effectively decrease symptom severity while broadening treatment reach.

Zainal NH, Soh CP et al. (2024). Do the effects of internet-delivered cognitive-behavioral therapy (i-CBT) last after a year and beyond? A meta-analysis of 154 randomized controlled trials (RCTs). *Clinical Psychology Review* 114, 102518. doi: 10.1016/j.cpr.2024.102518. **Summary**: Meta-analyses show durable symptom relief extending beyond 12 months for diverse conditions treated with i-CBT, reinforcing its long-term viability as a front-line intervention.

Traumatic Brain Injury

Bruce SL, Cooper MR et al. (2025). The Relationship Between Concussion and Combat History and Mental Health and Suicide Ideation Among United States Military Veterans – A Pilot Study. *Brain Sciences* 15(3), 234. doi: 10.3390/brainsci15030234. **Summary**: Pilot study links concussion and combat exposure histories to elevated depression, anxiety, and suicidal ideation, underscoring integrated screening for head injury and mental health in veteran populations.

Brickell TA, Ivins BJ et al. (2025). A Dyad Approach to Understanding Relationship Satisfaction and Health Outcomes in Military Couples Following Service Member and Veteran Traumatic Brain Injury. *Frontiers in Psychiatry* 16, 1465801. doi: 10.3389/fpsyt.2025.1465801. **Summary**: Dyadic analyses reveal that relationship satisfaction buffers physical and psychological health consequences following TBI, emphasizing couple-based rehabilitation to strengthen interpersonal functioning and improve recovery trajectories.

Congressional Budget Office (2012). The Veterans Health Administration's Treatment of PTSD and Traumatic Brain Injury Among Recent Combat Veterans. https://www.cbo.gov/publication/42969. **Summary**: Investigates the scope of VA care provided to servicemembers with PTSX and TBI.

Diaz-Arrastia R, Kochanek PM et al. (2014). Pharmacotherapy of Traumatic Brain Injury: State of the Science and the Road Forward: Report of the Department of Defense Neurotrauma Pharmacology Workgroup. *Journal of Neurotrauma* 31(2). doi.org/10.1089/neu.2013.3019 **Summary**: Summarizes existing pharmacological interventions for TBI, and addresses gaps in current knowledge.

Gordon ML and Agee B (2023). Addressing the dual burden: Treatment outcomes for traumatic brain injury (TBI) and post-traumatic stress disorder (PTSD). The Millennium Health Centers, Inc. Veterans-TBI Project, 1–10. **Summary**: Analyzes treatment outcomes for veterans suffering from both TBI and PTSX.

Karr JE, Rippey CS et al. (2025). Traumatic Brain Injury in US Veterans: Prevalence and Associations with Physical, Mental, and Cognitive Health. *Archives of Physical Medicine and Rehabilitation* 106(4), 537–547. doi: 10.1016/j.apmr.2024.11.010. **Summary**: Nationwide survey estimates TBI prevalence and links injury severity to poorer physical, cognitive, and mental health, informing screening priorities for veterans with comorbid traumatic stress.

Kitaj M and Goff DC (2024). Why Do Veterans Not Respond as Well as Civilians to Trauma-Focused Therapies for PTSD? *Harvard Review of Psychiatry* 32(4), 160–163. doi: 10.1097/HRP.0000000000000400. **Summary**: Examines the factors contributing to reduced treatment efficacy in veterans compared to civilians and highlights the unique stressors and complexities often faced by service members that can impede therapy outcomes.

Loane DJ and Faden AI (2010). Neuroprotection for traumatic brain injury: translational challenges and emerging therapeutic strategies. *Trends in Pharmacological Sciences* 31(12):596-604. doi: 10.1016/j.tips.2010.09.005. **Summary**: Reviews ongoing difficulties in translating TBI neuroprotective research into clinical practice, and surveys novel approaches poised to improve patient outcomes.

Minen MT, Mahmood N et al. (2024). Treatment Options for Posttraumatic Headache: A Current Review of the Literature. *Current Pain and Headache Reports* 28(4), 205–210. 10.1007/s11916-023-01199-y. **Summary**: Pharmacologic and non-pharmacologic interventions for posttraumatic headache; examines the complexities of comorbid conditions like PTSX and suggests integrated treatment approaches.

Porcu P, Barron AM et al. (2016). Neurosteroidogenesis Today: Novel Targets for Neuroactive Steroid Synthesis and Action and Their Relevance for Translational Research. *Journal of Neuroendocrinology* 28(2). doi: 10.1111/jne.12351. **Summary**: Examines the mechanisms of neurosteroid synthesis and examines their therapeutic significance for neuroinflammatory disorders including TBI and PTSX.

Radtke FA, Chapman G et al. (2017). Modulating Neuroinflammation to Treat Neuropsychiatric Disorders. *BioMed Research International* vol. 2017, Article ID 5071786, pp. 1–21. https://www.hindawi.com/journals/bmri/2017/5071786/. **Summary**: Derives a model of neurological inflammation and its critical role in neuropsychiatric disorders like PTSX, and suggests novel therapeutic approaches targeting the neuroinflammatory cascade.

Reddy DS and Estes WA (2010). Neurosteroids: Endogenous Role in the Human Brain and Therapeutic Potentials. *Progress in Brain Research* 186:113–137. doi: 10.1016/B978-0-444-53630-3.00008-7. **Summary**: Explores role of neurosteroids in modulating brain function and their potential as therapeutic agents for managing mood and cognition in neuropsychiatric disorders.

Sarris J, Murphy J et al (2016). Adjunctive Nutraceuticals for Depression: A Systematic Review and Meta-Analyses. *American Journal of Psychiatry* 173(6):575-87. doi: 10.1176/appi.ajp.2016.15091228. **Summary**: Identifies and evaluates nutraceuticals (e.g., omega-3s, folate) used alongside conventional antidepressant treatments, and highlights their potential to improve clinical outcomes in mood and stress-related conditions.

Schiepers OJ, Wichers MC and Maes M (2005). Cytokines and Major Depression. *Progress in Neuropsychopharmacology and Biological Psychiatry* 29(2):201–217. 10.1016/j.pnpbp.2004.11.003. **Summary**: Reviews evidence linking elevated proinflammatory cytokines to depression, suggesting immune-targeted interventions could be relevant to stress-related injuries.

Vagal Nerve Stimulation

Chen Z and Liu K (2025). Mechanism and Applications of Vagus Nerve Stimulation. *Current Issues in Molecular Biology* 47(2):122. doi: 10.3390/cimb47020122. **Summary**: Details the biological mechanisms of Vagus Nerve Stimulation (VNS) and its wide-ranging clinical applications, providing a foundational understanding of how modulating this nerve influences physiological and neurological processes.

Noble LJ, Meruva VB et al. (2019). Vagus nerve stimulation promotes generalization of conditioned fear extinction and reduces anxiety in rats. *Translational Psychiatry* 12(1):9-18. doi: 10.1016/j.brs.2018.09.013. **Summary**: Demonstrates that vagus nerve stimulation, paired with extinction training reduces fear and anxiety in rats, suggesting relevance for post-traumatic stress injuries.

Powers MB, Hays SA et al. (2025). Vagus nerve stimulation therapy for treatment-resistant PTSD. *Brain Stimulation* 18(3):665–675. doi: 10.1016/j.brs.2025.03.007. **Summary**: Evaluates the safety and efficacy of vagus nerve stimulation in individuals with treatment-resistant post-traumatic stress injuries.

Shiramatsu TI, Ibayashi K et al (2025). Vagus Nerve Stimulation Modulates Information Representation of Sustained Activity in a Layer-Specific Manner in the Rat Auditory Cortex. *Frontiers in Neural Circuits* 19:1569158. doi: 10.3389/fncir.2025.1569158. **Summary**: Suggests a mechanism by which neuromodulation can reshape sensory processing and brain circuitry.

Vabba A, Suzuki K et al (2025). The Vagus Nerve as a Gateway to Body Ownership: taVNS Reduces Susceptibility to a Virtual Version of the Cardiac and Tactile Rubber Hand Illusion. *Psychophysiology* 62(3):e70040. doi: 10.1111/psyp.70040. **Summary**: Demonstrates that non-invasive Vagus Nerve Stimulation (taVNS) influences interoception and body ownership, potentially explaining how autonomic regulation can ground individuals and reduce symptoms of dissociation common in trauma.

Virtual Reality for PTSX Therapy

Diemer J, Kothgassner OD et al. (2024). [VR-supported therapy for anxiety and posttraumatic stress disorder: current possibilities and limitations]. *Der Nervenarzt* 95(3), 223–229. doi: 10.1007/s00115-023-01570-9. **Summary**: Reviews the applications of virtual reality in treating anxiety and PTSX, examines current technological capabilities, potential clinical benefits and noted constraints.

Drop DLQ, Vlake JH et al. (2025). Effect of an intensive care unit virtual reality intervention on relatives' mental health distress: A multicenter, randomized controlled trial. *Critical Care* 29(1), 62. doi: 10.1186/s13054-025-05281-2. **Summary**: Evaluates the impact of ICU-specific virtual reality interventions on reducing symptoms of anxiety, depression, and post-traumatic stress among relatives of intensive care patients.

Lee M, Jang S et al. (2025). Virtual reality-based cognitive behavior therapy for major depressive disorder: An alternative to pharmacotherapy for reducing suicidality. *Yonsei Medical Journal* 66(1), 25–36. doi:10.3349/ymj.2024.0002. **Summary**: Investigates virtual reality cognitive behavior therapy as a non-pharmacological treatment for major depressive disorder.

Loucks L, Rizzo A and Rothbaum BO (2025). Virtual reality exposure for treating PTSD due to military sexual trauma. *Journal of Clinical Psychology* 81(2), 81–92. doi: 10.1002/jclp.23750. **Summary**: Explores the effectiveness of tailored virtual reality exposure therapy in treating PTSX specifically resulting from military sexual trauma, highlighting significant therapeutic outcomes.

Montesano A and Seinfeld S. (2025). Virtual reality in psychotherapy: A three-dimensional framework to navigate immersive clinical applications. *Journal of Clinical Psychology* Advance online publication. doi: 10.1002/jclp.70004. **Summary**: Presents a three-dimensional framework guiding clinicians in effectively integrating virtual reality into psychotherapy, emphasizing tailored strategies for therapeutic immersion and personalized treatment approaches.

Sim A, McNeilage AG et al. (2024). Impact of healthcare interventions on distress following acute musculoskeletal/orthopaedic injury: a scoping review of systematic reviews. *British Medical Journal Open* 14(7):e085778. doi: 10.1136/bmjopen-2024-085778. **Summary**: Maps a range of interventions designed to reduce psychological distress in individuals recovering from orthopaedic injuries, identifying both effective strategies and further neccessary issues.

Wankhede NL, Koppula S et al. (2025). Virtual reality modulating dynamics of neuroplasticity: Innovations in neuromotor rehabilitation. *Neuroscience* 566, 97–111. doi: 10.1016/j.neuroscience.2024.12.040. **Summary**: Explores how VR interventions reshape neuroplastic processes in neuromotor rehabilitation, and examines emerging evidence for improved recovery outcomes in both acute and chronic conditions.

Wiederhold BK and Wiederhold MD (2025). Virtual reality therapy combined with physiological monitoring provides effective treatment, with objective metrics, for post-traumatic stress disorder. *Expert Review of Medical Devices* 22(2), 117–119. doi:10.1080/17434440.2025.2454930. **Summary**: Demonstrates how combining virtual reality therapy with physiological monitoring effectively treats PTSX, providing objective metrics for therapeutic progress and clinical validation.

Wu JY, Tsai YY et al. (2025). Digital transformation of mental health therapy by integrating digitalized cognitive behavioral therapy and eye movement desensitization and reprocessing. *Medical and Biological Engineering and Computing* 63(2), 339–354. doi: 10.1007/s11517-024-03209-6. **Summary**: Details the convergence of digital tools with established psychotherapeutic methods, and offers a framework to optimize and personalize mental-health interventions like CBT and EMDR.

Zeka F, Clemmensen L et al. (2025). The Effectiveness of Immersive Virtual Reality-Based Treatment for Mental Disorders: A Systematic Review With Meta-Analysis. *Acta Psychiatrica Scandinavica* 151(3):210-230. doi: 10.1111/acps.13777. **Summary**: Provides quantitative synthesis of immersive VR interventions for various PTS injuries.

About the Authors

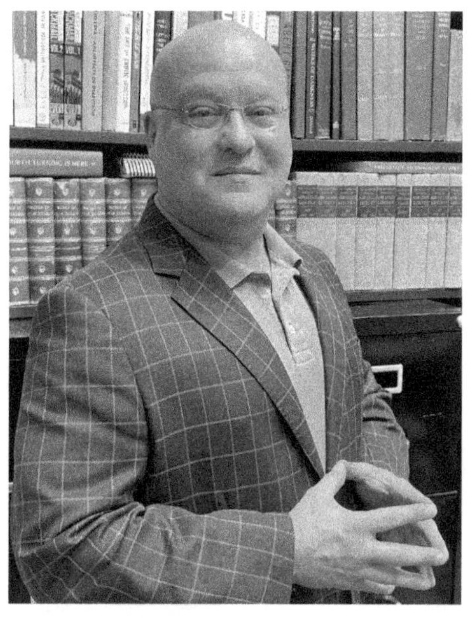

Dino Garner is a former biophysicist, Army Ranger, corp merc and military aviation photographer. He is a *New York Times* bestselling editor, author and ghostwriter of more than 50 books, including the Pulitzer-Prize-nominated books, *AEROMASTERS: Celebrating a Century of the American Fighter Pilot*, Vol. I and *SILENT SCARS, BOLD REMEDIES: Cutting-Edge Care and Healing from Post-Traumatic Stress Injuries.*

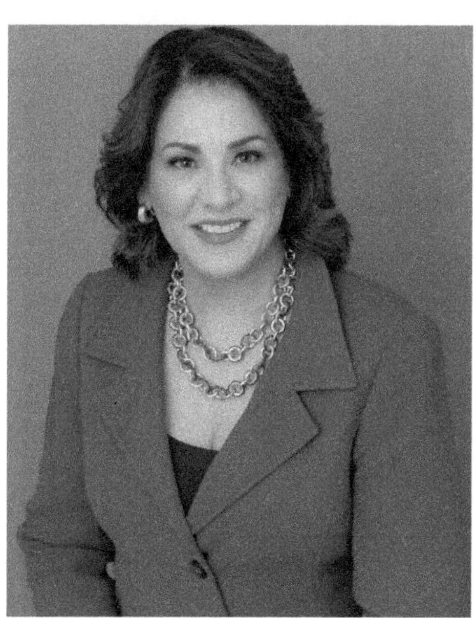

Liz Fetter is the author of "The Gift of Old-World Authenticity" in the bestselling book *The Keys To Authenticity* by Jack Canfield. A former technology CEO and consultant, she currently serves on public company boards. She is co-author of *AEROMASTERS* and *SILENT SCARS, BOLD REMEDIES*, and is also developing several new books.

Also from AIOS

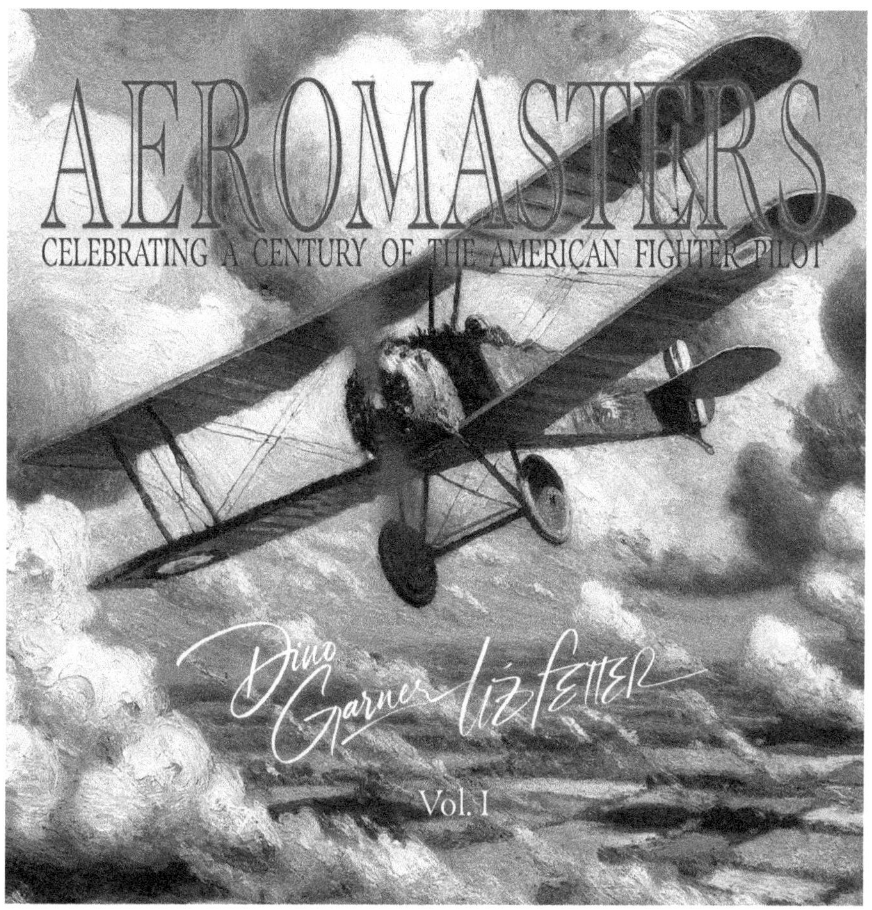

AEROMASTERS: Celebrating a Century of the American Fighter Pilot, Vol. I, offers an immersive and sensory-rich journey into the world of fighter aviation. Readers are transported inside the cockpit where they can almost smell the jet fuel and sweat, hear the laughter in the squadron bar, taste the tradition of Jeremiah Weed, and feel the intense pressure of a 9-G break turn. The authors' artistic essays and moving stories capture the essence of military fighter aviation, growing up in a fighter atmosphere, and the relentless pursuit of dreams.

Each tribute includes official portraits, flight wings, unit patches, and a history of heroic acts, providing a visual and narrative testament to the valor of U.S. fighter pilots and Air Force PJs.

Available on Amazon.com and from FrontierInsightsLLC.com.

"An unparalleled literary and visual masterpiece of American history."
—General John Jumper
17th Chief of Staff, US Air Force

"*AEROMASTERS: Celebrating a Century of the American Fighter Pilot* is an outstanding tribute to American fighter pilots and the profound impact they have had on the course of history . . . From the dogfights of World War I to the cutting-edge aerial tactics of modern-day conflicts, AEROMASTERS captures the evolution of fighter aviation and its critical role in shaping the world we live in today . . . This book also serves as a vital bridge to America's young people, offering them a window into the lives and legacies of those who have played a pivotal role in building and protecting this great nation."
—Lt Gen Dave "Zatar" Deptula
USAF (Ret.), F-15 Eagle Fighter Pilot
Dean, Mitchell Institute for Aerospace Studies

"Few authors have the deep understanding of fighter pilots, much less the passion to tell their stories in a way that captures not only what they did but also who they are. Dino Garner and Liz Fetter have both the knowledge and the passion to accurately tell the stories as well as capture the unique qualities of this amazing group called fighter pilots. In their landmark work *AEROMASTERS*, they have created the most comprehensive volume I've seen on this subject . . . If you are a fighter pilot like me or someone simply interested in stories of heroism, daring and fun, this book is for you! Fight's On!"
—Maj Gen Joe "Solo" Kunkel
US Air Force Fighter Pilot

"Captain Lance P. Sijan, my brother, served as an Air Force fighter pilot during the Vietnam War and became a POW following a premature explosion beneath his F-4C Phantom II. *AEROMASTERS: Celebrating a Century of the American Fighter Pilot* includes a poignant four-page homage to Lance that moved me deeply. I last saw him in 1967 when I was 13 years old, yet he continues to be my enduring hero. *AEROMASTERS* is a remarkable testament to the bravery and commitment of America's aviators. It stands out not only for its artistic flair, creativity and meticulous attention to detail, but also for its rarity in historical publications . . . *AEROMASTERS* is a breathtaking celebration of our heroes—a genuine masterpiece!"
—Janine Sijan
Executive Director, Lance P. Sijan Foundation

"A breathtaking masterpiece! *AEROMASTERS* is a stunning work of passion as told through the mind, eyes and heart of one of the most remarkable human beings on this planet . . . A++ to this fabulous work of art and storytelling."
—Matt Lum
President, VIDA Wealth Partners Inc.
World Adventurer and Lifelong Aviation Enthusiast

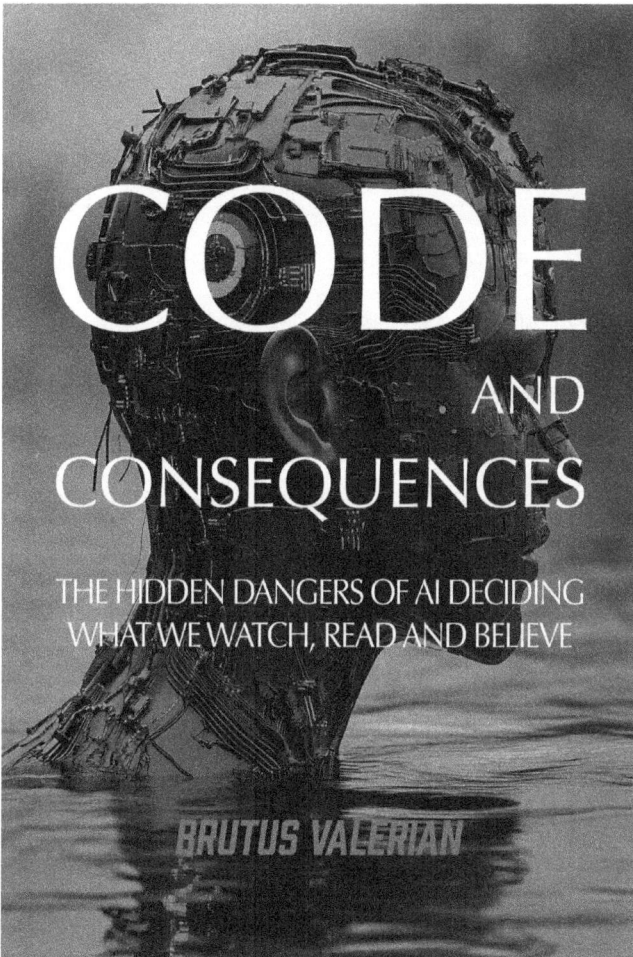

Generative AI has become one of the most transformative technologies of our time. This comprehensive guide unpacks how AI systems create text, images, and media that can rival human outputs, while also uncovering inherent risks like misinformation, privacy breaches, and employment shifts.

With clarity and depth, each chapter navigates intellectual property concerns, biases in training data, environmental footprints, and the regulatory hurdles shaping AI's future. Drawing on the latest research, this book offers insights into the profound impact on creativity, labor, and society—equipping readers with practical strategies for harnessing GenAI's advantages, mitigating its potential harms, and ensuring ethical progress worldwide.

eBook available on Amazon.com.

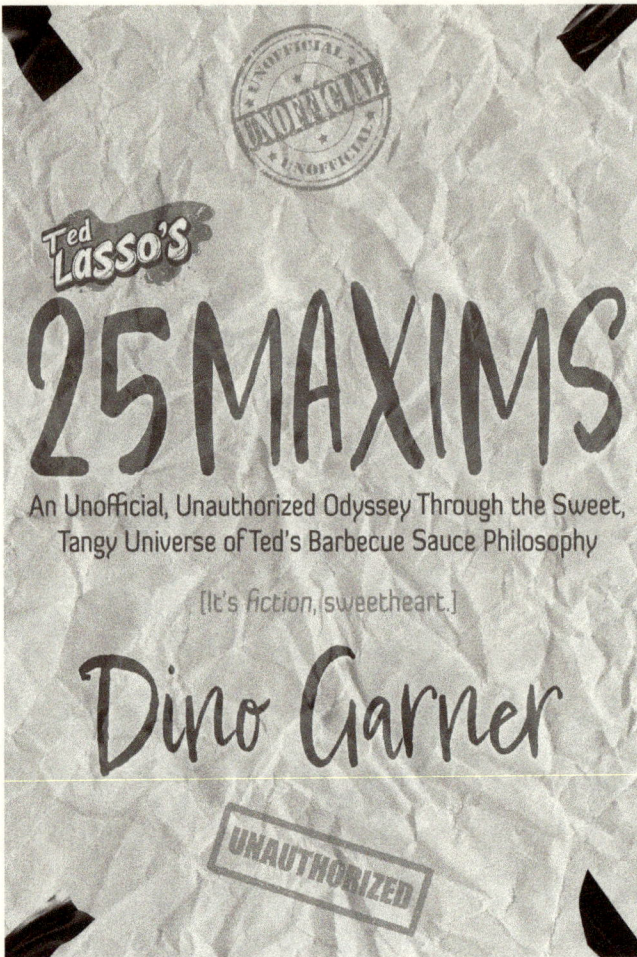

A big shout-out to the brilliant minds behind Ted Lasso, the people who first inspired this unofficial and unauthorized tribute to America's favorite barbecue-sauce philosophy. My wish is that you glean the unstoppable optimism, unwavering empathy, and gentle humor that this fictional hero embodies, weaving them into your life in ways that bring kindness and hope to those around you.

Let's honor the concept of positivity and forward-focused thinking that has brightened countless hearts on and off the pitch. I invite you to continue with clarity and open minds—secure in the knowledge that you journey forward ethically, with pure intentions, and with the unwavering conviction that all of us can discover fresh hope if we "dare to believe in belief," a principle so central to this book's spirit.

Coming December 2025 to Amazon.com.

Index

A

B

C

D

E

F

G

H

I

J

K

L

M

N

O

P

Q

R

S

T

U

V

W

Y

Z

www.ingramcontent.com/pod-product-compliance
Lightning Source LLC
Chambersburg PA
CBHW031135020426
42333CB00013B/394

* 9 7 8 1 7 3 7 3 8 8 0 8 1 *